Pediatric and Adolescent Urologic Imaging

Lane S. Palmer • Jeffrey S. Palmer
Editors

Pediatric and Adolescent Urologic Imaging

Springer

Editors
Lane S. Palmer, MD, FACS, FAAP
Hofstra North Shore LIJ School of Medicine
New Hyde Park, NY
USA

Division of Pediatric Urology
Cohen Children's Medical Center of New York
Long Island, NY
USA

Jeffrey S. Palmer, MD, FACS, FAAP
Pediatric and Adolescent Urology Institute
Cleveland, OH
USA

ISBN 978-1-4614-8653-4 ISBN 978-1-4614-8654-1 (eBook)
DOI 10.1007/978-1-4614-8654-1
Springer New York Heidelberg Dordrecht London

Library of Congress Control Number: 2013957139

Printed on acid-free paper

Springer is part of Springer Science+Business Media (www.springer.com)

This book is dedicated to our parents, whose love, support, dedication, sacrifices, and example have enabled their children to be the best that they could become. We thank them both.

Jeffrey S. Palmer, MD, FACS, FAAP

In addition, the loving support and understanding of my wife and children allows me the opportunity to work on projects, such as this one, aimed at helping others.

Lane S. Palmer, MD, FACS, FAAP

Foreword

Since I began practicing pediatric uroradiology almost 40 years ago, there have been many dramatic changes, not only in the diagnosis and treatment of abnormalities of the urinary tract of the fetus, infant, and child but also changes in the training of the people who do the diagnosing and the treating. Some of these changes are obvious and are the result of advances in medicine, but some are cultural and may be more subtle. I will mention but a few of these changes here.

Vesicoureteral reflux was thought by many to be secondary to infection or secondary to obstruction at the bladder neck or in the urethra, leading to many unnecessary operations. Vesicoureteral reflux is now known to be primary, the result of abnormality or immaturity at the ureterovesical junction, and reflux often resolves spontaneously as the child grows. It was not known that reflux is often familial and that it is rare in black children. And it was also not widely appreciated, as it is now, that reflux is a dynamic phenomenon that sometimes only occurs with voiding.

Another advance in the understanding of the child's urinary tract concerns the so-called megacystis-megaureter association. This is a condition in which the massively enlarged bladder was thought to be the cause of the dilatation of the ureters. Reduction cystoplasty (with incidental reimplantation of the refluxing ureters) was a common method of treatment. Then we learned that the massive reflux, with constant recycling of refluxed urine, was the cause of bladder enlargement. Reimplantation of the ureters, with cessation of the reflux, usually results in the gradual return of the bladder to normal size.

The ability to detect hydronephrosis and other abnormalities of the urinary tract in the asymptomatic fetus by prenatal ultrasound means that the infant can be evaluated and treated if necessary electively after delivery and not as an emergency only after he or she becomes ill, as was often the case 40 years ago. Prenatal detection of a urinary tract abnormality, such as posterior urethral valves in the male fetus, affords the pediatric urologist the opportunity to meet expectant parents before the baby is born, to provide advice and reassurance, and to establish a plan for postnatal management.

Prenatal detection and postnatal evaluation of the infant with a multicystic dysplastic kidney (MCDK) revolutionized the treatment of the child with this anomaly. Before prenatal detection was possible, most MCDKs were removed when detected. A healthy infant would be found to have a mass in his or her flank during a routine physical examination. An excretory urogram would show a normal, hypertrophied contralateral kidney and no visible kidney on the side of the mass. At the time of the almost inevitable operation, a MCDK would be found and the kidney would be removed. Since the introduction and widespread use of routine prenatal ultrasound, most MCDKs are detected in utero. The diagnosis is confirmed after delivery and the affected kidney is left in situ. No operation or other treatment is needed. The fluid in the cysts often resorbs and the affected kidney shrinks and sometimes becomes invisible on follow-up ultrasound examinations. It took awhile for this radical change in treatment to be disseminated and accepted.

Prenatal detection of hydronephrosis has also changed our understanding and hence management of primary megaureter. When I began practicing pediatric uroradiology, a patient with this condition would usually present with pyelonephritis in the first few years of life. Since the infant or child was sick and since imaging would show an underlying anatomic abnormality, virtually all such children underwent excision of the distal ureteric segment and reimplantation of the ureter, with ureteral tapering when needed. Now, however, hydronephrosis can be detected in the fetus and the infant evaluated, electively, soon after delivery and kept free from infection. As a result of this change in management, we have been able to see that the natural history of this abnormality, without surgery, is often spontaneous improvement and even resolution, and many if not most children with primary megaureter never need an operation.

Chronic renal failure used to be the most common cause of death in patients with neurogenic dysfunction of the bladder (so-called neurogenic bladder) associated with myelomeningocele. Now, after evaluation of the affected neonate by both the pediatric urologist (using urodynamic testing for neurourologic evaluation) and pediatric radiologist, appropriate treatment is instituted and maintained, and there need not be any renal deterioration at all. When I was a medical student, I was taught that if one "contaminated" the bladder of a patient with neurogenic dysfunction by catheterization, the patient would be doomed to a lifetime of intractable bladder infections. Now, one of the cornerstones of management of such a patient is clean, intermittent catheterization.

Forty years ago, exstrophy of the bladder was diagnosed at the time of birth, and the child was treated with either bladder closure at 3 or 4 years of age or urinary diversion, usually by means of ureterosigmoidostomy. Now, exstrophy is usually diagnosed prenatally by ultrasonography and sometimes magnetic resonance imaging as well; prenatal counseling can be provided, and complete primary repair can be undertaken, often in the neonatal period.

In the early 1970s, there were few pediatric urologists. Pediatric urologic surgery was usually performed by either "adult" urologists or by pediatric surgeons. If a rare person in North America wanted special training in pediatric urology, he usually went to England for a year of training with a mentor. Today, pediatric urology is practiced by men and women (a significant change, note the gender of the coauthors of this book), who have been trained in a pediatric urology fellowship in the United States or Canada, for one or more years after their general urology training. The same fellowship training model and "gender equality" have also occurred in pediatric radiology.

Another area of significant change, clearly shown by this book, is the working relationship between the pediatric radiologist and his or her pediatric urology colleague. In the past, each group worked separately, with little knowledge or appreciation of the other group's needs and concerns. It is gratifying for me, as this book clearly shows, to see how the practitioners of each specialty now often work together as a team, to the great advantage of each other, to each specialty, and of course to the care of the infant and child.

When I began, there was little knowledge of or concern for the deleterious effects of radiation from diagnostic imaging. Recently, greater knowledge of the potentially damaging effects of repeated doses of radiation from diagnostic procedures has become much better understood and disseminated. This understanding, and the need to address it, is the subject of the "Image Gently" campaign begun by the Society of Pediatric Radiology and of Chapter 7.

Still another area of significant change, the last one I will mention, is the recognition of the need for psychological support for the young patient and his or her family. When I was in training, I met Emma Plank. She had begun a unique training program for young women, teaching them how to work with children and their parents in the hospital, to try to make the time there more understandable and less scary. They were called Play Ladies. They are now called Child Life Specialists and they are an integral part of most children's hospitals, especially in radiology and urology.

Our ability in pediatric urology and uroradiology to understand, to diagnose, and to treat pediatric urologic problems has grown tremendously in the past four decades. Children worldwide are better for it. Some things, however—the embryology, anatomy, and physiology of the urinary tract and what can go wrong—have not changed. And, something else has not changed. It is the need to treat the young patient and his or her parents with dignity, concern, and sympathy and to provide the infant and the child with the most up-to-date diagnostic and therapeutic care, in a cost effective way, always striving to do things better and above all "to do no harm."

Robert L. Lebowitz, MD
Professor of Radiology, Emeritus
Boston Children's Hospital and Harvard Medical School
Boston, MA, USA

Preface

A vast number of children and adolescents in the United States are evaluated yearly for genitourinary conditions by radiographic testing, including ultrasonography, voiding cystourethrography, radioisotope renography, computerized tomography, and magnetic resonance imaging. Collaborative care of genitourinary conditions by the pediatric urologist and radiologist assists in the care of these patients. Historically, a multidisciplinary approach to several such conditions (e.g., myelomeningocele) has improved the care of these patients. It is in this spirit that we decided upon editing *Pediatric and Adolescent Urologic Imaging*, a unique comprehensive reference with each chapter written by both pediatric urologists and radiologists.

This combined-specialty evaluation of each topic through both radiographic images and corresponding clinical information will allow the clinician to integrate the radiographic imaging to the clinical data and the radiologist to have a broader clinical basis by which to interpret the imaging studies. Other health practitioners (i.e., primary care providers, general urologists, general radiologists, midlevel providers, and health professionals in training) will also find this book as a key reference.

The chapters are arranged into two parts to allow for easy access to the information. The first part, "Radiology Principles," provides the background information on the five more common radiographic tests (ultrasound, computerized tomography, magnetic resonance imaging, voiding cystourethrography, and nuclear medicine imaging) along with a history of pediatric urologic imaging and a discussion on radiation safety. The other part is entitled "Clinical Imaging." In this section, the authors integrate the lessons from the first section into the discussion of different urologic conditions based on genitourinary anatomy (kidney, ureter, bladder, urethra, adrenal gland, and scrotum) as well as the unique aspects of prenatal imaging, urolithiasis, interventional radiology, exstrophy-epispadias complex, trauma, and other urologic conditions.

Our goal is to edit a textbook written by the pediatric urologist and radiologist for pediatric urologists and radiologists. Upon completion of this text, it is our sincere hope that the reader will have both the pediatric urologist and radiologist perspectives of urologic imaging of children and adolescents.

Long Island, NY, USA — Lane S. Palmer, MD, FACS, FAAP
Cleveland, OH, USA — Jeffrey S. Palmer, MD, FACS, FAAP

Contents

Contributors

Liza M. Aguiar, MD Department of Urology, The Warren Alpert Medical School of Brown University, Hasbro Children's Hospital, Providence, RI, USA

Carol E. Barnewolt, MD Department of Radiology, Harvard Medical School, Boston, MA, USA

Division of Ultrasound, Department of Radiology, Children's Hospital Boston, Boston, MA, USA

Laurence S. Baskin, MD Department of Urology, University of California, San Francisco, CA, USA

Richard D. Bellah, MD Perelman School of Medicine, University of Pennsylvania, Philadelphia, PA, USA

Department of Radiology, The Children's Hospital of Philadelphia, Philadelphia, PA, USA

Jane E. Benson, MD Robert T. Jeffs Division of Pediatric Urology, Johns Hopkins University School of Medicine, Baltimore, MD, USA

David A. Bloom, MD Division of Pediatric Urology, Department of Urology, University of Michigan, Ann Arbor, MI, USA

Mark Cain, MD Riley Hospital for Children, Indianapolis, IN, USA

Anthony A. Caldamone, MD Department of Urology, The Warren Alpert Medical School of Brown University, Hasbro Children's Hospital, Providence, RI, USA

Douglas A. Canning, MD Division of Urology, Department of Surgery, The Children's Hospital of Philadelphia, Philadelphia, PA, USA

Division of Urology, Department of Surgery, Perelman School of Medicine, University of Pennsylvania, Philadelphia, PA, USA

Jessica T. Casey, MS, MD Department of Urology, Northwestern University Feinberg School of Medicine, Chicago, IL, USA

Marc Cendron, MD Department of Urology, Children's Hospital Boston, Harvard Medical School, Boston, MA, USA

Earl Y. Cheng, MD Division of Urology, Ann and Robert H. Lurie Children's Hospital of Chicago, Northwestern University Feinberg School of Medicine, Chicago, IL, USA

Christina B. Ching, MD Urologic Surgery and Pediatrics, Division of Pediatric Urology, Monroe Carell Jr. Children's Hospital at Vanderbilt, Nashville, TN, USA

Jeanne S. Chow, MD Department of Urology, Harvard Medical School, Boston, MA, USA

Department of Radiology, Boston Children's Hospital, Boston, MA, USA

Ronald A. Cohen, MD Diagnostic Imaging, Children's Hospital and Research Center, Oakland, CA, USA

Lee Kathleen Collins, MD Division of Pediatric Radiology, Department of Radiology, Long Island Jewish Hospital, New Hyde Park, NY, USA

Gabriella L. Crane, MD Diagnostic Imaging, Monroe Carell Jr. Children's Hospital at Vanderbilt, Nashville, TN, USA

Jimena Cubillos, MD Division of Pediatric Urology, Department of Urology, University of Rochester School of Medicine and Dentistry/Strong Memorial Hospital, Rochester, NY, USA

Heather N. Di Carlo, MD James Buchanan Brady Urological Institute, The Johns Hopkins Children's Center, Baltimore, MD, USA

Robert T. Jeffs Division of Pediatric Urology, Johns Hopkins University School of Medicine, Baltimore, MD, USA

James S. Donaldson, MD Radiology, Department of Medical Imaging, Ann and Robert H. Lurie Children's Hospital of Chicago, Northwestern University Feinberg School of Medicine, Chicago, IL, USA

Lori Landau Dyer, MD Department of Urology, Pediatric Urology, New York Medical College, Valhalla, NY, USA

Carlos R. Estrada Jr., MD Department of Urology, Harvard Medical School, Boston Children's Hospital, Boston, MA, USA

Ronnie G. Fine, MD Division of Pediatric Urology, Cohen Children's Medical Center of New York, New Hyde Park, NY, USA

Hofstra North Shore-LIJ School of Medicine, New Hyde Park, NY, USA

John P. Gearhart, MD, FAAP James Buchanan Brady Urological Institute, The Johns Hopkins Children's Center, Baltimore, MD, USA

Robert T. Jeffs Division of Pediatric Urology, Johns Hopkins University School of Medicine, Baltimore, MD, USA

Steven G. Gilbert, PhD, DABT Institute of Neurotoxicology and Neurological Disorders, Seattle, WA, USA

Department of Environmental and Occupational Health Sciences, School of Public Health and Community Medicine, University of Washington, Seattle, WA, USA

Richard W. Grady, MD Department of Urology, The University of Washington School of Medicine, Seattle, WA, USA

Division of Pediatric Urology, Department of Surgery, Seattle Children's Hospital, Seattle, WA, USA

Kavita Gupta, BA, MD Division of Urology, Department of Surgery, The Children's Hospital of Philadelphia, Philadelphia, PA, USA

Cornelia K. Kaminsky, MD Pediatric Radiology, Children's Hospital Los Angeles, Los Angeles, CA, USA

Division of Pediatric Radiology, Department of Radiology, Keck School of Medicine of USC, Los Angeles, CA, USA

Boaz Karmazyn, MD Department of Radiology and Imaging Sciences, Riley Hospital for Children at IU Health, Indianapolis, IN, USA

Martin Kathrins, MD Division of Urology, Department of Urology, Children's Hospital of Philadelphia, Philadelphia, PA, USA

Division of Urology, Department of Surgery, University of Pennsylvania Health System, Philadelphia, PA, USA

Nina Klionsky, MD Department of Imaging Sciences, Pediatric Imaging, University of Rochester School of Medicine and Dentistry/Strong Memorial Hospital/Golisano Children's Hospital, Rochester, NY, USA

Chester J. Koh, MD Division of Pediatric Urology, Texas Children's Hospital/Baylor College of Medicine, Houston, TX, USA

Kate H. Kraft, MD Division of Pediatric Urology, Department of Urology, University of Michigan, Ann Arbor, MI, USA

Jon C. Kralik, MD Department of Radiology, University of Minnesota, Minneapolis, MN, USA

Aaron J. Krill, MD Division of Urology, Department of Surgery, Virginia Commonwealth University Medical Center, Richmond, VA, USA

Lesli M. LeCompte, MD Division of Pediatrics, Department of Radiology, Westchester Medical Center, New York Medical College, Valhalla, NY, USA

Massoud Majd, MD, FACR Section of Nuclear Medicine, Department of Radiology, Children's National Medical Center, Washington, DC, USA

Radiology and Pediatrics, George Washington University School of Medicine, Washington, DC, USA

Kathleen McCarten, MD Department of Pediatric Radiology, The Warren Alpert Medical School of Brown University, Hasbro Children's Hospital, Providence, RI, USA

Lesli Nicolay, MD Division of Pediatric Urology, Department of Urology, Loma Linda University Medical Center, Loma Linda, CA, USA

Christopher J. Palestro, MD Department of Radiology, Hofstra North Shore-LIJ School of Medicine, Hempstead, NY, USA

Division of Nuclear Medicine and Molecular Imaging, North Shore Long Island Jewish Health System, Manhasset & New Hyde Park, NY, USA

Jeffrey S. Palmer, MD, FACS, FAAP Pediatric and Adolescent Urology Institute, Cleveland, OH, USA

Lane S. Palmer, MD, FACS, FAAP Hofstra North Shore-LIJ School of Medicine, New Hyde Park, NY, USA

Division of Pediatric Urology, Cohen Children's Medical Center of New York, Long Island, NY, USA

Robert P. Payne, MD, FRCSC Department of Urology, Stanford University School of Medicine, Stanford, CA, USA

John C. Pope IV, MD Urologic Surgery and Pediatrics, Division of Pediatric Urology, Monroe Carell Jr. Children's Hospital at Vanderbilt, Nashville, TN, USA

Derek Prabharasuth, MD Department of Urology, New York Medical College, Valhalla, NY, USA

Dana C. Rice, MD Department of Urology, George Washington University School of Medicine, Washington, DC, USA

Richard C. Rink, MD, FAAP, FACS Pediatric Urology, Riley Hospital for Children at IU Health, Indianapolis, IN, USA

Jeanne Choi Rosen, MD Division of Pediatric, Department of Diagnostic Radiology, Cohen Children's Hospital, North Shore Long Island Jewish Medical Center, New Hyde Park, NY, USA

H. Gil Rushton, MD, FAAP Division of Pediatric Urology, Children's National Medical Center, Washington, DC, USA

Urology and Pediatrics, George Washington University School of Medicine, Washington, DC, USA

Manojkumar Saranathan, PhD Department of Radiology, Stanford University School of Medicine, Stanford, CA, USA

Bruce J. Schlomer, MD Department of Urology, University of California, San Francisco, CA, USA

F. Glen Seidel, MD, FAAP, FACR Department of Radiology, Pediatric Radiology, Lucille Packard Children's Hospital, Stanford, CA, USA

Linda Dairiki Shortliffe, MD, FAAP Department of Urology, Stanford University School of Medicine, Stanford, CA, USA

Aseem R. Shukla, MD Department of Surgery, Pediatric Urology, Children's Hospital of Philadelphia, Philadelphia, PA, USA

Department of Surgery (in Urology), Perelman School of Medicine, University of Pennsylvania, Philadelphia, PA, USA

Konrad M. Szymanski, MD, MPH Pediatric Urology, Riley Hospital for Children at IU Health, Indianapolis, IN, USA

Duong D. Tu, MD Department of Urology, Harvard Medical School, Boston Children's Hospital, Boston, MA, USA

Shreyas Vasanawala, MD, PhD Body MRI, Department of Radiology, Stanford University School of Medicine, Stanford, CA, USA

Dana A. Weiss, MD Division of Urology, Department of Surgery, The Children's Hospital of Philadelphia, Philadelphia, PA, USA

Benjamin Whittam, MD Riley Hospital for Children, Indianapolis, IN, USA

Katie Willihnganz-Lawson, MD Department of Urology, University of Minnesota Medical Center, Minneapolis, MN, USA

Department of Pediatric Urology, University of Minnesota Amplatz Children's Hospital, Minneapolis, MN, USA

Benjamin Yuh, MD Department of Urology, USC Institute of Urology, Keck School of Medicine of USC, Los Angeles, CA, USA

Part I

Radiology Principles

History of Pediatric Urologic Imaging

1

Kate H. Kraft and David A. Bloom

The Beginnings: Plain Films and Cystography

The story of genitourinary tract imaging is a coincidence of art, technology, and epistemology. Urinary tract visualization began with da Vinci (1452–1519) and Vesalius (1514–1564) who transformed observations of anatomic dissections into drawings (Fig. 1.1). This work was useful for education but hardly practical for the real-time practice of medicine. Photographic technology was a huge boon to medical education as well and quickly extended its impact to the therapeutic arena [1].

Modern genitourinary tract imaging, however, resulted from the union of two milestone medical specialties. Urology was the first deliberately specified subspecialty in medicine, as evidenced in the oath of Hippocrates. Those who have taken that oath since 450 BC accept responsibility for almost all aspects of healthcare and swear that they "will not cut for stone" but rather should defer that practice to "specialists in that art." Bladder stones have been a persistent plague for children and adults throughout human history until recent times. Itinerant lithotomists offered surgical treatments throughout most of the ensuing 2.5 millennia after Hippocrates, although left little evidence of their work aside from the oath and subsequent allusions to their existence and practice. Herbalists, midwives, acupuncturists, and other practitioners plied their techniques and trades over those centuries, but in the orthodoxy of Western medicine, other specialties did not emerge until the second half of the nineteenth century.

Even from its primitive start, lithotomy was heavily dependent on technology. One can easily imagine little progress in the technology of knives and other instruments occurred in the time between Hippocrates and the Industrial Revolution. Only as the second half of the nineteenth century proceeded toward the turn of the next century did science and technology produce precision and ingenious instruments such as the lithotrite and optical endoscopes that allowed a new iteration of the lithotomist. Genitourinary surgery, or urology as it came to be called, moved well beyond lithotomy to investigate and treat all sorts of genitourinary pathology with safe and tolerable access to deep interiors of the human body.

Coupled to this new iteration of urology was the discovery of Wilhelm Conrad Roentgen in 1895. His X-ray pictures utilizing the Crookes tube allowed a new level of diagnostic opportunity in the human body. The tipping point was quickly appreciated as in the following year, 1,000 papers were published related to the new modality [2]. That first image of the ring finger of Roentgen's wife initiated bone visualization, and it was only a short step of imagination to investigate the urinary tract. On July 11, 1896, within a

K.H. Kraft, MD • D.A. Bloom, MD (✉)
Division of Pediatric Urology, Department of Urology, University of Michigan, 1500 E. Medical Center Drive, SPC 5330, 3875 Taubman Center, Ann Arbor, MI, USA
e-mail: kraftk@med.umich.edu; dabloom@umich.edu

L.S. Palmer, J.S. Palmer (eds.), *Pediatric and Adolescent Urologic Imaging*,
DOI 10.1007/978-1-4614-8654-1_1, © Springer Science+Business Media New York 2014

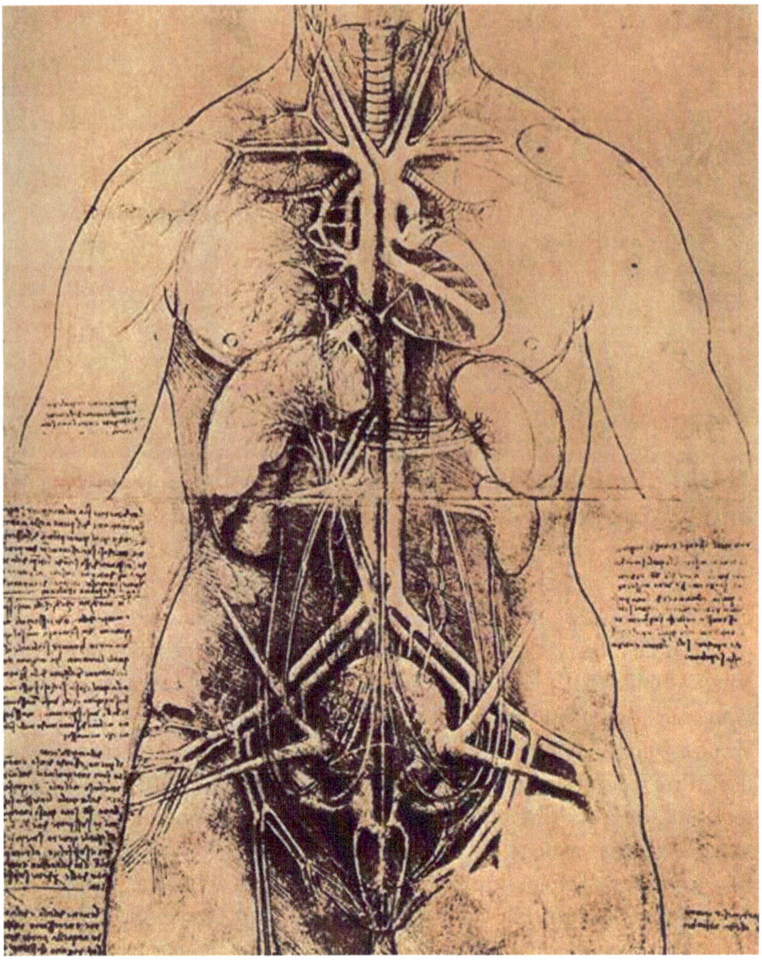

Fig. 1.1 The principal organs and vascular and urinogenital systems of a woman, c. 1507 by Leonardo da Vinci

year of Roentgen's pivotal discovery, Dr. John Macintyre of Glasgow reported the X-ray demonstration of a renal stone [3]. The length of the exposure was 12 min, and a subsequent operative procedure confirmed presence of the stone.

X-ray was not readily adopted as a solution to identifying urinary calculi due to the technical limitations of equipment available at the time. The low output and lack of intensifying screens required exposure times of at least ten minutes, and only large radiopaque calculi could be detected. Variable tube output and scattered radiation weakened image quality [4]. Fenwick in 1897 utilized intraoperative X-ray exposure of a kidney to try to localize a stone but was unsuccessful. In the same year, Tuffier passed a catheter with a metal stylet into the ureter under X-ray to define its course radiologically [5]. This was more of a novelty than any clinical value, although Klose in 1904 demonstrated a duplex ureter by using two styleted catheters [6]. Also in 1904, Keller filled a bladder with air to demonstrate a diverticulum via X-ray [7]. Air and carbon dioxide proved difficult in distinguishing the urinary tract from bowel gas. In 1905 Voelcker and von Lichtenburg, urologically oriented surgeons from Germany and Budapest, reported positive clinical experience with collargol, a colloidal silver material, for cystography via intravesical injection [8]. The director of the General Electric Research Laboratory, William D. Coolidge, invented an X-ray tube with an improved cathode that offered a much more exact and controlled output of the X-ray by 1913 [9]. The Coolidge tube was a major contribution to the developing field of radiology, and its basic design is still used today.

Retrograde Pyelography

Retrograde is a word of distinguished provenance having early been used, if not invented, by Shakespeare. In *Hamlet* (1599–1602), Claudius tries to dissuade his nephew (and stepson) the prince from returning to school in Wittenberg, saying of that intent:

> It is most retrograde to our desire
> And we beseech you, bend you to remain
> Here in the cheer and comfort of our eye…

In *All's Well that Ends Well* (1604–1605), Helena says, "When he was retrograde, I think, rather." Although a less memorable quote, Helena's comment still gives a full sense of the term. Astronomy as a field also uses the term, most usually in relation to orbiting planets and their moons. Thus, eight planets in our solar system orbit the sun in one direction called "prograde" (counterclockwise as viewed from the pole star, Polaris), while Venus and Uranus have retrograde orbits.

Medicine did not embrace the term "retrograde" until after 1906 when Voelcker and von Lichtenburg described a happy marriage between Mr. Roentgen's pictures and urology as they passed a cystoscope into the bladder, catheterized a ureter, and injected a contrast agent so as to "shoot" a retrograde pyelogram and visualize the upper urinary tract [10]. The material injected, 2 % collargol, was a colloidal silver solution they had previously employed for cystography. Stronger solutions, of Argyrol and 5 % silver iodide, caused toxic damage to the ureters and kidney. At some point, the term "retrograde" came into the picture. Other agents such as air, carbon dioxide, and various heavy metal compounds were utilized as agents to delineate the upper urinary tract under X-ray.

Uhle and Pfahler wrote a paper in 1910 that suggested bismuth paste or dense fluids "cast a shadow" [11]. Bismuth, however, was insoluble and its salts were toxic. Thorium nitrate-citrate visualized well but was somewhat irritative and seemed to become toxic after standing. In 1918, Cameron introduced a sodium and potassium iodide contrast material but abandoned the potassium due to toxicity [12]. The resulting 13.5 % sodium iodide became the standard for retrograde pyelography with its minimal toxicity, good visualization, and isotonicity with urine. A variety of other materials including lithium iodide, colloidal thorium dioxide, and Lipiodol did not find enduring places in the investigational armamentarium.

Intravenous Pyelography

Organic iodides proved the most versatile contrast agents for genitourinary imaging. In 1923, Osborne noticed opacification of the urinary tract in patients with syphilis treated with sodium iodide [4]. In the same year, Rowntree used 10 % sodium iodide orally as well as intravenously. Imaging quality was elusive at the contrast volumes that were safe. A young American urologist named Moses Swick introduced a safe and effective form of iodide called uroselectan. Swick had gone to Germany in 1928 to work with Leopold Lichtwitz, a professor of medicine in Hamburg, where he studied an experimental antimicrobial called Selectan-Neutral, a double iodide compound that had been used to treat urinary tract infections. The compound originally was developed in 1923 by Arthur Binz, professor of chemistry in Berlin, in attempts to create agents with minimal toxicity for treating spirochetal and trypanosomal diseases [13]. Given the utility of iodated compounds in urinary tract imaging, Swick attempted to use the agent for human infections as well as for urography but was deterred by the side effects and marginal quality of images. Trying to find a better form of the contrast material and desiring to work with a larger patient population, Swick transferred his investigations to Berlin, where he worked in the urology clinic of Alexander von Lichtenburg. In 1929, he developed a new compound called Uroselectan with a single iodine atom attached to a 5-carbon pyridine ring. This was soluble enough and nontoxic in rabbits, dogs, and finally humans. When injected intravenously, this agent outlined the urinary tract clearly and give birth to the intravenous pyelogram (IVP) [13–15].

Toxic issues of ego and priority cloud the story. Although the creation of Uroselectan seems to have been created by Swick, von Lichtenberg claimed ownership of the innovation. Swick won initial recognition, presenting his work at the Ninth Congress of the German Urologic Society in Munich during which he outlined steps in the discovery of Uroselectan as well as how to perform intravenous urography with the new contrast agent. After Swick's presentation, von Lichtenburg delivered a paper that listed Swick as coauthor and described their clinical experience with Uroselectan in 84 patients [16].

Swick returned to New York in 1929, where he worked as a urologist at the Mount Sinai Hospital. Mount Sinai's Chief of Radiology Leopold Jaches presented a sensational paper at the 81st session of the AMA Section on Urology. Leading off the ensuing published discussion of the paper, Leopold Lichtwitz said, "Pyelography by way of excretion is an old desire." The subsequent debate included Binz, who stated, "Sodium-2-oxo-5-iodo-pyridine-N-acetate, in its present form, was made in 1927, long before Dr. Swick came to Germany. Its selection by me for the purpose of intravenous urography was not due to the suggestions of Dr. Swick but was an answer to clinical principles which had been agreed on by Professor von Lichtenburg and me, before Professor von Lichtenburg's trip to America last year." On the other hand, Swick told a different version of the story and stated, "The full data concerning these conferences [with Binz] and other matters here discussed will be presented by me tomorrow before the Section on Urology" [13, 17].

Swick cried foul finding himself barred from the 1930 American Urological Association meeting program even though von Lichtenburg was invited to discuss the principles of intravenous urography. Over the next 35 years, Swick did not receive the recognition he believed was deserved. Victor Marshall, professor of urology at Cornell, led efforts for the Section on Urology of the New York Academy of Medicine to award Swick the distinguished Valentine Medal in 1965. Introductory remarks referred to the three decades of frustration Swick suffered in being overlooked for his contributions to his field, and apologies were subsequently forwarded to Swick from a number of prominent leaders in the AUA [13, 18, 19].

Triiodinated contrast media were developed in the 1950s: acetrizoate sodium (Urokon) in 1955, diatrizoate sodium (Hypaque), methylglucamine salt (Renografin), and iothalamate meglumine (Conray) [4]. These agents became routinely used intravenously, making the IVP the cornerstone of urologic imaging for both adults and children at the time. Radiology departments might perform 15–30 IVPs a day, and in most institutions several radiography rooms were solely dedicated to IVPs [20]. Abdominal compression was routinely implemented to distend the calyces and ureters [21]. If an IVP or retrograde pyelogram suggested presence of a renal parenchymal mass, nephrotomography was commonly performed as a separate study the following day [22]. A scout tomogram was followed by a large dose of contrast material injected rapidly through a large-bore IV with 5 mm thick tomographic sections of the kidney in anteroposterior and oblique views. If the findings implied presence of a simple cyst, with smooth margins and a thin rim, then no further images were obtained. Otherwise, a flush aortogram with selective arteriogram would be performed [20]. Bosniak showed that IVP without tomography often missed renal masses [23].

Percutaneous Nephrostogram and Interventional Radiology

Before cross-sectional imaging became routinely available, percutaneous aspiration with contrast injection of renal cysts was used to characterize renal masses seen on IVP or angiography. Diagnostic percutaneous renal puncture was described by Knut Lindblom in 1952 [24], and percutaneous trocar nephrostomy for hydronephrosis was performed by Willard E. Goodwin in 1955 [25, 26]. It was not until nearly 3 decades later in 1981 that Peter Alken reported percutaneous stone surgery [27].

In the 1970s and 1980s, percutaneous antegrade pyelography became reserved for the study of the hydronephrotic collecting system that could not otherwise be sufficiently evaluated by ultrasound, IVP, or nuclear renography. Percutaneous puncture of the kidney in an infant or child was usually performed with a combination of sedation and local anesthesia. The needle was placed in the dilated collecting system under ultrasonic or fluoroscopic guidance, and the pelvicaliceal system was opacified with injection of contrast followed by fluoroscopic spot films. The antegrade pyelogram was sometimes combined with a pressure-flow study (the Whitaker test) to assess the presence of obstruction within the upper urinary tract [28, 29].

Voiding Cystourethrography

In 1944 upon observing that no reports in the radiology literature described arthrography in children, Brodny and Robins stated, "When sufficient experience has been gained, urethrography will be found as valuable for the study of lower urinary tract disease as pyelography is for the diagnosis of renal pathologic lesions" [30]. They sought to identify the ideal contrast medium to opacify the bladder and urethra and yield sufficient anatomical information. Over the prior four decades, several preparations had been introduced but were imperfect. These included metallic salts, halogen salts, iodized oils, and intravenous urographic media. Solutions of silver salts required such high concentrations for adequate radiopacity that they often resulted in toxicity and local tissue injury. Aqueous suspensions of insoluble barium or bismuth salts provided adequate opacification, but insoluble particles remaining in the bladder required copious irrigation for removal to prevent future calculus formation. Concentrated solutions of sodium and potassium iodides and bromides were irritating, and more dilute solutions did not opacify the urinary tract adequately. Additionally, the poor viscosity of these solutions made them impractical for urethrography. In 1923, Lipiodol was introduced as a nonirritating contrast medium that opacified the lower urinary tract sufficiently. A halogenated oil, iodochloral, later offered similar results. Brodny and Robins performed studies with both media and found two flaws in their use: (1) globules of oil form in the bladder in the presence of urine and make it difficult to outline the base of the bladder and (2) they posed risk of oil embolism in the presence of epithelial lesions [30]. The intravenous contrast media introduced for IVP were adapted for cystourethrography because these substances were considered nonirritating, nontoxic, and well tolerated if absorbed in the bloodstream. They lacked viscosity, however, so attempts were made to thicken these agents with glucose or acacia [31]. Despite this, the agents flowed too rapidly through the urethra to obtain acceptable images.

In 1947 Brodny and Robins introduced rayopake as a superior contrast medium for cystourethrography. It consisted of an organic compound containing iodine diethanolamine to render it soluble in water and a polymeric form of polyvinyl alcohol to increase the viscosity. Rayopake outlined the genitourinary tract clearly, did not form globules when mixed with urine or water, had adequate viscosity for performing urethrography, did not produce emboli, and did not irritate the urethral epithelium [30].

Despite safe, well-tolerated contrast solutions, evaluation of the lower urinary tract by means of VCUG took several decades for acceptance. After promoting their choice of contrast agent for cystourethrography, Brodny and Robins emphasized the utility of both retrograde and voiding cystourethrography in evaluating boys with suspected urologic disorders. Until they published their series of pediatric cystourethrographic studies in 1948, the merits of this study in children had not been sufficiently recognized [32]. A typical investigation of urinary tract pathology in children mid-century included IVP followed by endoscopy under general anesthesia. Because most parents and pediatricians did not wish to subject a child to a general anesthetic if the IVP was considered normal, IVP became the blanket test for evaluating the entire urinary tract. Direct radiologic investigation of the lower urinary tract was avoided for a number of reasons: (1) the difficulty of performing a voiding cystourethrogram on children, (2) fear of radiation exposure to the gonads, and (3) lack of appreciation for the value of a VCUG among clinicians at the time [33]. Radionuclide cystography was introduced in 1959 [34] and was considered by some superior to VCUG because it allowed quantitation of parameters affecting bladder function and could more adequately evaluate the filling and emptying of the bladder [35].

In the early to mid-1960s, VCUG became more accepted as a major diagnostic tool in pediatric uroradiology. Today VCUG is the principal examination used for the study of the bladder and urethra in children and considered the standard for detecting vesicoureteral reflux. The retrograde urethrogram is the primary urographic study for demonstrating the details of abnormalities in the male urethra below the level of the sphincter.

Ultrasonography

Black-background real-time ultrasound became standard in the late 1970s. Digital scan converters allowed for obtaining images quickly, and soon ultrasonography became the gold standard for differentiating solid from cystic renal lesions, making nephrotomography and arteriography second line in the evaluation of renal masses [20, 36]. Ultrasonography changed the approach to the imaging of the urinary tract in the child, leading to decreased utilization of IVPs by the late 1970s [37]. Whereas IVP was once the first-line test for the exploration of pediatric urological diseases, ultrasound soon became the preferred form of imaging. The reduced risk of ionizing radiation, contrast reactions, and iatrogenic complications made ultrasound ideal for evaluating newborns, infants, and children as well as the fetal urinary tract in utero [38]. In the early 1980s, the lack of all risk was not completely proven, so ultrasound was still used in moderation, especially in pregnancy [39, 40].

With improvement in ultrasonographic imaging over the last 30 years, more facile detection of urologic abnormalities in the antenatal period has changed the practice of pediatric urology. Detection of clinically significant antenatal hydronephrosis helps the pediatric urologist plan treatment, if indicated, in the neonatal period as well as determine whether fetal intervention is warranted. Antenatally detected urologic diagnoses may lead to a prenatal visit between parents and the pediatric urologist, helping to establish rapport and provide reassurance prior to delivery [41, 42].

Ultrasonography has also afforded us an accessible, inexpensive, and safe way to follow young patients after delivery and understand the natural history of urologic problems. For example, before antenatal ultrasound, patients with primary obstructed megaureter typically did not present until later in life with symptoms of pyelonephritis. Of those with megaureter now detected antenatally, we know that approximately 80 % will have spontaneous resolution of hydronephrosis over time and not require intervention, but those that persist or progress can be repaired [43]. Antenatal detection of hydronephrosis on ultrasound has also resulted in the early elective detection of vesicoureteral reflux with VCUG. While such information is debated by some authorities, we believe that early recognition of vesicoureteral reflux can preempt reflux nephropathy in many children [44].

Early detection and the ability to follow the multicystic dysplastic kidney (MCDK) with ultrasonography has also transformed the management of this condition in that previously almost all MCDKs were removed upon discovery. Now most are found with antenatal imaging, and the pathognomic criteria for diagnosis have arisen from characteristics seen on ultrasound, including the presence of noncommunicating cysts varying in size. Serial ultrasound has proven that the majority of MCDKs involute over time with no need for nephrectomy [45, 46].

Antenatal ultrasonography has also allowed uroradiologists and pediatric urologists to characterize the actual prevalence of certain congenital conditions. Based on imaging, we now know that the most common antenatally detected urologic abnormality is ureteropelvic junction obstruction (UPJO), followed closely by megaureter, VUR, and renal duplication. Fortunately, boys with posterior urethral valves (PUV) represent only a small percentage of antenatal hydronephrosis [47]. Due to early detection of UPJO with antenatal ultrasound, the prevalent etiology has shifted from extrinsic to intrinsic obstruction. Before routine antenatal imaging, the majority of pediatric patients with UPJO would present when older with symptoms of obstruction as was once called Dietl's crisis. Now infants with an intrinsically narrowed UPJ segment are found before they present with symptoms. Today only a small percentage of these patients present later in life. Because of early detection, now those with extrinsic compression comprise the majority of symptomatic cases of UPJ typically seen in older children [48].

Bladder exstrophy was formerly diagnosed at birth, limiting the ability to provide antenatal counseling to parents, plan delivery, and prepare for closure in the OR. Now with antenatal sonography this rare anomaly may be detected before birth, providing an advantage to both parents and providers to prepare them for future intervention. A much more common application of ultrasonography initially described by Miskin et al. has revolutionized imaging of the testes, particularly with use of color Doppler to assess testicular flow and gray scale to evaluate testicular masses, torsion, or inflammation [49, 50].

Nuclear Imaging

Nuclear medicine imaging surfaced in the 1960s and was initially performed with a rectilinear scanner and 131 iodohippurate sodium (Hippuran 131) to demonstrate renal function more than to evaluate renal anatomy. In the next decade, the Anger gamma camera replaced the rectilinear scanner; technetium-based isotopes such as Tc-diethylenetriaminepentaacetic acid (DTPA) and Tc-dimercaptosuccinic acid (DMSA) came into use [51]. These agents had a much shorter half-life and more favorable photopeak for imaging, so both renal anatomy and function could be effectively studied [20]. The primary benefit of nuclear medicine techniques was seen in the limited pharmacologic, toxic, osmotic, allergic, and hemodynamic effects associated with radiotracers as compared to contrast agents. In the late 1970s and early 1980s, several studies highlighted the utility of DMSA in detecting renal scarring, particularly in children with a known history of urinary tract infection. The IVP and renal ultrasound were surpassed by DMSA, in providing a distinction between normal and abnormal renal tissue [52, 53]. By the late 1980s a few medical institutions routinely employed nuclear medicine methods to investigate genitourinary pathology in children, but soon thereafter nuclear imaging became more routinely available and came into wide use by pediatric urologists.

Computerized Tomography

Computerized tomography (CT) was originally developed in the 1970s and went through a number of iterations before it became the standard for assessing renal masses, diagnosing renal inflammatory disease, and evaluating renal trauma in the 1980s [54–58]. Cross-sectional imaging began to replace IVP as the primary imaging modality to assess renal pathology in the early 1990s and effectively extended to three-dimensional imaging of the arterial system. Smith et al. first described noncontrast CT to evaluate patients with renal colic, allowing quick assessment without use of contrast agents and better sensitivity for radiolucent stones as compared to IVP [59]. CT urography has become the preferred imaging method over the last 15 years for assessing the upper tracts in hematuria workup [60]. While CT scan may be the study of choice in certain clinical scenarios, we believe it should be used very sparingly in children since radiation doses from CT are cumulative over the life of an individual [61, 62].

Magnetic Resonance Imaging

Urologic magnetic resonance imaging (MRI) entered the urologic armamentarium in the early 1980s and became readily available by the end of the decade [63–66]. This is particularly useful in patients with adverse reactions to iodinated contrast, although at its beginning the modality was too slow and expensive for routine use. For evaluating children with renal disease, MRI was initially deemed a limited study, and recommendations were made that it be used as an adjunct to other imaging modalities such as ultrasound [67]. In 1991 Sigmund et al. described RARE (Rapid Acquisition with Relaxation Enhancement) MRI in children, a technique thought to delineate the upper tract so well as to replace the IVP and other routine studies at the time. However, due to the lack of information RARE MRI could provide with respect to renal function and vesicoureteral reflux, in addition to its cumbersome methodology and restricted availability, it did not become a substitute for all other imaging studies [68]. Just over a decade later, advances in MR urography (MRU) including gadolinium as a contrast agent allowed for a sophisticated study with detailed anatomical information as well as functional assessment of the kidney and lower urinary tract [69, 70]. Attempts have been made to correlate MRU findings with those seen on diuretic renography, but a lack of standardized protocols results in limited accuracy and reproducibility among various institutions to date, although this will surely improve.

Future Directions

Pediatric uroradiography has evolved enormously over the last century, yet the search for the ideal imaging study continues. A number of special considerations in genitourinary imaging are unique to the pediatric population, such as cumulative risks of exposure to ionizing radiation, occasional need for general anesthesia, and stress surrounding catheterization and immobilization. Imaging techniques that eliminate radiation, restraint, sedation, and anxiety yet provide good functional and anatomic detail will win the day. Voiding urosonography, for example, is a radiation-free imaging method that not only provides radiographic information about the presence and grade of vesicoureteral reflux but may ultimately be more sensitive than VCUG [71]. While the list of developments in imaging over the past several decades is long, pediatric uroradiology continues to advance rapidly, providing pediatric and radiologists alike with a number of tools to facilitate exceptional urologic care for children.

In few aspects of medicine is the link between the basic sciences (physics, chemistry, biology) and practical application to human health as visible and fruitful as in the story of genitourinary imaging. That link between the metaphoric "bench and bedside" is contingent upon information science, technology, an educated workforce, and entrepreneurial enterprise in a free society. Pediatric urologic imaging is a classic case study of the human mind over matter.

References

1. Halajian EB, Wheat TA, Bloom DA. Arpad G Gerster, MD and the first photographic surgical textbook. J Am Coll Surg. 2006;203(1):116–23.
2. DiSantis DJ. Early American radiology: the pioneer years. AJR Am J Roentgenol. 1986;147(4):850–3.
3. Macintyre J. Photography of renal calculus. Lancet. 1896;2:118.
4. Oyen R, Gryspeerdt S, Baert AL. The history of uroradiology. J Belg Radiol. 1995;78(5):291–4.
5. Tuffier T. Sonde ureterale opaque. In: Duplay SE, Reclus P, editors. Traite de Chirurgie, vol. 7. Paris: Masson; 1897. p. 412–13.
6. Klose B. Radiographie eines durch das Kystoskop diagnostizierten Falles von kompletter Ureterenverdopplung. Deutsche Zeitschrift f Chirurgie. 1904;72:614–17.
7. Gillies CL, Kerr HD. The roentgen diagnosis of lesions of the lower urinary tract. Radiology. 1936;26: 286–94.
8. Voelcker F, von Lichtenburg A. Die Gestalt der menschlichen Harnblase im Roentgenbilde. Muenchener Medizische Wochenschrif. 1905;52(33):1576–8.
9. Coolidge WD. A powerful roentgen ray tube with a pure electron discharge. Phys Rev. 1913;2:409–30.
10. Voelcker F, von Lichtenburg A. Pyelographie Röntgenographie des Nierenbeckens nach Kollargolfüllung. Muenchener Medizische Wochenschrif. 1906;53: 105–6.
11. Uhle AA, Pfahler GE, Mackinney WH, Miller AG. XIII. Combined cystoscopic and roentgenographic examination of the kidneys and ureter. Ann Surg. 1910;51(4):546–51.
12. Cameron DF. Aqueous solutions of potassium and sodium iodide as opaque mediums in roentgenography: a preliminary report. JAMA. 1918;70:754–5.
13. Elkin M. Stages in the growth of uroradiology. Radiology. 1990;175(2):297–306.

14. Swick M. Intravenous urography by means of the sodium salt of 5-iodo-2-pyridon-n-acetic acid. JAMA. 1930;95:1403.
15. Pollack HM. Uroradiology. In: McClennan BL, editor. Radiology Centennial. Reston: Radiology Centennial; 1996. p. 195–253.
16. von Lichtenburg A, Swick M. Clinical test of uroselectan. Klin Wochenschr. 1929;8:2089–91.
17. Jaches L. Intravenous urography (Swick method). JAMA. 1930;95:1409–12.
18. Melicow MM. Presentation of the fourth Ferdinand C. Valentine Medal and award to Moses Swick. Bull N Y Acad Med. 1966;42(2):123–7.
19. Swick M. The discovery of intravenous urography: historical and developmental aspects of the urographic media and their role in other diagnostic and therapeutic areas. Bull N Y Acad Med. 1966;42(2): 128–51.
20. Goldman SM, Sandler CM. Genitourinary imaging: the past 40 years. Radiology. 2000;215(2):313–24.
21. Daughtridge TG. Ureteral compression device for excretory urography. Am J Roentgenol Radium Ther Nucl Med. 1965;95(2):431–8.
22. Evans JA, Dubilier Jr W, Monteith JC. Nephrotomography; a preliminary report. Am J Roentgenol Radium Ther Nucl Med. 1954;71(2):213–23.
23. Bosniak MA. Nephrotomography: a relatively unappreciated but extremely valuable diagnostic tool. Radiology. 1974;113(2):313–21.
24. Lindblom K. Percutaneous puncture of renal cysts and tumors. Acta Radiol. 1946;27(1):66–72.
25. Goodwin WE, Casey WC, Woolf W. Percutaneous trocar (needle) nephrostomy in hydronephrosis. JAMA. 1955;157(11):891–4.
26. Palapattu GS, Bloom DA, Smith RB, Boxer RJ. Willard E. Goodwin: educator, innovator and pioneer. J Urol. 2004;172(1):40–4.
27. Alken P, Hutschenreiter G, Gunther R, Marberger M. Percutaneous stone manipulation. J Urol. 1981;125(4): 463–6.
28. Ben-Ami T, Lebowitz RL. Pediatric uroradiology. In: Retik AB, Cukier J, editors. Pediatric urology, vol. 14. Baltimore: Williams & Wilkins; 1987. p. 12–62.
29. Tchetgen MB, Bloom DA. Robert H. Whitaker and the Whitaker test: a pressure-flow study of the upper urinary tract. Urology. 2003;61:253–6.
30. Brodny ML, Robins SA. The use of a new viscous water-miscible contrast medium rayopake for cystourethrography. J Urol. 1947;58(3):182–4.
31. Flocks RH. Roentgen visualization of the posterior urethra. J Urol. 1933;30:711–36.
32. Brodny ML, Robins SA. Urethrocystography in the male child. JAMA. 1948;137(17):1511–17.
33. Burrows EH, Allen RP. Urethral lesions in infancy and childhood studied by micturition cystourethrography. Br J Radiol. 1964;37:187–99.
34. Winter CC. A new test for vesicoureteral reflux: an external technique using radioisotopes. J Urol. 1959; 81(1):105–11.
35. Conway JJ. Radionuclide cystography. Contrib Nephrol. 1984;39:1–19.
36. Ophir J, Maklad NF. Digital scan converters in diagnostic ultrasound imaging. Proc IEEE. 1979;67(4): 654–64.
37. Lebowitz RL, Ben-Ami T. Trends in pediatric uroradiology. Urol Radiol. 1983;5(3):135–47.
38. Slovis TL, Perlmutter AD. Recent advances in pediatric urological ultrasound. J Urol. 1980;123(5): 613–20.
39. Jacobson-Kram D. The effects of diagnostic ultrasound on sister chromatid exchange frequencies: a review of the recent literature. J Clin Ultrasound. 1984;12(1):5–10.
40. Martin AO. Can ultrasound cause genetic damage? J Clin Ultrasound. 1984;12(1):11–9.
41. Lebowitz RL. Paediatric urology and uroradiology: changes in the last 25 years. BJU Int. 2003;92 Suppl 1:7–9.
42. Lebowitz RL, Teele RL. Fetal and neonatal hydronephrosis. Urol Radiol. 1983;5(3):185–8.
43. McLellan DL, Retik AB, Bauer SB, et al. Rate and predictors of spontaneous resolution of prenatally diagnosed primary nonrefluxing megaureter. J Urol. 2002;168(5):2177–80; discussion 2180.
44. Paltiel HJ, Lebowitz RL. Neonatal hydronephrosis due to primary vesicoureteral reflux: trends in diagnosis and treatment. Radiology. 1989;170(3 Pt 1): 787–9.
45. Bloom DA, Brosman S. The multicystic kidney. J Urol. 1978;120(2):211–15.
46. Wacksman J, Phipps L. Report of the multicystic kidney registry: preliminary findings. J Urol. 1993;150(6):1870–2.
47. Brown T, Mandell J, Lebowitz RL. Neonatal hydronephrosis in the era of sonography. AJR Am J Roentgenol. 1987;148(5):959–63.
48. Rooks VJ, Lebowitz RL. Extrinsic ureteropelvic junction obstruction from a crossing renal vessel: demography and imaging. Pediatr Radiol. 2001;31(2):120–4.
49. Miskin M, Bain J. B-mode ultrasonic examination of the testes. J Clin Ultrasound. 1974;2(4):307–11.
50. Miskin M, Buckspan M, Bain J. Ultrasonographic examination of scrotal masses. J Urol. 1977; 117(2):185–8.
51. Blaufox MD. The role of nuclear medicine: a historical perspective. In: Blaufox MD, editor. Evaluation of renal function and disease with radionuclides: the upper urinary tract. Basel: Karger; 1989. p. 2–11.
52. Bingham JB, Maisey MN. An evaluation of the use of 99Tcm-dimercaptosuccinic acid (DMSA) as a static renal imaging agent. Br J Radiol. 1978; 51(608):599–607.
53. Merrick MV, Uttley WS, Wild SR. The detection of pyelonephritic scarring in children by radioisotope imaging. Br J Radiol. 1980;53(630):544–56.
54. Hoffman EP, Mindelzun RE, Anderson RU. Computed tomography in acute pyelonephritis associated with diabetes. Radiology. 1980;135(3):691–5.

55. Rauschkolb EN, Sandler CM, Patel S, Childs TL. Computed tomography of renal inflammatory disease. J Comput Assist Tomogr. 1982;6(3):502–6.
56. Lee JK, McClennan BL, Melson GL, Stanley RJ. Acute focal bacterial nephritis: emphasis on gray scale sonography and computed tomography. AJR Am J Roentgenol. 1980;135(1):87–92.
57. Federle MP, Kaiser JA, McAninch JW, Jeffrey RB, Mall JC. The role of computed tomography in renal trauma. Radiology. 1981;141(2):455–60.
58. Sandler CM, Toombs BD. Computed tomographic evaluation of blunt renal injuries. Radiology. 1981; 141(2):461–6.
59. Smith RC, Rosenfield AT, Choe KA, et al. Acute flank pain: comparison of non-contrast-enhanced CT and intravenous urography. Radiology. 1995;194(3): 789–94.
60. Perlman ES, Rosenfield AT, Wexler JS, Glickman MG. CT urography in the evaluation of urinary tract disease. J Comput Assist Tomogr. 1996;20(4):620–6.
61. Frush DP, Donnelly LF, Rosen NS. Computed tomography and radiation risks: what pediatric health care providers should know. Pediatrics. 2003;112(4): 951–7.
62. Johnson EK, Faerber GJ, Roberts WW, Wolf Jr SJ, Park JM, Bloom DA, Wan J. Are stone protocol computed tomography scans mandatory for children with suspected urinary calculi? Urology. 2001;78(3): 662–6.
63. Damadian R. Tumor detection by nuclear magnetic resonance. Science. 1971;171(3976):1151–3.
64. Pettigrew RI, Avruch L, Dannels W, Coumans J, Bernardino ME. Fast-field-echo MR imaging with Gd-DTPA: physiologic evaluation of the kidney and liver. Radiology. 1986;160(2):561–3.
65. Hricak H, Crooks L, Sheldon P, Kaufman L. Nuclear magnetic resonance imaging of the kidney. Radiology. 1983;146(2):425–32.
66. Newhouse JH. Urinary tract imaging by nuclear magnetic resonance. Urol Radiol. 1982;4(2–3):171–5.
67. Dietrich RB, Kangarloo H. Kidneys in infants and children: evaluation with MR. Radiology. 1986; 159(1):215–21.
68. Sigmund G, Stoever B, Zimmerhackl LB, et al. RARE-MR-urography in the diagnosis of upper urinary tract abnormalities in children. Pediatr Radiol. 1991;21(6):416–20.
69. Perez-Brayfield MR, Kirsch AJ, Jones RA, Grattan-Smith JD. A prospective study comparing ultrasound, nuclear scintigraphy and dynamic contrast enhanced magnetic resonance imaging in the evaluation of hydronephrosis. J Urol. 2003;170(4 Pt 1): 1330–4.
70. Grattan-Smith JD, Perez-Bayfield MR, Jones RA, et al. MR imaging of kidneys: functional evaluation using F-15 perfusion imaging. Pediatr Radiol. 2003; 33(5):293–304.
71. Papadopoulou F, Anthopoulou A, Siomou E, Efremidis S, Tsamboulas C, Darge K. Harmonic voiding urosonography with a second-generation contrast agent for the diagnosis of vesicoureteral reflux. Pediatr Radiol. 2009;39(3):239–44.

Principles of Ultrasound

2

Jeanne Choi Rosen, Lesli Nicolay, and Jeffrey S. Palmer

Introduction

Ultrasound is the most common imaging modality to study the genitourinary system in the pediatric population. While advances in other technologies further the ability to image the genitourinary tract, ultrasound has remained the imaging study of choice as it is noninvasive and involves no ionizing radiation, and the images are acquired quickly, in multiple planes in real time, without the need for sedation. There are portable units also available for clinical use. Ultrasound is a very advantageous imaging modality particularly for the young child, whose potential lack of cooperation may not allow a second chance to obtain imaging of the possible abnormality. It is also a relatively more cost-efficient imaging modality, as compared to CT scan and MRI. As significant numbers of prenatal ultrasounds are performed, many genitourinary abnormalities are being incidentally identified, requiring postnatal confirmation. The postnatal ultrasound has proven invaluable in identifying those patients for which additional imaging studies such as voiding cystourethrogram (VCUG), nuclear renography, CT, and MRI are indicated. Many children may need serial studies throughout the childhood to follow an abnormality, such as hydronephrosis. Ultrasound can also help identify patients where no further imaging workup is necessary. It has been also proven to be invaluable in the assessment of the acutely ill patient, being very highly sensitive and specific for certain diagnoses and can provide image guidance for procedures.

Background of Ultrasound

Ultrasound images are obtained by the interaction of sound waves with tissues and fluid. The term ultrasound is used as the frequency of the sound waves utilized is above the level which the human ear can detect—above 20 kHz. Ultrasound has its history in the development of SONAR, which means Sound Navigation and Ranging. Sound waves were used to help localize depth, such as structure in a lake. The piezoelectric effect was discovered in the late 1880s by the Curie brothers. With the advent of SONAR, new concepts of the physics of sound waves were being explored and new uses discovered. In 1955, Dr. Ian McDonald, seeing the application of ultrasound in the military,

J.C. Rosen, MD
Division of Pediatric, Department of Diagnostic Radiology, Cohen Children's Hospital, North Shore Long Island Jewish Medical Center, Second Floor, New Hyde Park, NY 11040, USA
e-mail: jchoiros@nshs.edu

L. Nicolay, MD
Division of Pediatric Urology, Department of Urology, Loma Linda University Medical Center, Loma Linda, CA, USA
e-mail: linicolay@gmail.com

J.S. Palmer, MD, FACS, FAAP (✉)
Pediatric and Adolescent Urology Institute, Cleveland, OH, USA
e-mail: jeffreypalmermd@gmail.com

L.S. Palmer, J.S. Palmer (eds.), *Pediatric and Adolescent Urologic Imaging*,
DOI 10.1007/978-1-4614-8654-1_2, © Springer Science+Business Media New York 2014

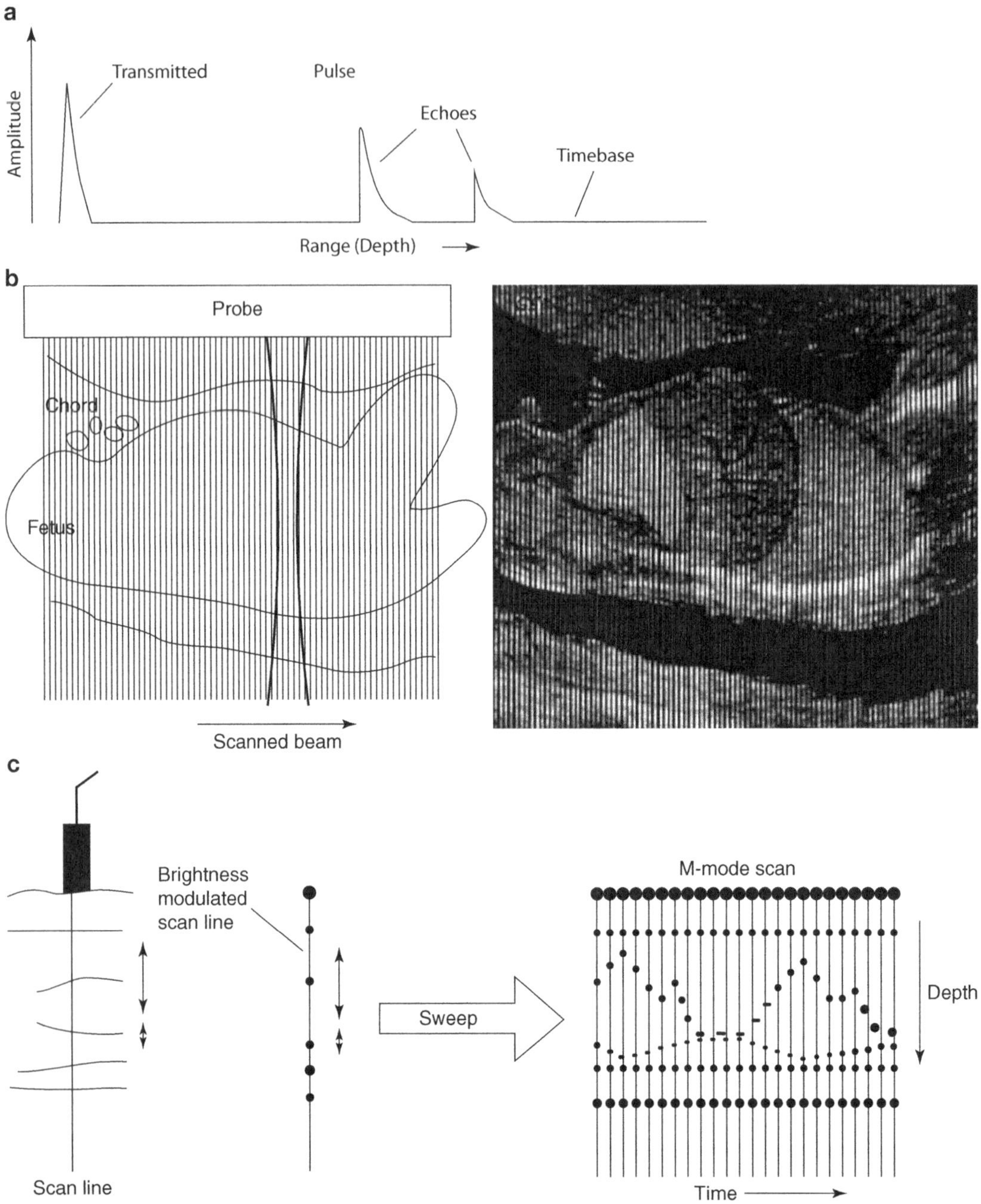

Fig. 2.1 (**a**) An example of an A-mode scan. The received echo amplitude is plotted against time of transmission which is proportional to the depth. (**b**) In B-mode, the received echoes are displayed as a series of dots of varying brightness creating a two-dimensional image. (**c**) In M-mode, a diagram is created by graphing the received echoes on a plot of depth versus time (From Whittingham [2]. Reprinted with permission from Elsevier Limited)

worked with several individuals to develop this technology for obstetrical and gynecologic patients. There were handful of indications for ultrasound in medical imaging, but its use was limited by the technology of the period.

The basic ultrasound unit is composed of a transmitter, a transducer, an image display, and image storage system. There are three common types of sonographic image display used today (Fig. 2.1):

A-mode (amplitude mode) ultrasound obtains echoes along a specified depth axis. After propagation through the tissues, the echoes that are returned are graphically displayed with the amplitude of the echo versus time. This appears on the screen as spikes along a horizontal line. This mode is particularly useful in situations that knowledge of the depth of the interface is desired and can be used therapeutically [1].

B-mode (brightness mode) ultrasound converts the received echoes into a series of dots of varying brightness, creating a two-dimensional grayscale image [2]. Early B-mode scanners required a patient to be placed in an immersion bath. In 1962, three men—Joseph Holmes, William Wright, and Ralph Meyerdirk—developed the compound contact B-mode scanner, revolutionizing ultrasound imaging in health care. Several more advances in B-mode scanners were developed in the 1970s.

When real-time capability was developed in B-mode, this became the dominant form of medical sonography. Real-time B-mode obtains information to create two-dimensional images that are used for the majority of medical imaging. For a given plane, multiple piezoelectric crystals are arrayed, and sound waves are sent and received and are then integrated to produce a grayscale image. The spectrum of grayscale brightness that is displayed for each received echo corresponds to the amplitude of the wave. The beam is rapidly and continuously reproduced and received to provide a dynamic, real-time image [1].

M-mode (motion mode) ultrasound obtains a series of B-mode signals, which are then displayed along a time axis, allowing for evaluation of the motion of a structure [1]. Therefore, at specific known depths from the transducer, the echoes are translated as motion of that structure. Short segments of the data can be stored digitally and played back instantly. Most common uses for this mode would be for analyzing movements of the heart or in obstetrics to isolate the beating heart of a fetus.

Basic Concept of Ultrasound

The ultrasound wave is produced by applying short burst of alternating electrical current to special crystals known as piezoelectric crystals, housed in the transducer, also known as a probe (Fig. 2.2). The electric current causes heating and polarizing of the lead atoms that are loosely bound within a crystal matrix. The crystal will then expand and contract, converting electrical energy into an acoustic wave. This phenomenon of converting electric energy into a pressure/sound wave energy and vice versa is known as the piezoelectric effect. Today these elements are commonly made from ceramic materials [3, 4].

The frequency of the wave produced is dependent on the pulses of electrical current and the plate thickness of the piezoelectric material. Typical frequencies of ultrasound waves, i.e., transducers used in urological exams, are between 2.0 and 15 MHz, which are above the limits of human hearing. These acoustic waves are transmitted into the patient by the transducer, with the aid of a coupling gel, when the transducer is placed on the body. The efficiency of this process is improved by the presence of an impedance barrier, the rubber surface present on the transducer. These sound waves can then be reflected, refracted, scattered, or absorbed by the body.

The ultrasound wave is affected by the physical characteristics of the tissue through which it is propagated and then reflected. As the wave travels through the body, ultrasound echoes are received by the transducer. These echoes are then converted back into electric energy, which are then processed and translated into an image on the screen.

The Principles and Physics of Ultrasound in the Body

The ultrasound wave is a mechanical wave. Its movement through tissue causes oscillation of the tissue in a longitudinal direction, propagating the mechanical wave. As the ultrasound wave moves through different types of tissues, i.e., density, the elements of the tissue will oscillate higher or lower in relation to its ambient state, without net motion.

Frequency

The number of waves or pulses occurring in time, i.e., seconds, and is expressed in Hertz

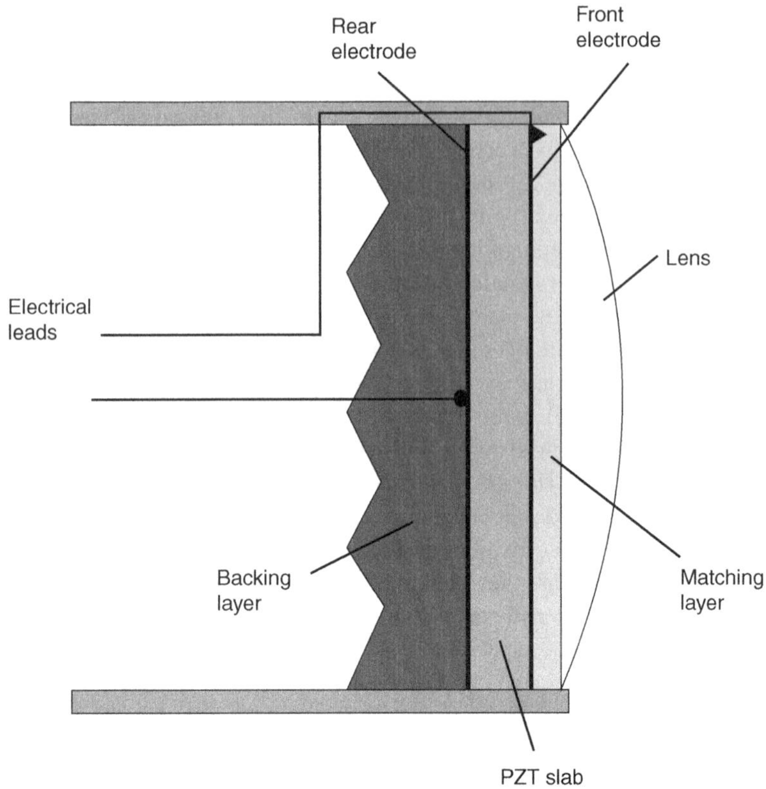

Fig. 2.2 The basic components of an ultrasound probe (From Whittingham [2]. Reprinted with permission from Elsevier Limited)

(Hz). Wavelength (λ) describes the physical space that one pulse length occupies. Frequency and wavelength are inversely related because of their relationship to velocity (velocity = frequency × wavelength). A higher frequency will result in a shorter wavelength and vice versa. For ultrasound imaging, the general ultrasound tissue velocity or speed is given as a constant (c) at 1,540 m/s [5, 6].

Assuming constant velocity (c), the depth (D) at which the interface occurred can be calculated as D = c/2 x (time from pulse generated to echo-detection). The number 2 reflects that the wave traveled from the transducer to a point and the sound wave traveled back from that point, prior to being received by the transducer [4].

Amplitude

The maximum height or size that the wave travels in the positive or negative direction. The clinical significance of the wave amplitude is that it corresponds to the energy contained in the mechanical wave. Energy is equal to the amplitude squared. In clinical terms of the grayscale image, the amplitude affects the pixel brightness so that a greater amplitude wave produces pixels that are brighter [4].

Reflection

There are two types of wave reflections that occur and are received by the transducer that demonstrate clinical significance, specular echo and scatter echo.

When the transducer sends and receives a wave that is reflected off a smooth/flat surface, perpendicular to the angle of the moving sound wave, the echo is considered a specular or mirror-like echo. The angle of reflection will be equal to the angle of incidence keeping with Snell's Law. This type of echo, the specular echo, is characteristically reflected with the highest intensity strength and directionality. Specular echoes are seen from the linings of hollow viscera, blood vessels, fascial planes, organ capsules, skin, and gas or bone surfaces. To help correct for the speckling characteristic seen in some tissues, a technique called compounding can be used. Compounding sends sound waves into the tissue from multiples angles. Sending compound waves enables better image contrast by combining specular echoes, so they are more likely to be detected which results in minimizing speckling.

When sound waves are reflected off surfaces with irregularities, and the irregularities are similar in size to the wavelength of the sound wave, the energy of the wave is dispersed in all directions. This is known as scatter. The scatter echo returning to the transducer is therefore weaker and typically only detectible if several of the scattered wavelets are superimposed to produce an additive effect. Scattering accounts for the textured appearance of a tissue type, which is a result of an interference pattern, and is referred to as speckling. This property gives parenchyma such as the liver or testicles their characteristic appearance and makes them distinguishable from other structures. However, it should be noted that there is a spectrum between specular echoes and scattering with most tissues demonstrating properties that fall between the two extremes.

Rarefaction

It should also be stated that when a sound wave pulse is sent from the transducer, the wave does not necessarily propagate in a uniform and linear manner. Rather, the wave pulse becomes distorted as it travels through the tissue medium with some areas of the pulse having higher frequency components or harmonics corresponding to areas with increasing density of the medium. A portion of the wave would then travel faster than the rarefaction component of the wave which travels slightly slower. Rarefaction artifacts can occur therefore at the interface of two types of tissue as the angle of the sound wave is no longer linear. This can be seen at tissue interfaces such as fat and soft tissue or at soft tissue fluid interfaces. In the latter, the part of the beam that does not pass through the fluid is less intense that those traveling through the fluid structure. The difference in distortion is dependent on the initial sound wave intensity. The higher the acoustic power, the stronger the harmonics, and therefore a greater difference between the weaker sections of the wave frequency can occur. Stronger areas of the beam are typically located in the central section of the wave beam. Additionally, since it takes a few cycles to ramp up the intensities, frequencies are also weaker within the first few millimeters of tissue penetrated. Machines that filter out and select for a particular frequency produce a better image with improved contrast and counteract this distortion.

Absorption

The energy from the sound wave stimulates the tissue particles to move, enabling the sound wave to be transmitted as an acoustic vibration. If the tissue particles move in a cohesive and organized manner, then the vibration is transmitted efficiently. However, if the particle movement becomes chaotic and disjointed, then the sound wave will become chaotic, and the energy from the sound wave will be lost and converted into heat. When sound wave energy is lost by this method, it is referred to as absorption. Absorption is greater when the percentage of large particles in the tissue is increased; thus, the tissue has a greater viscosity. Similarly, absorption is dependent on the frequency of the sound wave with greater absorption occurring with higher frequencies. Per 1 cm depth of sound wave penetration, 1 dB is lost per 1 MHz transmitted. Thus, the higher the frequency, the more decibels are lost per centimeter of tissue causing the potential depth of penetration to be decreased. Since the speed of the sound wave traveling through soft tissues is constant, the time delay of the reflected sound wave can be used to calculate the depth of reflected image.

Attenuation

Anytime energy is lost and not returned to the transducer it is referred to as attenuation.

Absorption is only one type of attenuation and was explained in the previous paragraph. Another type of attenuation occurs when the sound wave is reflected or refracted in such a way that the wave is unable to be returned in the same plane as to be detected by the receiving transducer. When a sound wave crosses an interface between two different tissues, some of the wave's energy is reflected. The degree or proportion of the energy in the wave that is reflected is dependent on the change in the tissue density across that interface, also known as the impedance mismatch.

Typically, only a small percentage of reflection occurs with interfaces of similar tissues (<10 %). However, a tissue-gas interface leads to almost complete reflection of the wave and with tissue-bone or tissue-calculus interfaces resulting in almost 60–75 % of the wave being reflected. When this degree of reflection occurs, an acoustic shadow is then created. The acoustic shadow prevents visualization of structures deep to this interface as there had been almost complete reflection of the sound wave. The dark band is caused as the tissue absorbs the sound wave faster than the background, and the area deep to the highly attenuating region appears dark. Fat, gas, and calcifications are especially associated with shadowing (Fig. 2.3). Calcifications that are smaller than 5 mm will demonstrate shadowing when higher-resolution transducers are used. Similarly, aggregates of fine calcifications can shadow if their size and density is sufficiently high. Another type of shadowing is known as edge shadows or edge artifact that appears as fine, dark lines extending deep to curved surfaces. These are commonly seen in isolated cysts or at the edge of a testis (Fig. 2.4).

In contrast, there can be increased transmission when waves are less attenuated, such as transmission of sound waves through a simple cyst. The posterior wall of the cyst can artificially appear hyperechoic. This is known as through transmission (Fig. 2.5).

Acoustic Impedance

This occurs at the interface of two tissue types, i.e., tissues with different densities. Part of the wave will be reflected and part will continue longitudinally through the tissues. The more different the tissues at the interface, the greater the contrast of the image obtained versus those of similar tissue density.

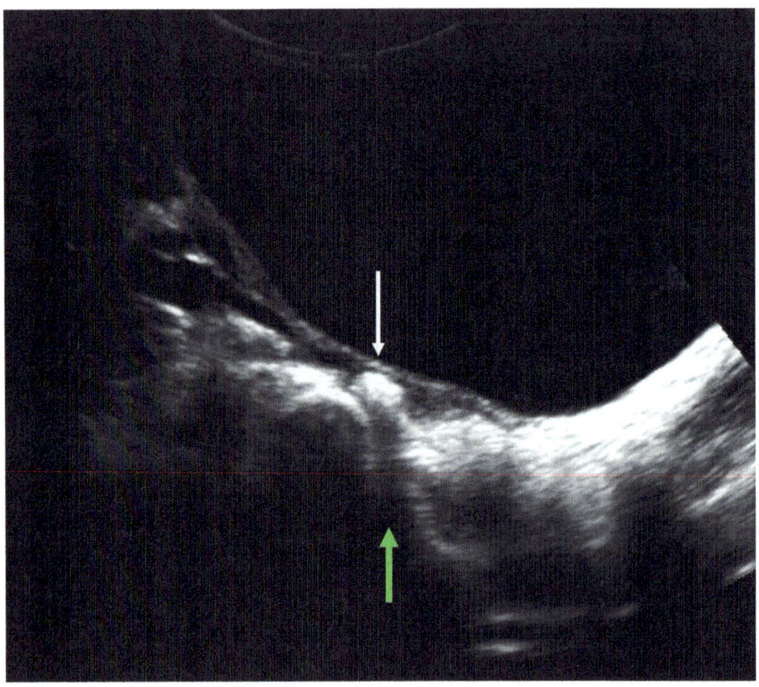

Fig. 2.3 Arrow pointing to a calculus (*white arrow*) in the distal right ureter demonstrating the phenomenon known as shadowing (*green arrow*)

Acoustic Intensity

This is defined as the power per unit area of the ultrasound pulse. The more ultrasound waves concentrated in a smaller area, the more the intensity of the sound waves and the more detailed the image. The larger the cross-sectional energy, the less intensity per unit area, the lower the amplitude.

Resolution

This is defined as the ability to distinguish two objects that are in close proximity to one another. There are two types of resolution, axial resolution and lateral resolution, which are important in generating the image.

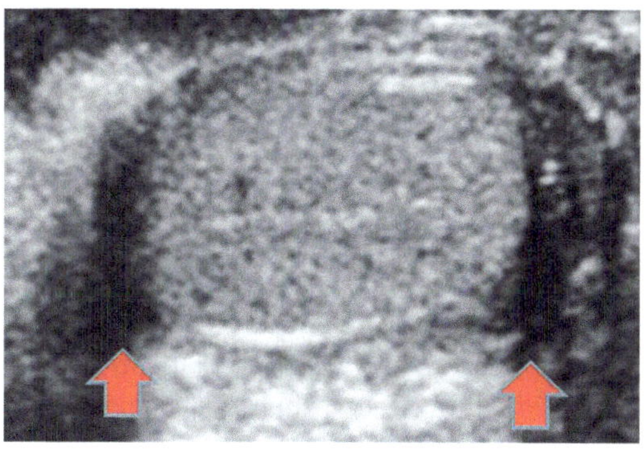

Fig. 2.4 Edge artifact is demonstrated on both the superior and inferior edges of this testis (*red arrows*)

Axial resolution is the ability to differentiate between objects that are in the direction of the traveling wave or in front of one another. This property is dependent on the frequency of the sound wave. A higher frequency results in better image resolution due to the shorter sound wavelength, allowing for differentiation of objects that are close to each other. However, higher frequencies have more rapid attenuation as it passes through tissues, and resolution therefore is limited by depth.

Lateral resolution is the ability to identify two separate objects that are next to each other. This characteristic is dependent on both the focus width of the ultrasound wave beam and the transducer. The narrower beam of focus for a particular depth enables better lateral resolution. For a larger beam of focus, i.e., scanned field of view, the acoustic intensity is less resulting in less amplitude and less resolution. Remember also the average velocity of a wave in human tissues is given as constant at 1,540 m/s, and a change in frequency equals a change in wavelength [5, 6]. This ultimately affects the depth of resolution. At higher frequencies, shorter wavelengths are produced allowing better resolution of more superficial structures. For deeper structures, longer wavelengths are required with

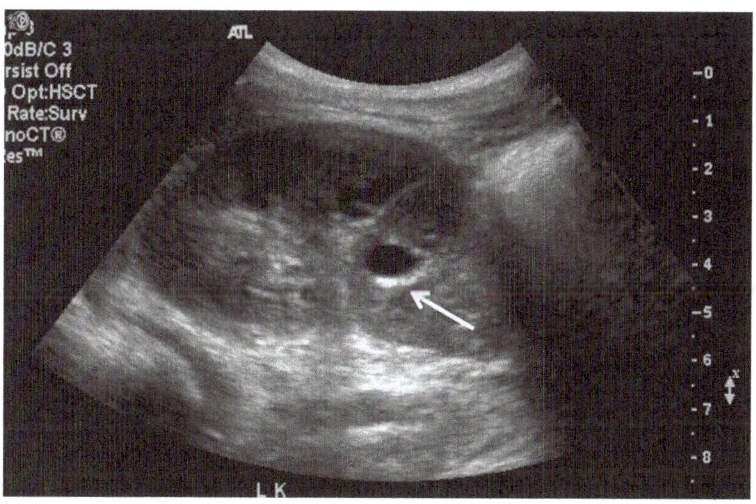

Fig. 2.5 Cyst in left kidney mid pole demonstrates the phenomenon of through transmission (*arrow*)

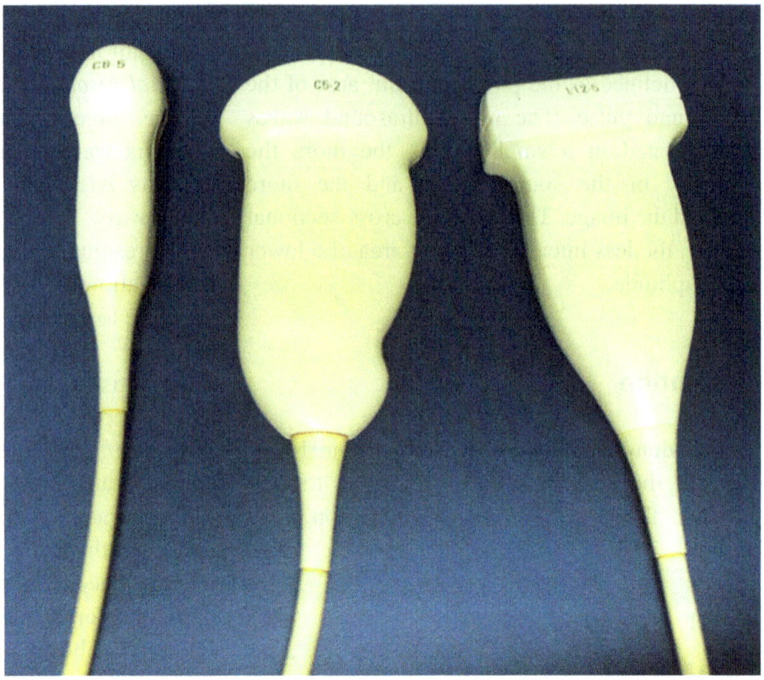

Fig. 2.6 Three of the more commonly used transducers

lower frequencies resulting in poor resolution. Typically for imaging structures such as the testicles or pediatric kidney, a higher frequency such as >7.5 MHz is used. But, for deeper structures such as the adolescent or adult kidney, 3.5–5 MHz is preferred.

The Transducers

There are many types of transducers available, each with its own advantages and disadvantages that make it uniquely suitable for various clinical applications of tissue imaging (Fig. 2.6). There are two general types of transducer classifications: mechanical and electronic steering. The mechanical types, of which there are two, rotating and oscillating, require the beam to be swept to image. The electronic steering transducers generate the beam sweep electronically by activating the crystal elements sequentially. The transducers used for conventional day-to-day imaging in the medical field are of the electronically steered category. The electronically steered transducers typically have a bandwidth of frequencies, such as 3–5 MHz or 6–15 MHz.

Electronically arrayed probes are the most common type of probe and are beneficial due to their compact size without moving parts. They contain an array of transducer elements but currently are limited to using frequencies below 15 MHz. Most linear and curvilinear probes can consist of 128–256 narrow transducer elements; however, only approximately 30 adjacent elements will be used to send a pulse at one time [2]. After the pulse is transmitted and received, the beam steps the array by dropping an element from the end and adding an element to the opposite end. Focusing at the depth of the scanning plane is achieved by firing of the outer elements in the group earlier than the central elements. The receiving of the focused beam is automatically controlled to match the depth of the echo. For initial reception, only 2–4 elements are used for closer targets, but as the target is deeper, the number of elements used to receive the returning echoes is increased.

Phased array probes scan in a sector field of view. Typically, phased arrays contain an average of 128 narrow transducer elements, which are all used at one time for scanning the plane. After the initial transmission and reception, the beam is steered at a new angle, and the elements are fired at varying times to enable all elements to arrive at the same time at the targeted focus [2, 3]. A new focus automatically advanced along the scan line after each transmission.

Modern array probes typically combine both techniques of steeping and steering the firing elements. Trapezoidal or virtual curvilinear scans are examples of such probes. They have a field of view similar to that of the curvilinear probed but without the disadvantage of the convex face.

Linear array transducers produce sound waves parallel to each other and produce a rectangular image. The width of the image and number of scan lines are the same at all tissue levels. This has the advantage of good near-field resolution. These typically have higher frequency bandwidths such as 9 or 6–15 MHz [3].

Sector transducers also known as vector array transducers have a small footprint and create a fanlike image that is narrow near the transducer and increase in width with deeper penetration. It is widely used in echocardiography but has been proven to be very useful scanning abdominal organs in small infants, such as the kidneys.

Curvilinear array transducers can be thought of as a combination of the linear and sector transducers. The probe emits sound waves as a diverging field of view, as wide as the linear array at the surface but fanning out with increasing depth. These often have frequencies of 2–5 MHz, as the advantage of a larger field of view is at a greater depth from the probe. The density of the scan lines decreases with increasing distance from the transducer.

There are also multiple tools at the disposal of the sonographer on the machine—slider posts to control gain, the ability to add focal zones, control the frequency within the dynamic range of the transducer, zoom in on an image, and change the depth to mention a few.

Despite significant advances in ultrasound technology, there are limitations to achieving optimal resolutions at greater depths. These limitations prompted the development of intracavitary probes such as transrectal probes for imaging the prostate and endovaginal probes for gynecological examinations. As these probes are now in much closer proximity to what were traditionally deep structures from an anterior abdominal wall approach, they are typically able to operate at frequencies between 7 and 15 MHz and provide high-resolution images as the depth of penetration has been decreased [1, 3].

Overview of Common Ultrasound Real-Time B-Mode Imaging

Grayscale Ultrasound

Grayscale real-time B-mode is the most commonly used mode of ultrasonography. A two-dimensional image consisting of variations of gray coloration (brightness) is dependent on the amplitude of the reflected sound wave. Strong echoes or large amplitude waves will be represented by shades near the white end of the spectrum, and weak echoes or waves having small amplitudes will correspond to shades in the black part of the spectrum. The position of the pixel is determined by the time it takes for the sound wave to be reflected back to the transducer. With experience, practitioners are able to decipher normal and abnormal patterns of echogenicity for the specific structures and tissues.

Doppler Ultrasonography

Continuous wave Doppler enables motion to be captured such as blood cells traveling in vessels or particles of urine flowing into the bladder seen as ureteral jets. The principle of capturing motion is derived from the knowledge that sound wave frequency will be changed based on the direction and velocity of moving objects relative to the observer, a phenomenon known as the Doppler shift. The frequency of the reflected wave will be greater than the original frequency when contacting an object moving towards the transducer. Similarly, the reflected wave frequency will be smaller when contacting an objection moving away from the transducer. In continuous wave Doppler, therefore, the moving structure will reflect the beam at different frequencies, which

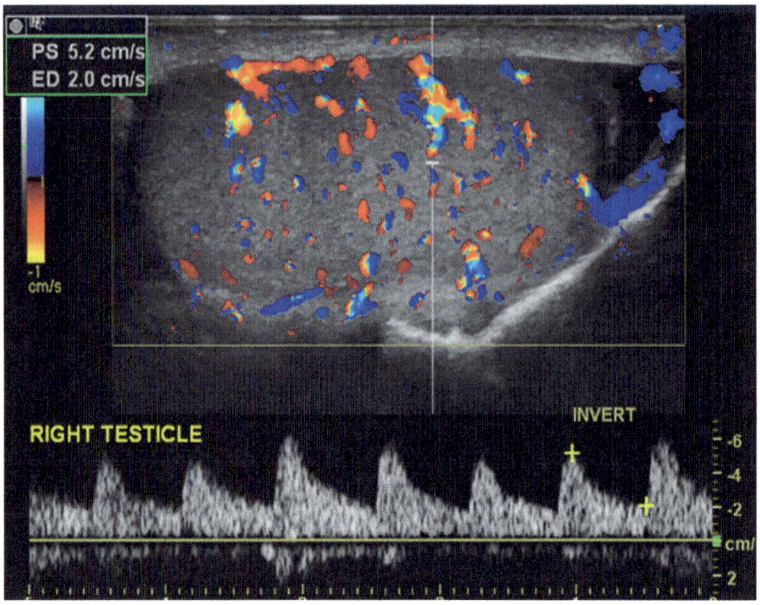

Fig. 2.7 Pulsed wave Doppler with *color image* aiding the placement of the sampling window to obtain an arterial tracing in a testicle. The flow is towards the transducer with the spectral waveform displayed above the baseline

are received by a parallel array of crystals. This then can be processed into an audible sound, with those of lower frequency registering a lower pitch/sound and higher frequencies a higher pitch/sound. Motion moving both towards and away from the transducer can be differentiated with color Doppler by assigning colors (conventionally blue and red) to objects moving towards and away from the transducer that is then superimposed on the grayscale image.

Duplex Ultrasound

Pulsed color wave Doppler occurs when pulses of sound are transmitted and received by the same transducer. This allows for the ability to assess depth of where the signal originated [7]. This limits the ability to assess very fast moving objects accurately. When employing pulse wave color Doppler, a small sample is interrogated, i.e., a "gated" sample. The B-mode scan image may have to be periodically updated when in pulse wave mode to verify gate placement. The sample window or gate can be wider or more focused as needed. The wider the gate, however, the less chance to detect small amounts of flow (Fig. 2.7).

Spectral Doppler refers to the graphic display of the changing velocities by a spectrum analyzer to aid in ease of interpretation. The spectral graph represents velocity on the vertical axis and time on the horizontal axis. Furthermore, the direction of flow towards the transducer is displayed above the baseline, and flow away from the transducer is depicted below. This can be done both for pulse wave and continuous color Doppler. The auditory signal again is processed so that one would hear a lower pitch hum sound for a slower moving vascular structure such as a vein as compared to the higher pitch variability sound of an artery (Fig. 2.8).

Power Doppler is another type of Doppler mode. Rather than assessing direction of flow or velocity, this mode assesses only intensity of signal. This is to aid for detection of blood flow in very small vessels and can be helpful also when optimal angles of insonation cannot be performed [7].

Attention to technique in the performance of Doppler imaging is paramount. The accuracy of the measured flow velocity is very dependent on the angle of the transmitted sound wave beam. The beam angle must measure the flow velocity at less than 90°, as the accuracy of the velocity is inversely proportional to the beam angle [7]. The reported error of a beam measured without an

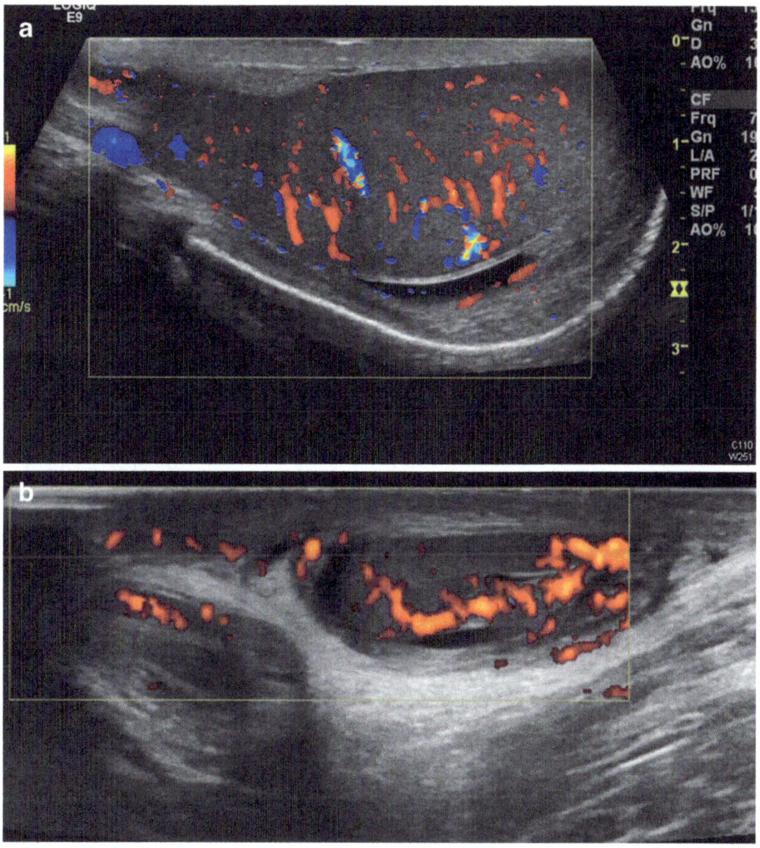

Fig. 2.8 (**a**) Color Doppler image of the testes. *Blue* represents flow away from the transducer; *red* represents flow to the transducer in a different patient (**b**) power Doppler image which does not reflect direction but only the presence of Doppler flow

angle (0°) to the flow is minimal; however, angles measured at 60° and greater from the flow have large amounts of error and should not be used [5]. Additionally, the technologist/physician must ensure that the appropriate scale, wall filter, and PRF (pulse repetition frequency) are utilized, dictated by the type of exam and indication to optimally obtain Doppler signal.

Methods to Improve Image Quality

There have been many advances in the mechanics of ultrasound, to enhance image quality. To discuss all of the various technologies is beyond the scope of this chapter, but the more common advances to improve image quality in use and being evaluated are as follows:

Time Gain Compensation: TGC refers to the process where the received signals are all uniformly preamplified by application of depth-dependent echo gain factors so that the end result is that essentially the same type of reflective structures, regardless of depth, will have the same level of brightness. This process compensates for the attenuation of sound waves of deeper structures, allowing for visualization of both near-field and far-field structures at the same time. This is known also as swept gain and depth gain compensation [4].

Tissue Harmonics: This process takes advantage of the natural creation of harmonic waveforms within the soft tissues of the body. It was discovered by accident from experiments with microbubble contrast agents in ultrasound. During those experiments, it was noted that the tissue would generate a multiple of the fundamental wave and these harmonic waveforms could be received by the transducer. Stronger harmonic signals were generated at greater tissue depths, i.e., farther from the skin surface. Therefore, there is less artifact present from near-field acoustic reflective surfaces. As these received signals are generated by the body, there is less tissue to travel through resulting in a better signal-to-noise ratio. The beam itself is also narrower than the fundamental beam resulting in superior lateral resolution in the far field as compared to the fundamental beam. These factors result in sharper imaging at greater depths. Due to limitations of most commercially available transducers, it is the second harmonic wavelength which is twice the wavelength of the fundamental, i.e., transmitted, wavelength that is utilized [4].

Spatial Compounding: This process obtains information from several different angles of insonation and combines them to produce a single image. For a linear transducer, the multiple parallel lines would be obtained in several orientations. The echoes of the multiple acquired signals in the different orientations are then averaged, and a compound image is generated. This leads to less artifact including speckle and noise, thereby improving resolution [4].

Chip Encoding: One way to overcome the limitation inherent to higher frequencies and maintain resolution for greater depths is to use a method to transmit coded pulses. Such pulses are produced for a longer duration, and the frequency of each pulse is increased to a peak during the generation of the pulse. A scanner is used to condense these long pulses down into shorter pulses by utilizing a matched decoding filter. The result of the conversion is improved spatial resolution at greater depths by reducing the signal-to-noise ratio [4].

Ultrasound Contrast Agents: These agents have been in use for some time in Europe and Japan and are gaining popularity in the United States, with several investigations under way [8]. These contrast agents consist of microbubbles of air or perfluorocarbon gas stabilized by a protein, lipid, or polymer shell. The half-life of the bubble is a few minutes, enough to assess blood flow in the lesions in the liver or kidney, for example. As the gas diffuse out of the bubble, the bubble itself dissolves. It has also been used to detect vesicoureteral reflux [9]. Although US contrast material has been approved for clinical use for cardiac diagnosis in the United States for a number of years, its use for other radiologic indications, including uroradiologic, is currently under investigation [8, 9].

Performing GU-Indicated Ultrasounds in Children

Ultrasound imaging is performed in children for the purposes of investigation, screening, or surveillance (Table 2.1). It is important for the ultrasound to be performed in a systematic and

Table 2.1 Indications for ultrasound in children

Renal and bladder
Investigation
Febrile urinary tract infection
Recurrent nonfebrile urinary tract infections
In utero anomaly of the urinary tract
Flank pain or renal colic
Palpable abdominal or pelvic mass
Hypertension
Hematuria
Proteinuria
Azotemia
Voiding dysfunction
Screening
Single umbilical artery
Family history of polycystic kidney disease
Hemihypertrophy
Syndrome associated with renal involvement (i.e., tuberous sclerosis, CHARGE, VACTERL, WAGR)
Surveillance
Hydronephrosis
Vesicoureteral reflux
Nephrolithiasis
Renal cystic disease
Neurogenic bladder disease (i.e., myelodysplasia)
Obstructive uropathy (i.e., posterior urethral valves)
Scrotal
Palpable or possible intrascrotal mass
Tumor (benign or malignant)
Spermatocele/epididymal cyst
Hernia
Hydrocele
Varicocele
Undescended testis
Testicular microlithiasis
Acute scrotal pain and/or swelling
Torsion of the spermatic cord
Torsion of the testicular appendages
Epididymo-orchitis
Henoch-Schonlein purpura

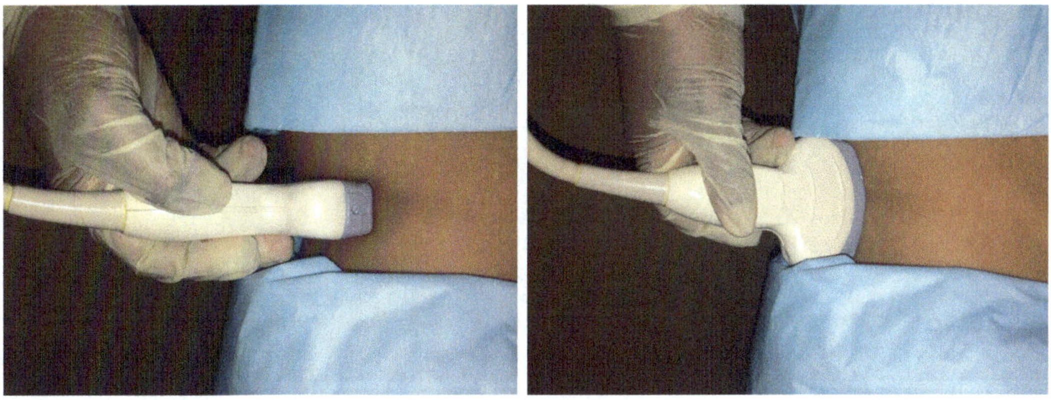

Fig. 2.9 Curvilinear ultrasound probe used during performance of a renal ultrasound. The probe is placed in the transverse (*left*) as well as sagittal (*right*) planes

standard fashion in order to yield a reproducible and clinically relevant study. While this principle is true for all imaging studies, it is particularly important in ultrasound as each study may vary with the skill and technique of the person performing the study.

Renal Ultrasound: The kidney is one component of a complete retroperitoneal ultrasound study. The other components include the abdominal aorta, origins of the common iliac arteries, the inferior vena cava, and any abnormalities encountered. The kidneys are imaged in both the longitudinal and transverse planes starting with the child in the supine position (Fig. 2.9). Asking the child to take a deep inspiration may improve visualization of the kidney, by causing it to move caudally below the ribs. In the young child or one who cannot follow such commands, a bolster placed under the flank or positioning the child on the side with the ipsilateral arm raised above the head may help open up the space between the ribs and the iliac crest which may allow for a better imaging window to access the kidney. If necessary, one can also try to image the child in the prone position to access the kidney between the ribs (Fig. 2.10). The right kidney is commonly imaged along the anterior axillary line, using the liver as an acoustic window. The left kidney is imaged along the mid- and posterior axillary lines, using the spleen as an acoustic window. Imaging is generally performed with a curved linear array probe using frequencies of 4–8 MHz for children under 18 months and 3.5–5 MHz probes for older children. The kidney's location, orientation, axis, size, echogenicity of parenchyma compared to the liver, and corticomedullary differentiation are documented (Fig. 2.11). Any abnormalities of contour, duplication of the collecting system, visualization of proximal ureter, and the presence of stones, hydronephrosis, cysts, or masses should be evaluated and described. The physician and technologist must be aware of the unique features of a neonatal kidney as compared to older children and adults. There are standard charts that can be referred to regarding mean renal length by age [3].

Bladder: The bladder is the major but not the only component of the pelvic ultrasound, which also includes the surrounding organs such as rectum, ovaries and uterus in girls, and prostate and seminal vesicles in boys. The bladder is imaged with the child in the supine position, commonly using a sector array probe using 4–8 MHz for children less than 18 months and curved array 3.5–5 MHz for older children. The bladder should be imaged in two orthogonal planes, traditionally transverse and longitudinal/coronal, with the bladder adequately distended. The bladder wall thickness is evaluated, as well as the intraluminal and extraluminal structures, noting if abnormalities such as dilated distal ureters, ureteroceles, abnormal echoes within the bladder, or a dilated proximal urethra known as the keyhole sign are present. Normal structures are documented as well such, as the uterus and ovaries, stool in rectum, and the prostate and seminal vesicles, and

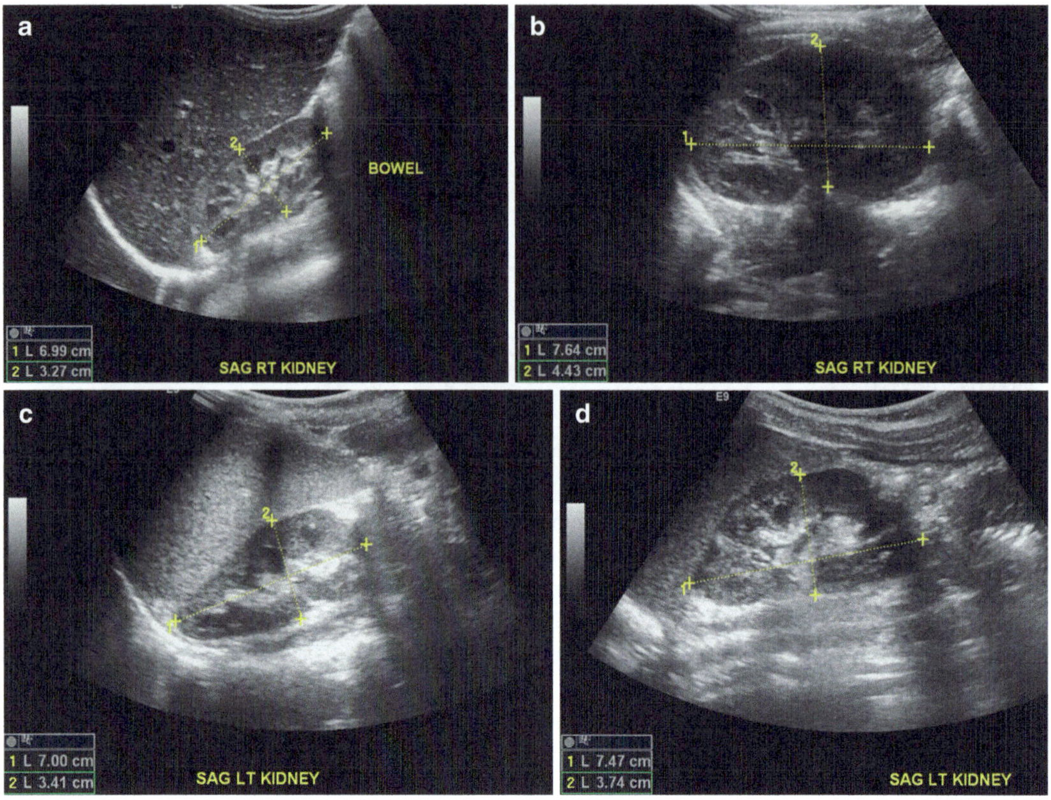

Fig. 2.10 Images (**a**) and (**c**) are obtained with pt in standard supine position with bowel gas obscuring portions of the kidneys. Same patient images (**b**) and (**d**) were obtained in the prone position with a bolster with improved visualization of the kidneys and more accurate measurements

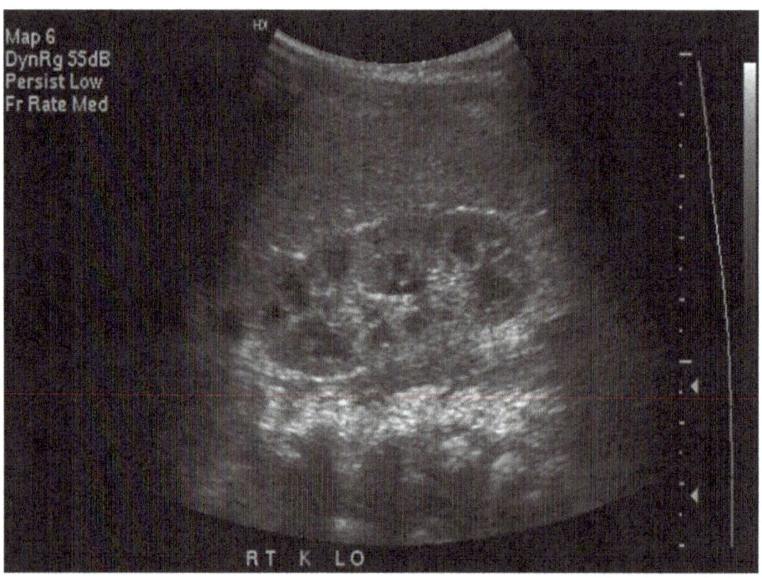

Fig. 2.11 Image of the right kidney in a child. There is corticomedullary differentiation with the medullary pyramids appearing as slightly darker triangular regions in the cortex. The renal sinus is more echogenic due to the presence of renal sinus fat

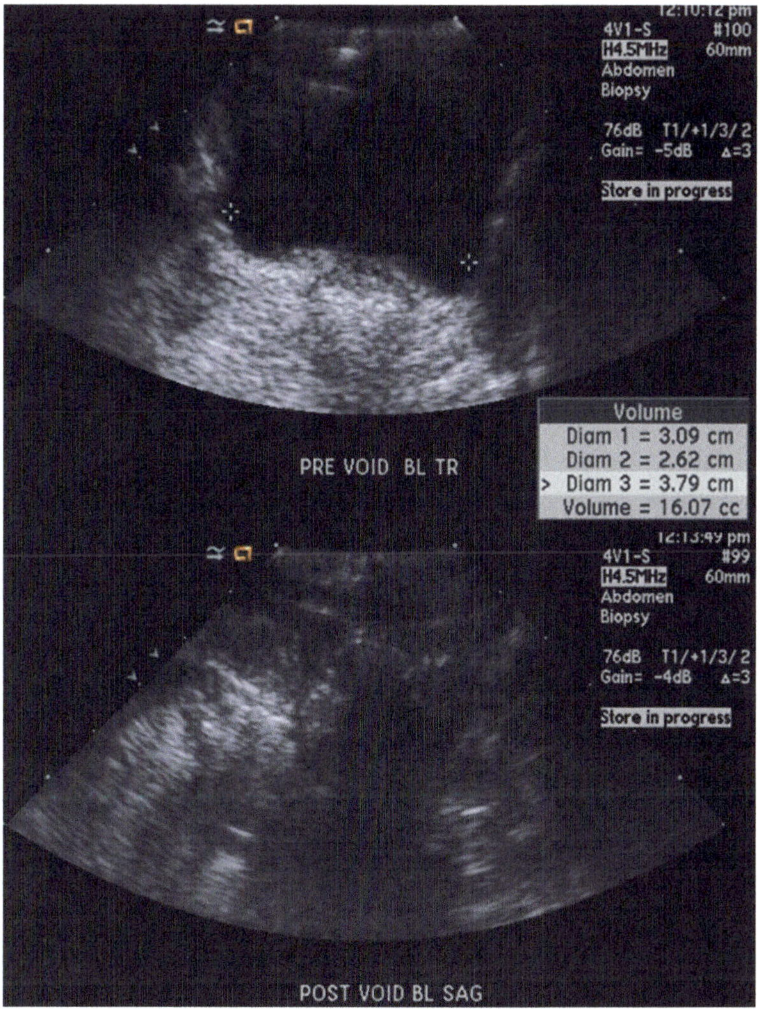

Fig. 2.12 Transverse images of the bladder. The *top image*, taken prior to voiding, demonstrates calculation of the ladder volume using three dimensions that can be related to expected bladder volumes for age. The *bottom image* demonstrates adequate emptying of the bladder of the same child

note is made if and how much free fluid is present posterior to the bladder. The transverse images are captured moving the probe caudally from the pubis to the umbilicus in 1–2 cm intervals. The longitudinal images are obtained moving from the midline in either direction at 1–2 cm intervals. Measurements recorded are the maximum height and width of the urine-distended bladder in the transverse plane and the length in the sagittal plane. Bladder volume can be determined by multiplying height, width, and length obtained by 0.65 – the standard formula of volume of an ellipsoid. Similarly, it is important to perform the study after voiding to assess the post-void residual or the presence of abnormalities suppressed by a distended bladder (Fig. 2.12). The color Doppler mode can be employed in the general region of the ureteral orifices along bladder floor to detect ureteral jets, i.e., efflux of urine into the bladder [1, 3] (Fig. 2.13).

Scrotum: The scrotal examine includes imaging of the testis, epididymis, and the spermatic cord and the scrotal wall. This evaluation is performed with the child in the supine position and the scrotum supported by a folded towel placed between the thighs. In older children and adolescents, the penis is positioned suprapubically and held in place with a second towel or by the patient. Scanning is performed using a high-frequency linear transducer such as 6–15 MHz. Both testes and epididymis should be compared together for size, echogenicity, and vascularity in the trans-

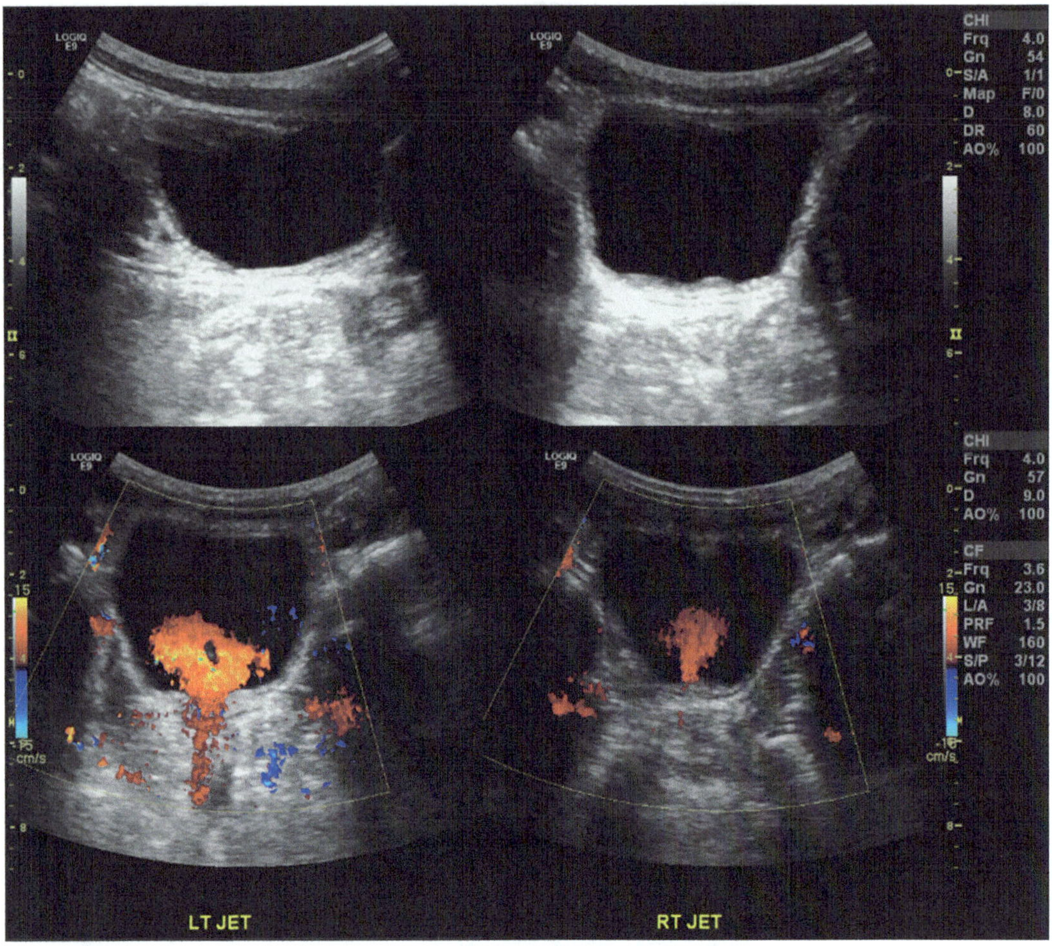

Fig. 2.13 Images of the bladder. Color Doppler can be employed to help identify ureteral jets

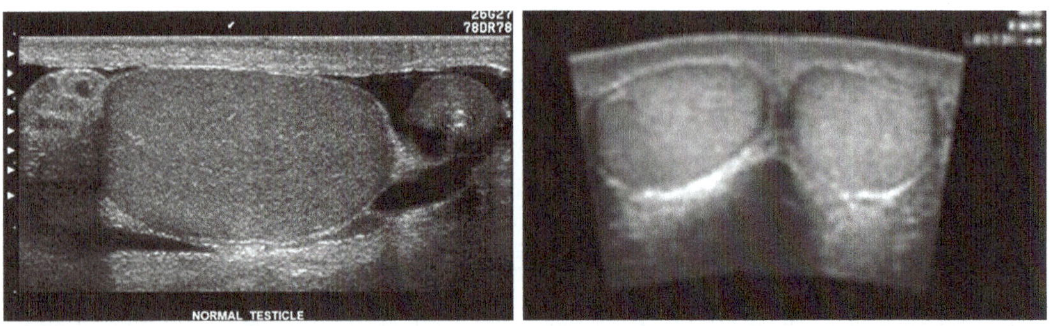

Fig. 2.14 Normal scrotal ultrasound. The *left image* demonstrates a sagittal view of the testis and the head and tail of the epididymis. The *right image* demonstrates a transverse view documenting the presence of two homogeneous testes

verse and longitudinal axis (Figs. 2.14 and 2.15). Note should be made of any abnormal echotexture, mass, and presence or absence of hydrocele or varicocele. Spectral Doppler analysis of the bilateral intratesticular vasculature should be performed when indicated. In patients presenting with acute scrotum, the asymptomatic side should be scanned first so that grayscale and color

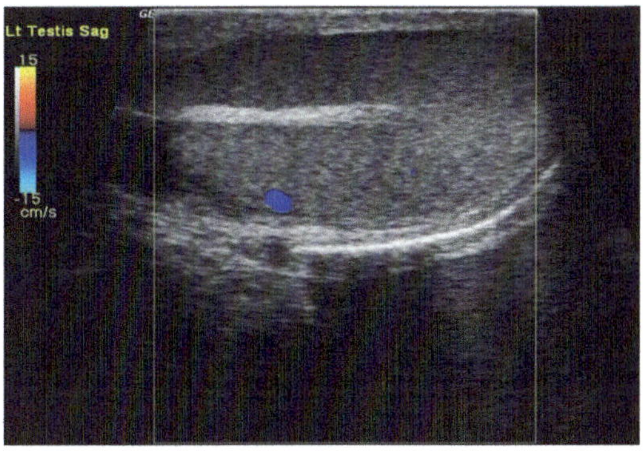

Fig. 2.15 Single longitudinal image through a testis with demonstration of the echogenic mediastinum and homogenous appearance to the testicular parenchyma

Doppler gain settings are set as the baseline for comparison to the affected side. It is important that the parameters for both color Doppler and spectral Doppler imaging are set appropriately in order to optimally evaluate the intratesticular vessels, which can be very challenging in the prepubertal patient. These parameters may need to be set at low PRFs and low wall filters in order to document blood flow [3]. If a varicocele is suspected, the exam should be performed during a Valsalva maneuver and/or by placing the child in the upright position to optimize the chance of detecting the venous distention.

References

1. Sanders RC. Clinical sonography: a practical guide. 2nd ed. Boston: Little Brown and Company; 1991.
2. Whittingham TA. Medical diagnostic applications and sources. Prog Biophys Mol Biol. 2007;93:84–110.
3. Siegel M. Pediatric sonography. 3rd ed. Philadelphia: Lippincott, Williams &Wilkins; 2002.
4. Hangiandreou N. B mode US: basic concepts and new technology. Radiographics. 2003;23:1019–33.
5. Gilbert BR. Office scrotal ultrasound. Part I: ultrasound anatomy, physical principles and ultrasound safety. AUA Update Ser. 2008;27(1):1–7.
6. Levitov A, Levitov A. Chapter 2. Physics of sound, ultrasound and Doppler effect and its diagnostic utility. In: Levitov A, Mayo P, Slonim AD, editors. Critical care ultrasonography. New York: McGraw Hill; 2009.
7. Boote E. Doppler US techniques: concepts of blood flow detection and flow dynamics. Radiographics. 2003;23:1315–27.
8. Brannigan M, Burns P, Wilson S. Blood flow patterns in focal liver lesions at microbubble-enhanced US. Radiographics. 2004;24:921–35.
9. Darge K. Voiding urosonography with ultrasound contrast agents for the diagnosis of vesicoureteric reflux in children. Pediatr Radiol. 2008;38(1):40–53.

Principles of Computerized Tomography (CT)

3

Cornelia K. Kaminsky, Benjamin Yuh, and Chester J. Koh

Introduction

While computerized tomography (CT) urography has been a mainstay for the imaging of the genitourinary (GU) tract in adults, it has been used less frequently in children due to concerns for the radiation dosages and the differing disease processes. Plain x-ray imaging, ultrasonography, voiding cystourethrography (VCUG), nuclear scintigraphy, and magnetic resonance (MR) urography continue to be the most commonly utilized diagnostic imaging methods for assessment of the pediatric genitourinary tract. However, as CT techniques have become more refined and the associated radiation dosages have continued to decrease, the use of CT urography in children appears to be expanding as well. Common indications for CT urography in children include the evaluation of urinary tract stones, tumors, urinary tract infections/inflammation, trauma, and hydronephrosis. In addition, the use of CT urography has been used to delineate anatomic variations associated with GU anomalies that are unable to be adequately assessed by the other modalities. Although functional assessment of the kidneys is possible with CT urography, its usage in children continues to be low due to the relatively high radiation dosages and because of MR urography's ability to evaluate the anatomy in a radiation-free manner. However, there remain a small number of infants and children who cannot be safely sedated for MR urography where CT urography may be a good alternative due to its excellent spatial resolution and short scan time requirements. In general, CT urography protocols in infants and children are based on body mass index, age, and weight to calculate contrast amounts and radiation dosages that are as low as possible in adherence to the "As Low As Reasonably Achievable" (ALARA) principles and "Image Gently" guidelines and the minimal use of multi-series imaging [1].

Radiation Dosages

The US FDA has recognized the risks of radiation exposure in children and currently recommends the reduction of unnecessary radiation exposure from medical imaging studies such as CT scans. Therefore, radiation exposure associated with GU tract imaging in children continues to worry

C.K. Kaminsky, MD
Pediatric Radiology, Children's Hospital Los Angeles, 4650 Sunset Blvd, MS#81, Los Angeles, CA 90027, USA

Division of Pediatric Radiology, Department of Radiology, Keck School of Medicine of USC, Los Angeles, CA, USA
e-mail: ckaminsky@chla.usc.edu

B. Yuh, MD
Department of Urology, USC Institute of Urology, Keck School of Medicine of USC, 1441 Eastlake Ave., Suite 7416, Los Angeles, CA 90089, USA

C.J. Koh, MD (✉)
Division of Pediatric Urology, Texas Children's Hospital / Baylor College of Medicine, 6701 Fannin St., Clinical Care Center, Suite 620, Houston, TX 77030, USA
e-mail: cxkoh@texaschildrens.org

L.S. Palmer, J.S. Palmer (eds.), *Pediatric and Adolescent Urologic Imaging*,
DOI 10.1007/978-1-4614-8654-1_3, © Springer Science+Business Media New York 2014

pediatric health care providers and parents and has led to a continuing effort to reduce radiation exposure in children to the minimal amounts necessary [2]. While the radiation dosage for a single plain abdominal x-ray (KUB) may range from 0.2 to 0.7 milliSieverts (mSv), excretory urography dosages range from 3 to 5 mSv [3]. The average radiation dosages for an unenhanced CT urogram are relatively low at 2–3 mSv on average, but they can be reduced to less than 1 mSv in many children. The radiation dosages for a two-phase CT urography with and without IV contrast can average 16 mSv, while those of a triple-phase CT urography can average 22 mSv. As a result, the usage of multiphase or functional CT urography in children is usually minimized, where functional assessment of the urinary tract, and especially the kidneys, is usually determined by other diagnostic modalities such as MR or nuclear scintigraphy. For select cases, CT urography is utilized when first-line diagnostic modalities are inconclusive.

CT Radiation Dosage Calculations

The reporting of CT dosages in children is now a legal requirement, and there are several methodologies in which CT radiation dosage calculations are performed. CTDI 100 is the CT radiation dosage measured in a phantom from a single axial scan over 100 mm in length within the ionization chamber. CTDIw is the average measured dosage at different locations in the axial scan plane since the dosage can be uneven within varying planes of tissue thickness:

$$\mathrm{CTDIw} = 1/3(\mathrm{CTDI100})\mathrm{center} + 2/3(\mathrm{CTDI100})\mathrm{surface}.$$

This is proportional to absorbed radiation dose independent of scan length. CTDIvolume (CTDIvol) is the dose variation in the Z plane related to spatial distance between adjacent scans and table speed, i.e., pitch, where pitch is the travel distance of the CT scanner table during a 360° rotation of the x-ray tube divided by x-ray beam collimation (equivalent to slice thickness). CTDIvol = CTDIw/pitch and is described in milligray (mGy) units. Therefore, when the pitch equals 1, then CTDIvol equals the CTDIw. Dose-length product (DLP) describes the length of the object being radiated and is proportional to the effective radiation dose. DLP = CTDIvol × length of radiated object and is described in mGy-cm units.

Multidetector CT (MDCT) Imaging

Multidetector CT (MDCT) imaging has been one of the most important recent advances in pediatric GU imaging [4]. Its short scan times have led to reductions in motion artifact and the avoidance of sedation. MDCT imaging also allows for the overlap of images from a single exposure, the reconstruction of images in different planes with creation of 3D projections, and the ability for precise timing of peak vascular and organ phase enhancement, which have led to major improvements in CT imaging for pediatric GU evaluation. As a result, MDCT imaging has greatly reduced the need for pediatric GU angiography. In addition, MDCT imaging provides subcentimeter resolution and therefore renders it more useful for pediatric GU tract imaging than MR imaging in this respect. Furthermore, bundled infants and children above 3 years of age can usually tolerate the short scans without the need for sedation, while children who may not be initially tolerant can often proceed through the short scan times with the help of parental coaching and avoid the need for sedation.

MDCT Technical Aspects

For MDCT imaging, the CT parameters should be set at ALARA (As Low As Reasonably Achievable) settings using weight or body mass index (BMI) criteria. The www.pedrad.org website can give up-to-date information on settings for a particular type of CT scanner. In general, patients less than 45 kg in weight need an 80 peak kilovoltage (kVp) dose setting, while larger patients need 100–120 kVp dose. The milliamperage (mAs) settings for abdominal CT imaging based on weight are as follows:

Weight <10 kg: 50 mAs
10–15 kg: 60 mAs
16–25 kg: 70 mAs
26–35 kg: 90 mAs
36–45 kg: 100 mAs
45 kg: >120 mAs

Since pitch is defined as the travel distance of the CT scanner table during a 360° rotation of the x-ray tube divided by x-ray beam collimation (equivalent to slice thickness), a patient's typical radiation dose will be inversely related to the pitch. Pitches of 1–2, where the table feed is greater than the collimation, lead to decreases in radiation dosage by 50 % but with associated loss of resolution. For a 16-row MDCT scanner, the collimation is 0.75–1.5 mm with a pitch of 1–1.5. For a 64-row MDCT scanner, the collimation is 0.63 mm–1.25 mm with pitch of 1–1.5. CT scan times are usually set at 0.5 ms or less such that CT urography which includes the abdomen and the pelvis has scan times of less than a minute and often take only a few seconds. Although the axial slice thicknesses are often 0.63 mm or less, the images are often reconstructed at a wider thickness between 2.5 and 5 mm, which decreases noise artifact. Multiplanar reconstruction (MPR) in coronal and sagittal planes can provide additional information on the anatomy. Occasionally, maximum intensity projections (MIP) can be performed in the coronal plane and can provide intravenous pyelogram-like images. Three-dimensional (3D) thick slab reconstruction including 3D thick slab MIP imaging can also be performed if further anatomic detail is necessary.

Nonionic intravenous contrast is generally preferred over ionic contrast, since it is associated with less discomfort at the injection site and less risks for allergic reaction, nausea, vomiting, and flushing. Intravenous contrast can be given by hand injection or mechanical power injector, with an injection rate of 3–4 ml/s with 20-gauge intravenous access and 1–1.5 ml/s with 24-gauge intravenous access. The intravenous contrast dose in general is 2 ml/kg up to 125 ml maximum. Oral contrast can be a negative contrast agent (dark appearing) such as water or Pedialyte or a positive contrast agent (dense appearing) such as diluted Gastrografin or nonionic IV contrast material mixed with liquids such as water, juice, Gatorade, or soda. The positive contrast is mixed such that 15–30 ml of contrast is added to a total liquid volume of 1,000 ml and then prescribed to the patient for oral consumption with volumes based on age. The oral contrast volume is preferably given at least 1–2 h before the scan and additionally about 15 min prior to the scan as follows:

<1-month-old: 60–90 ml initially followed by 30–45 ml
1-month-old to 1-year-old: 120–240 ml initially followed by 60–120 ml
1–5-year-old: 240–480 ml initially followed by 120–180 ml
6–12-year-old: 480–1,000 ml initially followed by 180–500 ml
>12 years old: 1,000 ml initially followed by 500 ml

For optimal CT urography, the patient should void just prior to the scan or undergo bladder catheterization to eliminate functional effects on the renal parenchyma and collecting system due to transmitted bladder pressure effects.

MDCT Imaging Phases

Noncontrast CT imaging is often utilized to detect urinary tract stones and for characterization of a kidney lesion (calcification, simple cystic fluid, proteinaceous fluid, solid, etc.). If a lesion is less than 5 mm in diameter, the determination of some lesions can be less sensitive. In addition, noncontrast CT imaging can be used for suspected bladder perforation to separate out radiodense fluid such as blood and other radiodense material from extravasated contrast during a CT cystogram study.

When intravenous contrast is used, there are usually four phases of contrast CT urography: the *arterial phase* begins between 15 and 25 s after the injection with delineation of the arteries. This phase can be programmed as a timed bolus or as a "bolus trigger" where the CT scanner begins scanning once the attenuation readings of the aorta hit a threshold value of 120 Hounsfield units (HU). In this phase, there may

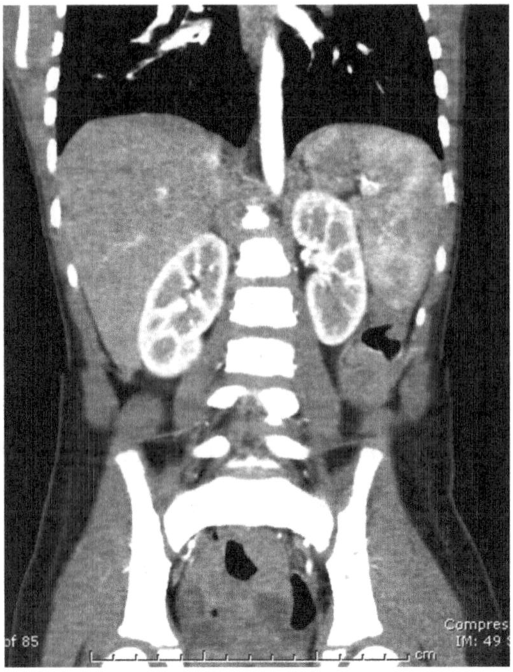

Fig. 3.1 Contrast CT image of the kidneys – early phase

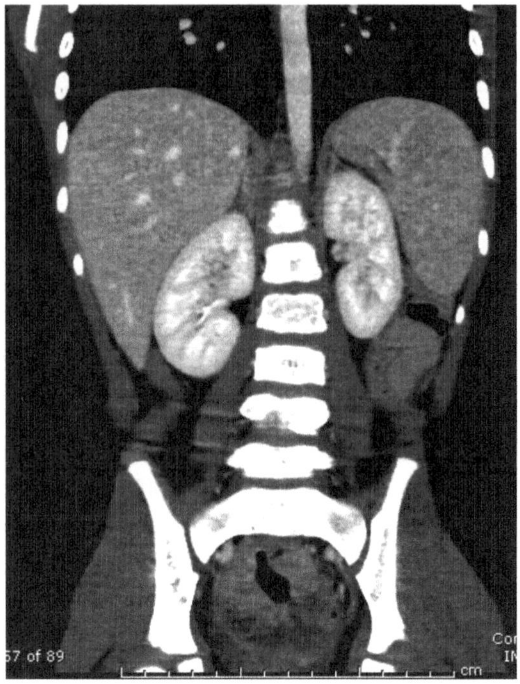

Fig. 3.2 Contrast CT image of the kidneys – late phase

be early renal cortex enhancement as well. The *corticomedullary phase* (cortical phase) begins approximately 30–40 s after the injection and corresponds with the late arterial phase with sharp cortical enhancement and visually nondetectable or minimal medullary enhancement (Fig. 3.1). This phase is used to assess veins, arteries, renal masses, cysts, infection, and trauma. However, it is not entirely reliable in visualizing some masses or infections, including fungal infections. The *nephrogenic phase* (medullary or tubular phase) begins approximately 75–120 s from the start of contrast injection and is the most reliable for the assessment of parenchymal lesions (Fig. 3.2). However, this phase may not allow detection of early enhancing lesions such as renal cell carcinoma foci or certain vascular malformations. In this phase, there is uniform parenchymal enhancement throughout the kidneys without excretion into the pelvicalyceal system. In addition, urothelial pathology can occasionally be appreciated during this phase as well as during the corticomedullary phase. The *excretory phase* occurs approximately 3–5 min after injection, but a longer scan time delay until 5–15 min after injection can be utilized to allow for improved visualization of the pelvicalyceal system and ureters. The parenchymal enhancement decreases during this phase, which is often helpful in assessing anatomic anomalies, obstructing lesions of the collecting system and ureters, noncalcified filling defects, and urothelial pathology.

Anatomy/Variations

Examples of CT imaging in the genitourinary tract have been included below. Subsequent chapters will provide further imaging details by organ system.

CT imaging of the GU tract usually involves the recognition of normal relevant anatomy and its variations. The renal margins may be smooth or lobulated (fetal lobulations) in areas of renicular fusion, where fetal lobulations can be differentiated from renal scarring in that they maintain their overall cortical thickness. The perinephric fat is generally minimal in children. The renal capsule usually cannot be separately identified from the rest of the renal tissue by CT.

The renal arteries branch from the aorta just below the superior mesenteric artery and split into its dorsal and ventral branches at the hilum. The renal veins are usually anterior to the arteries with the left renal vein coursing anterior to the aorta before reaching the inferior vena cava, although vascular anomalies are possible such as a retroaortic left renal vein anomaly or the "nutcracker" compression anomaly of the left renal vein between the superior mesenteric artery and the aorta which may be a source of hematuria. Prominent enhancing columns of Bertin that are identified as potential renal masses sonographically can be differentiated by CT as normal enhancing parenchyma. Though perinephric fat is usually minimal in children, it can become more prominent in children on steroid therapy, obese patients, immobile patients, patients with neuromuscular disorders, and patients with metabolic disorders. The perinephric fascia (Gerota's fascia) surrounds the space containing kidney, adrenal gland, renal pelvis, and proximal ureter. The posterior pararenal space is marked by the posterior renal fascia, psoas, and quadratus muscle, while the anterior pararenal space is bordered by the posterior parietal peritoneum, lateral conal fascia, and anterior renal fascia. The ureters course anteromedial to the psoas muscle in the abdominal cavity. In the pelvis, at a level just below the iliac vessel bifurcation near the level of the iliac crest, the ureters drape over the iliac artery initially and then course medial to the iliac vessels, which are medial to the iliopsoas muscle, before entering the trigone area of the bladder posteriorly.

Examples of Congenital Anomalies

CT can be very helpful in differentiating congenital anomalies of the kidneys, such as renal agenesis, renal ectopia, cross-fused kidneys, and renal aplasia/dysplasia in which there is small nonfunctioning poorly differentiated kidney tissue such as with an involuted multicystic dysplastic kidney (MCDK) (Fig. 3.3). With renal agenesis or ectopic kidneys, the adrenal gland appears elongated rather than lambda- or delta-shaped.

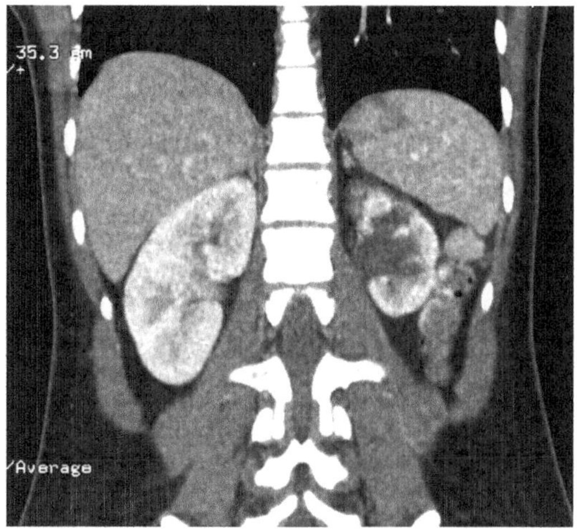

Fig. 3.3 Duplex left kidney with involuting upper pole system

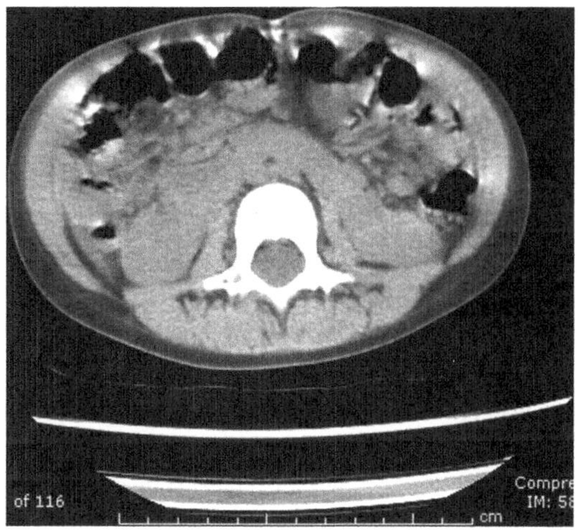

Fig. 3.4 Horseshoe kidney

Horseshoe kidney anomalies are most often associated with fusion at the lower poles by an isthmus of functional renal tissue or occasionally fibrous tissue (Fig. 3.4). The isthmus width is on average less than 1/3 the length of the kidney and is anteriorly located against the spine, which makes it prone to microtrauma and hematuria. The kidney location is still relatively within the renal fossa with the longitudinal axis of the kidney coursing laterally to medially opposite the normal axis. The renal pelvis is usually anteriorly oriented which can lead to hematuria from kidney trauma, uretero-pelvic (UPJ) obstruction, and occasional urinary

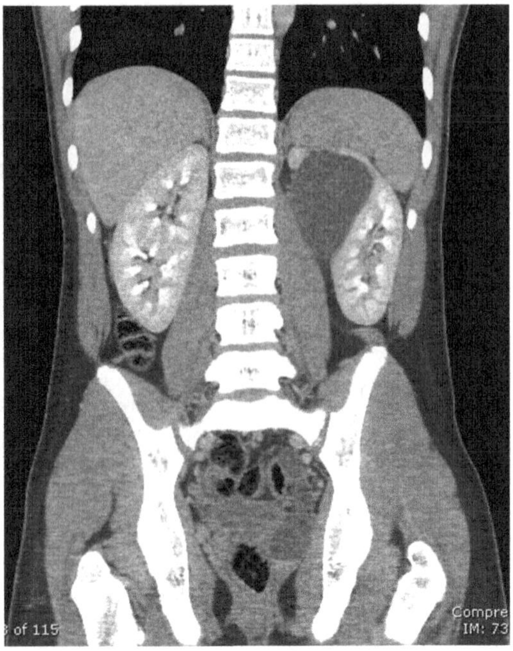

Fig. 3.5 Duplex left kidney with left upper pole hydronephrosis

stone formation. The arterial supply of the isthmus can be visualized with CT imaging and is often supplied by an accessory renal artery directly off the lower aorta below the main renal artery takeoff or occasionally a branch from an iliac vessel.

In addition, renal duplication anomalies are well visualized by CT imaging (Fig. 3.5). They are more commonly partial but can range from completely bifid renal pelvis to complete renal duplication with fusion of the duplicated ureters distally. Complete duplicated systems usually have ectopic ureteral insertion of the upper pole ureter inferomedial to the normal inserting lower pole ureter (Weigert-Meyer rule), and the upper pole system may be associated with a ureterocele. CT imaging can also delineate the ectopic insertion of a ureter to the vagina, seminal vesicles, epididymis, or urethra.

Urinary Stones/Nephrocalcinosis

While urinary stone formation is less common in children than in adults, CT is still used preferentially for its diagnosis [5]. Unenhanced CT's advantages over MRI include superior spatial resolution and the ability to visualize calcifications. CT's advantage over ultrasonography is its ability to visualize ureteral stones that can be obscured by bowel gas. CT can be used to assess presence, size, and location of stones, but it is also helpful in detecting the sequelae of urinary stones including hydroureteronephrosis, perinephric stranding with obstructed lymphatic drainage, renal enlargement, and urinoma.

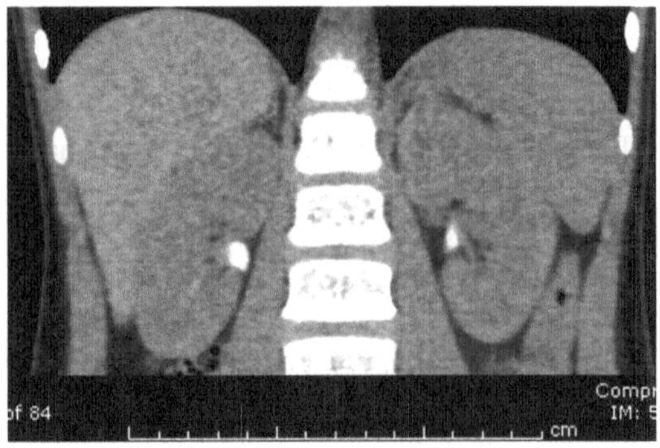

Fig. 3.6 Nephrocalcinosis

Nephrocalcinosis can be confirmed with unenhanced CT when ultrasonography has difficulty in separating renal hilar echogenic fat from nephrocalcinosis (Fig. 3.6) [6]. Faint or relatively dense medullary calcifications are easily seen by CT imaging, and CT imaging can demonstrate associated urinary milk of calcium depositions within the collecting system which are usually not appreciable by ultrasonography.

Pyelonephritis/Renal Scarring

Although CT is not generally used for the assessment of urinary tract infection/pyelonephritis, CT imaging occasionally is used to assess for complications of pyelonephritis including pyonephrosis and intrarenal/perirenal abscess [7]. Often CT imaging for the workup of generalized nonspecific abdominal pain can lead to an inadvertent demonstration of pyelonephritis. The CT findings of pyelonephritis are usually rounded and/or wedge-shaped low attenuation areas that are surrounded by normal tissue enhancement or a striated nephrogram appearance. The areas of low

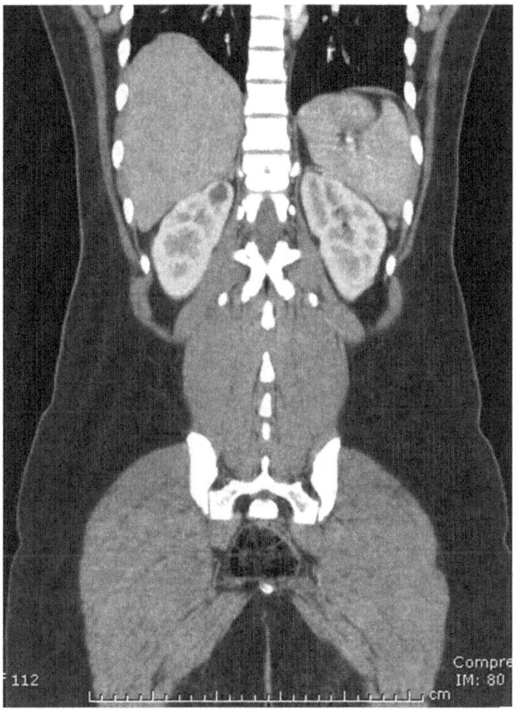

Fig. 3.7 Right upper pole kidney cyst

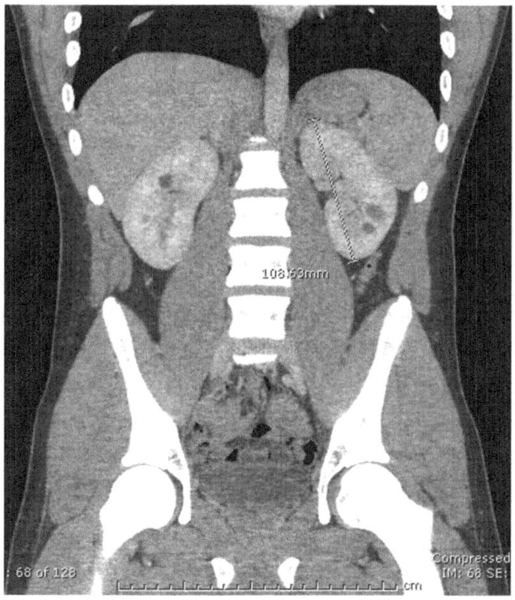

Fig. 3.8 Polycystic kidney

attenuation may be related to edema from infection and perhaps vasospasm. The affected kidney may be enlarged with possible urothelial thickening. The late sequelae of pyelonephritis from reflux nephropathy are also well demonstrated by CT with areas of renal scarring that may be focal and notched or more generalized with thinner cortex. These tend to be located at the poles of the kidney and are often seen with blunted/distorted calyces.

Kidney Cysts

Kidney cysts are rare in children and are usually related to a calyceal diverticulum, prior infection, prior trauma, or other cystic congenital and/or hereditary disease processes (Fig. 3.7). Many calyceal diverticular cysts can be seen with contrast filling on the delayed excretory phase during CT imaging. Simple cysts are usually lined with flattened epithelium and usually contain serous fluid with CT attenuation values of <20 Hounsfield units (HU). Occasionally, cysts can be hyperdense with attenuation values of 40–90 HU that is related to bleeding or infection. Some hyperdense cystic lesions may be related to malignant diseases in children such as renal cell carcinoma, although most cystic lesions in children are not malignant. The Bosniak classification system for renal cysts can generally be used to differentiate potential malignancy in children. Bosniak type 1 cysts are thin walled with less than 20 HU fluid attenuation values; Bosniak type 2 cysts have thin septations and calcifications or are central in location; Bosniak type 3 cysts contain thicker calcification and thicker septa and may have rim enhancement; and Bosniak type 4 cysts have much thicker walls/septa, possible calcifications, and enhancing solid tissue [8].

When children present with cysts and especially bilateral cysts, hereditary cystic disease etiologies should be considered, such as polycystic kidney disease (PCKD) (Fig. 3.8) or tuberous sclerosis. With tuberous sclerosis, the kidneys may contain multiple angiomyolipomas and cysts, but usually, one type is more dominant than the other. On CT imaging, the angiomyolipoma are usually subcentimeter in diameter and often associated with fatty attenuation. When they are extremely small, distinguishing between cysts and angiomyolipomas can be difficult. Since angiomyolipomas contain fat that may be slightly vascular, they can enhance slightly so that the Hounsfield unit readings can be mistaken for the readings of kidney cysts at less than 20 Hounsfield units and therefore not recognized as fat which generally produces negative Hounsfield unit numbers. Thin cut imaging and noncontrast CT correlation can help to differentiate between the two in this setting.

CT Vascular Imaging for the GU Tract

Imaging for renal vascular anomalies and diagnoses, such as renal artery stenosis, renal vein thrombosis, or trauma-associated renal artery occlusion, can be performed using CT angiograms as an alternative to MR imaging [9]. CT angiograms for vessel assessment are often performed in either the arterial phase or, more preferably, the late arterial/early venous phase to delineate both systems. The images are then reformatted in different planes as described previously.

CT imaging is also helpful in the assessment of arteriovenous fistula or other vascular malformations, where a dilated circuitous artery and vein that are entangled can be seen. Vascular imaging for transplanted kidneys can often be performed satisfactorily with CT angiograms instead of conventional angiograms, where the site of renal artery stenosis or kinking of vessels can be seen. CT imaging has the advantage of highlighting other potential complications from transplantation such as lymphoceles, urinomas, and hematomas.

Renal Masses

CT is the preferred imaging modality for assessing renal masses due to its superior spatial resolution, ability to show detailed vessel anatomy, calcifications, tumor extent, adjacent fat stranding that cannot easily be seen by MR, and superiority in detecting lung metastasis. Different phase contrast images also allow for improved tumor detection.

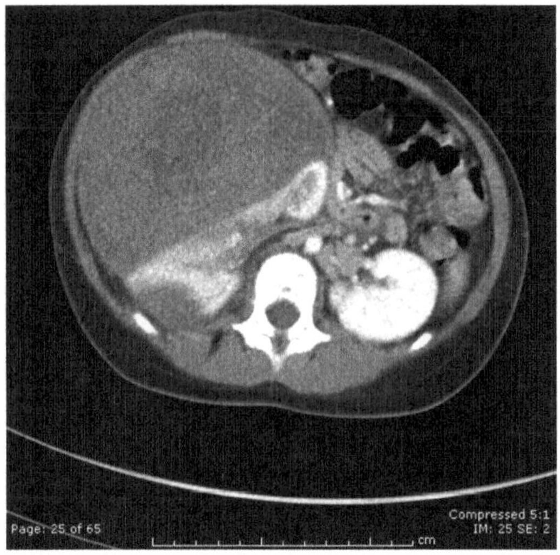

Fig. 3.9 Wilms tumor

For Wilms tumor (Fig. 3.9) or renal cell carcinoma, CT imaging can show the extent of the primary tumor and can be helpful for operative planning. Furthermore, vascular thrombi are delineated by CT imaging as low attenuation filling defects in the vessel, with a prolonged nephrogram and occasional collateral vessel filling with contrast. Nodal involvement can be detected and especially with newer helical MDCT scanners that can perform thinner slices [10].

Leukemias can appear by CT imaging as bilateral or unilateral nephromegaly since it can involve the kidneys asymmetrically, with possible loss of corticomedullary differentiation and/or focal areas of low attenuation with intravenous contrast due to lesser enhancement of leukemic mass clusters compared to the regular parenchyma [11]. Occasionally, the involvement can appear as striations and infiltration similar to the CT appearance of other nonspecific nephritis syndromes. Occasionally there is hydronephrosis from partial obstruction due to adjacent adenopathy.

Lymphomas may appear as masses that are usually homogeneous and hypoattenuated compared to normal parenchyma, with occasionally

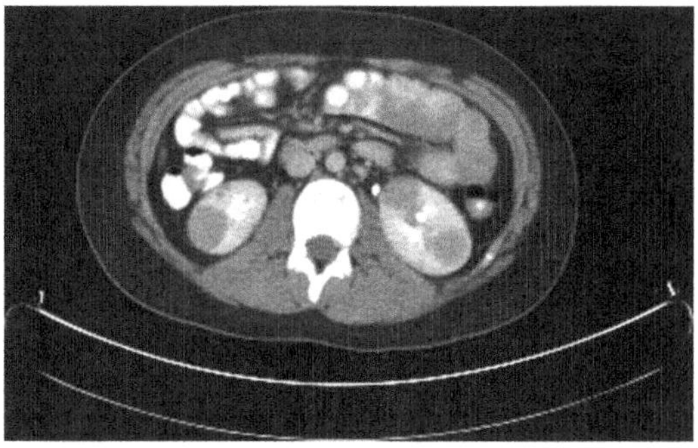

Fig. 3.10 Lymphoma

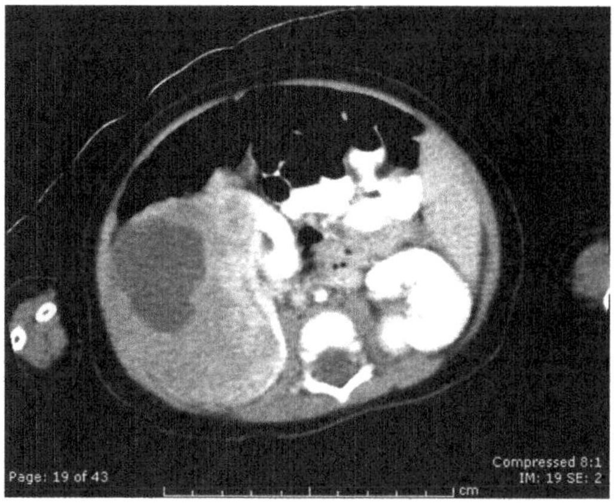

Fig. 3.11 Mesoblasticnephroma

heterogeneous necrosis or hemorrhage in large lesions (Fig. 3.10). Associated splenomegaly and other generalized adenopathy seen on CT can help in determining the diagnosis of lymphoma.

Angiomyolipoma, which is also known as renal hamartoma, contains mature fat, smooth muscle, and blood vessels and is seen in the majority of children with tuberous sclerosis. They also can be seen with neurofibromatosis and von Hippel-Lindau syndrome. While they can increase in size to appear like a large mass, they usually appear smaller and multifocal during childhood. More often these multifocal lesions appear as low attenuation foci that usually look like cysts on regular slice CT, but with thinner CT slice, technique can be delineated for the fatty tissues that they are [12]. While the attenuation of fat is usually less than zero HU, these lesions often appear to have attenuation values as high as 15–20 HU which is within the cystic fluid HU range. This occurs due to the fact that the fat is slightly vascular and enhances slightly with IV contrast though much less so than adjacent native kidney. Occasionally the attenuation may be slightly higher due to hemorrhage in it. Noncontrast CT thin slice images may be helpful in demonstrating the fat in the lesions better.

Mesoblastic nephroma, which is also known as fetal renal hamartoma, leiomyomatous hematoma, and mesenchymal hamartoma of infancy, is the most common renal tumor for infants under 4 months of age. It is considered a benign tumor with low mitotic rate but due to its dense spindle cells, usually appears hypoattenuated by contrast CT imaging with occasional areas of enhancement from noninvolved entrapped normal renal tissue (Fig. 3.11) [13]. It usually appears as a central tumor near the renal hilum but often can involve the majority of the kidney.

References

1. Shah NB, Platt SL. ALARA: is there a cause for alarm? Reducing radiation risks from computed tomography scanning in children. Curr Opin Pediatr. 2008;20(3):243–7. PubMed PMID: 18475090. Epub 2008/05/14. eng.
2. Yu L, Bruesewitz MR, Thomas KB, Fletcher JG, Kofler JM, McCollough CH. Optimal tube potential for radiation dose reduction in pediatric CT: principles, clinical implementations, and pitfalls. Radiographics. 2011;31(3):835–48. PubMed PMID: 21571660. Epub 2011/05/17. eng.
3. Dougeni E, Faulkner K, Panayiotakis G. A review of patient dose and optimisation methods in adult and paediatric CT scanning. Eur J Radiol. 2012;81(4):e665–83. PubMed PMID: 21684099. Epub 2011/06/21. eng.
4. Nievelstein RA, van Dam IM, van der Molen AJ. Multidetector CT in children: current concepts and dose reduction strategies. Pediatr Radiol. 2010;40(8):1324–44. PubMed PMID: 20535463. PubMed Central PMCID: 2895901.
5. Karmazyn B, Frush DP, Applegate KE, Maxfield C, Cohen MD, Jones RP. CT with a computer-simulated dose reduction technique for detection of pediatric nephroureterolithiasis: comparison of standard and reduced radiation doses. AJR Am J Roentgenol. 2009;192(1):143–9. PubMed PMID: 19098193.

6. Afschrift M, Nachtegaele P, Van Rattinghe R, Praet M, Voet D, Vanhaesebrouck P, et al. Nephrocalcinosis demonstrated by ultrasound and CT. Pediatr Radiol. 1983;13(1):42–3. PubMed PMID: 6844054.
7. Maturen KE, Blane CE, Strouse PJ. Computed tomographic diagnosis of unsuspected pyelonephritis in children. Can Assoc Radiol J. 2002;53(5):279–83.
8. Peng Y, Jia L, Sun N, Li J, Fu L, Zeng J, et al. Assessment of cystic renal masses in children: comparison of multislice computed tomography and ultrasound imaging using the Bosniak classification system. Eur J Radiol. 2010;75(3):287–92. PubMed PMID: 20594787.
9. Beier UH, John E, Lumpaopong A, Co JG, Jelnin V, Benedetti E, et al. Electron-beam CT as a diagnostic modality in pediatric nephrology and renal transplant surgery. Pediatr Nephrol. 2006;21(5):677–82. PubMed PMID: 16520947.
10. Lubahn JD, Cost NG, Kwon J, Powell JA, Yang M, Granberg CF, et al. Correlation between preoperative staging computerized tomography and pathological findings after nodal sampling in children with Wilms tumor. J Urol. 2012;188(4 Suppl):1500–4. PubMed PMID: 22910268.
11. Guillerman RP, Voss SD, Parker BR. Leukemia and lymphoma. Radiol Clin North Am. 2011;49(4):767–97, vii. PubMed PMID: 21807173.
12. Kim JK, Park SY, Shon JH, Cho KS. Angiomyolipoma with minimal fat: differentiation from renal cell carcinoma at biphasic helical CT. Radiology. 2004;230(3):677–84. PubMed PMID: 14990834.
13. Chaudry G, Perez-Atayde AR, Ngan BY, Gundogan M, Daneman A. Imaging of congenital mesoblastic nephroma with pathological correlation. Pediatr Radiol. 2009;39(10):1080–6. PubMed PMID: 19629463.

Principles of Magnetic Resonance Imaging (MRI)

4

Robert P. Payne, Manojkumar Saranathan, Shreyas Vasanawala, and Linda Dairiki Shortliffe

Introduction

Magnetic resonance imaging (MRI) is unique in its ability to provide anatomical *and* functional information. It does not involve ionizing radiation, making it much safer and appealing than other body imaging modalities such as CT, especially for use in a pediatric population. As a result, MRI has grown in popularity starting from the early 1980s. With more recent recognition from studies of atomic bomb survivors that increased risks of lifetime cancer exist even from relatively low-dosage radiation, MRI is becoming the modality of choice for imaging of complex anatomy in fetuses and children [1, 2].

MRI is well suited for urological imaging because it provides anatomical information with significantly better spatial resolution than nuclear renograms, in addition to functional information (Fig. 4.1). Pharmacological contrast agents (e.g., gadolinium chelates) used in MRI for angiography and quantification of renal function are much safer than iodinated contrast agents used in CT. Furthermore, these contrast agents exhibit very similar excretion properties as those of iodinated contrast agents and pharmacological agents used in nuclear medicine, enabling the use of quantitative modeling tools already developed for those other modalities. MRI has the ability to yield an array of semiquantitative and quantitative measures including renal and calyceal transit times, enhancement rates, time-to-peak estimates, separate measures of medullary and cortical function, single-kidney glomerular filtration rates (GFR), and even pixel-wise GFRs. Its safety and noninvasive properties make it ideal for obtaining renal functional data critical in pediatric urology.

Basics of Magnetic Resonance Imaging

Phenomenon of Nuclear Magnetic Resonance (NMR)

MRI and nuclear magnetic resonance spectroscopy (NMRS) are based on the phenomenon of nuclear magnetic resonance. All atoms with an odd number of protons and/or odd number of neutrons possess nuclear spin angular momentum and exhibit the phenomenon of magnetic resonance. There are many such nuclei in the body – ^{1}H, ^{13}C, ^{31}P – that exhibit this property,

R.P. Payne, MD, FRCSC
L.D. Shortliffe, MD, FAAP (✉)
Department of Urology,
Stanford University School of Medicine,
300 Pasteur Drive, Stanford, CA 94305-5118, USA
e-mail: lindashortliffe@stanford.edu

M. Saranathan, PhD
Department of Radiology,
Stanford University School of Medicine,
300 Pasteur Drive, Stanford, CA 94305-5118, USA

S. Vasanawala, MD, PhD
Body MRI, Department of Radiology,
Stanford University School of Medicine,
300 Pasteur Drive, Stanford, CA 94305-5118, USA

L.S. Palmer, J.S. Palmer (eds.), *Pediatric and Adolescent Urologic Imaging*,
DOI 10.1007/978-1-4614-8654-1_4, © Springer Science+Business Media New York 2014

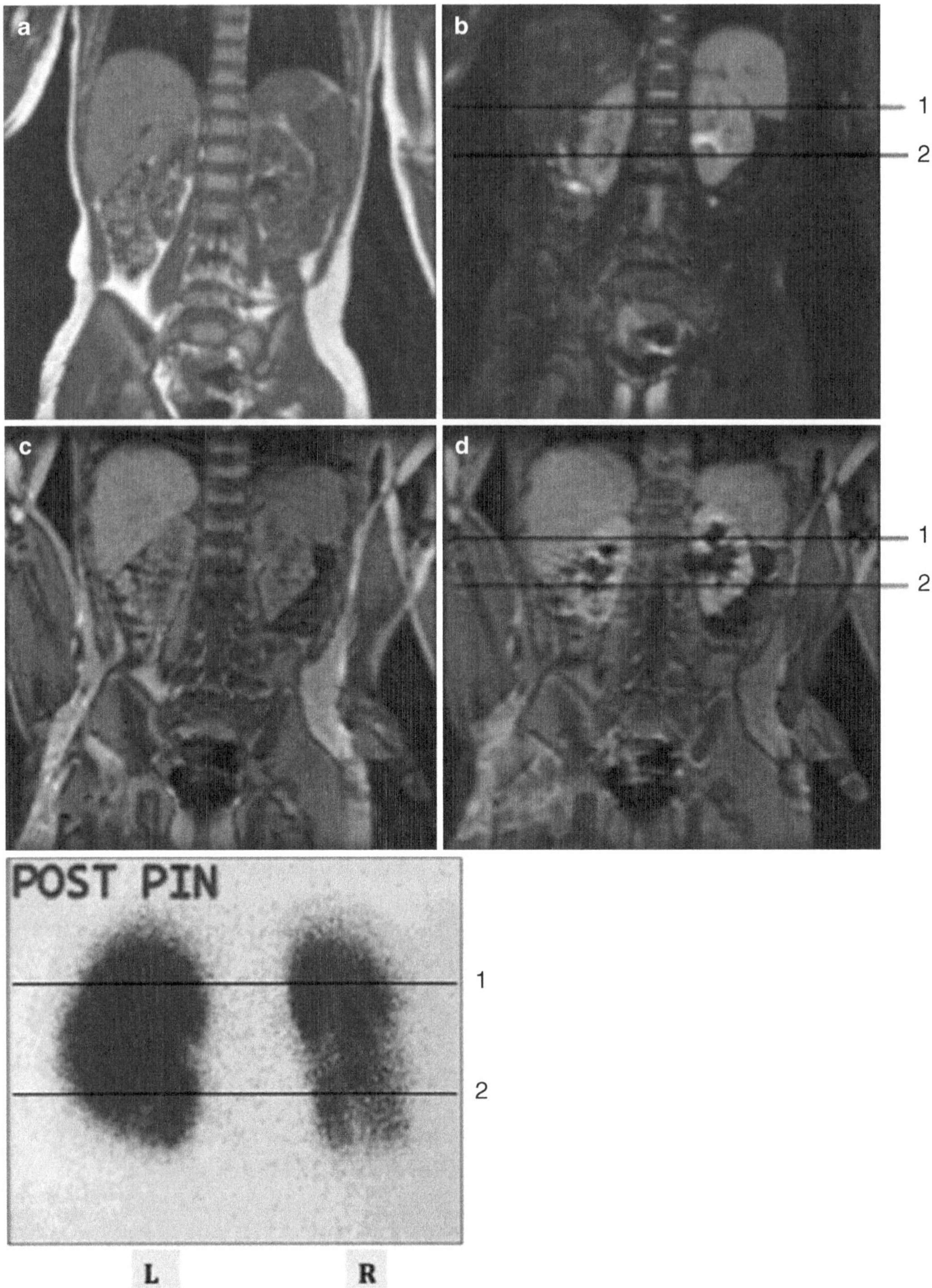

Fig. 4.1 (**a–d**) Magnetic resonance imaging (MRI) showing renal scars in a 3-year-old girl with reflux nephropathy. Dimercaptosuccinic acid (DMSA) radionuclide scan comparative coronal levels (*1*, *2*) are shown [37]

but we will restrict ourselves to the most abundant, i.e., the ^{1}H or proton, as it produces the largest signal and is most commonly used in clinical MRI. This section provides a brief introduction to the basics of NMR and MRI. For a more detailed coverage of the two areas, the reader is referred to books by Slichter and Nishimura [3, 4].

A proton can be thought of as a charged sphere spinning about its axis, which produces a magnetic field. These protons are most commonly referred to as spins in MRI. In the absence of any external magnetic field, the spins are randomly oriented in all directions, resulting in no net macroscopic magnetic field. When placed in a constant external magnetic field B_0, the spins align themselves parallel or antiparallel to B_0. There is a slight excess of spins aligned parallel to the B_0 field, resulting in a net magnetic moment M along B_0. This phenomenon is called *polarization*. Spins exhibit another phenomenon called *precession*. While spinning about their own axis, they also wobble around the B_0 field, analogous to the wobbling motion of a spinning top in a gravitational field. This precession frequency is called the *Larmor frequency*, which is the product of the external magnetic field B_0 and the gyromagnetic ratio γ, a constant for each nucleus. At 1.5 T, the Larmor frequency for protons is 63 MHz. Physically, this corresponds to a two-state split in energy levels when spins are placed in a magnetic field, with the energy difference between the states given by the Larmor frequency. When spins make transitions between the two energy levels, it results in absorption or emission of electromagnetic energy (photons) at the Larmor (resonance) frequency. This phenomenon is called *nuclear magnetic resonance (NMR)*.

NMR was first observed and described independently by Felix Bloch and Edward Purcell in 1946. It was soon used in chemistry to interrogate the structures of molecules and study other physical properties such as diffusion, but it was not until 1973 did Lauterbur make the first images by using principles of magnetic resonance in conjunction with linear gradients [5].

Signal Generation

The static B_0 field alone will not produce any useful measurable signal, as the system is in equilibrium. The net magnetic moment M has to be perturbed in order to observe it. This is done by the application of another radiofrequency (RF) magnetic field B_1 for a brief time interval τ and orthogonal to the static magnetic field B_0, which essentially transfers energy to the spins to cross the energy barrier between the two levels. The applied magnetic field is also at the Larmor frequency to elicit the resonance phenomenon. Physically, this can be thought of as applying a torque on M, which rotates it into a different plane, while M continues to precess about the resultant field. The angle θ by which M is rotated is called the *flip angle* in MRI. The magnetic moment M is usually rotated into the transverse plane orthogonal to the longitudinal B_0 field (i.e., 90° flip angle) to produce the largest signal. The orthogonal RF field B_1 is typically on the order of a fraction of a Gauss compared to the main magnetic field B_0 which ranges from 0.5 to 3 T for most whole-body human imaging systems. After a brief application of the RF field B_1, the net moment M, now in the transverse plane (x-y), continues to precess about B_0 and, by Faraday's laws of electromagnetic induction, induces a signal voltage in a coil placed in the transverse plane. In NMR spectroscopy and the early days of MRI, the RF coil used to produce the B_1 RF field was also used to receive this induced voltage signal, which is also at the Larmor frequency. In modern whole-body MRI systems, a "body coil" is used to produce a uniform B_1 excitation field, while local surface coil arrays are used for reception of the RF signal for increased sensitivity. Coils used for MRI signal reception are often tailored for the anatomy of interest. The nuclear magnetic resonance phenomenon including polarization, precession, and excitation is depicted pictorially in Fig. 4.2.

Any perturbed system tries to recover its equilibrium state – in this case, the equilibrium state is M being aligned with B_0. While precessing about B_0, the magnetization vector M exhibits

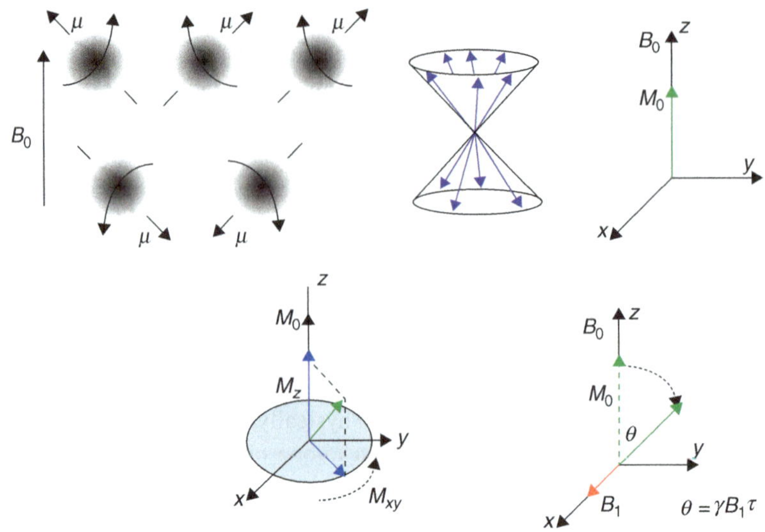

Fig. 4.2 The nuclear magnetic resonance phenomenon (clockwise) – protons abstracted as spinning spheres align themselves along or against a main magnetic field B_0 (polarization). They also process about the B_0 field and the vectors line up along the surface of a cone. The net effect is a resultant z magnetization M aligned along with B_0. When an external orthogonal radiofrequency field B_1 is applied along x, it causes M to tip away from the z-axis by a flip angle θ. The transverse component of M (M_{xy}) produces an induced voltage in a coil placed in the x-y plane and is the NMR signal

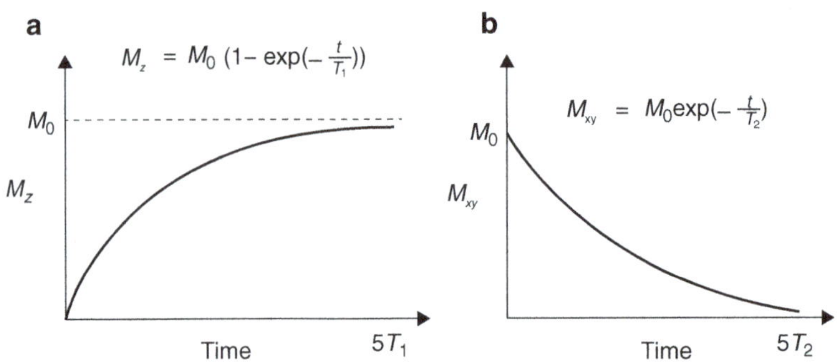

Fig. 4.3 Spin–lattice relaxation (T_1) and spin-spin relaxation (T_2) times – the parameter T_1 describes the recovery of the longitudinal magnetization M_z to its equilibrium value M_0, while T_2 describes the decay of the transverse magnetization M_{xy}. These parameters are different for different types of protons (e.g., protons in free water, bound water, and lipid) resulting in soft tissue contrast. The equations describing these relaxation times are also shown

two important properties that are the basis of image contrast in MRI – (1) the longitudinal component of M (M_z) grows exponentially with a time constant of T_1, referred to as spin–lattice relaxation time, and (2) the transverse component of M (M_{xy}) which is producing the MR signal decays exponentially with a time constant of T_2, referred to as spin-spin relaxation time. This is shown in Fig. 4.3. The equations governing the exponential behavior of these two components over time are called Bloch equations. Physically, T_1 refers to the transfer of energy from the excited spins to the lattice atoms, and T_2 refers to the loss of energy due to mutual interaction between the spins resulting in loss of phase coherence. The values of T_1 and T_2 differ for protons in different local magnetic environments and molecules giving rise to image contrast. For example, protons in lipid molecules exhibit a much shorter T_1 than free water protons in a cyst. The exponentially decaying signal induced by the coil is referred to as free induction decay (FID). T_1 also determines how often the experiment can be repeated, i.e., how often the B_1 RF pulse is applied and the time interval between applications of successive B_1 pulses is called *repetition time* (TR).

Image Formation

The application of an external RF field B_1 to tip the magnetic moment M to the transverse plane produces only a "one-dimensional" signal that contains no spatial information about the object being imaged. In order to achieve spatial discrimination, magnetic field gradients are used. The application of a magnetic field gradient G_x along the x-direction, for example, causes the main magnetic field B_0 to vary along x as B_0+xG_x, where x refers to the spatial coordinate. This causes spins along x to resonate in a range of frequencies centered around the Larmor frequency and linearly proportional to the distance of the spin from the isocenter of the bore (where the gradient strength is zero by design). By applying gradients along two directions x and y, a unique signal characterized by its unique frequency can be elicited as a function of x and y, which in essence is a two-dimensional image. In practice, a gradient is applied along the z direction to select a "slice." In order to separate signals with different frequency components, a Fourier transform is applied in the x-y dimension. *Magnetic field gradients can be applied along any direction, permitting image acquisition in arbitrary planes, a significant departure from the axial plane restriction of CT imaging.*

Image Contrast

The time between the application of a B_1 RF pulse and center of data acquisition is called *echo time* (TE). This parameter along with the sequence repetition time (TR) is a strong determinant of MRI image contrast. The spin–lattice and spin-spin relaxation times T_1 and T_2 along with the spin (or proton) density are different for protons in different molecules (e.g., fat, gray matter, white matter) and environments, generating soft tissue contrast. In the human body, typical values of T_2 are 10–50 ms and T_1 100–1,500 ms. By changing the TE and TR, differences in T_1, T_2, or proton density (PD) can be highlighted, giving rise to *T_1-weighted*, *T_2-weighted*, or *PD-weighted* images, the three most common types of images acquired in MRI. T_2-weighted sequences are characterized by long TR and long TEs, while *T1-weighted* sequences usually employ short TRs and short TEs. Proton-density weighting can be elicited using long TRs and short TEs, minimizing both T_1 and T_2 effects.

MRI Hardware

The main components of an MRI system are shown in Fig. 4.4. The main magnetic field B_0 is created by winding a superconducting material around a cylindrical bore, which also houses the patient table. The superconducting material enables the sustenance of high currents, which are needed for producing strong magnetic fields (1–3 T), typically used in modern whole-body MRI systems. The RF coil that produces the excitation RF B_1 field is also integrated into the bore. The MRI signal is typically sensed using RF coils with differing geometries, tailored to the body part being imaged. A torso phased-array receive coil for abdominal imaging is shown here. The spatially varying magnetic field gradients are also integrated into the bore and produced by winding wires around a core. These gradients are situated in a different layer in the bore than the superconducting windings, which produce B_0. The signal detected by the RF coils are filtered, amplified, digitized, and then processed to generate the final MRI image.

Magnetic Resonance Urography (MRU)

MRU refers to the class of MRI techniques that are used for noninvasive anatomical and functional imaging of the kidneys and the urinary tract. MRU is often classified as *static* (fluid) and *dynamic* (excretory) urography. Static fluid MRU is T_2-weighted and performed without any contrast injection, while dynamic or excretory MRU is performed after injection of a gadolinium-based pharmacological contrast agent using a *T1-weighted* MR imaging sequence. Friedburg

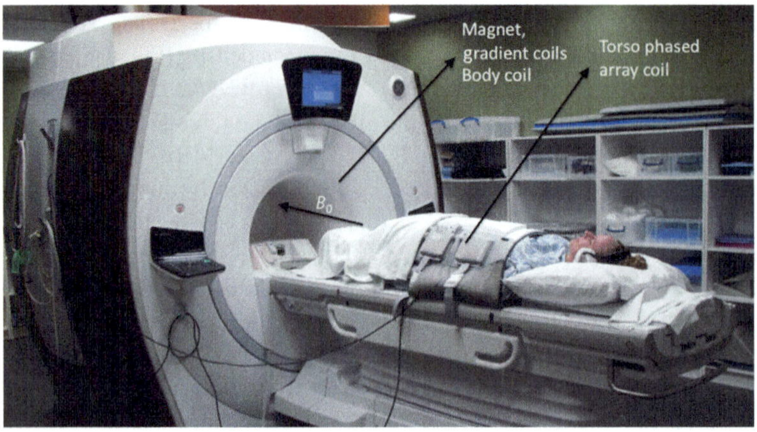

Fig. 4.4 A modern whole-body 3T MRI clinical scanner – the cylindrical bore houses the superconducting coil, which produces the main magnetic field (B_0), the gradient coils, as well as the body RF coil which excites the spins. MRI signal reception is performed using a torso phased-array coil designed for abdominal imaging and wrapped around the patient as shown (Image courtesy: Ann Sawyer, Stanford University)

and associates first applied MRI to urography using a strongly T_2-weighted sequence to delineate the efferent urinary pathways in 1987 [6]. In most situations, static and dynamic MRU provide complementary information, leading to a more accurate diagnosis.

Static MR Urography

Static MRU is very useful for characterization of fluid-filled and dilated structures such as hydronephrosis, megaureters, cysts, ureteroceles, and similar pathologies. While it is very useful for obtaining anatomic information in patients with dilated or obstructed collecting systems, it is not very useful for eliciting functional information, especially in non-dilated systems. Because gadolinium contrast agents cause concomitant reduction of T_2 relaxation times in addition to T_1, static MRU is performed *prior* to injection of gadolinium-based contrast agents. In static MRU, the long T_2 relaxation time of urine is exploited for achieving T_2-weighting [7, 8]. A pulse sequence with a long echo time (TE) is used to suppress signal from background tissue, which have shorter T_2 relaxation times. Fat suppression can also be used to further reduce background signal and improve conspicuity of structures of interest such as the ureters. In addition to thin section multi-slice 2D imaging, thick slab 2D imaging or even 3D T_2-weighted imaging sequences have been reported for use in static fluid MRU.

In order to minimize scan times and reduce motion artifacts from breathing and peristalsis, a half-Fourier single-shot imaging technique (called *single-shot fast spin echo* (SSFSE), *rapid acquisition with relaxation enhancement* (RARE), or *single-shot turbo spin* echo (TSE) by the main MRI vendors) is most commonly used in conjunction with breath-holding [8, 9]. Sometimes, respiratory gating is used to gate the acquisition to the quiescent period of the respiratory cycle and obviate the need for breath-holding. The use of respiratory-gated 3D spin echo sequences has also been reported but at the cost of increased scan times [10]. The use of variable refocusing flip angle 3D fast spin echo sequences (called *Cube*, *SPACE*, or *VISTA* by three of the main MRI vendors) can enable the use of long echo trains, which significantly reduces scan times. Three-dimensional imaging sequences enable the acquisition of volumes with thin section thicknesses, which can then be post-processed to yield maximum intensity projection (MIP) or volume rendered images for depiction of the entire urinary tract.

Dynamic MR Urography

Dynamic or excretory MRU is T_1-weighted and performed *after* administration of a gadolinium-based contrast agent to follow its time course of uptake and excretion. This information can then be used to generate quantitative metrics of renal

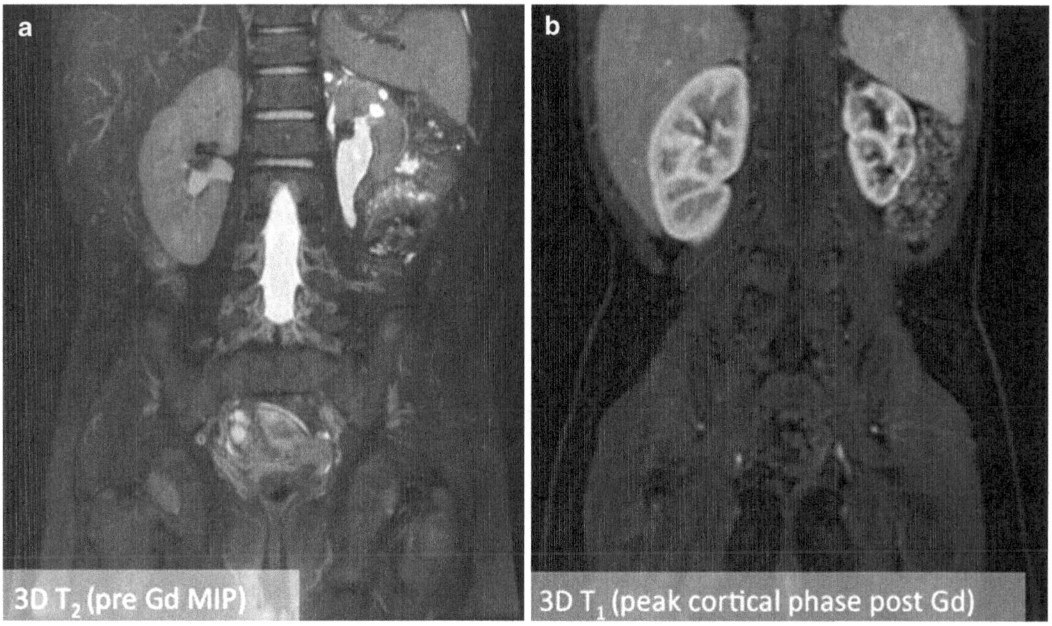

Fig. 4.5 An example of static MR urography (*left*) versus dynamic MR urography (*right*) images from a patient with a slightly atrophied left kidney and multiple cysts. The fluid-filled cysts are clearly visualized on the static 3D *T2-weighted* image, whereas the dynamic 3D T_1-weighted image acquired 30 s after injection of gadolinium contrast shows peak cortical enhancement and lack of cystic enhancement

function such as renal and calyceal transit times, differential renal function, single-kidney GFRs, and even GFR maps. Due to the high vascularity of tumors, T_1-weighted MRI is also used in the detection and characterization of malignancies. Dynamic MRU is more useful in non-dilated systems but requires minimal renal function for excretion and redistribution of the contrast material, often enhanced by using a diuretic such as furosemide. This also causes dilution and redistribution of the contrast agent for optimal image quality and minimizes any signal loss from contrast agent pooling [11, 12].

A 3D spoiled gradient-echo sequence with fat suppression is used repeatedly to capture the signal time course to filling and excretion of urine [11, 13, 14]. This sequence is referred to as *VIBE*, *THRIVE*, or *LAVA* by the main MRI vendors. Fat suppression improves ureter conspicuity as in static MRU. The urine signal is bright due to the T_1 shortening produced by the contrast agent in conjunction with the T_1-weighted pulse sequence, which renders background dark due its longer T_1. A coronal 3D acquisition can be used to image the kidneys, ureters, and the bladder in a single plane. This sequence is typically acquired in a breath-hold if possible or using respiratory gating. Figure 4.5 shows an example of static MR urography (left) and dynamic MR urography (right) on a patient with a smaller left kidney and multiple cysts. The fluid-filled cysts are clearly visualized on the static T_2-weighted image, whereas the dynamic T_1-weighted image shows the cortical enhancement and the lack of enhancement of the cysts. The dynamic 3D T_1-weighted sequence used respiratory triggering to acquire each 3D volume in about 12 s.

Contrast Agents

Gadolinium is a heavy metal in the lanthanide series and is widely used in MRI as an intravenous contrast agent after chelating it with various ligands, most commonly DTPA (Gd-DTPA), to render it safe. A paramagnetic ion with a large magnetic moment due to its seven unpaired electrons, even in very small amounts, gadolinium reduces the T_1 and T_2 of the water protons it comes in close proximity to. The amount of T_1 shortening is linearly proportional to the concentration of contrast agent present for the range of typical in vivo concentrations. Gadolinium chelates exhibit pharmacokinetic properties very similar to that of iodinated contrast agents – they disperse readily into intravascular and extracellular compartments and are excreted by glomerular filtration. The T_1-shortening property of Gd-DTPA and similar contrast agents make it attractive for T_1-weighted imaging. In dynamic MRU, imaging is performed repeatedly following administration of the contrast agent.

In order to extract quantifiable measures of renal function, the MRI signal intensity is used as a surrogate for contrast agent concentration. This approximation is valid only at low concentrations of gadolinium contrast typically 0.1 mmol/kg. In MRU, since urine can concentrate in structures especially when there is an obstruction, the gadolinium concentration can also become very high resulting in signal loss due to T_2* effects. As a result, concentrations as low as 0.025 mmol/kg are used. An accurate way of estimating the contrast agent concentration from MRI signal intensity is using the knowledge of T_1 prior to injection acquired using a T_1-mapping technique. The most commonly used T_1-mapping technique is to image using a pure T_1-weighted imaging sequence such as 3D spoiled gradient echo with multiple flip angles. The T_1 values can then be estimated using a parametric fitting. The change in T_1 can then be used to calibrate the contrast agent concentration, as the signal dependency on T_1 is known a priori [15].

Elements of a Typical MRU Examination

A typical MRU exam comprises of four main steps: (a) patient preparation, (b) data acquisition, (c) image processing, and (d) modeling. While the first two steps are absolutely essential to extract any functional information from the dynamic MRU examination, the last step of modeling is usually performed only if a fully quantitative parametric modeling is desired. The image-processing step is used to segment out the aorta, collecting systems, medulla, and cortex for the individual kidneys. These steps are summarized in Fig. 4.6. The segmented cortex and medulla for each kidney are depicted in different colors. After this segmentation step performed for the images at each time point, semiquantitative measures such as renal and calyceal transit times, volumes of the segmented compartments, relative signal enhancement curves, and differential renal function can be computed. The images can be processed further to extract single-kidney GFRs, medullary and cortical GFRs, or pixel-wise GFR maps using modeling techniques. Many groups use basic image processing to segment and extract semiquantitative parameters instead of modeling the contrast uptake using complex parametric models.

Patient Preparation

Patient preparation is a critical aspect to obtaining reliable MRU quality. Most subjects under 6 years of age require sedation or anesthesia. A recent serum creatinine should be sought to estimate GFR. At our institution, *a GFR less than 30 mL/min/m² precludes administration of gadolinium.* Intravenous access with at least a 22 gauge peripheral IV is required; with 20 gauge preferred in older children. Thirty minutes prior to the start of image acquisition, a 20 mL/kg intravenous bolus of saline or lactated Ringers is administered, though this may be decreased on a case-by-case basis in patients' cardiac or respiratory conditions that require restricted fluid intake. Once the bolus is complete, maintenance fluids of 10 mL/kg/h are continued until the completion of image acquisition. Additionally, a urinary bladder catheter is placed to ensure an empty bladder for physiologic reasons as well as to ensure the patient does not have to prematurely terminate the exam to void.

It is important that gadolinium contrast be diluted and dispersed in the collecting systems for optimal visualization as well as to minimize signal loss due to T_2* effects that can result from the pooling of gadolinium. As a result, dynamic MRU is almost always preceded by administration of a diuretic agent such as furosemide. This enhances the urinary flow and distribution of gadolinium within the collecting systems for optimal visualization.

Image Acquisition

Figure 4.7 summarizes a typical MRU protocol performed at our institution on a child with crossed fused renal ectopia. The top panel

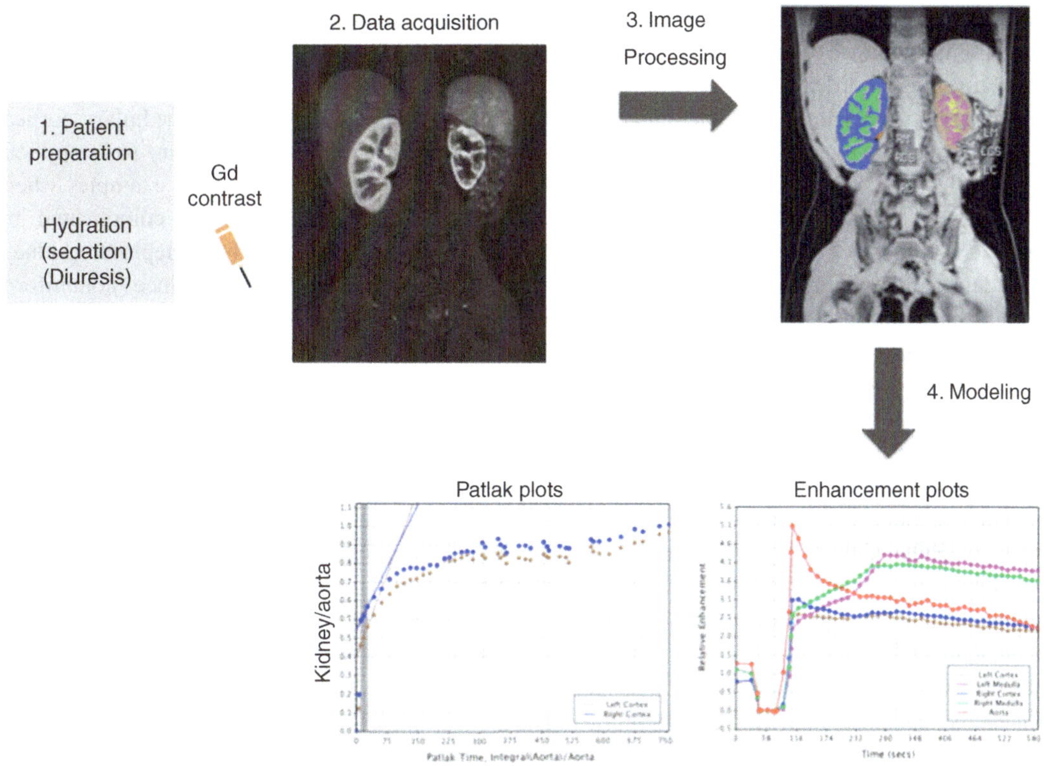

Fig. 4.6 Elements of a typical MRU exam illustrating the key steps of patient preparation, data acquisition (imaging), image processing, and modeling. The image-processing step is used to segment the kidney into medulla, cortex, and collecting system (*color coded* here) to generate separate cortical and medullary GFR measurements

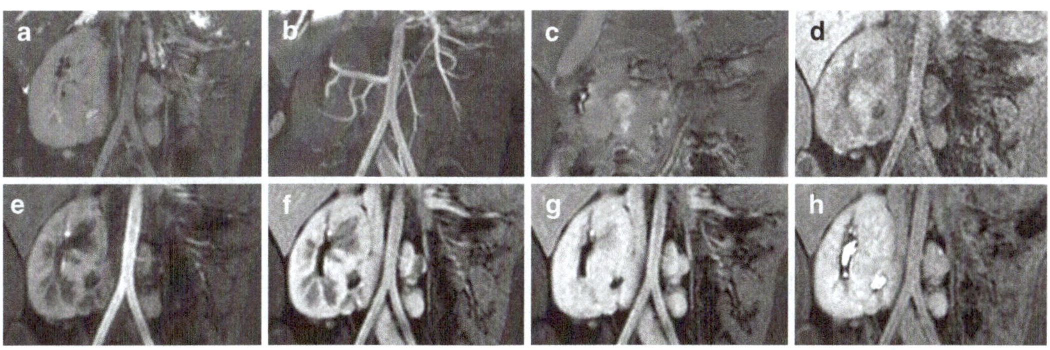

Fig. 4.7 Representative images from a typical MRU protocol performed at our institution on a child with crossed fused renal ectopia. Panels **a**–**c** show a 3D T_2-weighted image (**a**), a non-contrast angiography MIP image obtained using a 3D balanced SSFP sequence with an inversion recovery prep (**b**), a single frame from a multiphasic 2D balanced SSFP sequence (**c**). Pre-contrast (**d**) and post-contrast (**e**–**h**) phases from a respiratory-gated 3D T_1-weighted sequence with Dixon fat-water separation depict peak cortical enhancement (**e**), peak medullary enhancement (**f**), late enhancement, (**g**) and excretory phase with enhanced collecting system (**h**)

shows a 3D T_2-weighted image (a), a non-contrast angiography MIP image obtained using a 3D balanced SSFP sequence with an inversion recovery prep to suppress the background and venous signal (b) and a single frame from a multiphasic 2D balanced SSFP sequence (c). The remaining images (d–h) are from a respiratory-gated 3D *T1-weighted* sequence with Dixon fat-water separation obtained before injection of gadolinium contrast (d) and post-contrast (e–h) depicting peak cortical enhancement (e), peak medullary enhancement (f), late enhancement (g), and excretory phase with enhanced collecting system (h).

Image Processing

The data acquired in dynamic MRU is essentially a four-dimensional data set (i.e., a 3D volume as function of time). A number of quantitative metrics are extracted from these dynamic MRU images, which provide information about renal function. These metrics are computed pixel by pixel over the entire imaging volume or on the signal integrated over a user-specified *region of interest* (ROI). Commonly used metrics include *calyceal transit time* (CTT, the time taken for the contrast agent to reach the renal pelvis), *renal transit time* (RTT, the time between arrival of the contrast agent in the cortex and in the ureters), degree of enhancement (the maximum signal enhancement after injection of gadolinium contrast relative to the unenhanced signal expressed as a % and sometimes also calculated as a ratio to remove effects such as coil shading), time to peak (time taken to reach maximum degree of enhancement), maximal slope of enhancement, and differential renal function (maximum slope or area under the signal enhancement curve normalized by renal volume).

The features of interest in the 3D images are segmented first prior to extraction of parameters [16]. Simple image-processing techniques like image thresholding and more complex morphological operations like erosion and dilation are used to extract and label the aorta, left and right medullae, cortices, and the left and right collecting systems. These steps may be time-consuming requiring manual input for identification of the regions as well as readjustment if the image contrast is poor. Time-to-peak maps can assist in segmentation by identifying the image phase with the brightest signal in the region of interest and speed up the segmentation process. Signal from the aorta is used by most modeling-based approaches to compute the arterial input function. Medullary and cortical volumes can be computed for each kidney and used for normalization of split or differential renal function measures. In highly dilated or atrophied kidneys, it may not be possible to achieve this medullary-cortical segmentation, and it is customary to lump them together. Figure 4.8 shows two examples where the image segmentation was complicated by an atrophic kidney or a hydronephrotic kidney. Phased-array coils often produce nonuniform intensity variations across the image and can be corrected using vendor-supplied software, which removes any coil-induced variations in image intensity across the image.

Modeling

While semiquantitative measures such as degree of enhancement and transit times are useful metrics, a more complex pharmacokinetic model can be used to extract the GFR. A number of models, varying in complexity, have been developed. The most popular as well as simplest of the models is the *Patlak-Rutland model* which assumes a vascular space and a nephron space with no loss or transit of tracer from the nephron space as shown in Fig. 4.9 [17, 18].

Patlak-Rutland Model. This model estimates the GFR using the metrics: **a(t)**, the amount of contrast agent in the arteries at a given time (*t*); **V(t)**, contrast in the vascular space at that time; **N(t)**, contrast in the nephron space; **Vs**, the fraction of contrast that flows into the vascular space; **c** a constant of proportionality that represents the GFR; and **C(t)**, the total amount of contrast agent in the kidney at time *t*. We can write the following:

$$V(t) = V_s \times a(t) \qquad \frac{dN}{dt} = c \times a(t) \tag{4.1–4.2}$$

Furthermore, we assume

$$K(t) = V(t) + N(t) \tag{4.3}$$

Solving these three equations, we get

$$\frac{K(t)}{a(t)} = V_s + GFR\frac{\int a(s)\,ds}{a(t)} \tag{4.4}$$

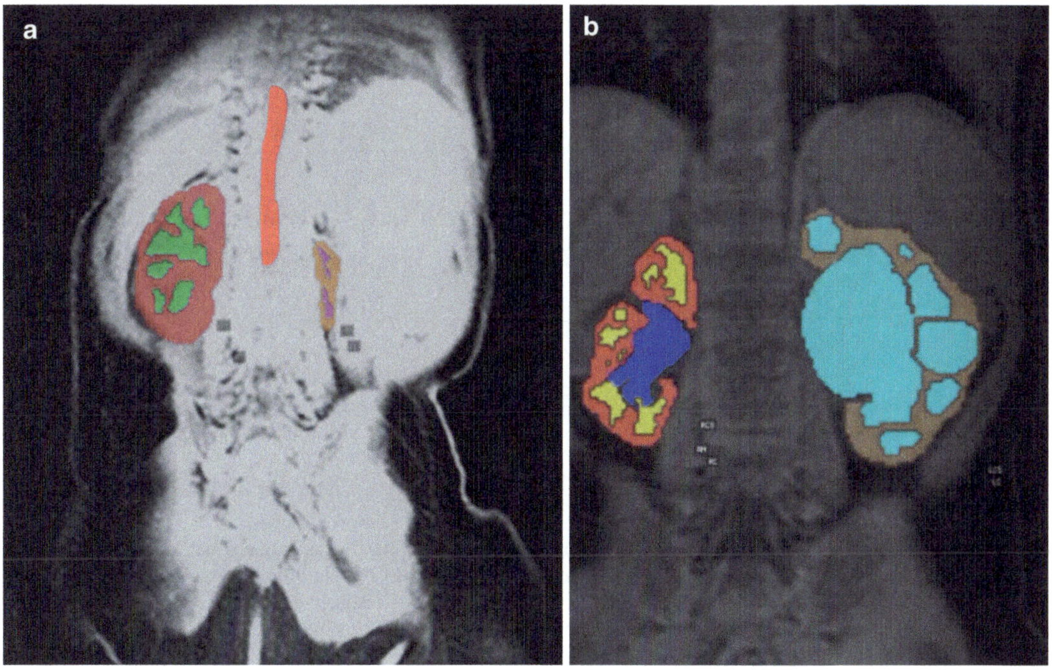

Fig. 4.8 Image segmentation results from a patient with an atrophic left kidney (*left*) and hydronephrosis (*right*), which make segmentation of the kidney into distinct cortical and medullary compartments difficult

Note that c has been replaced by the GFR, and the quantity $\frac{\int a(s)ds}{a(t)}$ is referred to as Patlak time. Equation 4.4 is plotted in Fig. 4.9, which is a classic Patlak plot. Note that the linearity of the curves no longer hold after the initial 1990s or so, due to the simplifying assumptions made in the Patlak-Rutland model. The initial slope of the curve is used and is a measure of GFR per unit volume, which is further corrected for volume, the *hematocrit* ratio (the volume % of red blood cells in the blood) and patient weight to yield a more accurate BSA-corrected GFR index. Note that this GFR index can be generated on a per-pixel basis to create a GFR map or generated for ROIs representing the left and right medullary and cortical compartments or the entire left and right kidneys, respectively.

The Patlak-Rutland model is a simple two-compartment model. More complex models have been proposed that incorporate outflow of contrast agent from the nephron space and take into account other anatomical features of the nephron such as proximal and distal tubules and the loops of Henle [19–21]. Figure 4.10 shows a comparison of the Patlak-Rutland model with a two-compartment and a three-compartment model, the latter accounting for outflow from the tubules. Preliminary results seem to indicate that the simpler Patlak-Rutland model performs more reliably than other more complex models, but this is an area of ongoing research [22].

Images from a typical pediatric MRU examination are shown in Fig. 4.11. Dynamic MRU was performed using a 3D T_1-weighted respiratory-gated sequence with a temporal resolution of 12 s per 3D volume. A pre-contrast phase and three post-contrast phases (peak cortical enhancement, peak medullary enhancement, and late excretory) are shown in panels a–d. A 3D MIP of the volume acquired 24 s after injection of contrast is shown in panel e, demonstrating the spatial and temporal resolution of the 3D dynamic sequence. A 3D MIP from a pre-contrast respiratory-gated 3D T_2 Cube acquisition is also shown in panel f,

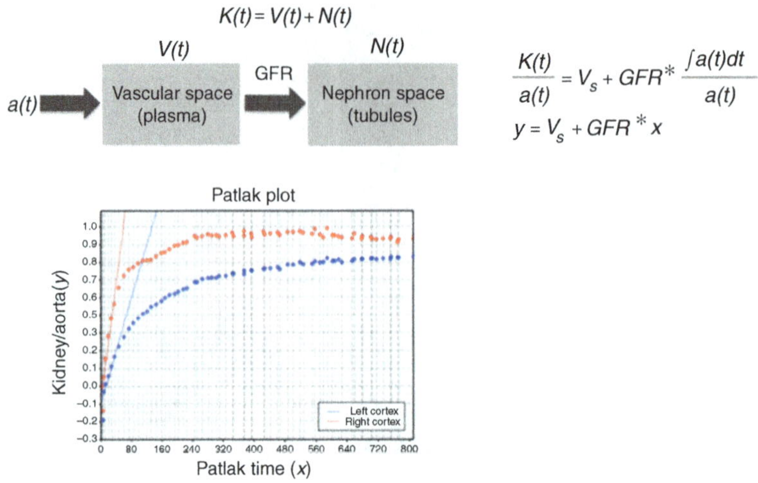

Fig. 4.9 The two-compartment Patlak-Rutland model accounting for vascular and nephron space (plasma and tubules). The equation on the *right* is linear, with the slope being equivalent to the GFR. The Patlak-Rutland plot estimated from data acquired on a patient with an atrophic left kidney is shown in the *bottom panel*. Note that the linearity of the Patlak model holds only for the initial points due to the simplifying assumptions made in the model. As a result, the initial slope (<90s typically) is used as the GFR estimate

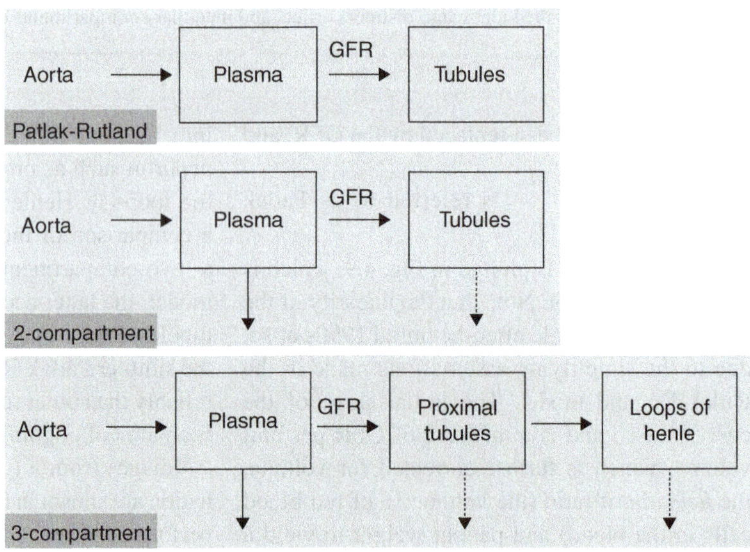

Fig. 4.10 The Patlak-Rutland model commonly used for generating GFR estimates shown (*top*) along with more complex pharmacokinetic models (*middle*, *bottom*) which model outflow from the renal tubules as well as take into account finer anatomical details (Adapted from Bokacheva [19])

illustrating the complementarity of the T_1 and T_2 acquisitions. The 3D data sets were segmented into left and right cortex, medulla, and collecting systems and analyzed using custom-developed software incorporated into OsiriX imaging software (Geneva, Switzerland). Relative signal enhancement plots of the aorta, left medulla and cortex, and right medulla and cortex are shown in Fig. 4.12a. The corresponding Patlak plots in Fig. 4.11b show a very subtle difference in initial slopes (which is a measure of GFR) between the left and the right cortex.

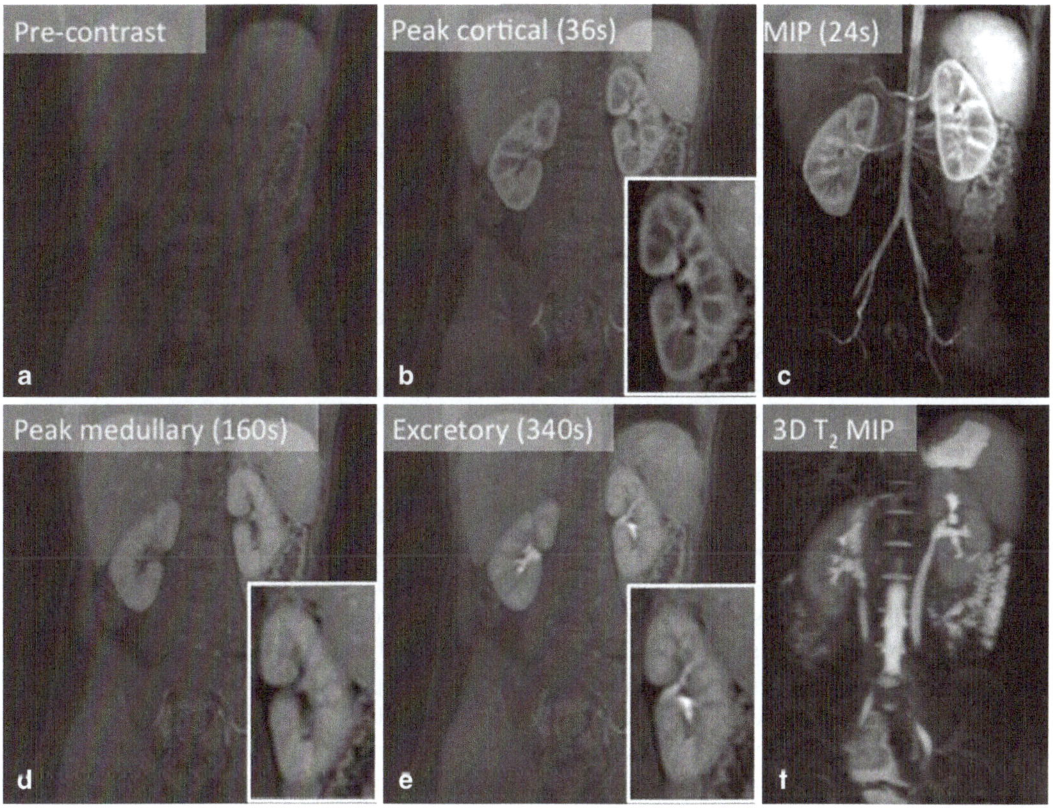

Fig. 4.11 Images from a typical MRU examination. A pre-contrast and three post-contrast phases acquired using a 3D respiratory-gated T_1-weighted sequence are shown in panels (**a–d**). A 3D MIP of the volume acquired 24 s after injection of contrast is shown in panel (**e**), demonstrating the high spatio-temporal resolution of the 3D dynamic sequence. A MIP from a pre-contrast respiratory-gated 3D T_2 Cube acquisition is shown in panel (**f**)

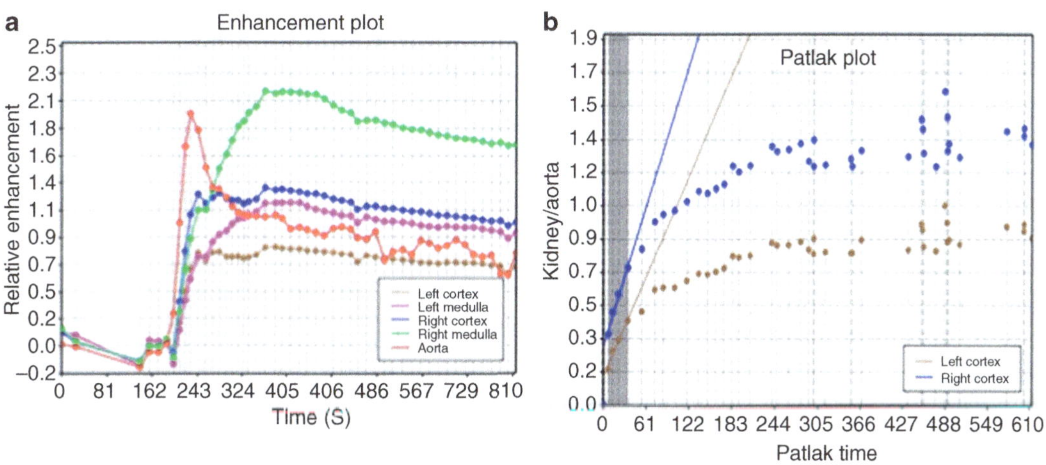

Fig. 4.12 Relative signal enhancement of the aorta, left cortex and medulla, and right cortex and medulla are shown in panel (**a**), and the corresponding Rutland-Patlak plots for the left and right cortex are shown in panel (**b**). These were generated from the dynamic 3D T_1 data shown in Fig. 4.11

Challenges and Limitations of Pediatric MRU

MRI also poses a number of technical challenges from motion sensitivity, contrast agent, and technical variable parameters. Since MRI is motion sensitive, sedation and/or anesthesia may be required in younger children to reduce and compensate for physiological anatomic motion due to respiration. Sedated subjects can be conveniently imaged using respiratory-gating techniques where the imaging acquisition is restricted to periods of respiratory quietus, typically end-expiration. The position of the diaphragm is monitored either mechanically using respiratory bellows that are wrapped around the abdomen or using a MR navigator echo that produces a one-dimensional image (cross-sectional profile) of the lung-liver interface. This position information can be used by the pulse sequence to gate the acquisition to the end-expiration period of the respiratory cycle. While the same technique can be applied to nonsedated subjects, the variability in breathing due to sleep apnea, hyperventilation, or irregular breathing patterns poses significant problems to the scan efficiency, prolonging scan times, and deteriorating image quality.

As already mentioned, gadolinium MRI signal intensity does not have a linear relationship with concentration except at very low doses, requiring additional corrections. Gadolinium-based contrast agents have also been implicated in nephrogenic systemic fibrosis that may occur when used in patients with severe renal insufficiency.

Finally, image signal-to-noise ratio (SNR), spatial coverage, and acquisition time are often conflicting variables in MRI, requiring careful optimization of the MRI protocol and sequence parameters. As in any dynamic MRI application, spatial resolution is traded with temporal resolution as only a finite amount of k-space coverage is possible in a given time interval. In order to quantify metrics of renal function such as the Patlak number accurately, it is desirable to keep the temporal resolution to 10 s or better [23]. This places restrictions on the spatial resolution and/or spatial coverage that can be achieved, which can limit segmentation of the medulla from the cortex both in cases of hypertrophy and atrophy. Moreover, depending on patient size, specialized radiofrequency coils may be required to optimize the signal-to-noise ratio. Parallel imaging techniques are increasingly being used to reduce scan time and optimize spatial and temporal resolution. They exploit the correlation between images generated by each coil element in a phased array and enable reduction in the amount of data that needs to be acquired to reconstruct an image (i.e., faster acquisition). Specially designed phased-array coils can improve image quality while permitting higher parallel imaging acceleration factors.

Clinical Indications

Genitourinary imaging in children is usually limited to disorders of the kidney, urinary collecting system, and testes. The general indications for imaging in pediatric and adolescent urology are typically related to (1) evaluation of symptoms such as urinary tract infection, hematuria, and abdominal or testicular masses or (2) evaluation of asymptomatic children with abnormal prenatal ultrasounds or incidental findings on radiologic studies performed for other reasons. The imaging studies selected in each case should guide and improve management by helping to give diagnosis, structure, and function. Also, the optimal imaging modality should provide comparative parameters to follow over time for potential prognosis. As a 3-dimensional imaging modality, MRI is an attractive alternative because it can potentially provide most of this information in a single study with the additional advantage that no ionizing radiation is used.

MRI was first used in pediatric urology over 25 years ago [24]. Since that time, sophisticated MR-based technologies have been developed to give precise anatomic and structural detail with high spatial resolution and simultaneous evaluation of organ function. MRI can be used to assess most genitourinary and testicular abnormalities and is rapidly becoming the imaging modality of choice when greater anatomic and functional detail is needed to assess complex anatomies and pathologies (Table 4.1). A specific advantage to

Table 4.1 Potential indications for MRI in pediatric urology

Hydronephrosis (complicated)
Ureteropelvic junction obstruction
Hydroureteronephrosis
Calyceal abnormality
Complex duplications of collecting system
Urinary tract infections (complicated)
Acute pyelonephritis/renal abscess
Renal scarring assessment
Vesicoureteral reflux
Renal masses
Staging of tumor volumes and metastatic evaluation
Tumor surveillance studies
Testes cancer
Initial staging and metastatic evaluation
Tumor surveillance
Renal transplantation
Donor assessment
Posttransplant renal failure
Ambiguous genitalia and complex pelvic anatomy
Bilateral and non-palpable testes
Complex fetal GU anomalies

MRI is the lack of exposure to ionizing radiation, which is particularly important in pregnant women, children, and those requiring serial 3-dimensional imaging. While past constraints related to MRI, including resource availability, imaging duration, and need for child immobilization with general anesthesia, has limited MRU clinical utility, current research is improving these issues and promises to make MRI the modality of choice for complex pediatric urologic situations.

Hydronephrosis

The most common urologic indication for imaging in infants and children is hydronephrosis, due in part to the increased use of prenatal imaging studies. Routine prenatal imaging using ultrasonography may lack full anatomic, functional, and prognostic information needed to guide early management decisions, and postnatal radiologic studies may be needed to determine whether or not surgical intervention is warranted. Compared to conventional imaging modalities, MRI is of great value in patients with complicated forms of hydronephrosis because of the anatomic and functional data that can be obtained.

Table 4.2 Classification of UPJ obstruction based on MRU-derived renal transit times compared to $t_{1/2}$ times obtained during diuretic renal scintigraphy [25, 26]

	Renal transit time (min)	$t_{1/2}$ (min)
Normal	≤4	≤15
Equivocal	4–8	15–30
Obstructed	≥8	≥30

Ureteropelvic Junction Obstruction (UPJO)

UPJO is a common cause of hydronephrosis in children, and the decision to intervene is based on the presence of symptoms (pain, hematuria, infections, stones) and/or when renal function or the degree of hydronephrosis worsens. Traditionally, diuretic renal scintigraphy has been used to measure renal function and drainage curves, and additional studies are often required to obtain reliable anatomic information. MRU, on the other hand, combines detailed renal anatomy with functional assessment when an imaging agent (gadolinium) is administered and followed as it transits the renal parenchyma and calyceal systems (i.e., referred to by some as renal and calyceal transit time, RTT, and CTT, respectively) (Table 4.2). RTT may be of limited value when assessing a poorly functioning kidney, especially in those with minimal urinary production. CTT has been used as an indicator of pathophysiologic obstruction and is influenced by both GFR and tubular reabsorption of urine [26].

Unlike other modalities, MRU has the ability to subcategorize obstructed kidneys (RTT ≥ 8 min) by renal function based on contrast dynamics seen in the renal parenchyma. As this means of evaluation focuses on renal rather than collecting system pathophysiologic changes, there is the possibility that prognostic information may be obtained. The severely damaged and decompensated kidney compared with a normal kidney will display asymmetrical nephrograms, dense and prolonged enhancement, and delayed calyceal transit times when subjected to the fluid and diuretic challenge.

MRU can also estimate the discrepant isolated renal GFR by Patlak-Rutland formulae (*vide supra see: Modeling*) and renal volume with the later a functional surrogate. This way of classifying obstruction may offer some ability to predict better which hydronephrotic kidneys would benefit most from early surgical correction in order to eliminate potential renal demise. Decompensated systems may have more significant improvements in renal function following successful pyeloplasty compared to compensated systems [27]. Further studies are needed to assess the potential prognostic implications of this MRU-derived classification system.

MRU offers high-resolution anatomic detail that is impossible from ultrasonography and nuclear renography, such as crossing vessels, and allows understanding of more complex diagnostic challenges and potential surgical planning (Fig. 4.13). Signs of obstructive nephropathy, such as small subcortical cysts, poor corticomedullary differentiation, decreased cortical signal intensity, and poorly defined or patchy nephrograms, are readily seen on MRU as well. These features represent areas of renal damage and impaired function, which are unlikely to improve with surgery.

Hydroureteronephrosis

Despite the high rate of spontaneous resolution, hydroureteronephrosis or megaureter is a finding that often leads to an extensive workup given the potential for obstructive or refluxing etiologies that require surgical correction in 30 % of children detected antenatally [28]. In order to select which patients would benefit from surgery versus conservative management, a thorough workup is mandatory which often includes ultrasonography, VCUG, and diuretic renal scintigraphy. Dilation of the upper urinary tract is well imaged with MRI by combining T_2-weighted and delayed post-contrast T1-weighted images that can delineate the entire anatomy of the ureter from the renal pelvis to its distal site of insertion. MRU has the added benefit of providing functional information and can classify megaureter as obstructed or nonobstructed (Table 4.2). As a single study, MRU provides the same information obtained from both ultrasound and diuretic renal scintigraphy in the workup of hydroureteronephrosis, without exposure to ionizing radiation [29]. As seen in Fig. 4.14, MRU can accurately identify the site of ureteric insertion and can reliably diagnose ureteral ectopia in both single and duplicated systems, even when markedly dilated or poorly functioning because of the 3-dimensional character of the modality [30].

Urinary Tract Infections

Acute Pyelonephritis

DMSA scintigraphy is considered the gold standard for the diagnosis of acute pyelonephritis despite its inability to reliably differentiate

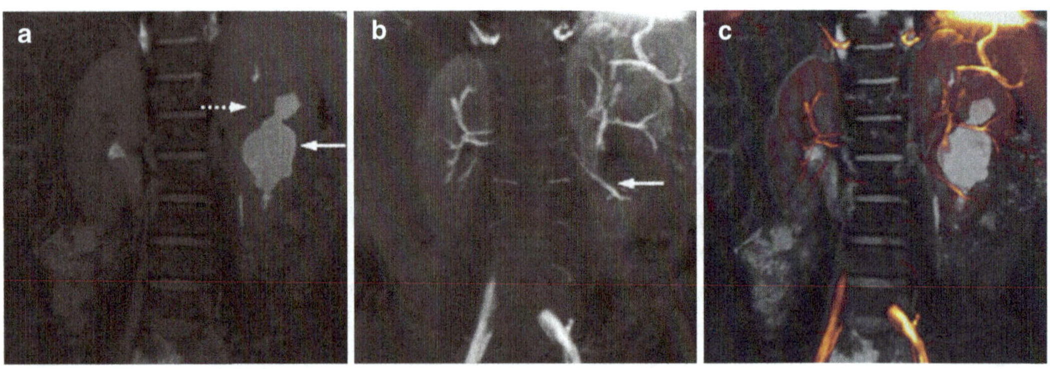

Fig. 4.13 A 6-year-old girl with duplicated left kidney and UPJO of lower pole moiety. (**a**) Thick slab maximum intensity projection (*MIP*) of fat-suppressed T_2-weighted sequence showing hydronephrosis of left lower pole moiety (*arrow*) and unobstructed upper pole ureter (*dotted arrow*). (**b**) Non-contrast MR angiogram using inflow inversion recovery demonstrating obstructing lower pole crossing vessel (*arrow*) (**c**) overlay images (**a**) in gray scale and (**b**) in color

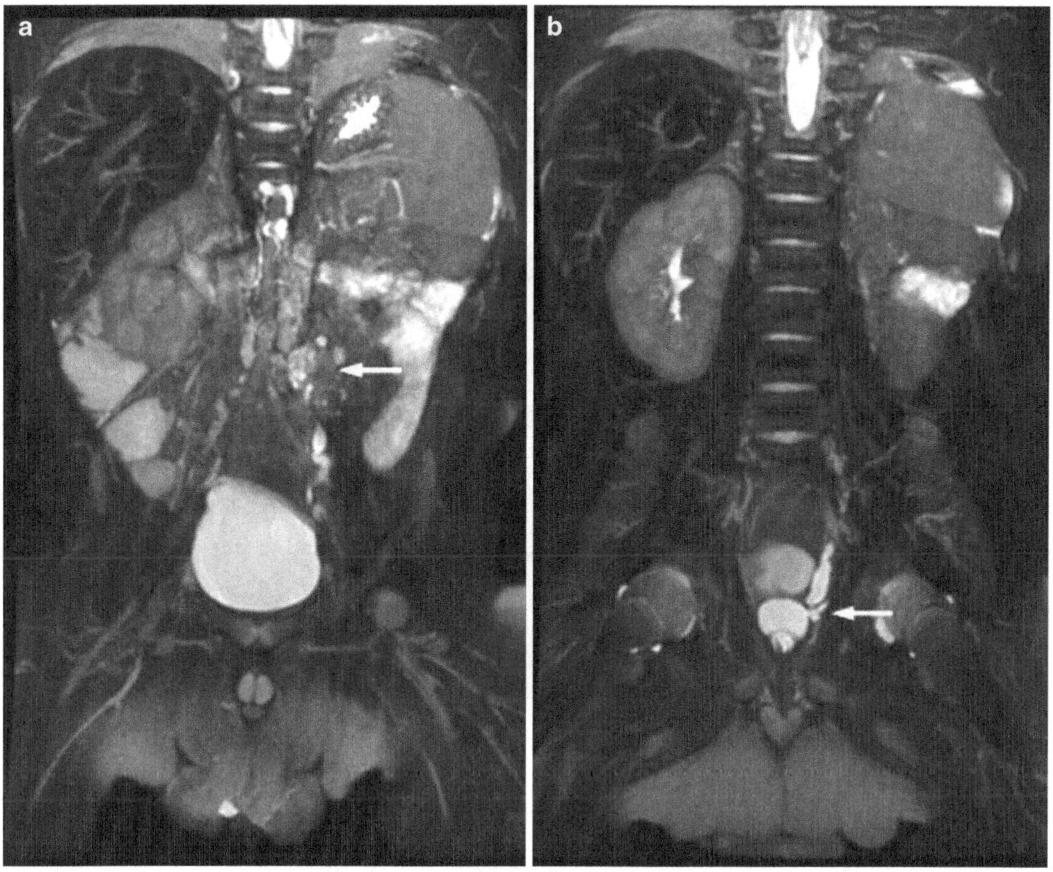

Fig. 4.14 T_2-weighted images of 18-month-old boy with (**a**) left multicystic dysplastic kidney (*arrow*) secondary to (**b**) an ectopic ureter seen inserting into posterior urethra above the sphincter (*arrow*)

between permanent and transient lesions. By analyzing multiple anatomic and functional parameters, MRU can more accurately characterize lesions of the renal parenchyma and can differentiate between acute pyelonephritis, acquired pyelonephritic scars, and areas of congenital renal dysplasia. It has been shown that MRI detects more pyelonephritic lesions compared to DMSA scanning and has a superior interobserver agreement. Lonergan et al. reported that the proportion of positive agreement between readers for the presence of acute pyelonephritic lesion was 0.85 and 0.57, and the negative agreement was 0.88 and 0.80 for MRI and renal scintigraphy, respectively [31]. A distinct and valuable advantage of MRU over DMSA is its ability to distinguish acute pyelonephritis from chronic renal scarring at the time of initial evaluation [32]. Using DMSA as the gold standard, a gadolinium-enhanced T_1 sequence from a MRU has a sensitivity of 100 % and a specificity of 78 % for the detection of renal scars [33].

During DMSA scans, acute pyelonephritis and renal scars are similarly characterized by areas of decreased uptake of the radionucleotide. However, because MRU can easily differentiate renal parenchyma from the background, these lesions can be further characterized based on their renal contours and signal intensities. Gadolinium-enhanced imaging sequences produce low signal intensity in normal kidneys, whereas areas of acute pyelonephritis display high signal intensity on a background of low signal intensity within the renal parenchyma (Fig. 4.15) [31]. Renal scars are seen on *T2-weighted* images as focal areas of parenchymal loss often associated with a deformed underlying calyx (Fig. 4.16), which

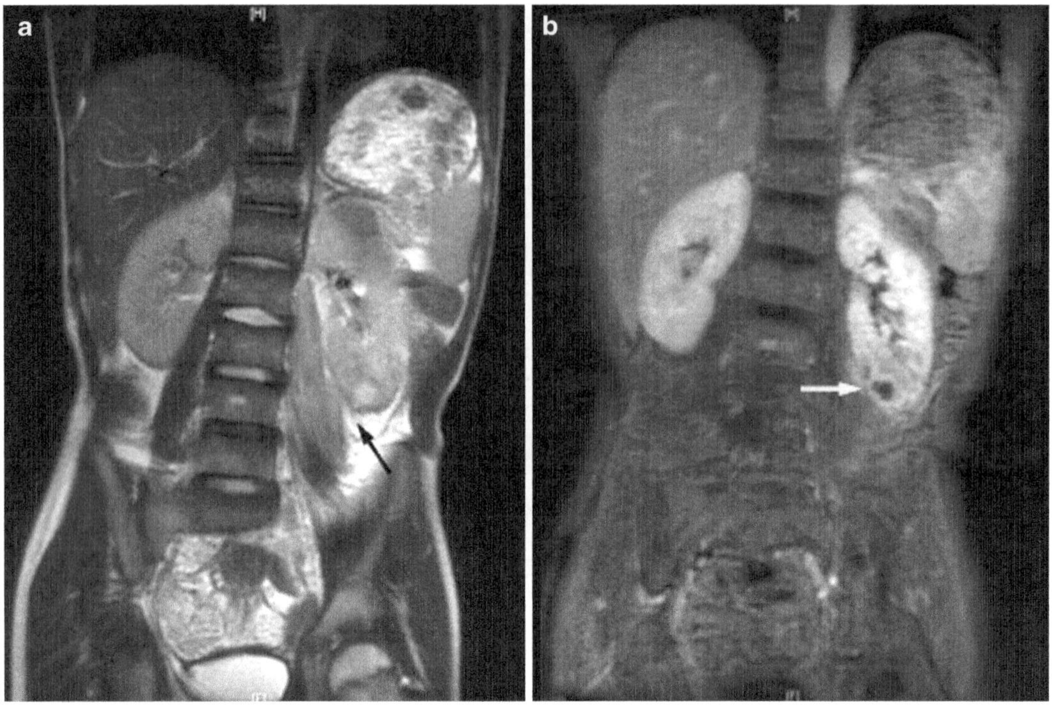

Fig. 4.15 An 8-year-old boy with febrile UTI and equivocal renal ultrasound. (**a**) T_2-weighted image showing high signal intensity in lower pole of left kidney and ipsilateral psoas muscle (*arrow*) consistent with an inflammatory process. (b) T_1-weighted gadolinium-enhanced image demonstrating renal abscess in lower pole of left kidney (*arrow*)

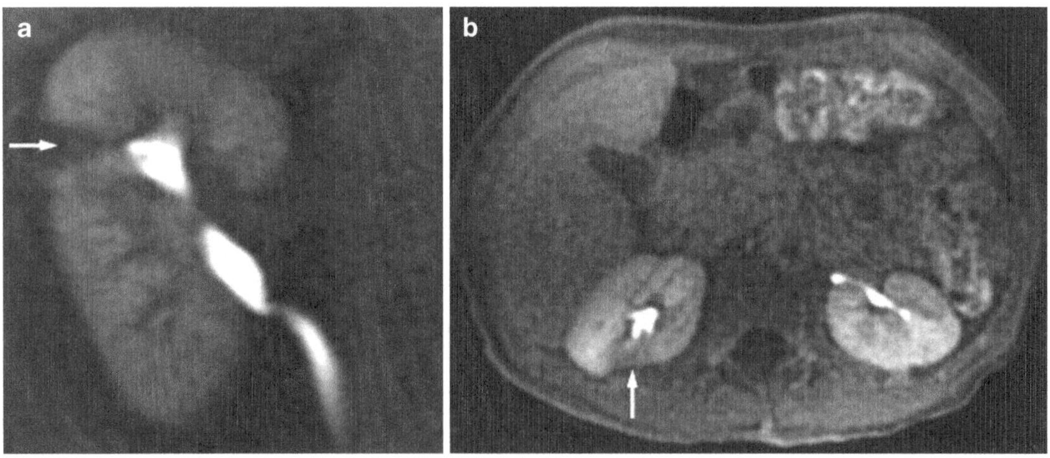

Fig. 4.16 (**a**) T_2-weighted pre-contrast image of the right kidney showing an upper pole segment with low signal intensity (*arrow*) and (**b**) T_1-weighted post-contrast image with decreased uptake of gadolinium in posterior upper pole segment (*arrow*) consistent with a postinfectious renal scar

results in an abnormal renal contour. Affected regions show no appreciable contrast enhancement. Recent technical advances have made it possible to capture the cortical phase of the dynamic post-contrast scan which appears to be the best sequence to identify cortical perfusion defects and may negate the need for longer inversion-recovery sequences [34].

Using the initial renal evaluation of a child with a febrile urinary tract infection (UTI) as the primary guide to subsequent urinary tract evaluation advocates for the use of DMSA scanning as the initial imaging study in order to identify those children at risk of progressive renal injury [35]. The same argument could therefore be made for using MRU as the initial radiological study in children with a documented febrile UTI as it can clearly identify those with renal involvement. Additionally, it can distinguish among acute pyelonephritis, renal scarring, and reflux nephropathy, which is not possible when using more traditional radiologic studies.

Vesicoureteral Reflux (VUR)

Currently, the gold standard investigation for detecting VUR is a voiding cystourethrogram (VCUG). The VCUG provides anatomic visualization of the bladder, any filling defects, and urethra, detects vesicoureteral reflux, and is the only modality that shows the calyceal detail to grade VUR during voiding. Despite its widespread use, a VCUG is associated with direct irradiation to the gonads of pediatric patients with exposures ranging from 0.7 to 1.1 mSv in boys and from 0.27 to 1.25 mSv in girls [36]. With the recent advent of near real-time magnetic resonance fluoroscopy, MRVCUG has been used and evaluated as a potential alternative to VCUG for the detection of VUR even though the voiding phase may not be obtained [37].

During this study, T_1-weighted images are analyzed before and after transurethral injection of gadolinium. When compared to conventional VCUG, Lee *et al.* found that MRVCUG has a sensitivity of 76 % and a specificity of 90 % for detecting VUR and demonstrated good concordance with grading [38]. With current MR technology, these inferior results are likely caused by the inherent difficulties of assessing the voiding phase during MR imaging because children may be under sedation or anesthesia and unable to void. Whether the MRVCUG becomes more clinically useful may depend upon future technological developments.

One of the added benefits of MR urography compared to VCUG alone in the workup of a child with VUR is that it can simultaneously image the kidneys to assess for the presence of reflux nephropathy and post-pyelonephritic scarring. Assessing the degree of renal damage and presence of significant reflux nephropathy in a child with VUR may alter management when deciding among the various treatment options, which can range from close follow-up to reconstructive surgery [39].

Renal Masses

While the initial imaging modality of choice for investigating a child with a renal mass is usually ultrasonography because it can effectively characterize the cystic and/or solid nature of the lesion, if malignancy is considered additional, more detailed imaging is usually required. Traditionally, CT has been employed in these patients to determine the precise origin of the mass, degree of local invasion, vascularity, and presence of local and distant metastases. Although CT scans are clinically useful, ionizing radiation exposure to children ranges from 3 to 20 mSv. Children with malignant renal masses may require serial body CT scans to assess for disease recurrence, increasing the known risks of secondary cancers from exposure to ionizing radiation [40].

The first indication to use MRI in the pediatric population was in children with Wilms' tumor [24]. These tumors are generally heterogeneous with variable signal intensities due to the cystic, hemorrhagic, and necrotic components that are often present (Fig. 4.17). Since its debut over 25 years ago, MRI has been increasingly used to diagnose, stage, monitor response to chemotherapy, and follow patients with Wilms' tumor [41]. CT and MRI are equally capable of detecting lymph node involvement (sensitivity 67 % and specificity 100 %) and perirenal tumor extension (sensitivity 60 % and specificity 90 %), which is critically important when determining if preoperative chemotherapy is needed [42]. Other studies have demonstrated that MRI is superior to CT for the detection of renal vein and IVC thrombus (100 % vs. 50 %) and for detecting synchronous

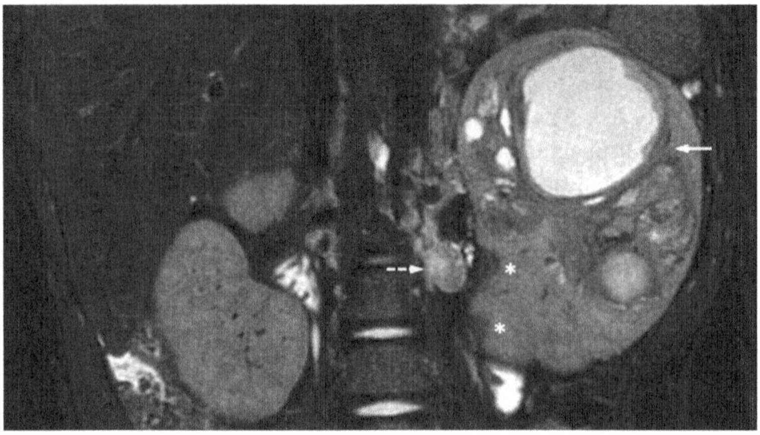

Fig. 4.17 A 3-year-old girl with a T_2-weighted image demonstrating large heterogenous and cystic mass in the upper pole of the left kidney encased by a low signal pseudocapsule consistent with Wilms' tumor (*solid arrow*). Perilobar nephrogenic rests are also seen in the lower pole of the ipsilateral kidney (*asterisks*), and hilar lymphadenopathy is present concerning for regional metastasis (*dotted arrow*)

bilateral Wilms' tumor (100 % vs. 87 %) [43, 44]. Since MRI does not expose patients to radiation and has been shown to be equivalent and in some instances superior to CT scanning, most institutions have adopted it as their primary imaging modality of choice for malignant renal masses.

Renal Transplantation

The evaluation of a potential living renal transplant donor is extensive and is designed to identify candidates with normal renal anatomy and function. Traditionally, this was accomplished by using multiple imaging modalities, including various combinations of ultrasonography, CT scanning, renal scintigraphy, and renal angiography [45]. Recently, MRI has been shown to serve as a cost-effective single study alternative to comprehensively assess the renal function and vessel morphology of potential living kidney donors [46].

MRI with or without gadolinium is an accurate method to assess for posttransplant renal failure and urologic complications following renal transplantation, but gadolinium is no longer administered as frequently due to concerns related to nephrogenic systemic fibrosis (NSF, see below) [47]. A recent study comparing *T2-weighted* and contrast-enhanced sequences for the evaluation of posttransplant renal failure has shown *T*2-weighted images without contrast to be as accurate (sensitivity 76 % and specificity 74 %) as contrast-enhanced MRU (sensitivity 86 % and specificity 83 %) while avoiding potential gadolinium-related toxicity [48].

Complex Fetal GU Anomalies

The recent interest in fetal MRI was sparked in 1994 when a 3-year follow-up study failed to show any harmful side effects in children imaged in utero, including hearing deficits [49]. It is important to note that gadolinium crosses the placenta and is not recommended in pregnant women. Rather, *T2-weighted* sequences and diffusion-weighted images are used to delineate dilated urinary tracts, characterize the renal parenchyma, and may predict renal function.

Fetal MRI is an accurate means of evaluating complex fetal urinary tract anomalies detected by prenatal ultrasound (Fig. 4.18). Kajbafzadeh et al. compared fetal MRI and prenatal ultrasonography with postnatal autopsy and surgical pathology results. This study found that fetal MRI was significantly more sensitive than ultrasound in the detection of fetal uropathies, 96 % vs. 58 %, respectively, and provided additional information in 33 % of cases [50]. MRI during pregnancy may characterize the cause of oligohydramnios in fetuses with genitourinary and/or pelvic and perineal pathology. Notably, information gained from fetal MRI in one study lead to a change in therapeutic approach in 33 % of newborns [51].

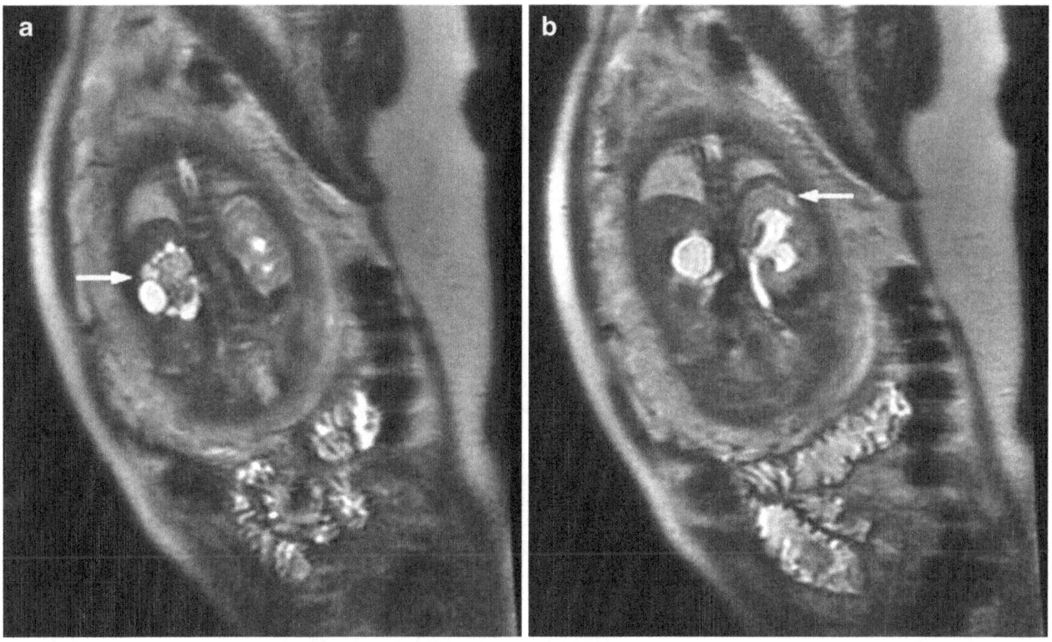

Fig. 4.18 A 25-year-old G5P2 carrying singleton fetus at 32 weeks' gestation with (**a**) left multicystic dysplastic kidney (*arrow*) and (**b**) right hydronephrosis with proximal ureteral dilation and small subcortical cysts (*arrow*) not seen on ultrasound consistent with obstructive nephropathy

Ambiguous Genitalia and Disorders of Sexual Development

Disorders of sexual development (DSD) include a spectrum of congenital anomalies in which the chromosomal sex differs from the phenotypic sex or when the phenotypic sex is ambiguous and not classifiable. Establishing a precise diagnosis in DSD is critically important since ambiguity often represents a social, psychological, and sometimes medical emergency, in the newborn. DSD can be subcategorized into four main groups which include disorders of gonadal differentiation, masculinized female (46, XX – *female pseudohermaphrodism often represented by congenital adrenal hyperplasia*), undermasculinized male (46, XY – *male pseudohermaphrodism, testicular feminization*), and ovotesticular syndrome (*true hermaphroditism*) [52]. Many of these children require abdominopelvic evaluation to identify the internal reproductive anatomy and gauge the functional potential of the genitalia and reproductive tract. Anatomic depiction of the internal genitalia is essential not only for gender assignment but, moreover, for planning surgical reconstructive procedures.

Ultrasound is typically the first radiologic examination obtained because is it a noninvasive, rapid way to detect the presence and location of the gonads and ductal structures. MRI can be used to identify and clarify abdominopelvic genital anatomy when ultrasonography is indeterminate (Fig. 4.19). MRI has been shown to accurately identify the uterus in 93 %, the vagina in 95 %, the penis in 100 %, the testis in 88 %, and the ovary in 74 %. MRI can also differentiate between a penis and a hypertrophied clitoris when the supporting penile structures are depicted, which include the bulbospongiosus muscle and posteriorly located transversus perinea muscle [53].

Rarely, MRI may be used to detect a potential undescended or abdominal testes. Ectopic gonads, testes, and immature ovaries are readily seen on MRI because they have an intermediate signal intensity on T_1-weighted sequences and a high signal intensity with an intermediate signal intensity surrounding the rim on T_2-weighted images [54].

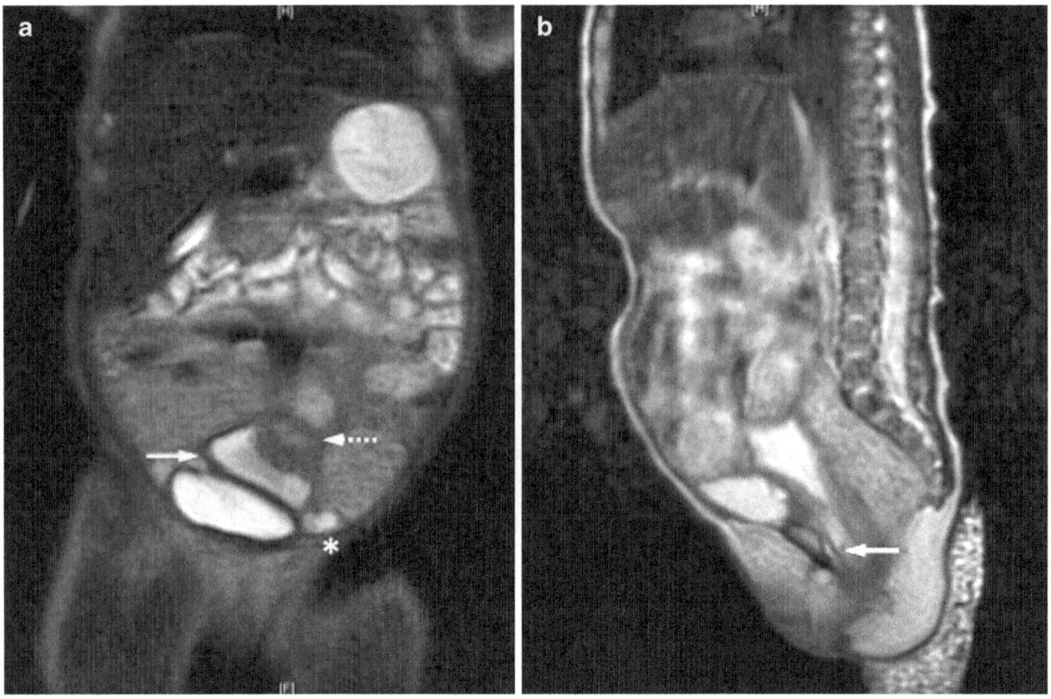

Fig. 4.19 T_2-weighted images of 12-month-old girl with ambiguous genitalia demonstrating (**a**) bifid bladder with common septum (*solid arrow*), uterus (*dotted arrow*), and ovary (*asterisk*). (**b**) Urogenital sinus with low urethral confluence (*arrow*)

When normal sized, these are bright and easily detected on MRI, and when absent, associated atrophic vessels may be seen (Fig. 4.20).

Clinical Contraindications and Limitations (Table 4.3)

End-Stage Renal Disease (Dialysis Dependent)

Gadolinium-enhanced MRI is specifically contraindicated in dialysis-dependent patients and those with renal failure (GFR <30 ml/kg/m^2) in association with inflammatory conditions (i.e., infection, surgery) because of the potential for NSF [55]. When gadolinium is contraindicated, T_2-weighted sequences can be used to assess the urinary tract.

Adverse Gadolinium Reactions

A previous history of allergic or anaphylactic reaction to gadolinium is an absolute contraindication for the use of gadolinium-based contrast agents (GBCA) during MRI. GBCAs are generally well tolerated in the pediatric population and rarely reported to cause adverse events. Most side effects are mild, such as headaches, nausea, and taste perversion. Mild reactions have been reported in up to 8 % of patients, and allergic reactions occur between 0.04 and 0.4 % of the time following gadolinium exposure [56]. Known allergy to iodine-based contrast agents does not preclude the use of GBCA.

Nephrogenic systemic fibrosis (NSF) is a rare condition involving fibrotic lesions of the skin and internal organs that has been associated with gadolinium exposure when administered with severe renal insufficiency [57]. There have been nine reported cases of NSF in the pediatric population that were linked to GBCA exposure [58, 59]. The incidence of NSF in the general population is less than 0.1 % but can occur in up to 3 % of patients with specific risk factors, including renal failure (acute or chronic), the use of certain forms of GBCA (i.e., gadodiamide), or exposure to high

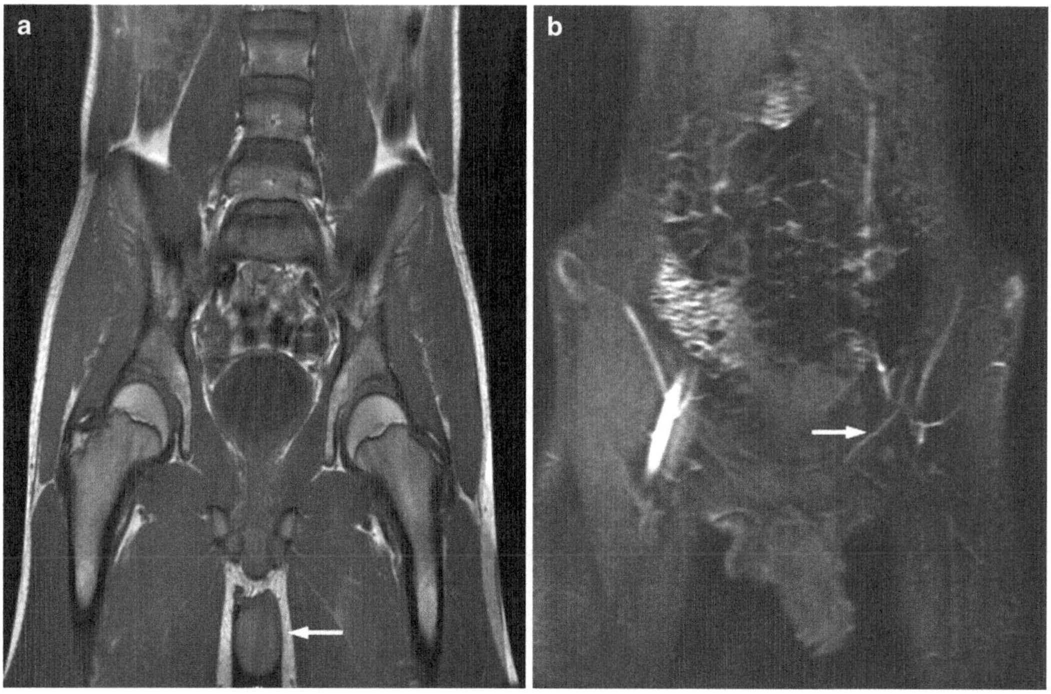

Fig. 4.20 A 13-year-old boy with solitary left testes and non-palpable right testes absent from birth. (**a**) T_1-weighted image demonstrating high signal intensity in solitary left testes locate in scrotum (*arrow*) and (**b**) T_2-weighted angiogram with well-developed gonadal vessels in left inguinal canal (*arrow*) and absence of gonadal vessels on the right

Table 4.3 Possible limitations and contraindications to MRI in pediatric urology

Absolute contraindications
- End-stage renal disease (dialysis dependent)
- Previous adverse gadolinium reactions
- Metallic foreign body
Relative contraindications
- Implantable medical device
- Renal failure (acute or chronic)
- Nephrolithiasis

doses of GBCA [60]. With the adoption of restrictive usage policies for gadolinium in the USA, the incidence of NSF has significantly decreased [55].

Metallic Foreign Bodies

MRI-induced heating is a recognized risk for implanted metallic devices as the radiofrequency field energy generated during MRI can be coupled into conducting metal (especially ferrous containing) and can cause severe device malfunction, injury, and imaging artifact in patients with pacemakers or orthopedic implants. Artificial urethral sphincters and titanium, cobalt-chromium, copper-based rods, surgical clips, and staples are usually compatible with MRI [61]. Some devices, such as ventriculoperitoneal shunts and drug delivery systems, are also compatible with MRI but may require reprogramming after exposure to the magnetic field [62].

References

1. Preston DL, Cullings H, Suyama A, Funamoto S, Nishi N, Soda M, et al. Solid cancer incidence in atomic bomb survivors exposed in utero or as young children. J Natl Cancer Inst. 2008;100(6):428–36.
2. Preston DL, Shimizu Y, Pierce DA, Suyama A, Mabuchi K. Studies of mortality of atomic bomb survivors. Report 13: solid cancer and noncancer disease mortality: 1950–1997. Radiat Res. 2003;160(4): 381–407.
3. Slichter CP. Principles of magnetic resonance. 3rd enl. and updated ed. Berlin/New York: Springer; 1990.
4. Nishimura DG. Principles of magnetic resonance imaging. San Francisco: Stanford University Press; 2010.

5. Lauterbur PC. Image formation by induced local interactions. Examples employing nuclear magnetic resonance. Clin Orthop Relat Res. 1973;244:3–6.
6. Friedburg HGWB, Hennig J, Frankenschmidt A, Hauenstein KH. Initial clinical experiences with RARE-MR urography. Urologe A. 1987;26:309–16.
7. Sigmund G, Stoever B, Zimmerhackl LB, Frankenschmidt A, Nitzsche E, Leititis JU, et al. RARE-MR-urography in the diagnosis of upper urinary tract abnormalities in children. Pediatr Radiol. 1991;21(6):416–20.
8. Aerts P, VanHoe L, Bosmans H, Oyen R, Marchal G, Baert AL. Breath-hold MR urography using the HASTE technique. Am J Roentgenol. 1996; 166(3):543–5.
9. Tang Y, Yamashita Y, Namimoto T, Abe Y, Nishiharu T, Sumi S, et al. The value of MR urography that uses HASTE sequences to reveal urinary tract disorders. Am J Roentgenol. 1996;167(6):1497–502.
10. O'Malley ME, Soto JA, Yucel EK, Hussain S. MR urography: evaluation of a three-dimensional fast spin-echo technique in patients with hydronephrosis. Am J Roentgenol. 1997;168(2):387–92.
11. Ergen FB, Hussain HK, Carlos RC, Johnson TD, Adusumilli S, Weadock WJ, et al. 3D Excretory MR urography: improved image quality with intravenous saline and diuretic administration. J Magn Reson Imaging. 2007;25(4):783–9.
12. Karabacakoglu A, Karakose S, Ince O, Cobankara OE, Karalezli G. Diagnostic value of diuretic-enhanced excretory MR urography in patients with obstructive uropathy. Eur J Radiol. 2004;52(3):320–7.
13. Nolte-Ernsting CCA, Bucker A, Adam GB, Neuerburg JM, Jung P, Hunter DW, et al. Gadolinium-enhanced excretory MR urography after low-dose diuretic injection: comparison with conventional excretory urography. Radiology. 1998;209(1):147–57.
14. Sudah M, Vanninen R, Partanen K, Heino A, Vainio P, Ala-Opas M. MR urography in evaluation of acute flank pain: T2-weighted sequences and gadolinium-enhanced three-dimensional FLASH compared with urography. Am J Roentgenol. 2001;176(1):105–12.
15. Rusinek H, Lee VS, Johnson G. Optimal dose of Gd-DTPA in dynamic MR studies. Magn Reson Med. 2001;46(2):312–16.
16. Jones TD, Kernek KM, Yang XJ, Lopez-Beltran A, MacLennan GT, Eble JN, et al. Thyroid transcription factor 1 expression in small cell carcinoma of the urinary bladder: an immunohistochemical profile of 44 cases. Hum Pathol. 2005;36(7):718–23.
17. Hackstein N, Heckrodt J, Rau WS. Measurement of single-kidney glomerular filtration rate using a contrast-enhanced dynamic gradient-echo sequence and the Rutland-Patlak plot technique. J Magn Reson Imaging. 2003;18(6):714–25.
18. Jones RA, Easley K, Little SB, Scherz H, Kirsch AJ, Grattan-Smith JD. Dynamic contrast-enhanced MR urography in the evaluation of pediatric hydronephrosis: part I, functional assessment. Am J Roentgenol. 2005;185(6):1598–607.
19. Bokacheva L, Rusinek H, Zhang JL, Lee VS. Assessment of renal function with dynamic contrast-enhanced MR imaging. Magn Reson Imaging Clin N Am. 2008;16(4):597–611.
20. Lee VS, Rusinek H, Bokacheva L, Huang AJ, Oesingmann N, Chen Q, et al. Renal function measurements from MR renography and a simplified multicompartmental model. Am J Physiol Renal Physiol. 2007;292(5):F1548–59.
21. Annet L, Hermoye L, Peeters F, Jamar F, Dehoux JP, Van Beers BE. Glomerular filtration rate: assessment with dynamic contrast-enhanced MRI and a cortical-compartment model in the rabbit kidney. J Magn Reson Imaging. 2004;20(5):843–9.
22. Buckley DL, Shurrab AE, Cheung CM, Jones AP, Mamtora H, Kalra PA. Measurement of single kidney function using dynamic contrast-enhanced MRI: comparison of two models in human subjects. J Magn Reson Imaging. 2006;24(5):1117–23.
23. Michaely HJ, Sourbron SP, Buettner C, Lodemann KP, Reiser MF, Schoenberg SO. Temporal constraints in renal perfusion imaging with a 2-compartment model. Invest Radiol. 2008;43(2):120–8.
24. Dietrich RB, Kangarloo H. Kidneys in infants and children – evaluation with MR. Radiology. 1986; 159(1):215–21.
25. Grattan-Smith JD, Jones RA. MR urography in children. Pediatr Radiol. 2006;36(11):1119–32; quiz 228–9.
26. Kass EJ, Majd M, Belman AB. Comparison of the diuretic renogram and the pressure perfusion study in children. J Urol. 1985;134(1):92–6.
27. Little SB, Jones RA, Grattan-Smith JD. Evaluation of UPJ obstruction before and after pyeloplasty using MR urography. Pediatr Radiol. 2008;38:S106–24.
28. Chertin B, Pollack A, Koulikov D, Rabinowitz R, Shen O, Hain D, et al. Long-term follow up of antenatally diagnosed megaureters. J Pediatr Urol. 2008;4(3):188–91.
29. Wildbrett P, Langner S, Lode H, Abel J, Otto S, Hosten N, et al. Impact of magnetic resonance urography and ultrasonography on diagnosis and management of hydronephrosis and megaureter in paediatric patients. Afr J Paediatr Surg. 2012;9(2):122–7.
30. Staatz G, Nolte-Ernsting CC, Haage P, Tacke J, Rohrmann D, Stollbrink C, et al. [Gadolinium-enhanced T(1)-weighted MR urography versus T(2)-weighted (HASTE) MR urography in children]. Rofo. 2001;173(11):991–6.
31. Lonergan GJ, Pennington DJ, Morrison JC, Haws RM, Grimley MS, Kao TC. Childhood pyelonephritis: comparison of gadolinium-enhanced MR imaging and renal cortical scintigraphy for diagnosis. Radiology. 1998;207(2):377–84.
32. Weiser AC, Amukele SA, Leonidas JC, Palmer LS. The role of gadolinium enhanced magnetic resonance imaging for children with suspected acute pyelonephritis. J Urol. 2003;169(6):2308–11.
33. Chan YL, Chan KW, Yeung CK, Roebuck DJ, Chu WCW, Lee KH, et al. Potential utility of MRI in the evaluation of children at risk of renal scarring. Pediatr Radiol. 1999;29(11):856–62.

34. Grattan-Smith JD, Little SB, Jones RA. Evaluation of reflux nephropathy, pyelonephritis and renal dysplasia. Pediatr Radiol. 2008;38 Suppl 1:S83–105.
35. Herz D, Merguerian P, McQuiston L, Danielson C, Gheen M, Brenfleck L. 5-year prospective results of dimercapto-succinic acid imaging in children with febrile urinary tract infection: proof that the top-down approach works. J Urol. 2010;184(4 Suppl):1703–9.
36. Leibovic SJ, Lebowitz RL. Reducing patient dose in voiding cystourethrography. Urol Radiol. 1981;2(2):103–7.
37. Rodriguez LV, Spielman D, Herfkens RJ, Shortliffe LD. Magnetic resonance imaging for the evaluation of hydronephrosis, reflux and renal scarring in children. J Urol. 2001;166(3):1023–7.
38. Lee SK, Chang Y, Park NH, Kim YH, Woo S. Magnetic resonance voiding cystography in the diagnosis of vesicoureteral reflux: comparative study with voiding cystourethrography. J Magn Reson Imaging. 2005;21(4):406–14.
39. Chang SL, Caruso TJ, Shortliffe LD. Magnetic resonance imaging detected renal volume reduction in refluxing and nonrefluxing kidneys. J Urol. 2007;178(6):2550–4.
40. Pearce MS, Salotti JA, Little MP, McHugh K, Lee C, Kim KP, et al. Radiation exposure from CT scans in childhood and subsequent risk of leukaemia and brain tumours: a retrospective cohort study. Lancet. 2012;380(9840):499–505.
41. Belt TG, Cohen MD, Smith JA, Cory DA, McKenna S, Weetman R. MRI of Wilms' tumor: promise as the primary imaging method. AJR Am J Roentgenol. 1986;146(5):955–61.
42. Siegel MJ, Chung EM. Wilms' tumor and other pediatric renal masses. Magn Reson Imaging Clin N Am. 2008;16(3):479–97, vi.
43. Weese DL, Applebaum H, Taber P. Mapping intravascular extension of Wilms' tumor with magnetic resonance imaging. J Pediatr Surg. 1991;26(1):64–7.
44. Ritchey ML, Green DM, Breslow NB, Moksness J, Norkool P. Accuracy of current imaging modalities in the diagnosis of synchronous bilateral Wilms' tumor. A report from the National Wilms Tumor Study Group. Cancer Am Cancer Soc. 1995;75(2):600–4.
45. Mandelbrot DA, Pavlakis M, Danovitch GM, Johnson SR, Karp SJ, Khwaja K, et al. The medical evaluation of living kidney donors: a survey of US transplant centers. Am J Transplant. 2007;7(10):2333–43.
46. Rossi C, Boss A, Artunc F, Yildiz S, Martirosian P, Dittmann H, et al. Comprehensive assessment of renal function and vessel morphology in potential living kidney donors an MRI-based approach. Invest Radiol. 2009;44(11):705–11.
47. Cohnen M, Brause M, May P, Hetzel G, Saleh A, Grabensee B, et al. Contrast-enhanced MR urography in the evaluation of renal transplants with urological complications. Clin Nephrol. 2002;58(2):111–17.
48. Blondin D, Lanzman RS, Mathys C, Grotemeyer D, Voiculescu A, Sandmann W, et al. Functional MRI of transplanted kidneys using diffusion-weighted imaging. Rofo-Fortschr Rontg. 2009;181(12):1162–7.
49. Baker PN, Johnson IR, Harvey PR, Gowland PA, Mansfield P. A three-year follow-up of children imaged in utero with echo-planar magnetic resonance. Am J Obstet Gynecol. 1994;170(1 Pt 1):32–3.
50. Kajbafzadeh AM, Payabvash S, Sadeghi Z, Elmi A, Jamal A, Hantoshzadeh Z, et al. Comparison of magnetic resonance urography with ultrasound studies in detection of fetal urogenital anomalies. J Pediatr Urol. 2008;4(1):32–9.
51. Alamo L, Laswad T, Schnyder P, Meuli R, Vial Y, Osterheld MC, et al. Fetal MRI as complement to US in the diagnosis and characterization of anomalies of the genito-urinary tract. Eur J Radiol. 2010;76(2):258–64.
52. Wein AJ, Kavoussi LR, Campbell MF. Campbell-Walsh urology, editor-in-chief, Alan J. Wein; editors, Louis R. Kavoussi ... et al.. 10th ed. Philadelphia: Elsevier Saunders; 2012.
53. Secaf E, Hricak H, Gooding CA, Ho VW, Gorczyca DP, Ringertz H, et al. Role of MRI in the evaluation of ambiguous genitalia. Pediatr Radiol. 1994;24(4):231–5.
54. Gambino J, Caldwell B, Dietrich R, Walot I, Kangarloo H. Congenital disorders of sexual differentiation: MR findings. AJR Am J Roentgenol. 1992;158(2):363–7.
55. Altun E, Martin DR, Wertman R, Lugo-Somolinos A, Fuller 3rd ER, Semelka RC. Nephrogenic systemic fibrosis: change in incidence following a switch in gadolinium agents and adoption of a gadolinium policy–report from two U.S. universities. Radiology. 2009;253(3):689–96.
56. Hunt CH, Hartman RP, Hesley GK. Frequency and severity of adverse effects of iodinated and gadolinium contrast materials: retrospective review of 456,930 doses. AJR Am J Roentgenol. 2009;193(4):1124–7.
57. Altun E, Semelka RC, Cakit C. Nephrogenic systemic fibrosis and management of high-risk patients. Acad Radiol. 2009;16(7):897–905.
58. Cowper SE, Boyer PJ. Nephrogenic systemic fibrosis: an update. Curr Rheumatol Rep. 2006;8(2):151–7.
59. Grobner T. Gadolinium – a specific trigger for the development of nephrogenic fibrosing dermopathy and nephrogenic systemic fibrosis? Nephrol Dial Transplant. 2006;21(4):1104–8.
60. Abujudeh HH, Kaewlai R, Kagan A, Chibnik LB, Nazarian RM, High WA, Kay J. Nephrogenic systemic fibrosis after gadopentetate dimeglumine exposure: case series of 36 patients. Radiology. 2009;253(1):81–9.
61. Cerwinka WH, Kirsch AJ. Magnetic resonance urography in pediatric urology. Curr Opin Urol. 2010;20(4):323–9.
62. Lavinio A, Harding S, Van Der Boogaard F, Czosnyka M, Smielewski P, Richards HK, et al. Magnetic field interactions in adjustable hydrocephalus shunts. J Neurosurg Pediatr. 2008;2(3):222–8.

5 Principles of Voiding Cystourethrography (VCUG)

Jimena Cubillos and Nina Klionsky

Introduction

The voiding cystourethrogram (VCUG) is one of the most commonly performed studies in pediatrics. A VCUG is a fluoroscopic study that can assess the structure and function of the bladder and the structure of the urethra. It is frequently used in the evaluation of children with urinary tract infections to determine the presence of vesicoureteral reflux (VUR), bladder diverticula, complete bladder emptying, and to assess for possible bladder sphincter discoordination. VCUG is also performed in the evaluation of hydronephrosis, congenital renal anomalies, imperforate anus, cloacal abnormalities, disorders of sexual differentiation, trauma, and screening siblings for VUR. In addition, it provides information regarding the urethra and is used in diagnosing posterior urethral valves, urethral strictures, or suspicion of a duplicated urethra or other anomalies.

Vesicoureteral reflux (VUR) may lead to renal scarring. Neonates and infants are most susceptible, as the greatest risk of renal damage is during the first 2 years of life [1]. Reflux is the most common cause of antenatally detected hydronephrosis, accounting for up to 40 % of cases [2] and also is present in 30–50 % of children who present with a febrile UTI [3].

The study is performed in a fluoroscopic suite. The urinary bladder is catheterized and emptied. It is then filled with radiopaque contrast by gravity drip. At a minimum, images should include an early filling image, bilateral oblique images of the ureterovesical junction (UVJ) when the bladder is full, voiding images of the urethra, and post-void images of the kidneys and bladder. Depending on the child, the study can be performed with or without sedation. Careful technique is required to provide adequate images without exposing the child to unnecessary radiation.

Physics

The fluoroscopic equipment has several components: the x-ray generator, x-ray tube, collimator, filtration, grid, image intensifier, optical coupling, video camera, and the monitor as demonstrated in Fig. 5.1.

The x-ray generator allows for the selection of kilovolt peak (kVp) and tube current (mA) that is

J. Cubillos, MD (✉)
Division of Pediatric Urology, Department of Urology, University of Rochester School of Medicine and Dentistry/Strong Memorial Hospital/Golisano Children's Hospital, 601 Elmwood Ave., 656, Rochester, NY 14642, USA
e-mail: jimena_cubillos@urmc.rochester.edu

N. Klionsky, MD
Department of Imaging Sciences, Pediatric Imaging, University of Rochester School of Medicine and Dentistry/Strong Memorial Hospital/Golisano Children's Hospital, 601 Elmwood Ave., 648, Rochester, NY 14642, USA
e-mail: nina_klionsky@urmc.rochester.edu

L.S. Palmer, J.S. Palmer (eds.), *Pediatric and Adolescent Urologic Imaging*,
DOI 10.1007/978-1-4614-8654-1_5, © Springer Science+Business Media New York 2014

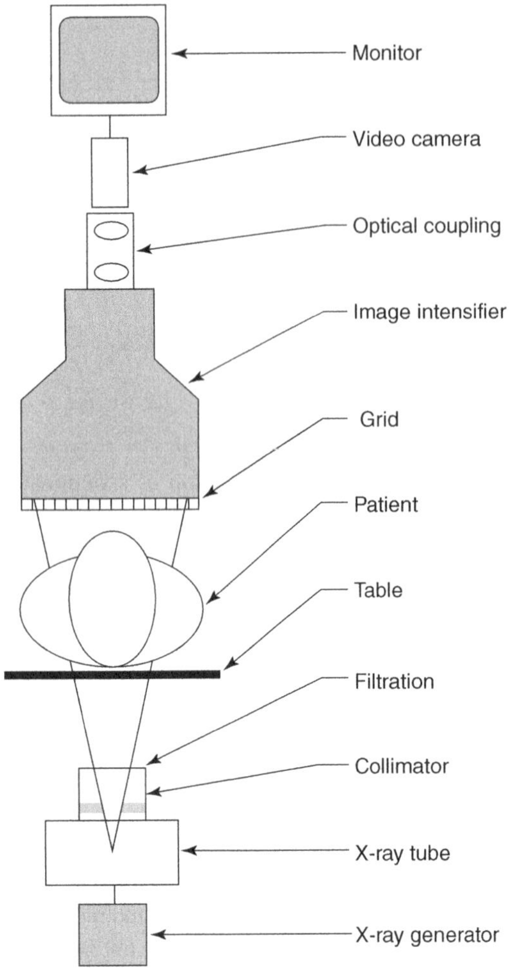

Fig. 5.1 Diagram shows the components of a fluoroscopic imaging chain [4] (Reprinted from Schueler [4]. With permission from Radiological Society of North America)

delivered to the x-ray tube. Generator types may be single phase, three phase, constant potential, and high frequency. Continuous or pulsed exposure is used to energize the tube. The main advantage of pulsed exposure is reduction in radiation exposure. There may be improvement in temporal resolution and decreased motion artifact. High-frequency generators provide superior exposure reproducibility and are the most compact and the cheapest, making them the most commonly used equipment [4].

The x-ray tube converts electrical energy produced by the generator into an x-ray beam.

The collimator defines the shape of the x-ray beam and limits the x-ray beam to the field of vision. The x-ray beam should be collimated to the area of interest to decrease the radiation to the tissue, therefore reducing the scatter produced and improving image contrast. When using collimation, it is important that the electronic collimation matches the manual collimation. Electronic collimation can mask critical information included on the image and cover up anatomy that is exposed [5].

Filters are used to attenuate low energy x-rays from the beam, which are absorbed by the patient but not transmitted to the image receptor. By absorbing these rays, filters aid in decreasing exposure to the patient.

Anti-scatter grids reduce the scattered x-rays reaching the image receptor, thereby improving the image contrast. However, this requires an increase in radiation exposure. Grids should be removed when performing studies where the scatter is low, particularly in pediatrics.

The image intensifier converts x-rays into a visible light image and amplifies the image brightness for better visibility [4]. Optical coupling distributes light from the image intensifier output window to a video camera and other image recording devices. A television system is used to view the image and a recording device stores the images.

Radiation Exposure and Radiation Safety

When using radiation, the ALARA principle, or *a*s *l*ow *a*s *r*easonably *a*chievable, should be implemented. This term was first used to refer to power plant and other radiation workers and has subsequently been applied to the medical imaging. Decreasing radiation exposure is especially important when children are involved as the radiation effects are cumulative, lifelong, and children are more sensitive to the effects of radiation. The linear no-threshold model of potential radiation damage means that any dose of radiation may cause some harm. Potential clinical effects of radiation exposure, in

Table 5.1 Potential clinical effects of radiation exposure

Skin effects	Threshold dose (Gy)	Time of onset
Early transient Erythema	2	2–24 h
Main erythema reaction	6	1.5 weeks
Temporary depilation	3	3 weeks
Permanent depilation	7	3 weeks
Dermal necrosis	>12	>52 weeks
Eye effects		
Lens opacity	>1–2	>5 years
Cataract	>5	>5 years

Reproduced from Connolly [6]. With kind permission from Springer Science and Business Media

addition to those of malignancies, are listed on Table 5.1.

When considering the use of radiation, first one should ask if there is a non-radiation alternative that can provide the information desired, such as ultrasound. For many of the indications for obtaining a VCUG, the answer is no. Next, one should focus on decreasing the amount of radiation exposure to the patient. This is where the ALARA principle is applied.

Three factors affect the radiation dose to health care workers as well as to the patient for any radiographic procedure: time, distance, and shielding.

Time refers to the duration the patient is under exposure. Radiation exposure is directly proportional to the duration of fluoroscopic time so one should be mindful of the amount of time exposures are collected. Having protocols in place for the timing and number of images obtained during a VCUG can decrease the amount of radiation administered. For example, for a routine VCUG, there is little value in obtaining images over the ureters during filling or voiding unless an abnormality is seen. Time is decreased by having experienced personnel perform the procedure and teach those who are learning. The use of stopwatches, alarm bells, or radio communication letting the operator know how long the machine has been used for can decrease the exposure time [6, 7]. Pulsed fluoroscopy reduces radiation exposure by decreasing the amount of time the beam reaches the patient compared with continuous fluoroscopy.

Distance refers to separation of the subject from the radiation source. Increasing distance decreases the radiation dose in an inversely proportional fashion. The radiographic exam table should be as far from the radiation source as possible, although this is a fixed distance in fluoroscopy. The patient should be as close as possible to the image intensifier to reduce the scatter, although this may need to be modified due to patient fright and inability to cooperate. A less cooperative patient can lead to increased exam and exposure time due to motion artifact, causing the need to repeat images.

Shielding not only benefits the patient but also reduces the intensity of the radiation reaching the worker [7]. Shielding refers to limiting the direction of the radiation source in the housing and to collimating the beam size to minimize the x-ray exposure and scatter; it may include using lead pads to protect parts of the patient not involved in the examination and includes leaded rooms and aprons to protect workers in and outside of the fluoroscopy room.

As mentioned previously, the use of grids should only be used when the body part thickness indicates their use (when body part thickness is more than 12 cm) and should be removed when not indicated [8], which is common in pediatrics.

A combination of features can markedly reduce the radiation exposure. By using low-frequency pulsed fluoroscopy, tight collimation, no magnification, and half-dose parameters, the reduction in effective dose can be as high as 90 % without sacrificing resolution [3, 6, 9]. Using high-quality image-capture technology can also reduce radiation dose [9, 10]. Modern techniques have decreased the radiation dose of fluoroscopic VCUGs from 100 times to 10 times the radiation dose compared to radionucleotide cystograms [3], although the radiation dose may vary with fluoroscopic VCUGs pending the number of images obtained.

Digital Fluoroscopy

As technology continues to advance, digital fluoroscopy is becoming the mainstay. Digital radiology uses x-ray sensors bonded onto thin-film transistor integrated circuits to instantaneously convert the image stored on the sensor to a visible digital image [11]. This can be either through direct detection, converting the x-rays into an electronic charge, or indirect, by converting the x-rays into light and then converting the light into an electronic charge. In film, optical density on the film is used as an exposure indication. With digital images, overexposed images are not as easily identified as underexposed images, resulting in unknowingly increased radiation exposure [8]. Underexposed images are easily identified by increased noise. However, overexposed images are sharp, and exposure cannot be assessed visually. Up to 43 % of pediatric digital images are overexposed [11]. Feedback on the exposure is provided by the exposure indicator at the image receptor. It is influenced by the part thickness, artifacts, source-to-image distance, collimation, grids, centering, image plate size, and equipment and detector design [8]. There is a tendency towards exposure creep, the gradual increase in the technician's selected exposure to obtain better quality images, as technicians need to repeat underexposed images [8]. In some areas, there is a trend towards exposure slide, where the radiologist accepts a nosier image until the image cannot be interpreted and needs to be repeated [5]. As a result, periodic checks by tracking exposure index and deviation index should be performed on a regular basis to assess for appropriate exposure.

Other challenges in digital imaging include the lack of standardization among vendors, lack of pediatric specific educational material and techniques, inability to use automatic exposure control in smaller children, and limitations of collimation and shielding of unnecessary body parts in smaller children [5]. Vendors of different machines have different exposure indicators; they have variable nomenclature and nonstandard units for reference values. In addition to the values being different, they may also be in inverse order so that the values may increase for overexposure for one manufactured and decrease for another [5]. Lastly, values provided may be inaccurate or uninterpretable in small children as indicated in Table 5.2. Technicians may be working with various types of machines in a given work day, making it more difficult to determine the amount of radiation being provided. These challenges are depicted on Table 5.3.

Table 5.2 Technical factors that can affect the exposure indicator (EI)

Technical factors
Size of detector/image receptor matched to patient size
Collimation and field size in relation to patient's body parts
Metal implants in patients (scoliosis rods, metal plates, screws, pacemakers)
Gonadal shield

Reproduced from Goske [5]. With kind permission from Springer Science and Business Media

Despite these challenges, there are many advantages to digital radiography. The last image taken can be saved without having additional radiation exposure [3], post processing allows the radiologist to analyze various anatomical sites without needing additional images, the images can be stored and retrieved without losing image quality, and they can be accessed by various providers throughout a network.

Technical Considerations

Timing of VCUG

VCUGs needed for evaluation of a congenital anomaly can be obtained at any time. When a VCUG is necessitated following a urinary tract infection, previous recommendations were to delay the study by several weeks to allow the inflammatory process to resolve, as this may lead to detection of transient reflux secondary to ureteral dilation and inflammatory changes at the UVJ if performed too early [13, 14]. In addition, there also were concerns that if a VCUG is performed during an active infection, it may prolong the UTI or lead to bacterial dissemination and possibly sepsis [15]. Spencer [15] performed

Table 5.3 Suggested guidelines for QC action based on estimated incident exposure (conventional CR system for an "equivalent" speed class = 200)

Fuji (S No.)	Agfa (IgM)	Kodak(exposureindex)	Detector exposure estimate (mR)	Indication
>1,000	<1.45	<1,250	<0.20	Underexposed: repeat
1,000–601	1.45–1.74	1,250–1,549	0.2–0.3	Underexposed: QC exception
600–301	1.75–2.04	1,550–1,849	0.3–0.7	Underexposed: QC review
300–150	2.05–2.35	1,850–2,150	0.7–1.3	Acceptable range
149–75	2.36–2.65	2,151–2,450	1.3–2.7	Overexposed: QC review
74–50	2.66–2.95	2,451–2,750	2.7–4.0	Overexposed: QC exception
<50	>2.95	>2,750	>4.0	Overexposed: repeat if necessary

Reprinted from Williams et al. [12]. With permission from Elsevier

Abbreviations: *IgM* log of median exposure, *QC* quality control, *S number* sensitivity number

a retrospective review of VCUGs obtained over a 5-year period in all children admitted with a febrile UTI. Children were divided into two cohorts: those with an early VCUG, performed within the week of diagnosis after appropriate antibiotics had been initiated (67 patients), and those with a late VCUG, performed more than 1 week after diagnosis (65). All patients were followed for a period of 5 years after discharge to assess for complications. The incidence and severity of VUR were similar in the two groups. The early group showed no sign of worsening illness after the test was performed and had similar ED and hospital admissions rate as the late group. One hundred percent of the patients in the early group had their VCUGs done vs. 77 % in the late group ($p = 0.005$). These findings suggest that VCUGs can be obtained safely after appropriate antibiotics have been instituted and that compliance rates are better when the test is performed early, especially if it performed during an acute hospitalization. This could also be beneficial for children with recurrent episodes of pyelonephritis, who may only reflux during an active infection.

Patient Preparation

VCUGs are considered to be one of the most stressful urologic studies performed for both patients and parents [9, 16] with up to 27 % of patients experiencing severe distress [17] and 71 % of children experiencing serious or severe distress or panic on the Groningen Distress Rating Scale [16]. Distress may be secondary to the catheterization, but also may be related to fear of the unknown. Unexpected stress is more anxiety provoking and more difficult to deal with than anticipated or predicted stress [9]. Srivastava et al. [18] found that parents anticipated their child would experience more fear than they observed ($p = 0.04$), tended to anticipate that their child would suffer more distress than observed ($p = 0.08$), and anticipated that their child would suffer far more distress after the VCUG than they observed ($p < 0.01$). There was a significant correlation between the parents' anxiety and their perception of the severity of their child's fear ($r = 0.52$, $p = 0.009$), distress ($r = 0.48$, $p = 0.017$), and pain ($r = 0.50$, $p = 0.01$) during the procedure.

Preparation of both the parent and the child via education can help decrease perceived anxiety and stress levels for the parents and the child [19, 20]. Education can be in the form of reading materials or videos. In some centers, children are given a tour and allowed to sit on the table while a doll is catheterized as the procedure is explained so they know what to expect and are given an opportunity to ask questions. After determining that VCUGs were one of the most stressful studies performed at their institution partly due to lack of information, Phillips et al. [16] sought to

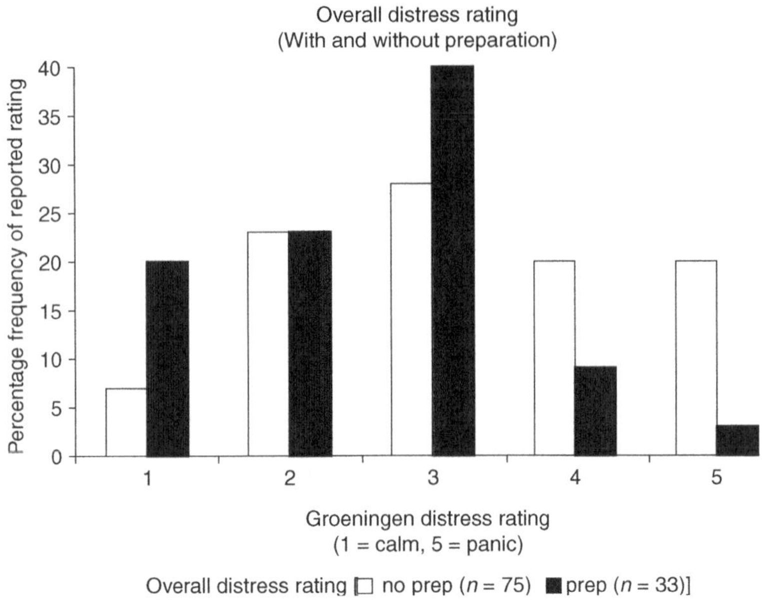

Fig. 5.2 Overall distress rating (with and without preparation) [16]. Legend: *White bar*, no prep ($n=75$); *black bar*, prep ($n=33$). Groningen Distress Rating Scale: *1*, calm; *2*, mild distress; *3*, serious distress; *4*, severe distress; *5*, panic (Reproduced from Phillips [16]. With kind permission from Wiley)

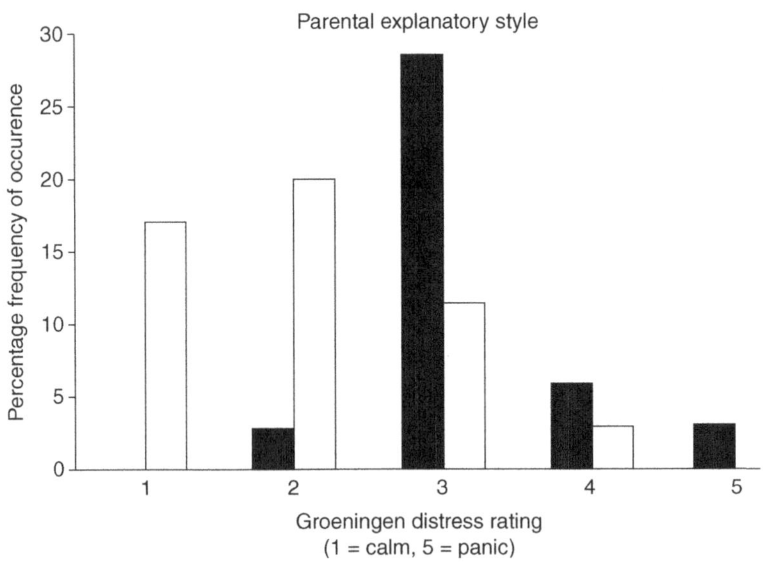

Fig. 5.3 Parental explanatory style [16]. Legend: *Black bar*, avoid/omit; *white bar*, describe in full. GDRS = *1*, calm; *2*, mild distress; *3*, serious distress; *4*, severe distress; *5*, panic (Reproduced from [16]. With kind permission from Wiley)

determine if better patient preparation would alleviate parental and patient distress. They had two intervention groups and compared their distress level to their historic controls. One intervention group was given a story book describing the procedure and expectations, while the second group was given the book as well as play therapy where they had the procedure explained with the aid of a gender appropriate doll. The child's distress was significantly reduced with preparation ($p=0.0026$) with a median distress score on the Groningen Distress Rating Scale of 2.5 in the preparation group vs. 3.3 in the controls (Fig. 5.2). Among the preparation group, children had lower distress scores when parents provided full disclosure compared to those where parents avoided or omitted upsetting details ($p=0.0025$) (Fig. 5.3). Between the two preparation groups, there was no difference in distress scores with the addition of play therapy.

During the procedure, a calm parent should be allowed to accompany the child as this decreases patient distress [16]. Parents can help their child by providing support and distracting them with toys, videos, balloons, etc. In addition, children depend on their parents to help them cope with stressful situations [16]. Children have been found to be more cooperative and calm with invasive procedures when supported by their parents and prompted to model coping behaviors [16]. The use of child life specialists when available is also recommended.

The Role of Sedation

Despite appropriate preparation, some patients may still exhibit high levels of distress when having a VCUG, particularly if they have had a previous negative experience such as prior catheterization or if there are other external circumstances. During these situations, sedation may be useful. There are several concerns regarding the use of sedation: cost, time, safety, and effects sedation can have on bladder dynamics. Herd found that the increased costs were related to the need for a recovery room and staff and that safety was excellent in the context of experienced staff with proper equipment and available emergency preparations [21]. In a randomized trial of sedation vs. placebo, sedation added approximately 60 min to the entire procedure, mostly as recovery time [22]. There was no significant difference in the filling or voiding phase, and there was no difference in the volume infused between the two groups [22]. VUR was identified in 16 % of children, without difference between the two groups ($p=0.31$).

Although the use of sedation increases the overall procedure time, sedation is useful in decreasing anxiety and distress among children older than 1 year and their parents. In a randomized double-blind controlled trial of oral midazolam 30 min prior to catheterization at a dose of 0.5 mg/kg vs. placebo, 61 % of children experienced serious or severe distress in the placebo vs. 16 % in the treatment group, with the NNT being 2.9 (Fig. 5.4) [22]. When the test was divided into parts (entering the room, catheterization, filling, voiding, and leaving the room), there were differences in distress detected at entering the room ($p=0.01$), filling ($p=0.0001$), and voiding ($p<0.0001$), and no difference detected at catheterization ($p=0.10$) and leaving the room ($p=0.18$) as depicted in Fig. 5.5. Both groups were provided educational pamphlets and offered play therapy prior to the procedure. In review of five comparative studies, the use of midazolam significantly lessened distress without affecting voiding dynamics or having adverse effects [21].

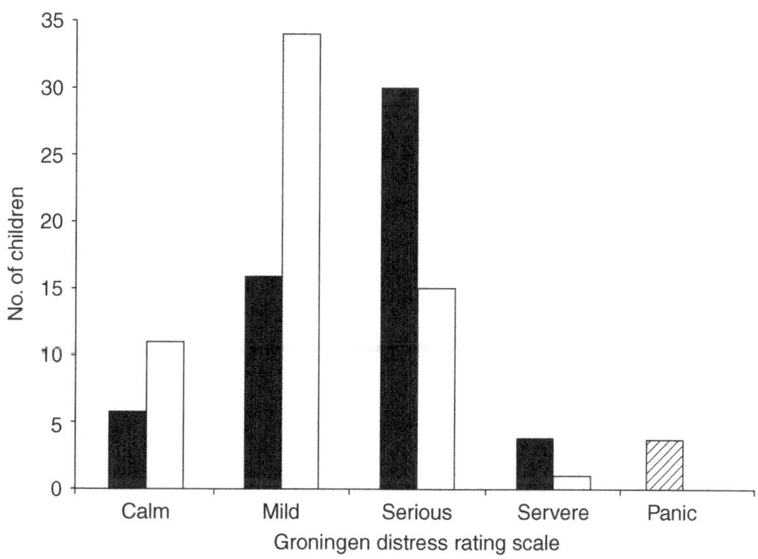

Fig. 5.4 Distress levels at any stage during voiding cystourethrography [22]. *Bar graph* shows peak distress score at any stage during voiding cystourethrography (VCU) ($n=117$). Fifty-six received placebo (*black bars*) and 61 received midazolam (*white bars*). *Striped box* represents four children – all of whom were in the placebo group – who failed to complete VCU due to panic (From Herd et al. [22]. Reprinted with permission from the American Journal of Roentgenology)

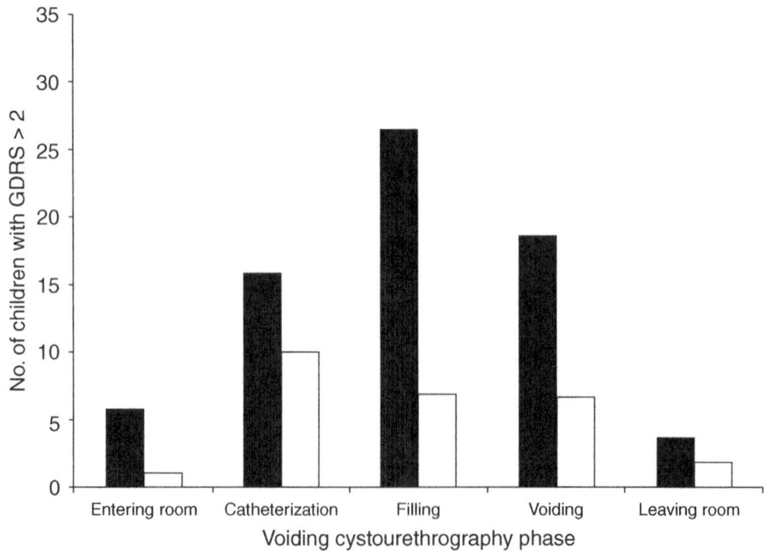

Fig. 5.5 Distress levels at different phases of a voiding cystourethrography [22] *Bar graph shows number of children (n = 117) who experienced serious or severe distress* (Groningen Distress Rating Scale [GDRS] score > 2) at each phase of voiding cystourethrography. Fifty-six received placebo (*black bars*) and 61 received midazolam (*white bars*) (From Herd et al. [22]. Reprinted with permission from the American Journal of Roentgenology)

Ferguson randomized children to midazolam 15 min prior to the procedure vs. placebo in a double-blind fashion and found no difference with the use of midazolam at decreasing anxiety in children or in their secondary outcomes of the degree of parental anxiety, health care professional perception, and post-procedure behavior outcomes [23]. It is possible that the differences may be secondary to a smaller sample size, decreased wait time to the procedure, or the use of different assessment tools.

The use of nitrous oxide and propofol has also been studied. In a retrospective study of the use of propofol, there was a decreased ability in children to completely void, which may interfere with the diagnosis of VUR [24]. Keidan et al. compared 50 % nitrous oxide in 23 children to 0.5 mg/kg oral midazolam in 24 children; there was no placebo group [21]. They did not find a significant difference in the two groups. There was a trend towards longer time to void in the nitrous group (15.3 min vs. 7.2 min), although this was not significant ($p = 0.8$), but those in the nitrous group had a faster recovery time (29 min vs. 63 min, $p < 0.001$). Zier used 70 % nitrous for catheterization only in 107 older children and compared this to 107 children without the use of sedation. FACES scale was 6 for the nonsedated group and 0 for the sedated group ($p < 0.001$) immediately after catheterization and the Brief Behavioral Distress Scores were 44 in the nonsedated group vs. 11 for the sedated group ($p < 0.001$) [21].

Overall, the use of sedation can help alleviate distress in older children and does not appear to affect bladder dynamics or detection of VUR. It is safe when used appropriately and with experienced staff in a setting where emergency protocols are set in place.

Catheterization

Catheterization of the urethra should be performed using strict aseptic technique. An 8 French feeding tube should be used instead of an indwelling catheter as having an inflated catheter balloon can be falsely mistaken for a ureterocele. For older children, a larger catheter can be used, and a smaller one for premature or very small infants. The catheter should be advanced no further than 1–2 cm after urine is obtained to prevent injury to the bladder or the formation of a knot in the tube. The catheter should be secured and a urine sample sent for aerobic culture and sensitivity, as up to 3 % can be positive for a urine infection [9]. Alternatively, a urine dip can be performed and cultures sent for those specimens that are positive for leukocytes and/or nitrites [9]. In uncircumcised newborns, the foreskin should not be forcefully retracted. It is imperative that the phallus not rest over a urinal, as this may cause external compression of the urethra giving a false impression of urethral obstruction. In boys, the external sphincter is the most common site of resistance. Applying gentle, steady posterior pressure can help advance the catheter into the bladder. Also, advancing the catheter when he takes a deep breath may facilitate placement. If he voids during catheter placement, maintain a hold of the catheter and continue to advance, since the urethra is open during voiding. In girls, good retractions of the labia with the aid of soft gauze can help visualize the meatus midline, just anterior to the vagina. Two percent lidocaine jelly can be used to decrease sensation in older children but needs to be placed several minutes prior to catheterization in order to take effect.

There is some debate as to whether the catheter should remain in or be removed during the voiding phase of the VCUG. The main concern about leaving the catheter in place is possibly missing posterior urethral valves (PUV). To address this question, Ditchfield et al. performed a retrospective study of the preoperative VCUGs performed in a consecutive series of 48 boys with cystoscopically proven PUV [25]. The VCUGs were independently reviewed by three radiologists. The catheter was left in place during voiding in 28 (58 %) and removed in 17 (35 %). Three patients (6 %) had the study performed with and then without a catheter. PUV were detected in 25 (89 %) of the 28 with a catheter and 15 (88 %) without the catheter. Five boys were found to have PUV on cystoscopy, but the VCUG did not have a dilated posterior urethra or "other evidence of obstruction." Of those 5 boys, 3 had the VCUG performed with a catheter, and 2 had it without a catheter. In the three boys that had the VCUG performed with and without the catheter, PUV were detected in both studies. Overall, there was no difference in the detection of PUV if voiding took place with or without a catheter as demonstrated on Table 5.4.

Table 5.4 Diagnostic findings of posterior urethral valves at voiding cystourethrography according to whether a catheter is in place during voiding

	No (%) of patients	Dilated posterior urethra (% of cases with finding)	Visible valves (% of cases with finding)
Catheter	28 (58)	25 (89)	19 (68)
No catheter	17 (35)	15 (88)	5 (29)
Both	3 (6)	3 (100)	3 (100)
Total	48 (100)	43 (90)	27 (56)

From Fernbach et al. [26]. Reprinted with permission from the American Journal of Roentgenology

There are several benefits to leaving the catheter in place during voiding: cyclic exams would not require re-catheterization, exams can be repeated if the results are equivocal or there are technical failures, and the bladder can be distended until the patient initiates voiding. In addition, if there is contrast remaining in the upper tracts, the bladder can be drained to determine if the residual contrast is due to continuous reflux or secondary obstruction [25, 26].

Contrast Media

Low-osmolar contrast material should be adequate. Dilute contrast is useful when trying to outline the presence of the ureterocele as concentrated contrast at large volume may obscure its detection. Taking into account the effects on the bladder and children's distress to cold (room temperature) contrast on children's distress and on the bladder, ideally the contrast material should be warm (body temperature). Receptors located within the bladder mucosa and trigone are responsible for a very sensitive cooling reflex [9]. They stimulate unmyelinated C-afferent fibers in the pelvic and pudendal nerves that consequently stimulate a detrusor contraction [27]. As a result, infusing the bladder with cold fluid can cause the bladder to empty at smaller volumes [9, 27]. This reflex is usually suppressed by 4 years of age [27]. When looking at distress levels in children under 1 year of age, 72 % of children having warm instillation had minimal distress vs. 48 % having cold instillation (Fig. 5.6) [27].

Contrast media should be infused slowly under gravity via the catheter and not injected

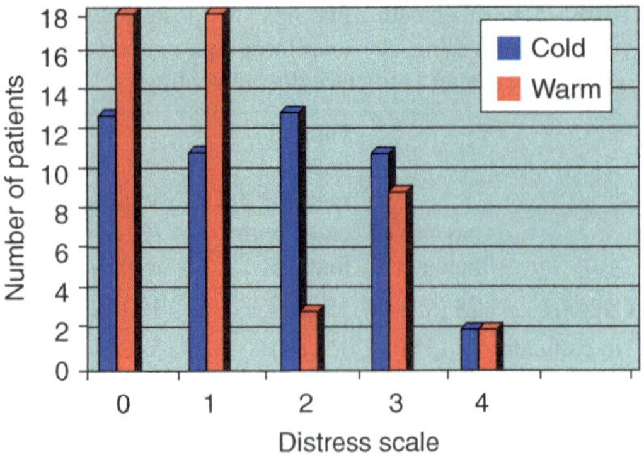

Fig. 5.6 The variation in perceived distress using warm or cold contrast medium [27]. Scale = *0*, no distress; *1*, flinching during infusion only; *2*, mild dress, crying < 50 % of examination; *3*, moderate distress, crying > 50 % of examination; *4*, severe distress, crying throughout the examination (Reprinted from Goodman et al. [26]. With permission from Elsevier)

under pressure. This will decrease bladder spasms and also is less likely to cause transmucosal absorption and subsequent potential contrast reaction [9, 26]. As bladder capacity is reached, the flow may slow down, stop, or even reverse [26]. Some advocate filling the bladder at a rate of 2 ml/kg/min at a pressure of 40 cmH_2O [28]. However, there are no universal protocols regarding the instillation of contrast. Palmer surveyed 41 institutions regarding their methodology [29]. The majority of discrepancy between institutions was on the height of the contrast material and on the formula used to estimate bladder capacity (EBC) in children less than 2 years of age. There was a 90 % consistency rate on infusing the contrast material under gravity, using feeding tubes or catheters without the balloon inflated, using non-diluted contrast, allowing parents in the room, and removing the catheter at the onset of voiding [29]. The Koff formula [EBC (mL) = (age + 2) × 30)] is commonly used to estimate bladder capacity in children greater than 2 years of age. Twelve percent of the institutions surveyed stopped infusing at EBC. However, younger children tend to have larger bladder sizes than predicted, and some children reflux at volumes larger than predicted [28, 29]. In addition, children with voiding or bladder dysfunction may have larger than expected bladder capacity. As a result, stopping the infusion at EBC instead of at the start of voiding may lead to false negatives and may miss important clinical information. If voided volumes are lower than expected, one should consider refilling the bladder [26] as VUR may not be detected if the bladder is underdistended.

Images

No universal protocols exist regarding the performance of a VCUG. As previously stated, images should include (a) an early filling image, (b) bilateral steep oblique images of the ureterovesical junction (UVJ), including the trigone or the presumed location of the distal ureters, when the bladder is full, (c) voiding images of the urethra, and (d) post-void images of the kidneys and bladder. Additional views of the bladder and kidneys during repeated filling and voiding can detect subtle abnormalities, such as intermittent VUR. If reflux is present, delayed images of the kidneys can determine how well the system drains. The scout image, if performed, should include assessment of the spine and pelvis looking for spinal dysraphism, sacral agenesis, scoliosis, or other abnormalities as seen in Fig. 5.7. Masses, stones, or foreign bodies may be seen. Figure 5.8 depicts large renal calculi seen on the scout film. Colonic gas pattern and volume of stool should be assessed as constipation may play a significant role in the underlying urologic problem.

Early fill AP coned down view of the bladder may detect a ureterocele, as seen on Fig. 5.9, or a filling defect that may represent a bladder mass, clot, or other pathology. Correct catheter placement should be confirmed during this phase of the study.

The full bladder is evaluated with steep oblique images, coned to the posterior bladder and trigone, and the expected location of the distal ureters (Figs. 5.10 and 5.11). These images evaluate

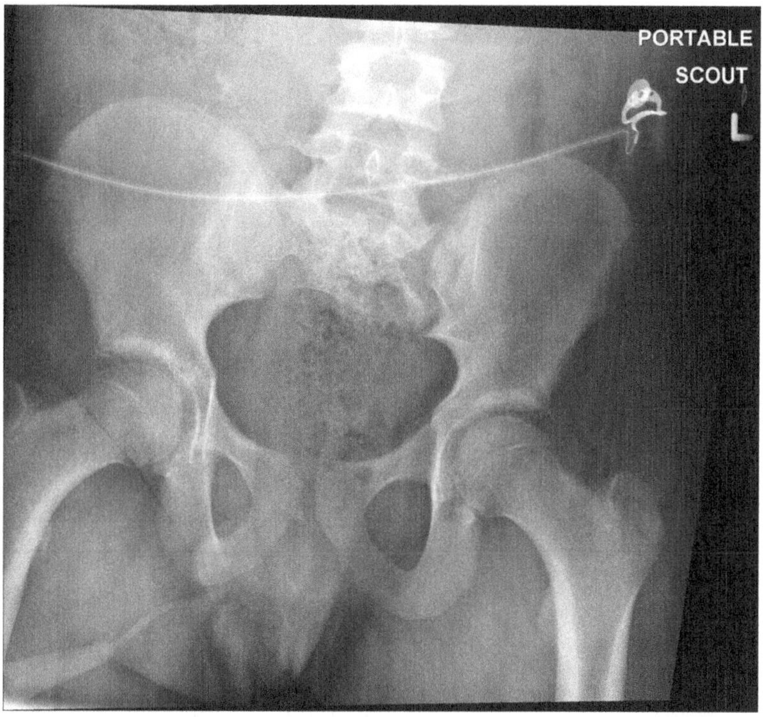

Fig. 5.7 Scout film demonstrating sacral agenesis in a boy with a neurogenic bladder

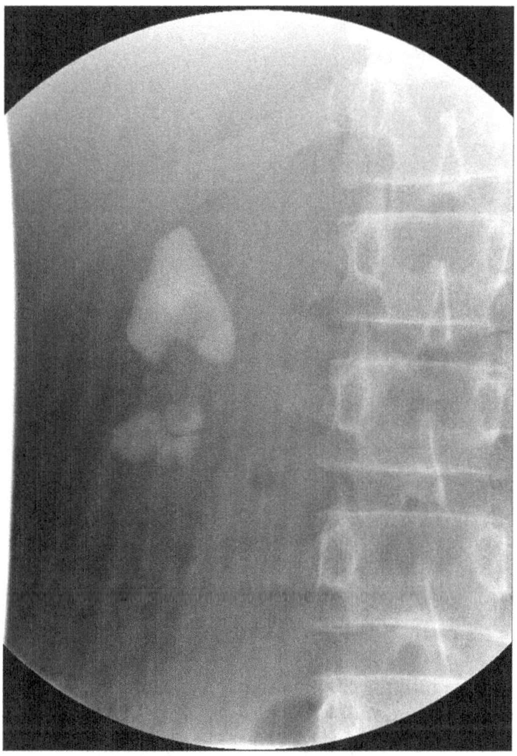

Fig. 5.8 Scout film with large renal stones

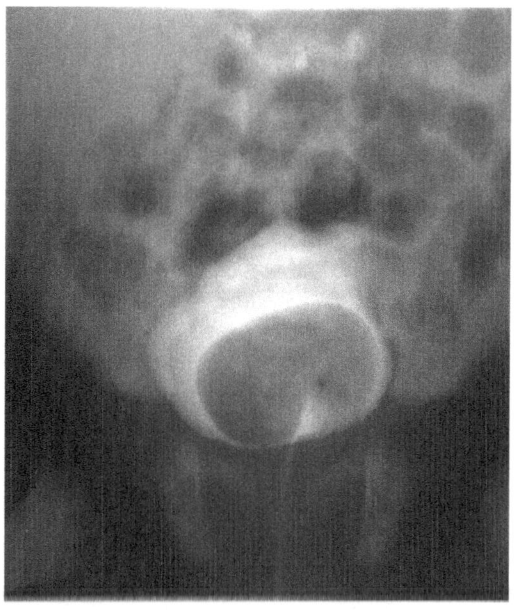

Fig. 5.9 Large ureterocele seen in an infant with a history of hydronephrosis

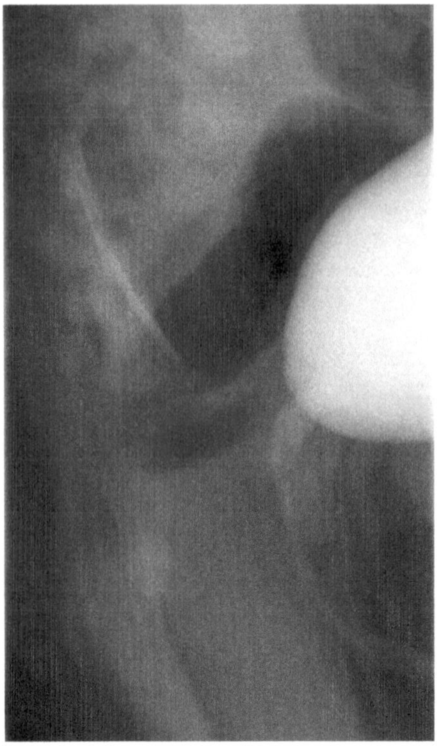

Fig. 5.10 Oblique film demonstrating no evidence of reflux on the right

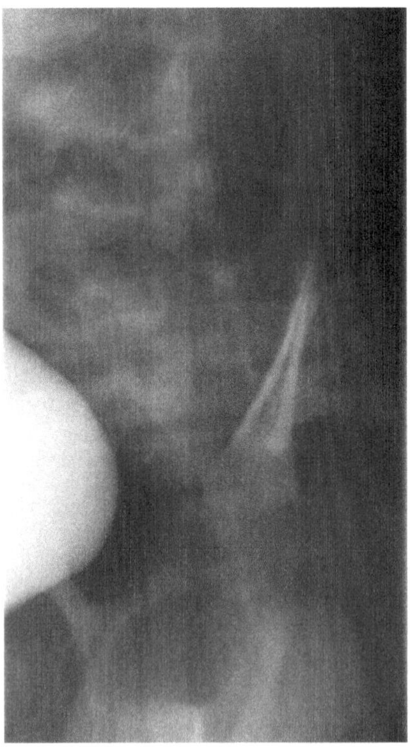

Fig. 5.11 Oblique film showing no evidence of reflux on the left

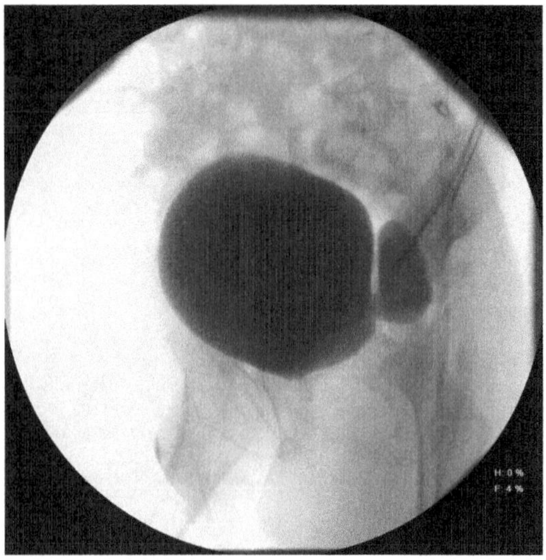

Fig. 5.12 Oblique view demonstrating a diverticulum. Diverticula may be congenital or may be secondary to high-pressure voiding or a neurogenic bladder

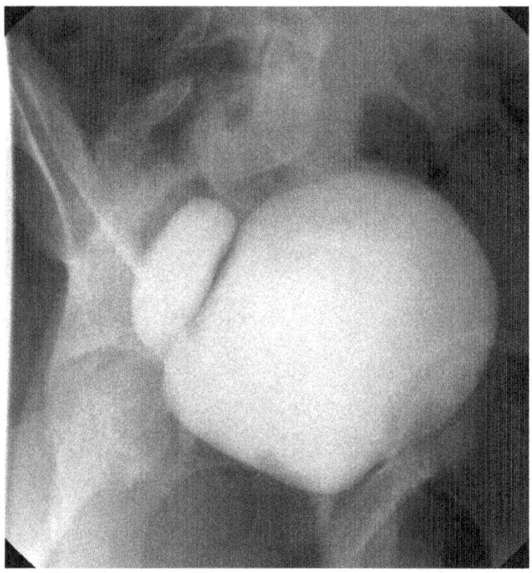

Fig. 5.13 Oblique image demonstrating a bladder diverticulum

for low grade VUR, everting ureteroceles, diverticula, or other bladder anomalies (Figs. 5.12, 5.13, 5.14, 5.15, and 5.16). Additional assessments include bladder capacity, contour, presence of trabeculations, and emptying capability [26]. Figure 5.17 demonstrates a classic appearance of a neurogenic bladder with high-grade VUR.

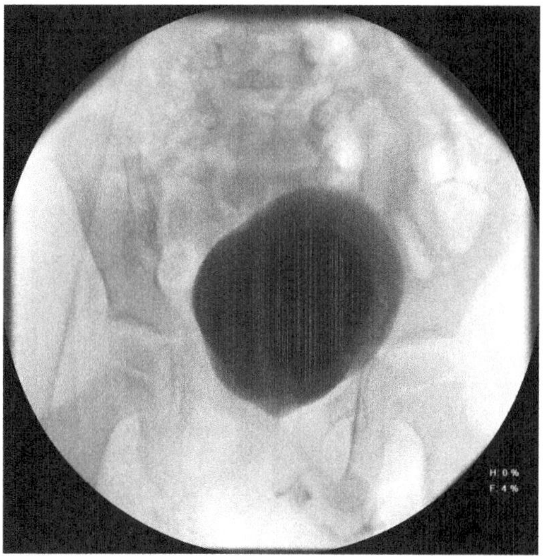

Fig. 5.14 AP view of a bladder diverticulum. With more concentrated contrast, the diverticulum could be missed in this view

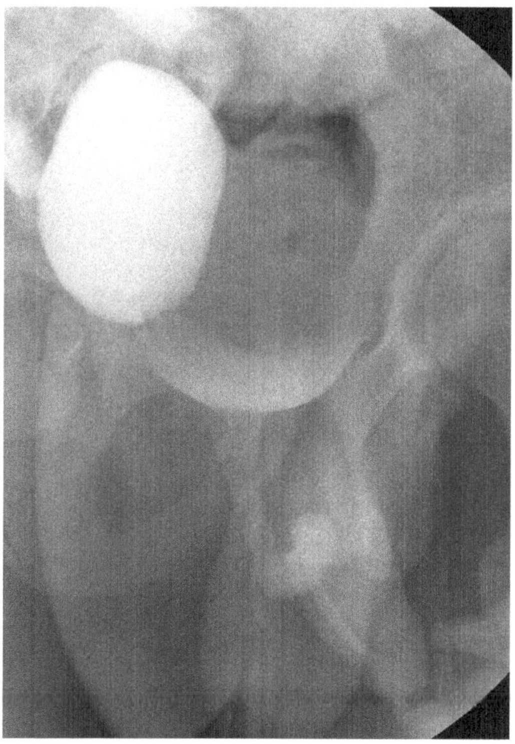

Fig. 5.15 Voiding image demonstrates filling of a diverticulum during voiding with a rim of contrast seen at the base of the bladder

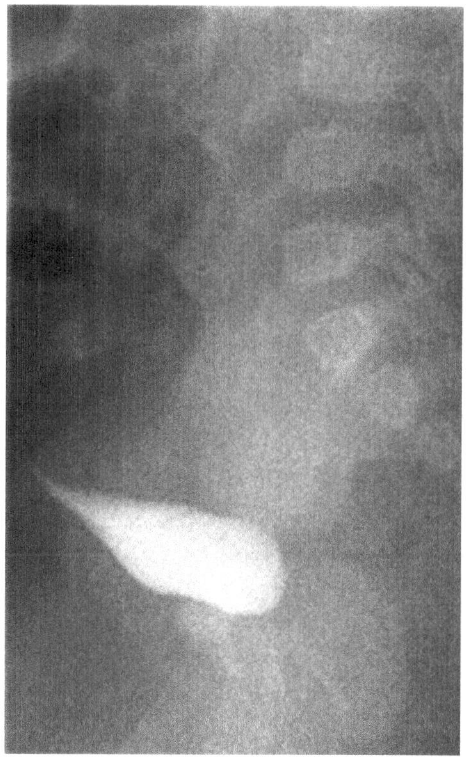

Fig. 5.16 Patent urachal sinus

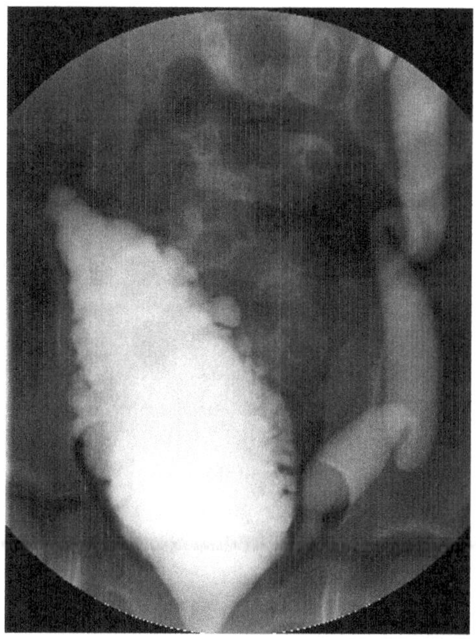

Fig. 5.17 Neurogenic bladder demonstrating a classic Christmas tree appearance secondary to trabeculations and sacculations. The refluxing ureter is dilated and tortuous

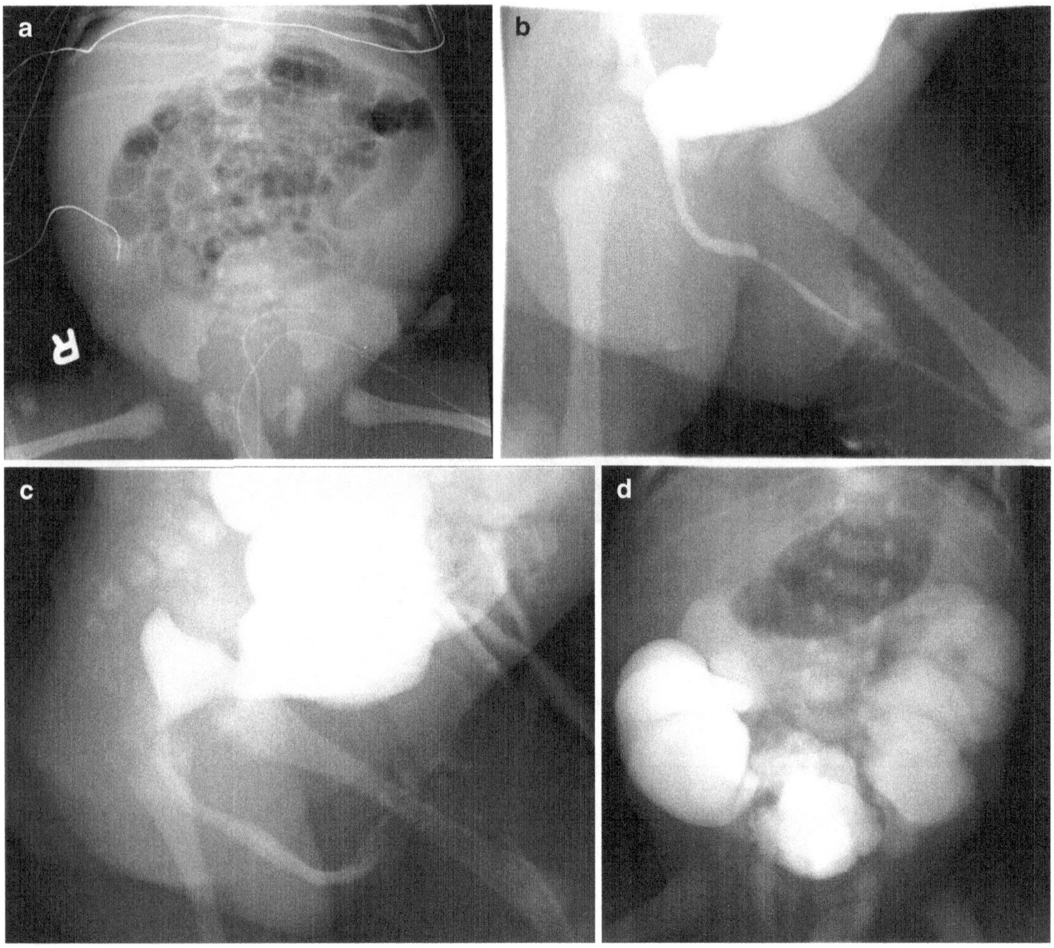

Fig. 5.18 (**a**) Scout film of a patient with Eagle-Barrett (Triad) syndrome demonstrated a protuberant abdomen and flared ribs. (**b** and **c**) Voiding images of a two patients with Eagle-Barrett demonstrating a patent urethra with a dilated posterior urethra and an enlarged smooth bladder with trabeculations. (**d**) Post-void images demonstrating massive VUR with incomplete emptying in a patient with Eagle-Barrett syndrome. Eighty-five percent of patients with Eagle-Barrett syndrome will have VUR [2]

Other bladder anomalies may be demonstrated as seen on Fig. 5.18, taken of a child with Eagle-Barrett syndrome and Fig. 5.19, taken of a child with a common urogenital sinus.

If present, VUR should be reported based on the International Reflux Study Committee's classification (Table 5.5, Figs. 5.20, 5.21, 5.22, 5.23, 5.24, 5.25, and 5.26). The grade of reflux is determined on the most severe VUR seen, which usually, but not always, coincides with the peak of voiding [2]. Insertion site of the refluxing ureter as well as the timing of VUR should be stated as this may have prognostic implications, as seen on Figs. 5.27 and 5.28. High-resolution renal images should be obtained pre- and post-void to assess for VUR, especially if no obvious reflux is seen on fluoroscopically saved images. Reflux is most likely to occur during voiding. Approximately 20 % of reflux will be missed if voiding does not occur [26]. Intrarenal

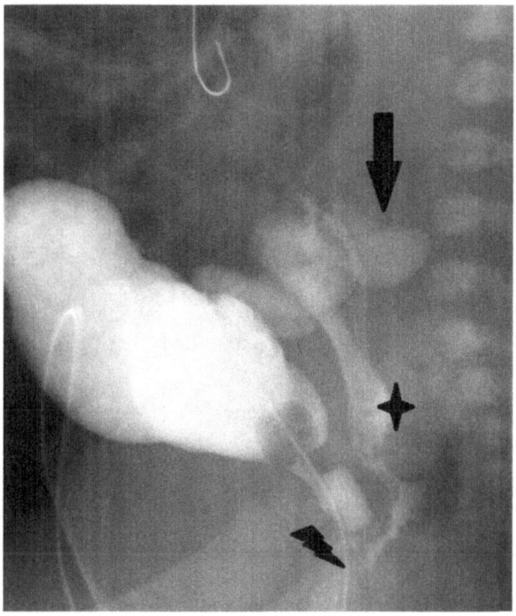

Fig. 5.19 VCUG obtained in a child with a common urogenital (*UG*) sinus. The *thick arrow* indicates associated VUR. The *lightning bolt* demonstrates the common UG sinus. The *Star* depicts contrast entering the vagina

Table 5.5 International Reflux Study Committee's grading of vesicoureteral reflux

Grade I	Reflux into the ureter only
Grade II	Reflux into a non-dilated ureter and pelvicalyceal system
Grade III	Reflux into a mild or moderately dilated ureter and collecting system with no or very minimal blunting of the fornices
Grade IV	Reflux into a moderately dilated ureter and system with blunting of the fornices but preservation of the papillary indentations
Grade V	Reflux into a grossly dilated ureter and system with loss of the papillary indentation

reflux may be demonstrated on VCUGs. This is demonstrated by contrast seen within the renal parenchyma in addition to the collecting system. This should be reported as it has prognostic implications for renal scarring, hypertension, and long-term renal function (Fig. 5.29).

Voiding images should be obtained in an anterior oblique position for males and AP or oblique position for females (Figs. 5.30 and 5.31) [26]. During voiding, the caliber of the urethra should be evaluated as well as the presence of VUR. Figure 5.32 demonstrates posterior urethral valves in a boy with a history of bilateral hydronephrosis. He had bilateral VUR with rupture of a calyx on the right, causing a right-sided urinoma, as seen on Fig. 5.33. Other urethral anomalies include urethral duplication and megalourethras as seen in Figs. 5.34 and 5.35.

Coordinated voiding between the bladder neck and external sphincter and the caliber of the bladder neck should be assessed, particularly in girls and patients with a neurogenic bladder. Figure 5.36 demonstrates a spin top urethra seen in female with dysfunctional voiding, and Fig. 5.37 demonstrates some reflux of contrast in the vaginal vault. This is frequently seen in infants, and in older patients may be a sign of vaginal trapping of urine during voiding, which could be a source of recurrent urinary tract infections.

Post-void images of the kidneys in an AP view are obtained to assess for VUR. These images should be performed soon after the patient stops voiding, even if the bladder has not completely emptied. Quickly draining vesicoureteral reflux may be missed, if the patient is allowed to void in the restroom instead of on the table or there are

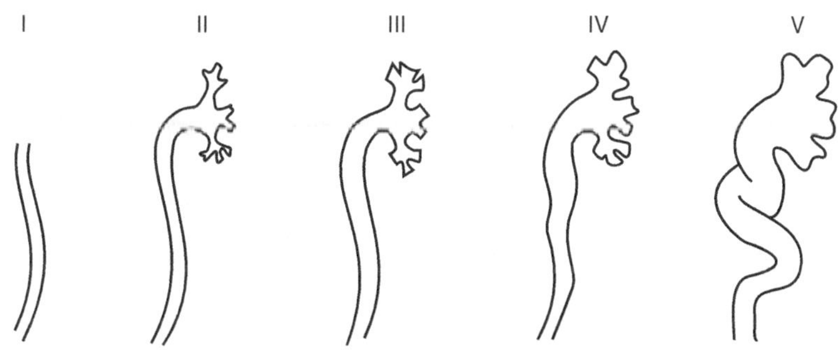

Fig. 5.20 International Reflux Study Committee's grading of vesicoureteral reflux

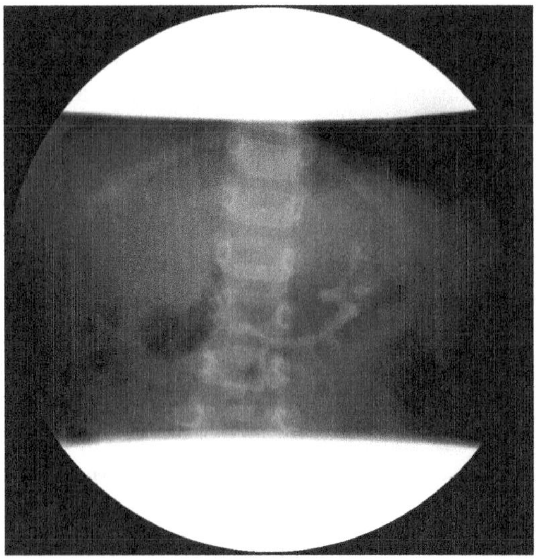

Fig. 5.21 Grade II left VUR

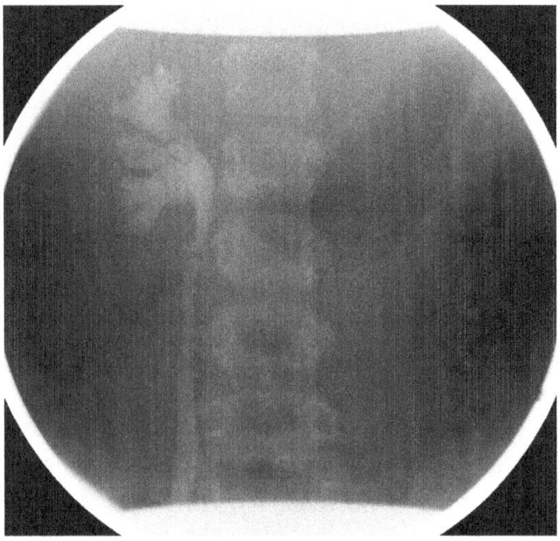

Fig. 5.22 Grade III right VUR

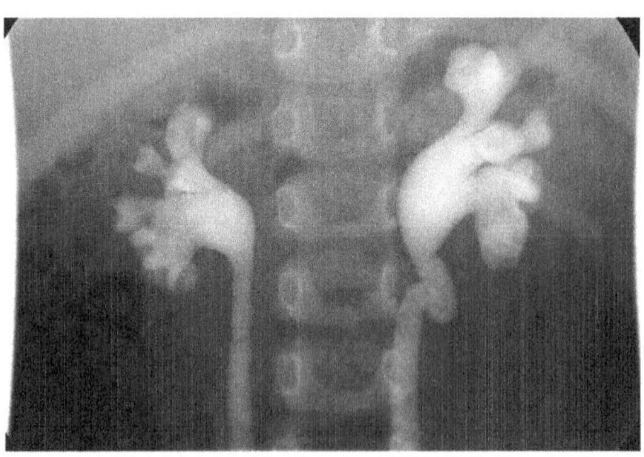

Fig. 5.23 Bilateral grade IV VUR, worse on the left with stool seen in the colon

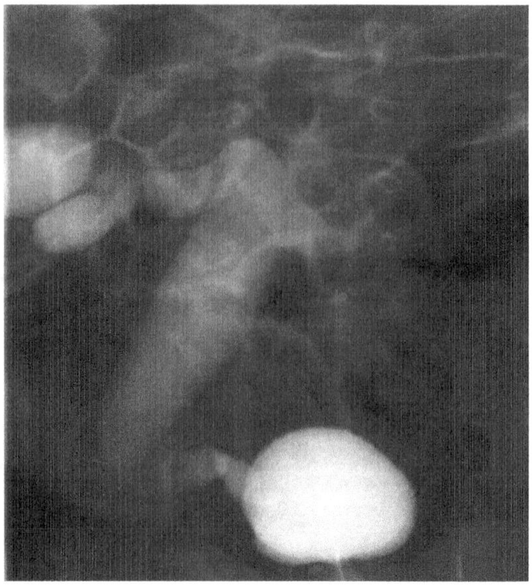

Fig. 5.24 VUR into the right tortuous lower pole ureter and calyces. Note dilution of contrast in a dilated ureter by retained unopacified urine

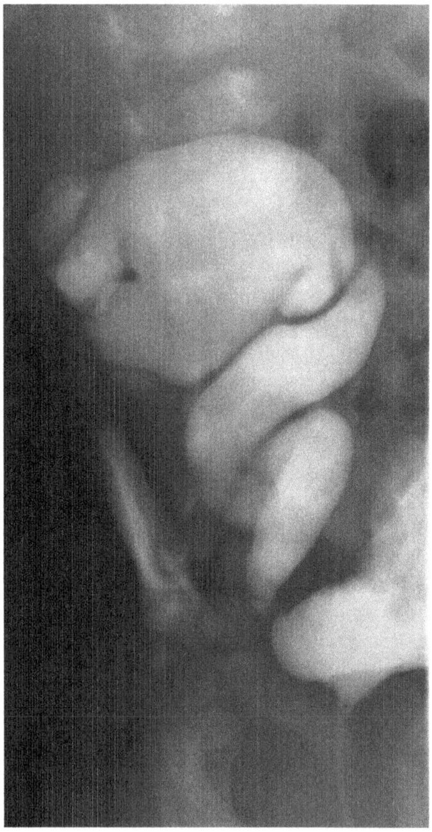

Fig. 5.25 Grade V right lower pole VUR

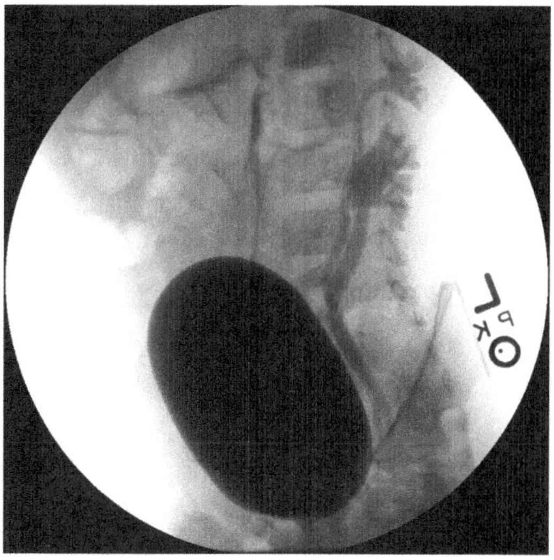

Fig. 5.26 Grade I right VUR with left VUR into a duplicated system

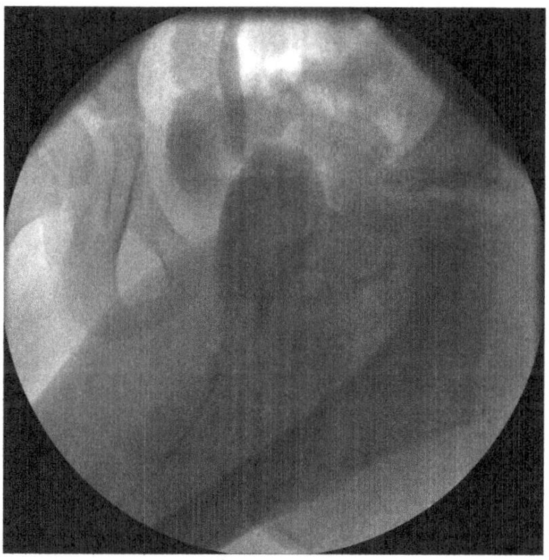

Fig. 5.27 Catheter inadvertently placed in the vagina opacifying a normal appearing vagina with a refluxing ectopic right ureter

other delays in obtaining the post-void images. If high-grade VUR, grades IV or V, is present, then delayed images should be performed approximately 15 min after voiding to assess for underlying UPJ or UVJ obstruction (Fig. 5.38).

In addition, post-void bladder images assess for complete emptying. It is important to note that the majority of infants do not empty to completion

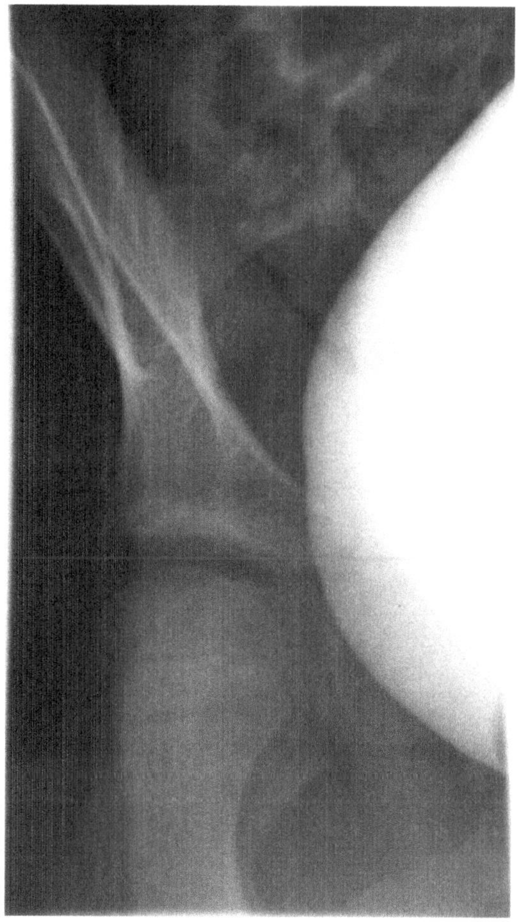

Fig. 5.28 Views of the bladder in the same patient as Fig. 5.27, demonstrating no evidence of VUR from the urinary bladder

[32]. If the patient double voids, repeat post-void images of the kidneys and bladder should be obtained. It is important to note the presence of contrast in the vagina (Fig. 5.37) which could be normal pooling artifact from supine voiding, but might account for symptoms of post void wetness, vaginitis, or false-positive bacterial growth in non-catheterized urine samples.

Cyclic VCUG

Cyclic VCUGs entail having the bladder fill and having the patient void several times. When performing a cyclic VCUG, most will leave the catheter in place. Repeat images of the bladder

Fig. 5.29 Intrarenal reflux demonstrated by the *arrows* (Reproduced from Kanumakala et al. [30]. With permission from BMJ Publishing Group LTD)

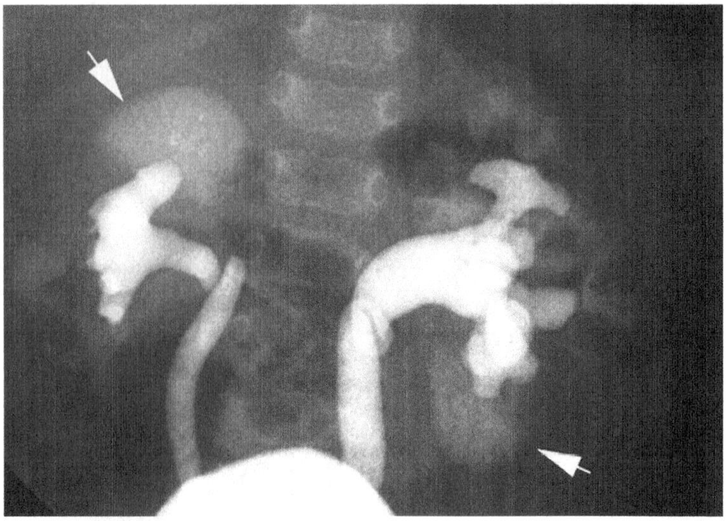

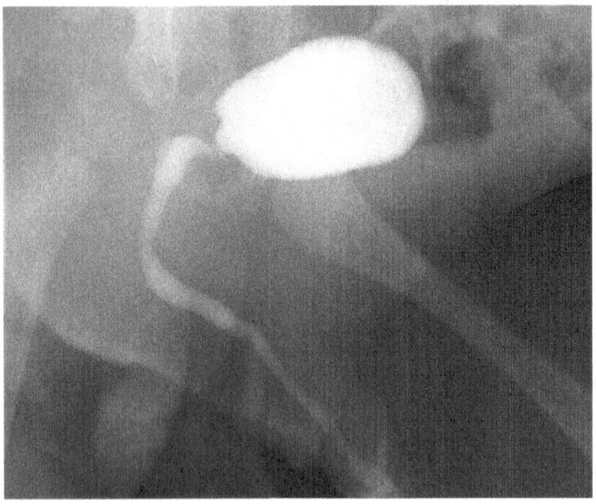

Fig. 5.30 Normal male urethra

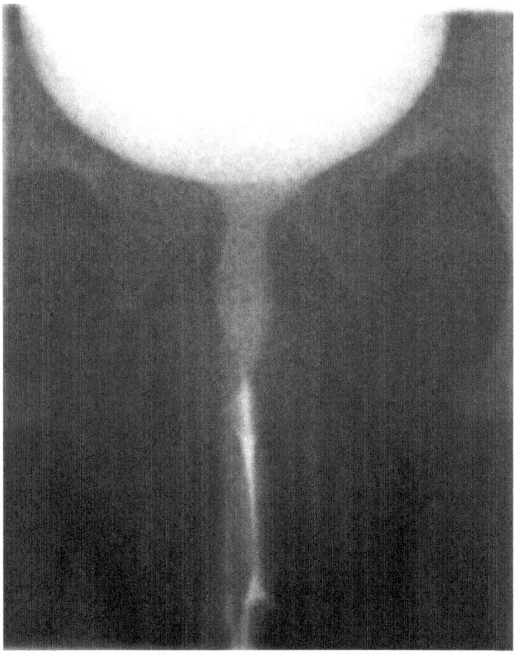

Fig. 5.31 Normal female urethra

and kidneys during voiding and post-void are performed. As VUR can be intermittent, cyclic studies increase the yield of detecting VUR up to 20 % [9, 33], most of which have been grade II or higher. In addition, the grade of VUR detected may be higher on the second cycling phase [9, 33]. Cyclic studies are encouraged for children under the age of 5 years, in children in whom VUR is suspected, or in patients with a suspected ectopic ureter [34]. Also, cyclic studies should be performed in children who spontaneously void at low volumes, as this may be secondary to bladder spasms, and the child may reflux at higher volumes in a normal physiologic state. If an ectopic ureter is draining into the bladder neck, it may first need to empty prior to seeing contrast material refluxing into the ureter, and only minimal contrast may reflux. This contrast may be further obscured by vaginal reflux. If a second voiding cycle is not performed, this refluxing ureter may be missed. Several cycles and having the patient in an oblique position may increase the changes of detecting the refluxing ectopic ureter [34].

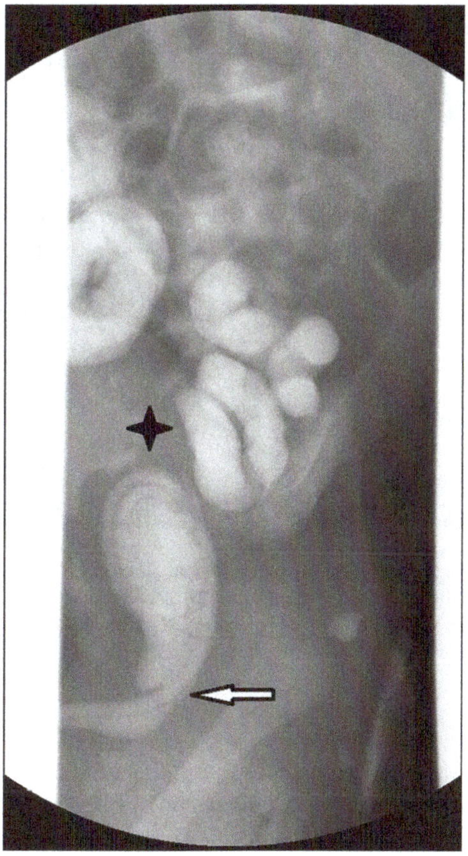

Fig. 5.32 Post-void image in a patient with posterior urethral valves. Typical findings of a dilated, elongated posterior urethra with a filling defect at the level of the obstruction are demonstrated by the *arrow*. The catheter is curled in the posterior urethra. The bladder is empty demonstrated by the *star* and there is bilateral VUR

Complications

VCUGs are generally a low-risk procedure. One of the main considerations includes radiation exposure as stated previously. Catheter-related complications include dysuria, perineal discomfort, urinary retention, hematuria, creation of a false passage, perforation, or knotting of the catheter that may require surgery. In addition, catheters may be placed in the vagina, ureteral orifice, prostatic utricle, or a ureterocele leading to misinformation [35]. Instrumentation may cause a urinary tract infection and rarely lead to sepsis [36]. There may be an allergic reaction to latex or to the contrast material if it is absorbed.

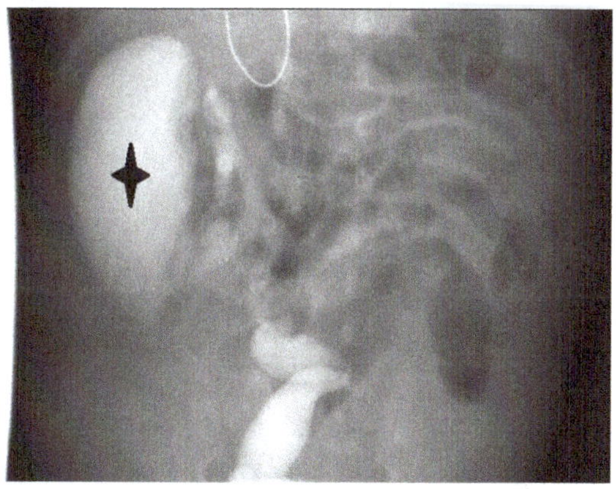

Fig. 5.33 Urinoma (*star*) due to a calyceal rupture in the same patient with VUR secondary to posterior urethral valves

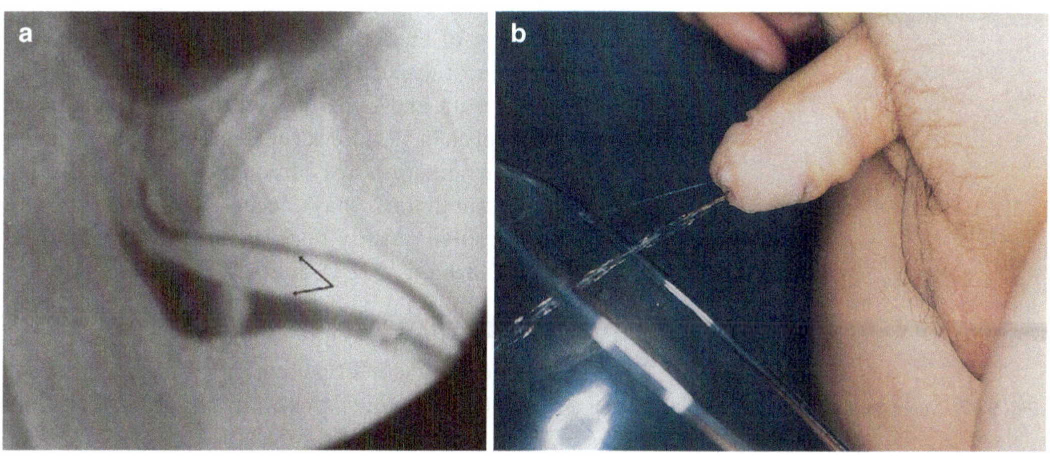

Fig. 5.34 (**a**) VCUG demonstrates contrast traveling through a complete urethral duplication (*two arrows*) (Reprinted from Palmer [31]. With permission from Elsevier). (**b**) Clinical photograph obtained in a 13-year-old boy during voiding shows complete urethral duplication (Reprinted from Berrocal et al. [2]. With permission from Radiological Society of North America)

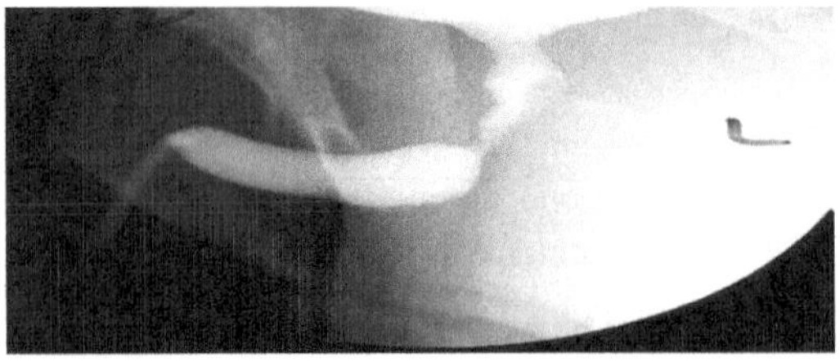

Fig. 5.35 Saccular-type megalourethra (Reprinted from Palmer [31]. With permission from Elsevier)

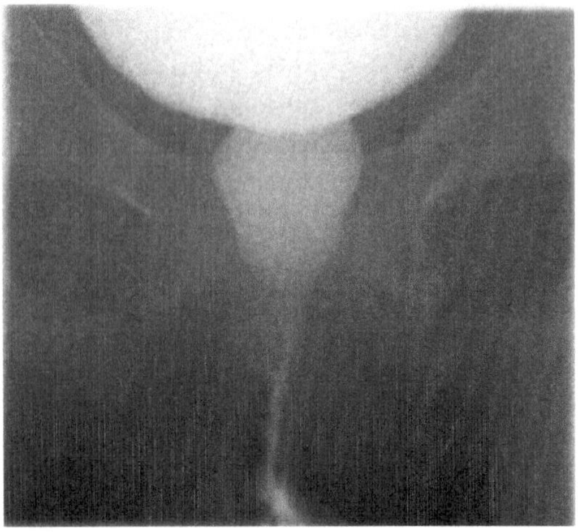

Fig. 5.36 Spin top urethra associated with dysfunctional voiding

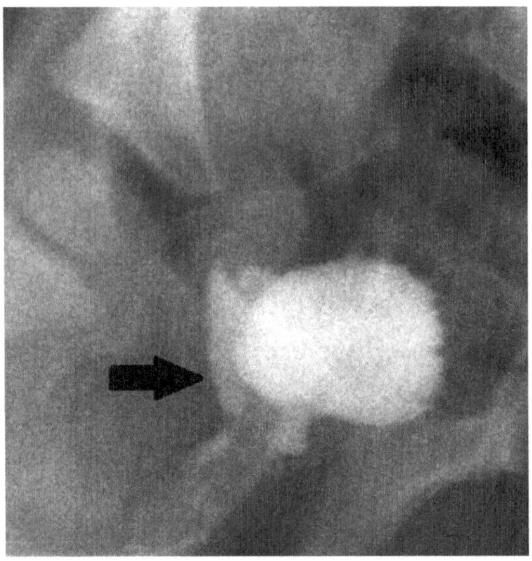

Fig. 5.37 Vaginal reflux of contrast depicted by the arrow

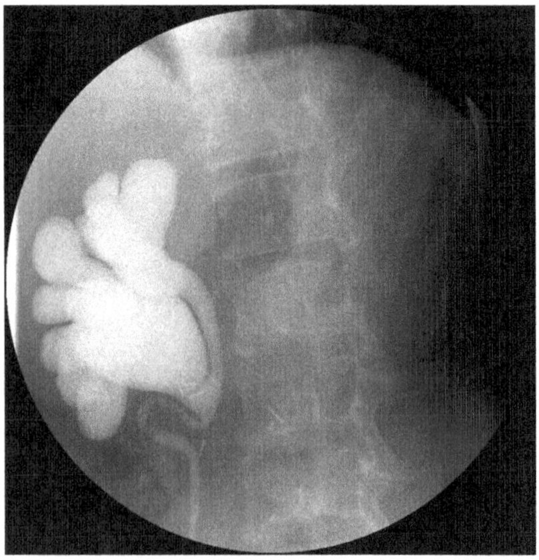

Fig. 5.38 VUR into a bifid system. There is "J hooking" of the ureter at the level of the UPJ with a disproportionally dilated renal pelvis to the ureter suggestive of an underlying UPJ obstruction

Special considerations should be made in patients with a spinal cord injury to avoid autonomic hyperreflexia (dysreflexia), which is potentially fatal. Autonomic hyperreflexia can occur in patients with a lesion above the sympathetic outflow, which is usually around T6 but has been reported as low as T10. There is a sympathetic surge secondary to a noxious stimulus below the level of the lesion. As a result of this surge, patients may have flushing of the face and body above the lesion and sweating. Cardiac symptoms include bradycardia and hypertension that can cause headaches or if more severe, cerebral hemorrhaging or seizures. Less frequently tachycardia and arrhythmias may occur. Symptoms usually resolve quickly once the stimulus is removed. During a VCUG, the noxious stimulus is frequently a full bladder. If these symptoms occur, the study should be aborted and the bladder drained. In patients with a known history of autonomic hyperreflexia, prophylaxis and proper monitoring should be instituted if the study is absolutely necessary.

Conclusion

VCUGs are one of the most commonly performed imaging studies in children. They have a low complication rate and provide information on structure and function. Modern techniques and judicial use of radiation have significantly reduced the overall radiation exposure. Although still considered one of the most distressing studies, proper patient preparation and the use of sedation, when needed, can help lower distress levels in both the child and their parents.

Key Points

- When using radiation, the ALARA principle, or *a*s *l*ow *a*s *r*easonably *a*chievable, should be implemented
- Quality assurance measurements should be implemented to assess for appropriate exposure levels in digital imaging
- VCUGs can be safely performed during a urinary tract infection once appropriate antibiotics have been initiated
- Appropriate patient and parental preparation can decrease distress associated with the study. When appropriate, sedation can be used without significantly affecting test results
- Ideally, contrast media should be at body temperature to decrease patient distress and inadvertent early detrusor contractions causing the bladder to empty at lower volumes
- Cyclic VCUGs should be performed in children under the age of 5 years, those in whom VUR or ectopic ureters is suspected, and in those with spontaneous voiding at volumes less than expected for age
- Complications are low. Special considerations should be implemented in patients at risk for autonomic hyperreflexia (dysreflexia)

References

1. Belman BA. A perspective on vesicoureteral reflux. Urol Clin North Am. 1995;22(1):139–50.
2. Berrocal T, Lopez-Pereira P, Arjonilla A, Gutierrez J. Anomalies of the distal ureter, bladder, and urethra in children: embryologic, radiologic, and pathologic features. Radiographics. 2002;22(5):1139–64.
3. Lee RS, Diamond DA, Chow JS. Applying the ALARA concept to the evaluation of vesicoureteral reflux. Pediatr Radiol. 2006;36 Suppl 2:185–91.
4. Schueler BA. The AAPM/RSNA physics tutorial for residents: general overview of fluoroscopic imaging. Radiographics. 2000;20(4):1115–26.
5. Goske MJ, Charkot E, Hermann T, John SD, Mills TT, Morrison G, Smith SN. Image gently: challenges for radiologic technologist when performing digital radiology in children. Pediatr Radiol. 2011;41:611–19.
6. Connolly B, Racadio J, Towbin R. Practice of ALARA in the pediatric interventional suite. Pediatr Radiol. 2006;36 Suppl 2:163–7.
7. Bevelacqua JJ. Practical and effective ALARA. Health Phys. 2010;98 Suppl 2:S39–47.
8. Moore QT, Don S, Goske MJ, Strauss KJ, Cohen M, Herrmann T, MacDougall R, Noble L, Morrison G, John SD, Lehman L. Image gently: using exposure indicators to improve pediatric digital radiology. Radiol Technol. 2012;84(1):93–9.
9. Agrawalla S, Pearce R, Goodman TR. How to perform the perfect voiding cystourethrogram. Pediatr Radiol. 2004;34:114–19.
10. Bazopoulos EV, Prassopoulous PK, Damilakis JE, Raissaki MT, Megremis SD, Gourtsoyiannis NC. A comparison between digital fluoroscopic hard copies and 105-mm spot films in evaluating vesicoureteric reflux in children. Pediatr Radiol. 1998;28(3):162–6.
11. Racadio JM, Connolly B. Image gently, step lightly: practice of ALARA in pediatric interventional radiology. http://www.pedrad.org/associations/5364/ig/index.cfm?page=596
12. Williams MB, Krupinski EA, Strauss KJ, Breeden 3rd WK, Rzeszotarski MS, Applegate K, Wyatt M, Bjork S, Seibert JA. Digital radiography image quality: image acquisition. J Am Coll Radiol. 2007;4(6):371–88.
13. Andrich MP, Majd M. Diagnostic imaging in the evaluation of the first urinary tract infection in infants and young children. Pediatrics. 1992;90(3):436–41.
14. McDonald A, Scranton M, Gillespie R, Mahajan V, Edwards GA. Voiding cystourethrograms and urinary tract infections: how long to wait? Pediatrics. 2000;105(4):e50.
15. Spencer JD, Bates CM, Mahan JD, Niland ML, Staker SR, Hains DS, Schwaderer AL. The accuracy and health risks of a voiding cystourethrogram after a febrile urinary tract infection. J Pediatr Urol. 2012;8(1):72–6.

16. Phillips DA, Watson AR, MacKinlay D. Distress and the micturating cystourethrogram: does preparation help? Acta Paediatr. 1998;87:175–9.
17. Robinson M, Savage J, Steward M, Sweeney L. The diagnostic value, parental and patient acceptability of micturating cysto-urethrography in children. Ir Med J. 1999;92(5):366–8.
18. Srivastava T, Betts G, Rosenberg AR, Kainer G. Perception of fear, distress, and pain by parents of children undergoing a micturating cystourethrogram: a prospective study. J Paediatr Child Health. 2001; 37:271–3.
19. Zelikovsky N, Rodrigue JR, Gidcz CA, Davis MA. Cognitive behavioral and behavioral interventions help young children cope during a voiding cystourethrogram. J Pediatr Psychol. 2000;25(8):535–43.
20. Salmon K, Pereira JK. Predicting children's response to an invasive medical investigation; the influence of effortful control and parent behavior. J Pediatr Psychol. 2002;27(3):227–33.
21. Herd DW. Anxiety in children undergoing VCUG: sedation or no sedation? Adv Urol. 2008; 498614.
22. Herd DW, McAnulty KA, Keene NA, Sommerville DE. Conscious sedation reduces distress in children undergoing voiding cystourethrography and does not interfere with the diagnosis of vesicoureteric reflux: a randomized controlled study. AJR Am J Roentgenol. 2006;187(6):1621–6.
23. Ferguson GG, Chen C, Yan Y, Royer ME, Campigotto M, Traxel EJ, Coplen DE, Austin PF. The efficacy of oral midazolam for decreasing anxiety in children undergoing voiding cystourethrogram: a randomized, double-blind, placebo controlled study. J Urol. 2011;185(6 Suppl):2542–6.
24. Merguerian PA, Corbett ST, Cravero J. Voiding ability using propofol sedation in children undergoing voiding cystourethrograms: a retrospective analysis. J Urol. 2006;176(1):299–302.
25. Ditchfield MR, Grattan-Smith JD, de Campo JF, Hutson JM. Voiding cystourethrography in boys: does the presence of the catheter obscure the diagnosis of posterior urethral valves? AJR Am J Roentgenol. 1995;164:1233–5.
26. Fernbach SK, Feinstein KA, Schmidt MB. Pediatric voiding cystourethrography: a pictorial guide. Radiographics. 2000;20(1):155–68.
27. Goodman TR, Kilborn T, Pearce R. Warm or cold contrast medium in the micturating cystourethrogram (MCUG): which is best? Clin Radiol. 2003;58: 551–4.
28. Kogan BA, Giramonti K, Feustel PJ, Lin WY. Bladder volume on voiding cystourethrogram correlates with indications and results in male infants. Urology. 2011;77:458–62.
29. Palmer BW, Ramji FG, Snyder CT, et al. Voiding cystourethrogram – are our protocols the same? J Urol. 2011;186:1668.
30. Kanumakala S, Kalidasan V, Kenney I. Intra-renal reflux. Arch Dis Child. 2004;89:692.
31. Palmer LS. Pediatric urologic imaging. Urol Clin North Am. 2006;33:409–23.
32. Sillen U. Bladder function in healthy neonates and its development during infancy. J Urol. 2001;166: 2376–81.
33. Papadopoulou F, Efremidis SC, Oiconomou A, Badouraki M, Panteleili M, Papachristou F, Soteriou I. Cyclic voiding cystourethrography: is vesicoureteral reflux missed with standard voiding cystourethrography? Eur Radiol. 2002;12(3):666–70.
34. Canning DA, Lambert SM. Chapter 115. Evaluation of the pediatric urology patient voiding cystourethrography. In: Campbell-Walsh urology. 10th ed. Philadelphia: Elsevier Saunders; 2012. p. 3067–84.
35. Rathaus V, Konen O, Shapiro M, Grunebaum M. Malposition of catheters during voiding cystourethrography. Eur Radiol. 2001;11(4):651–4.
36. McAlister WH, Cacciarelli A, Shackelford GD. Complications associated with cystourethrography in children. Radiology. 1974;111(1):167–72.

6 Principles of Nuclear Medicine Imaging

Aaron J. Krill and Christopher J. Palestro

Nuclear medicine imaging makes use of compounds labeled with small quantities of radioactivity, called tracers, that emit gamma rays detected by a gamma camera. All the nuclear medicine procedures utilized by pediatric urologists provide valuable diagnostic and functional information. Renal perfusion can be quantified which allows for accurate estimates of glomerular filtration rate (GFR). The renal cortex can be imaged very precisely, and any areas of decreased or absent tracer uptake that would signify hypoperfusion from acute pyelonephritis, renal dysplasia, or renal cortical scarring are clearly shown. Renal handling and clearance of radiotracer can also be used to estimate split, or differential, renal function and urinary drainage and can aid in the diagnosis of obstruction. Ischemia associated with testicular torsion can be differentiated from inflammation. The one procedure that fails to provide functional information is direct radionuclide cystography (DRC) which, however, offers a method to detect vesicoureteral reflux that is comparable to fluoroscopic voiding cystourethrography (VCUG) (Table 6.1).

The success of radionuclide renal imaging depends on several factors, including: (1) plasma protein binding and thus volume of distribution of the tracer; (2) rapid delivery to and selective uptake of the tracer by the target organ, e.g., the kidneys, versus the "background"; (3) photon attenuation by fluid collections and surrounding organs; (4) renal function; and (5) technical aspects such as selection of the region of interest (the organs to be evaluated) as well as selection of an appropriate background area.

In general, radionuclide image resolution is diminished compared to, while the radiation dose is similar or often lower than other radiologic imaging modalities such as the conventional VCUG, intravenous pyelography (IVP), and CT scanning. Unlike standard radiology, radiation

Table 6.1 Common uses of nuclear studies in pediatric urology

Estimation of renal plasma flow (GFR/global renal function)
Evaluation of renal cortical lesions (pyelonephritis, scarring)
Estimation of differential renal function (DRF)
Evaluation of urinary drainage, diagnosis of renal obstruction
Evaluation and surveillance of vesicoureteral reflux
Determination of testicular blood flow in cases of suspected testicular torsion

A.J. Krill, MD (✉)
Division of Urology, Department of Surgery, Virginia Commonwealth University Medical Center, 1200 East Broad St., Suite 7205, 980118, Richmond, VA 23298-0118, USA
e-mail: akrill@mcvh-vcu.edu

C.J. Palestro, MD
Department of Radiology, Hofstra North Shore-LIJ School of Medicine, Hempstead, NY, USA

Division of Nuclear Medicine and Molecular Imaging, North Shore Long Island Jewish Health System, 270-05 76th Ave., Manhasset & New Hyde Park, NY 11040, USA
e-mail: palestro@lij.edu

L.S. Palmer, J.S. Palmer (eds.), *Pediatric and Adolescent Urologic Imaging*, DOI 10.1007/978-1-4614-8654-1_6,

dosage depends primarily on the amount of radioactivity administered. Patient exposure is independent of the number of images obtained, and this allows for almost unlimited "real-time" dynamic imaging which can be important when determining time-dependent processes, such as sporadic vesicoureteral reflux or renal drainage. Administered activity (radiotracer dosage) guidelines can be found in the Society of Nuclear Medicine website (www.snm.org).

Radiopharmaceuticals

Radiopharmaceuticals for evaluation of the kidneys are classified into three general categories: cortical agents, tubular agents, and glomerular agents.

Cortical Agents

^{99m}Tc-Dimercaptosuccinic acid (DMSA) is extensively bound to plasma proteins (90 %), and very little is taken up by red blood cells (0–5 %) [1]. A small amount is glomerularly filtered [2, 3], but this tracer accumulates predominantly in the proximal convoluted tubules. Up to half of the injected activity is retained in the kidneys at 2 h and 70 % at 24 h postinjection [1, 4]. The highest-quality images are obtained about 2–4 h postinjection. These characteristics of DMSA make it an ideal imaging agent for the renal cortex to detect and define pyelonephritis, and renal cortical scarring and to assess the size, shape, and position of the kidneys, and to provide a reasonable estimate of split renal function. Due to its complex renal clearance, DMSA is not useful for estimating global renal function or GFR [5]. Similarly, it is not useful for evaluating urinary drainage because only a small fraction is eliminated in the urine (6 % at 1 h, 25 % at 14 h) [1]. DMSA has been used to aid in localization of renal ectopia, but abdominopelvic ultrasonography may obviate the need for this [6]. ^{99m}Tc-Glucoheptonate, another agent used for renal cortical imaging, is no longer available.

Tubular Agents

These agents are excreted principally through the tubules.^{99m}Tc-Mercaptoacetyltriglycine (MAG3) is the only approved tubular agent available for use in the United States. It is largely bound to plasma proteins (up to 90 %) with minimal (1–2.3 %) binding to red blood cells. This results in a significantly reduced volume of distribution and a high target to background ratio which translates into improved image quality and increased utility in younger patients [7–9].^{99m}Tc-MAG3 is rapidly extracted and secreted by the proximal renal tubules, in a manner qualitatively similar to that of orthoiodohippurate. Renal uptake is reduced by poor function. Up to 70 % of the injected dose is eliminated within 30 min, and by 3 h, up to 90 % can be recovered in the urine [7, 10]. ^{99m}Tc-MAG3 can be used quantitatively or qualitatively for evaluating obstructive uropathy, renovascular hypertension, and renal allografts and has been used to approximate effective renal plasma flow (ERPF) measurement. However, ^{99m}Tc-MAG3 slightly underestimates split renal function when compared directly to ^{99m}Tc-DMSA. This effect was magnified when there was a large difference in function between kidneys but never exceeded 4.3 % [11]. Some authors also have used it for cortical imaging [12, 13].

Glomerular Agents

^{99m}Tc-Diethylenetriaminepentaacetic acid (DTPA) is excreted predominantly by glomerular filtration and can be used to measure GFR. Like ^{99m}Tc-MAG3, ^{99m}Tc-DTPA can be used to assess renal blood flow and function, renal allografts, suspected renovascular hypertension, and obstructive uropathy [14, 15]. Its renal extraction fraction, however, is only about 20 %, compared to 40–50 % for ^{99m}Tc-MAG3 (K). Renal excretion is significantly affected by reduced renal function and performs inferior to ^{99m}Tc-MAG3 in patients with poor renal function and in suspected obstruction [16, 17]. It is not a good agent for renal cortical imaging because of its relatively rapid excretion.

Iodine-125 iothalamate is used exclusively for the nonimaging assessment of GFR. The glomerular agents ^{131}I-orthoiodohippurate and ^{123}I-orthoiodohippurate, once the mainstay of radionuclide renal studies, are no longer available in the United States.

Radiation Dosimetry

In recent years, much has been written regarding radiation dose limitation, specifically the concept of "ALARA – as low as reasonably achievable." This has led authors to favor imaging modalities that do not utilize ionizing radiation whenever possible, such as ultrasonography or magnetic resonance imaging. In situations where this is not feasible or when US or MRI does not perform as well as nuclear or radiographic studies, one needs to choose the study that offers the greatest diagnostic information and with the least radiation exposure.

The majority of nuclear studies, with the exception of cystography, carry a significant radiation burden (Table 6.2). In most cases, nuclear medicine studies used in pediatric urology offer similar or less radiation than other comparable imaging modalities. An exception would be scrotal scintigraphy, whose nonnuclear imaging counterpart is Doppler. ^{99m}Tc-DMSA renal cortical imaging, because of its selective tubular uptake and delayed excretion, provides one of the higher effective radiation doses. This is similar to that of IVP but offers greater sensitivity and specificity [18]. Radionuclide cystography, due to the relatively short period of time and distribution limited mostly to the bladder, provides a much lower effective dose [19] than contrast voiding cystourethrography (VCUG). However, strides have been made in reducing the radiation exposure during VCUG by limiting fluoroscopy time and technical refinements of the instrumentation. The use of grid-controlled pulsed fluoroscopy decreases radiation doses across all age groups by 10–50 % compared to continuous fluoroscopy with an effective dose comparable to that of DRC [19, 20].

GFR Measurement

Traditionally, GFR has been determined by clearance of a substance that is (1) completely filtered by the glomerulus; (2) not synthesized, destroyed, reabsorbed, or secreted by the renal tubule; (3) physiologically inert; and (4) not bound to plasma

Table 6.2 Estimated total body radiation dosimetry (effective dose) for various radiologic and nuclear imaging studies

	Effective dose (mSv) 1 year of age	Effective dose (mSv) 5 years of age	Effective dose as a percentage of total annual atmospheric radiation exposure (%)
^{99m}Tc-**DMSA** cortical scintigraphy	0.8–0.9[a,b]	0.8–0.93[a,b]	25–3
^{99m}Tc-**MAG3** diuretic renography/ indirect radionuclide cystography	0.6–0.77[a,c]	0.6–1.49[a,c]	19–51
^{99m}Tc-**Pertechnate** direct radionuclide cystography	0.08[c]		2.5
^{99m}Tc-**Pertechnate** scrotal scintigraphy *without thyroid blockade*	1.4–1.9[a,c]	1.4–1.9[a,c]	45–61
Intravenous pyelogram (**IVP**) *with grid*	1.0[b]	1.2[b]	32–38
Voiding cystourethrogram (**VCUG**)	0.45–0.89[d,e]	0.45–0.72[d,e]	14–28
Voiding cystourethrogram (**VCUG**) *with GCPL*	0.053–0.069[d]		1.7–2.2

[a]Gadd et al. [88]
[b]Smith et al. [18]
[c]Stabin [19]
[d]Fotakis et al. [89]
[e]Ward et al. [20]

proteins [21]. Agents such as inulin, urea, and creatinine have been used to measure GFR. While inulin clearance is generally acknowledged as the gold standard, it has limited clinical utility as it must be continuously infused and requires multiple timed blood samples. *^{99m}Tc-DTPA*, however, despite having minimal protein binding, meets the above criteria and requires only one injection [22].

GFR can be estimated via DTPA scintigraphy with serial timed plasma samples or via a camera-only method, which is less cumbersome, requires less time, and does not involve blood sampling. Briefly, DTPA is drawn up into a syringe, a 1-min preinjection measurement of the amount of radioactivity in the syringe is made, it is rapidly injected intravenously, a 1-min postinjection measurement of the empty syringe is made, and serial images of both kidneys are acquired at 1-min intervals between 1 and 3 min postinjection. The 2–3-min interval is the best time for GFR measurement. Both total and fractional GFR can be estimated. The entire duration of the study is less than 10 min.

The camera-only technique was described by Gates who compared DTPA measurements of GFR to 24-h creatinine clearance values obtained for each patient. There was an excellent linear correlation (r^2>0.9) between the two measurements across a wide range (1–113 mL/min) of renal function. The DTPA study was repeated 24–48 h later, and a remarkable correlation coefficient (99 %) with the first study confirmed the technique's reproducibility [23]. Some studies suggest that ^{99m}Tc-DTPA is not reliable for estimating GFR in young children [24, 25]. Chandhoke et al. reported significant inaccuracy in estimation of GFR when compared to clearance of continuously infused iothalamate in children. They postulated that this may be due to the fact that the adult renal depth correction used in the Gates method may not be applicable to children [26].

Renal Cortical Scintigraphy

The very high uptake of ^{99m}Tc-DMSA by the pars recta of the proximal tubules and its minimal glomerular filtration and loss in the urine allows for detailed images of the renal cortex (Fig. 6.1). Traditionally, ^{99m}Tc-DMSA cortical imaging has been used to delineate areas of cortical hypoperfusion that accompany acute pyelonephritis and also to demonstrate renal scarring from prior infections. Lesions associated with acute pyelonephritis appear as areas of photopenia, with preservation of the normal renal contour. In contrast, renal cortical scars appear as

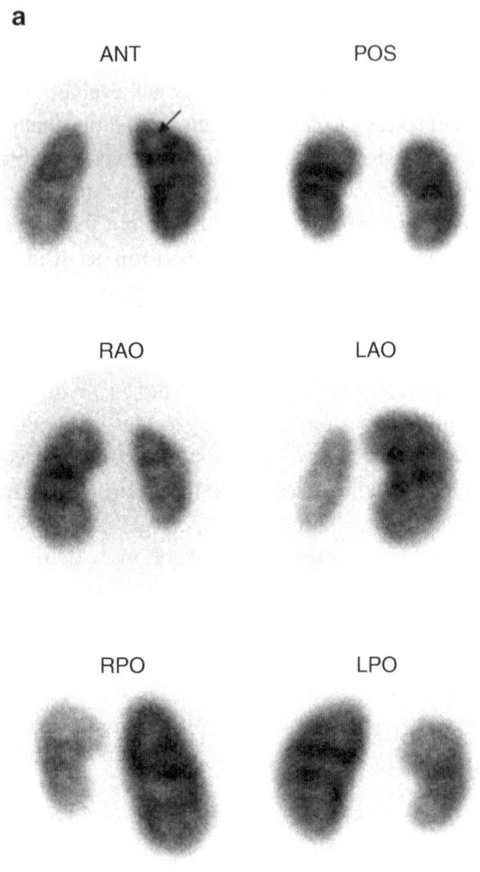

Fig. 6.1 Normal DMSA renal cortical study. (**a**) There is homogeneous distribution of activity throughout both kidneys on the pinhole images. The discrete round areas of decreased activity (*arrow*) are the calyces. The pinhole collimator distorts apparent organ size, which is why in some of the views, one kidney appears larger than the other. The coronal SPECT images (**b**) demonstrate homogeneous distribution of activity throughout the cortex of both kidneys. Note that unlike their appearance on the pinhole images, the kidneys are similar in size (With respect to the orientation of the SPECT images, the anterior most aspect of the kidneys is in the upper left image, and the posterior most aspect is in the lower right image)

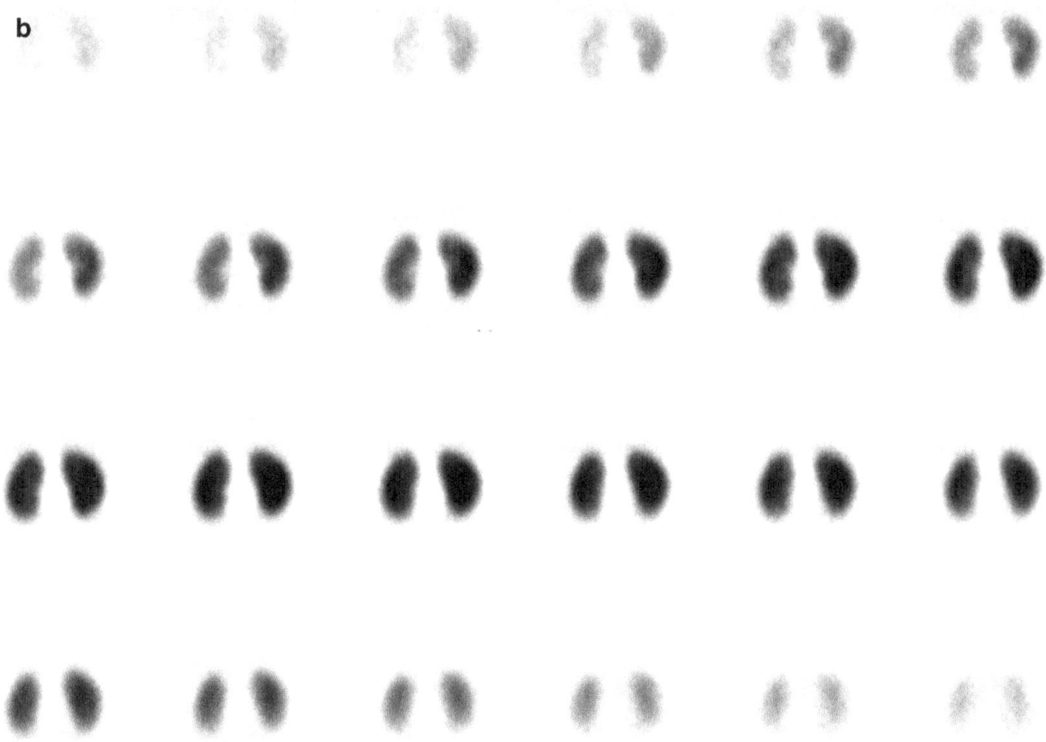

Fig. 6.1 (continued)

wedge-shaped areas of photopenia which distort the renal contour (Fig. 6.2). This information can aid in surgical planning and has been proposed to identify patients who should be screened for vesicoureteral reflux, the so-called top-down approach [27, 28].

^{99m}Tc-DMSA cortical scintigraphy also can provide information about differential renal function (Fig. 6.3). However, because it is filtered to a small degree, and blood clearance occurs over a period of hours, variations in renal DMSA uptake are not always equivalent to true variations in function. Thus, ^{99m}Tc-DMSA should not be used to estimate absolute renal function or GFR [29].

Description of Technique for ^{99m}Tc-DMSA Cortical Scintigraphy

In an effort to standardize reporting and methodology for renal cortical scintigraphy, several consensus statements and procedure guidelines have been issued, but there is still some variation in the timing of image acquisition (1.5–4 h postinjection), the need for sedation, type of views (planar and pinhole magnification vs. SPECT), and reporting of results [30, 31]. For clarity, the described technique is that of the Society of Nuclear Medicine Guideline publication in 1997, with some recent modifications by Zeissman et al. [31]. Single-photon emission computed tomography (SPECT) imaging will be described separately as there is considerable disagreement as to its utility versus standard planar and pinhole magnification images and also serious difficulties in multicenter standardization [31–34].

A large or standard field of view gamma camera equipped with a parallel-hole high-resolution collimator and/or a pinhole collimator with a 4 mm aperture is recommended. The patient is placed supine for parallel-hole imaging and prone for pinhole imaging. Imaging can begin at 1.5–2 h postinjection, although superior image quality is obtained by waiting at least 4 h [31, 35]. Classically, images are acquired in the posterior and the left and right posterior oblique planes.

Differential function is calculated from the posterior planar view using the parallel-hole collimator. Background correction can be undertaken by selecting a region of interest (ROI) around both kidneys in the planar projection and then drawing circumferential background regions approximately 2 pixels in width and 2 pixels away from the kidney. Acquisition time for the images varies by technique, with pinhole magnification requiring fewer counts (150,000 vs. 300,000) but longer acquisition time than the parallel-hole collimator (10 min vs. 5 min). For pinhole images, the kidney should fill approximately 2/3 of the field of view. In cases of significant hydronephrosis, furosemide can be given and/or delayed images can be performed up to 24 h after injection of radiotracer.

Various techniques have been described to adequately image the cortex; most centers rely on pinhole magnification to properly delineate renal scarring and acute pyelonephritis. These images should be correlated with other imaging modalities such as ultrasonography and voiding cystography, when available. A sample grading protocol used in the RIVUR trial is described in Table 6.3 in which the renal cortex is divided into numbered segments and severity graded by the quantity of segments involved [31].

SPECT Versus Standard Planar/Pinhole Imaging

Single-photon emission computed tomography, or SPECT, provides a panoramic multi-image view of both kidneys versus the standard three views of planar and pinhole magnification. Some suggest that SPECT is more sensitive and easier to interpret than planar and pinhole images. Other disagree contending that SPECT is less specific than planar and pinhole imaging. In an international multicenter survey of nuclear medicine experts, SPECT was performed routinely by only 22 % of respondents and seldom performed by 45 % of respondents and never used by 33 % of the respondents [30]. Further complicating matter is the absence of an accepted standard technique, with several authors reporting a range of projections (60–120) and varying increments of scanning time [35–37].

Interobserver Variability in SPECT and Planar ^{99m}Tc-DMSA Cortical Scintigraphy

^{99m}Tc-DMSA planar imaging has been shown to have excellent interobserver agreement in several reports using various measures. Consensus opinion regarding "normal" and "abnormal" among expert observers was 93.5 % and 90.5 %, respectively [38, 39]. While the reliability and reproducibility of planar and pinhole imaging is well established, little has been published on SPECT

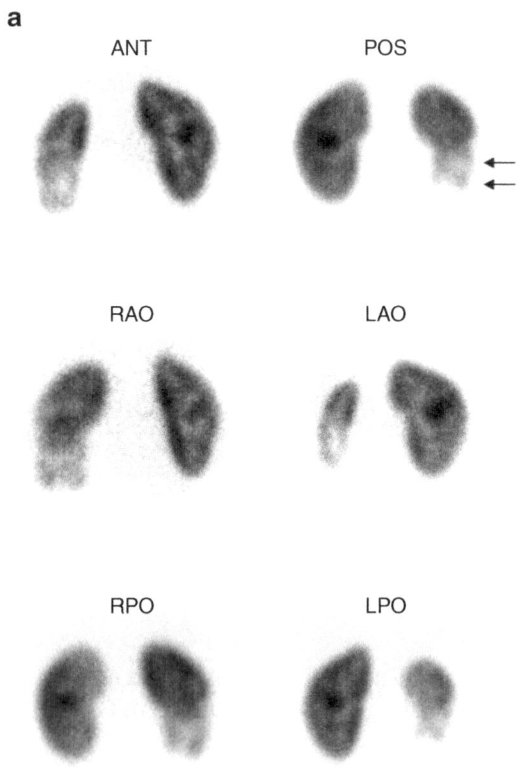

Fig. 6.2 Renal cortical scarring. Pinhole images (**a**) demonstrate an area of decreased tracer uptake with associated cortical volume loss (*arrow*), in the lower pole of the right kidney. On the coronal SPECT images (**b**), the right lower pole abnormality is equally well seen. In addition, the right kidney is smaller than the left

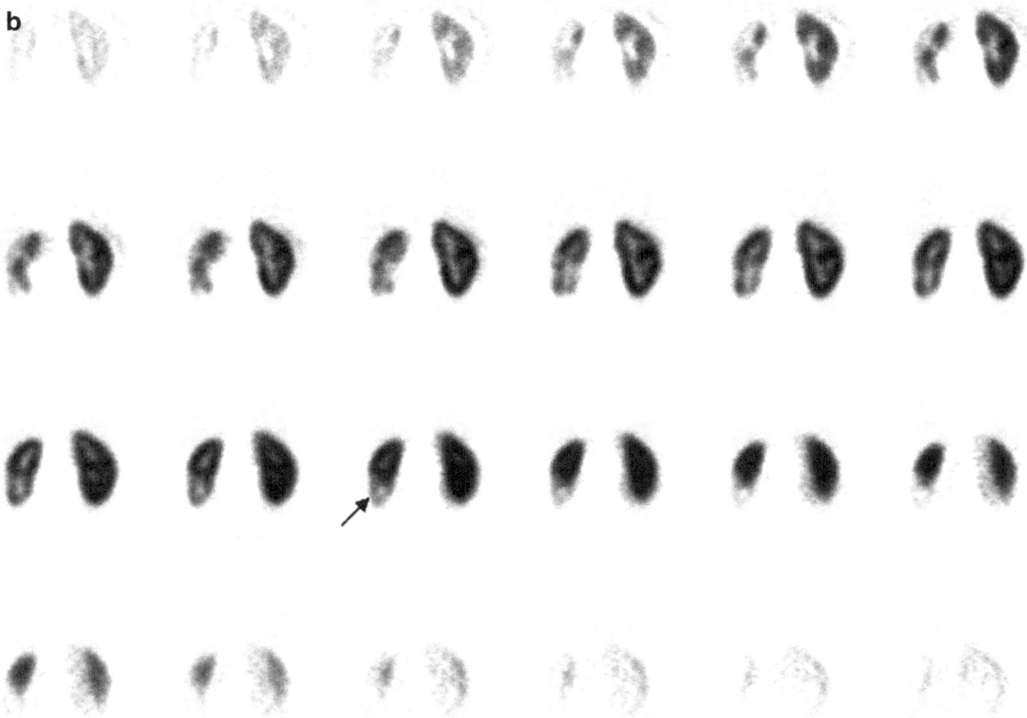

Fig. 6.2 (continued)

interobserver agreement, and the absence of a standard acquisition protocol hinders accurate comparisons among studies. Craig et al. suggest decreased reproducibility and interobserver agreement in interpretation of SPECT images compared to planar images [40]. Cost also can be a factor; by one estimate, SPECT costs up to 36 % more to perform than planar imaging. This is presumably due to longer image acquisition times and a possible greater need for sedation [41].

SPECT Versus Planar/Pinhole Magnification Imaging Animal Models

In comparison to standard planar and pinhole imaging, SPECT is comparable, possibly at the expense of decreased specificity and higher false-negatives. The performance of standard planar and pinhole magnification DMSA cortical imaging in the diagnosis of acute pyelonephritis has been widely investigated, and most authors agree on a sensitivity around 90 % and specificity between 90 and 100 % [42, 43].

Craig et al. report the results of a meta-analysis of published animal trials evaluating the overall ability of ^{99m}Tc-DMSA cortical scintigraphy to diagnose acute pyelonephritis. He initially found an *average sensitivity of 84 %* and an *average specificity of 88 %*; however, after correcting statistical errors and excluding some unusable data, there were no significant difference between SPECT and planar imaging [41].

In one elegantly designed study correlating histopathology and cortical scintigraphy in piglets, Majd et al. directly compared SPECT and pinhole imaging for detection of pyelonephritis 1–10 days after infection. After evaluating all zones of pyelonephritis over the entire time period, SPECT carried a sensitivity of 91 % vs. 86 % for pinhole imaging but was less specific, 82 % vs. 95 % compared to planar imaging.

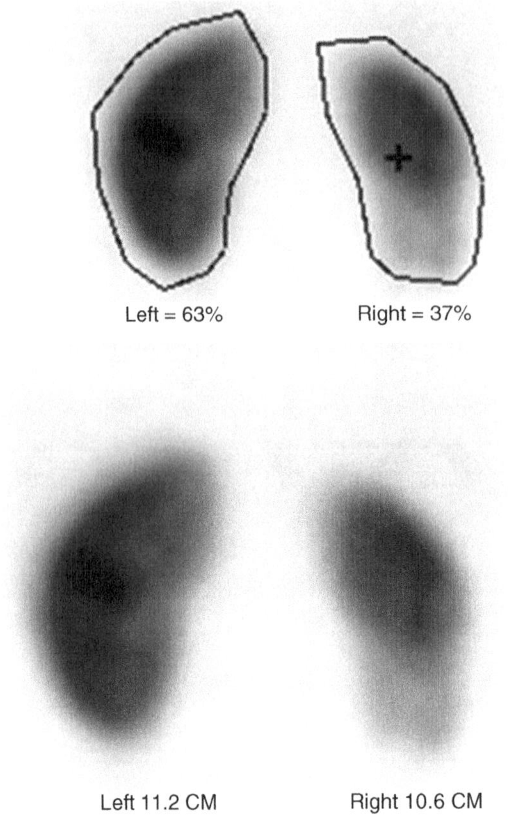

Fig. 6.3 When performing renal cortical scintigraphy, it also is possible to determine differential (split) renal function and to measure renal size

Table 6.3 Sample grading system for renal cortical scarring in ^{99m}Tc-DMSA scans (Zeissman et al. [31])

Grade	Severity	Number of affected renal segments
0	Normal	0
1	Mild	1–2
2	Moderate	3–4
3	Severe	>4
4	Global atrophy	Diffuse scarring

Overall accuracy was similar for both techniques, 88 % for SPECT and 90 % for pinhole imaging (Table 6.4) [42].

Rossleigh et al. compared SPECT to standard planar imaging in the diagnosis of renal cortical scarring in a refluxing piglet model with post-study histopathologic confirmation. Each animal after VCUG-confirmed VUR and ^{99m}Tc-DMSA-confirmed pyelonephritis underwent another planar ^{99m}Tc-DMSA and SPECT scan 3 months later. They reported similar sensitivity, specificity, and overall accuracy between planar images, pinhole magnification, and SPECT (Table 6.5) [34].

SPECT Versus Planar Imaging for Detecting Pyelonephritis

There are several human studies demonstrating the ability of SPECT to detect more renal lesions in acute pyelonephritis and renal cortical scars than planar and pinhole imaging. Tarkington et al. compared the ability of SPECT and pinhole imaging to detect renal cortical defects of various etiologies in 33 children, about 60 % of who did not have UTI, VUR, or prior pyelonephritis. In this heterogeneous population, 63 % of the pinhole image studies read as "normal" were found to have cortical abnormalities on SPECT. They also found that SPECT "clarified or enhanced" the pinhole imaging in 71 % of the kidneys studied. Overall SPECT found 55 % more cortical defects than pinhole imaging [44]. Yen et al. compared SPECT to planar imaging in 27 infants and 17 children upon diagnosis of acute pyelonephritis and at 3 months posttreatment and found SPECT identified significantly more scarring than planar imaging (33 % vs. 9.5 %, $p<0.05$) at

Table 6.4 Detection of acute pyelonephritis in piglets (Majd et al. [42])

	Sensitivity (%)	Specificity (%)	Accuracy (%)
Pinhole magnification	90	95	92
SPECT	96	95	96

Table 6.5 Detection of post-pyelonephritis renal scarring in pigs (Rossleigh et al. [34])

	Sensitivity (%)	Specificity (%)	Accuracy (%)
Pinhole magnification	74	99	92
SPECT	59	98	87

3 months, particularly in the presence of high-grade VUR than those found using planar imaging [36]. The prospective data of Applegate et al. seem to confirm prior human studies that SPECT detects more "definite" lesions than pinhole and planar images. Cortical defects were classified as "possible" or "definite" and "single" or "multiple" as defined by a consensus of three blinded experts. However, they found that no technique was superior for detecting multiple as opposed to solitary defects [32].

SPECT Versus Planar/Pinhole Imaging Summary

Data from studies in human subjects seem to corroborate previous animal studies that demonstrate increased sensitivity with SPECT, but without histopathologic analysis, false-positives cannot be excluded with certainty. As such, the pooled data from the animal studies is slightly less impressive but probably more accurate than that reported in human subjects. Regardless of technique, the performance of ^{99m}Tc-DMSA renal cortical scintigraphy in the diagnosis of acute pyelonephritis and the detection of renal cortical scarring is excellent. At best, SPECT is slightly more sensitive than, and is comparable in specificity to standard pinhole imaging. It seems that the combination of SPECT and pinhole imaging may improve interobserver agreement and may be more useful than either test alone.

Description of Technique for Diuretic Nuclear Renography

In 1992 the Society for Fetal Urology and the Pediatric Nuclear Medicine Council released a consensus statement regarding performance of the "well-tempered diuretic renogram" in response to a lack of standardization of technique and interpretation of dynamic renal imaging. However, this protocol has not been adopted universally, and debate continues regarding such technical aspects as method of pretest hydration, need for urethral catheterization, timing of diuretic administration, and even the method of calculation of urinary drainage [45, 46].

Patient Preparation

The infant kidney continues to mature, and GFR continues to increase for the first year of life which is reflected in the child's ability to clear ^{99m}Tc-MAG3 from the plasma [47]. In general, diuretic renography should be performed after the child is at least 1 month of age to limit spurious prolongation of drainage and a potentially inadequate response to diuretic challenge due to immature renal tubules [46]. Oral hydration is encouraged, and IV hydration is provided as a 15 mL/kg bolus of D5 0.3NS or D5 0.25NS 15 min prior to injection of radiotracer. Maintenance intravenous fluid is provided throughout the study. A urethral catheter for constant bladder drainage decreases the radiation dose to the bladder wall and gonads and also minimizes impedance of antegrade flow of urine from the collecting system simulating delayed drainage.

Renogram Phase

^{99m}Tc-MAG3 is administered intravenously with the child placed in supine position and the gamma camera under the bed. The field of view should include the heart, kidneys, ureters, and the bladder. Digital images are collected at 20 s/frame, and analog images are recorded for 30 min with practitioner preference determining the timing. A typical renogram acquisition is 1- or 2-min image intervals for 30 min (Fig. 6.4).

For accurate estimation of split renal function during the renogram phase, care must be taken when selecting the region of interest (ROI). This can be done manually or with computer assistance in a semiautomated or fully automated fashion. Regardless, the ROI must encompass the entire kidney including the renal pelvis. The background ROI should be approximately 2 pixels wide and encircle the renal ROI. Acquisition time should be a minimum of 20–30 min. To calculate differential renal function (DRF), the total counts of the renogram curve for each kidney minus the background counts are calculated during the interval from 60 s post tracer injection until the appearance of activity in the collecting system. Usually this is within the first 60–120 s of the study. There are several methods used to estimate DRF, but the two most commonly employed are the *integral method* where area under the renogram curve is calculated and the *Rutland-Patlak plot* which relies on the mean slope of the ascending renogram curve. In most situations, both methods are thought to be equivalent [48].

Controversy exists over the so-called "supra-normal" functioning kidney, split renal function of ≥55 % in unilateral hydronephrotic kidneys, which has a prevalence of 4–21 % [49–53]. Various explanations have been proposed, including compensatory hyperfunction, artifact related to background correction [49, 53], or variation in the method of quantification of function [50, 54]. Reports of laterality are variable.

Diuretic Phase

Furosemide at a dose of 1 mg/kg (max 40 mg) for children <1 year and 0.5 mg/kg for children >1 year is given IV after completion of the renogram phase, usually at 20–30 min (F+20–30) or when

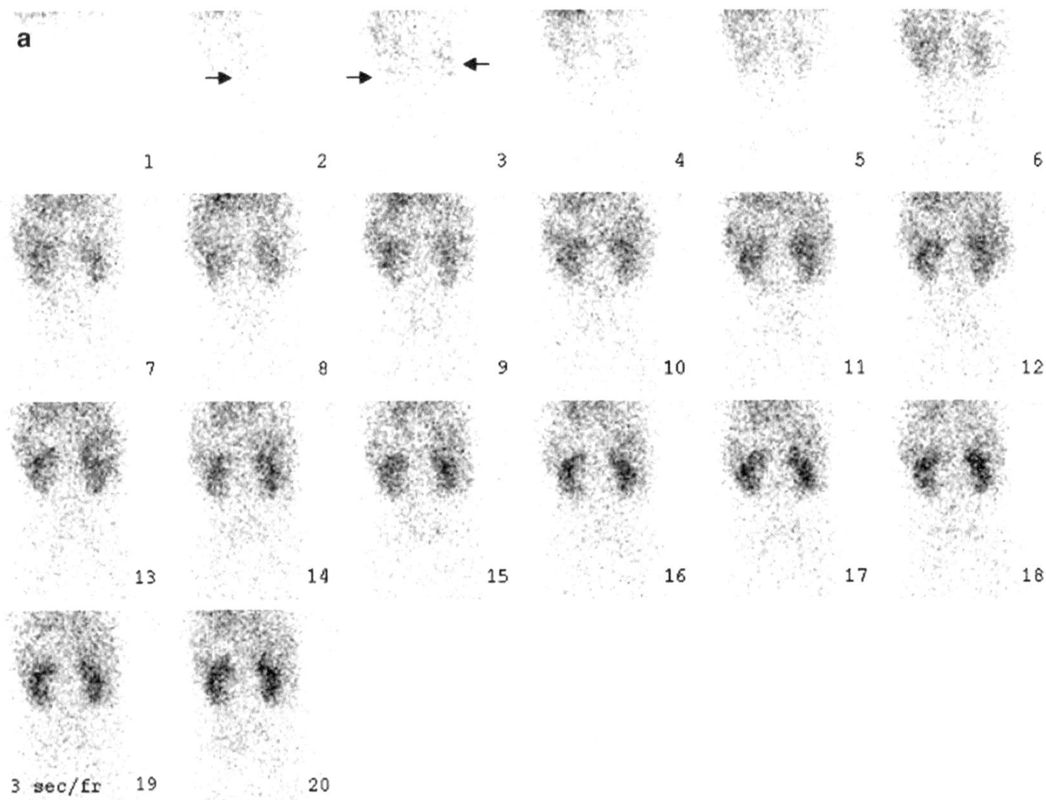

Fig. 6.4 Normal diuretic renography. On the flow phase (**a**) of the study, the abdominal aorta (*arrow*) appears in frame 2. The kidneys (*arrows*) are seen about 3 s later, in frame 3. Visualization of the kidneys within 2–3 s after visualization of the abdominal aorta generally is equated with normal renal perfusion. In the case of the renal transplant (not shown), the kidney should appear within 2–3 s after the iliac artery is seen. On the functional phase (**b**) of the study, the kidneys are similar in size, and there is prompt appearance of activity in the collecting systems and urinary bladder. Adequate hydration is important to the success of diuretic renography. Activity should appear in at least one of the collecting systems within 3–5 min after radionuclide injection. Alternatively bladder activity should appear within 10 min after injection. In this patient, activity is clearly seen in both collecting systems and the urinary bladder on frame 1 or about 3 min after injection

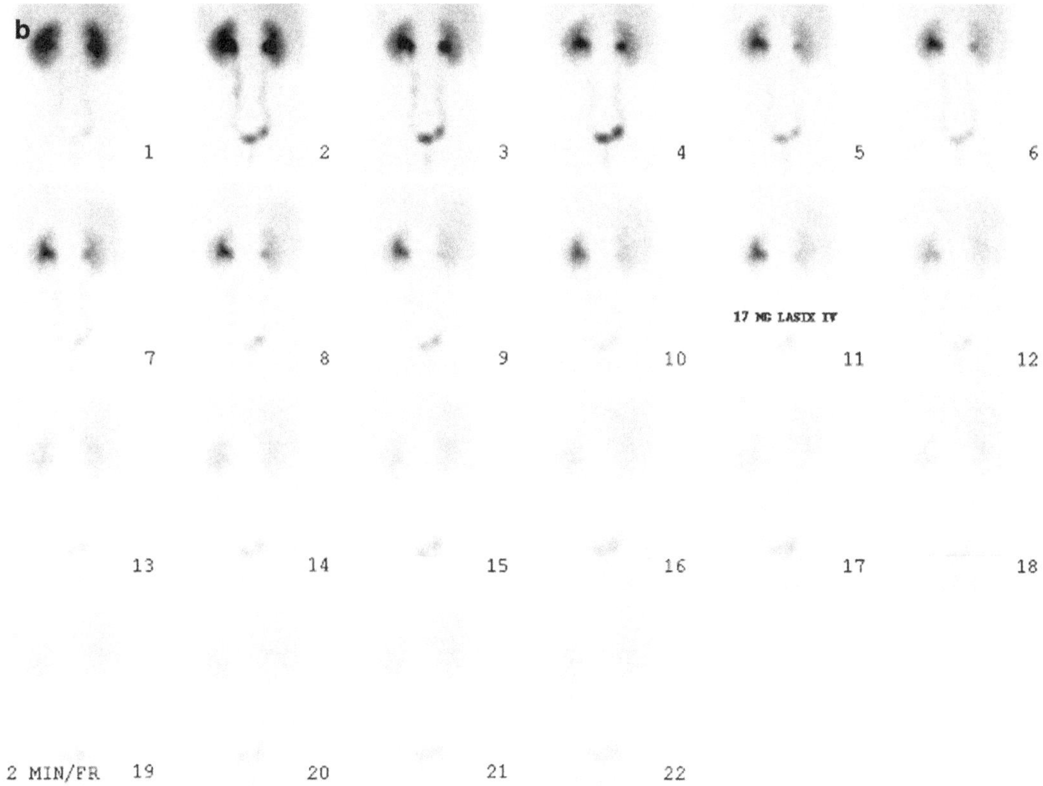

Fig. 6.4 (continued)

the collecting system is thought to be full. Other centers advocate simultaneous administration of tracer and diuretic (F0) in cases of known hydronephrosis [55]. To ensure uniform distribution of radiotracer throughout the collecting system, the child may be placed prone or in the sitting position to maximize drainage. In the setting of hydronephrosis, the ROI for the diuretic time-activity curve should only include the renal pelvis and collecting system. The background ROI should circumscribe the kidney excluding the hilum. For children with hydroureteronephrosis, the ROI for the diuretic time-activity curve should be placed around the dilated renal pelvis with a separate ROI circumscribing the ureter to the level of the UVJ making sure to exclude the urinary bladder.

Computer frame rates are recorded every 20 s for 40 min. Drainage can be calculated by determining the time it takes for half of the tracer activity to leave the collecting system after diuretic administration ($t_{1/2}$ washout), estimating output efficiency (OE), or calculating normalized residual activity (NORA) (Fig. 6.5).

Defining Renal Obstruction

The differentiation of antenatal hydronephrosis from significant renal obstruction that causes deterioration in function is by nature a retrospective diagnosis. Prior to the advent of routine antenatal ultrasound screening, most cases of UPJ or UVJ obstruction were detected later in life when patients developed symptoms. Since the 1970s, antenatal hydronephrosis has been commonly detected via ultrasound. Because this antenatally detected hydronephrosis (presumed urinary obstruction) is asymptomatic in the majority of cases, this poses a diagnostic and therapeutic dilemma for the pediatric urologist. Determining

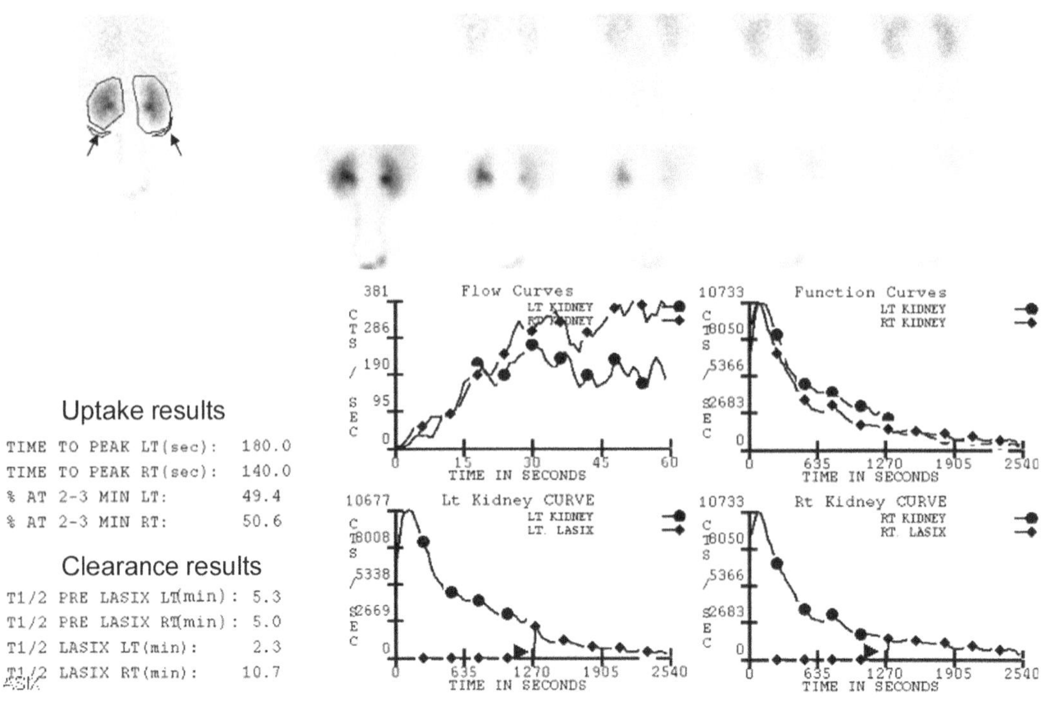

Fig. 6.5 Numeric data from the patient study illustrated in Fig. 6.4. The regions of interest drawn around the kidneys as well as the background regions (*arrows*) are shown in the *upper left image*. The *top left graph* is a representation of renal flow, and the *top right graph* represents renal function. The two graphs below are the individual functional curves of each kidney, with the *vertical bar* (*arrowheads*) indicating the time (approximately 21 min) at which diuretic was administered

which of these patients will require surgery and which will resolve has been challenging.

Historically, several diagnostic tests were used to predict obstruction, including IVP, and direct measures of renal pelvis pressure differentials (Whitaker test). Standard nuclear renograms followed, and renal transit times and/or visual analysis of renogram curves that tracked the passage of radiotracer through the kidney was used to define obstruction. Difficulties with poor image resolution and variations in patient hydration and a significant number of false-negative studies in hydronephrotic patients with delayed renograms without evidence of obstruction limited the usefulness of this technique.

O'Reilly et al. introduced the diuretic renogram (DRG) in the late 1970s in an effort to identify the children with dilated, nonobstructed collecting systems and separate them from children with true obstruction. The analysis of drainage curves was born, and various patterns of drainage were defined. The shape of a normal post-diuretic renal drainage curve was described as brisk and exhibited rapid elimination of tracer (*pattern I*). The "obstructive" pattern (*pattern II*) showed little response to the diuretic with a flat and sometimes rising drainage curve as activity continued to accumulate within the collecting system. A third pattern (*IIIa*) was described which revealed a normal and rapid response to diuretic even after a continually rising or plateau renogram curve. The fourth pattern (*IIIb*), thought to represent obstruction as well, was a rising or plateau renogram curve with no response to diuretic [56, 57].

To further characterize these patients, the concept of $t_{1/2}$ washout, or the time it takes for half of the radiotracer to drain after diuretic injection, was introduced. Three categories were created to stratify patients at risk: $t_{1/2}$ of less than 10 min, definitely normal; $t_{1/2}$ of 10–20 min, indeterminate; and $t_{1/2}$ greater than 20 min, obstructed (Figs. 6.6 and 6.7). Each of these parameters has significant shortcomings, and none have proven accurate enough to make the definitive diagnosis of obstruction in equivocal cases. Several authors have documented spontaneous resolution of hydronephrosis in children previously thought to be obstructed by drainage curve and $t_{1/2}$ washout [58–60].

Calculation of Halftime of Washout or $t_{1/2}$ Washout

The halftime for elimination of radiotracer beginning at the time of diuretic injection, or $t_{1/2}$ washout, has traditionally been the preferred way to define significant urinary obstruction [46, 61]. It is measured in minutes, with less than 10 min being thought of as normal or nonobstructed, 10–20 min as indeterminate, and greater than 20 min as significantly obstructed. Analysis begins at time *t* when the diuretic is administered, usually 20–30 min after injection of the radionuclide or when the collecting system is seen clearly. There is usually a short plateau and then a rapid decrease in activity that corresponds to diuretic response, which then plateaus as drainage of the radioactivity is completed. The shape of the drainage curve can supply useful information. Flat or rising curves are thought to represent obstruction. Use of the $t_{1/2}$ alone is troublesome, as it depends on several factors, including the state of hydration of the patient, the presence of significant hydronephrosis, and the amount of radioactivity at the time of diuretic injection and at the end point of the drainage phase. For example, in kidneys with

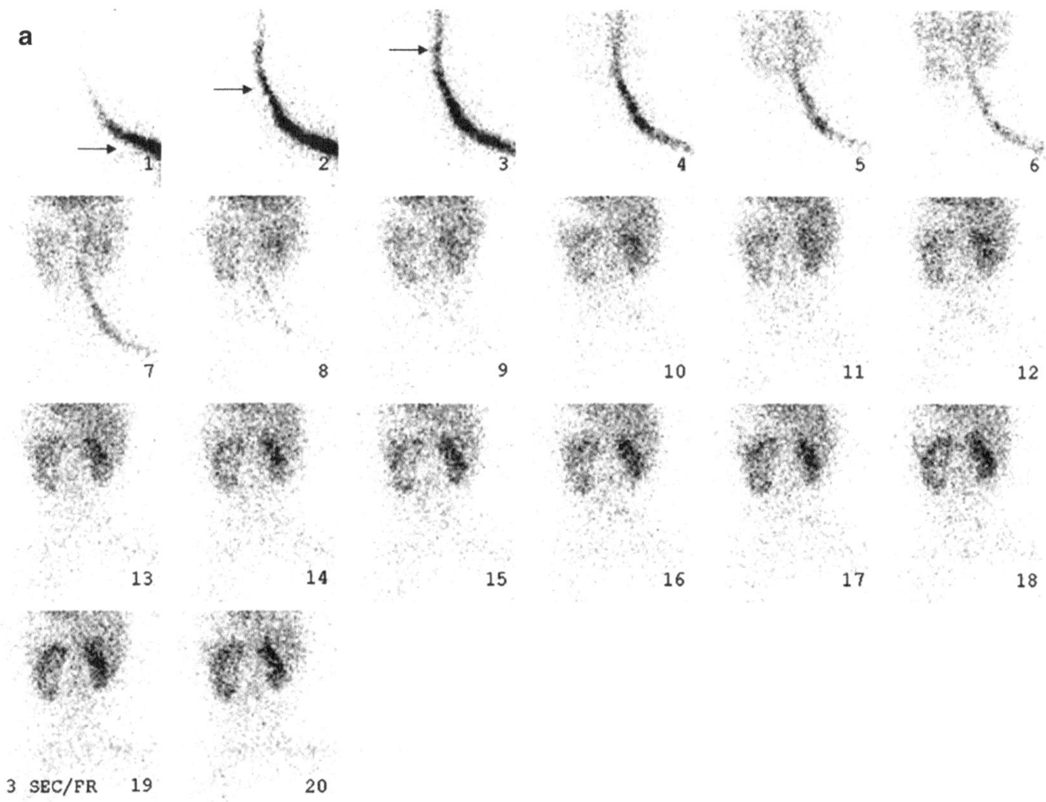

Fig. 6.6 Obstructed left kidney. Flow (**a**) and functional (**b**) images. On the initial images in the flow phase, it appears as if activity is moving retrograde in the aorta (*arrows*). The patient was injected in a lower extremity vein, and this actually is activity ascending through the inferior vena cava. The left kidney is considerably larger than the right. The right collecting system drains spontaneously prior to diuretic challenge, while there is little or no drainage from the left collecting system before or after diuretic challenge

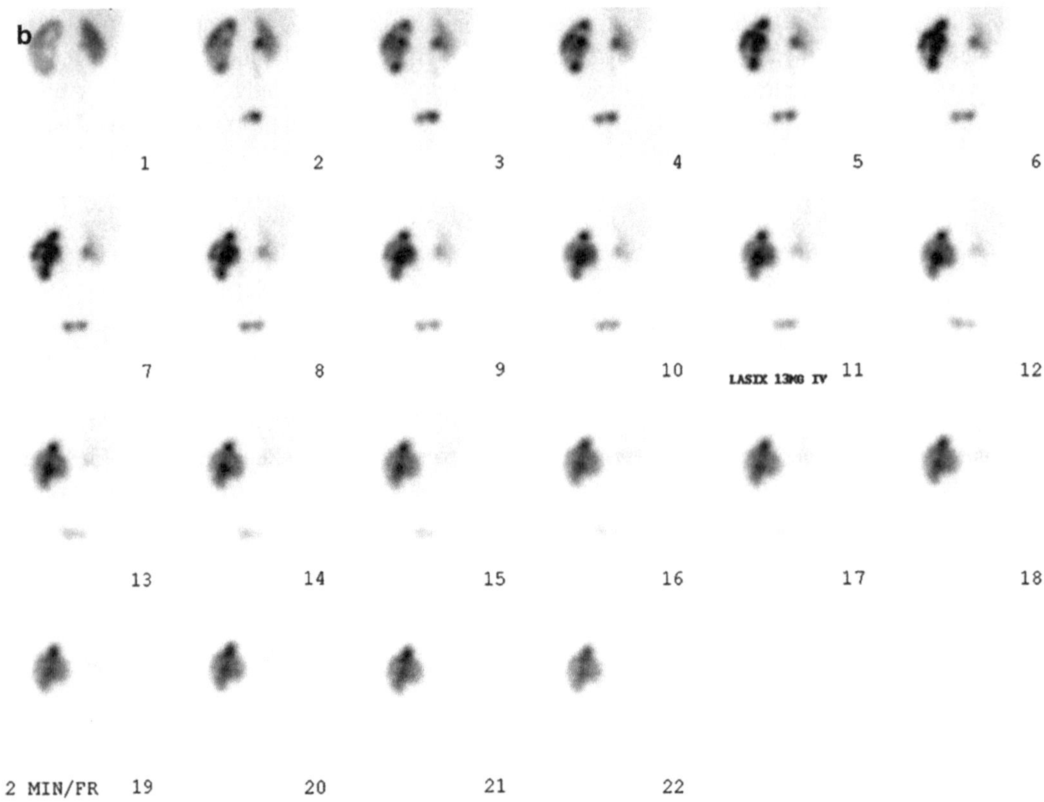

Fig. 6.6 (continued)

normal function with almost complete drainage before the diuretic injection, the drainage curve will be flat and the $t_{1/2}$ washout can be significantly prolonged even though drainage is normal. This underlies the importance of examining the drainage curve and not simply categorizing children by their $t_{1/2}$ washout values alone. As such, $t_{1/2}$ washout values should NOT be reported for kidneys that drain prior to diuretic administration (Fig. 6.7). While the $t_{1/2}$ washout is very useful for excluding obstruction in the setting of normal drainage, there is a significant portion of patients with indeterminate drainage values, and this can lead to diagnostic uncertainty.

Gravity-Assisted Drainage

The standard diuretic renogram is performed with the patient in the supine position. Patients who have nonobstructive significant hydronephrosis and those who have residual atonic renal pelvis after pyeloplasty often exhibit delayed $t_{1/2}$ in the "indeterminate" or "obstructed" range. Several authors suggest that renal drainage can also be positional, with possible improvement in renal drainage upon upright imaging [62, 63]. Wong et al. reported the effects of gravity-assisted drainage (GAD) in a mixed cohort of postoperative pyeloplasties, tapered ureteral reimplants, and children who were managed nonoperatively. GAD was performed by holding the child upright for 5 min after completion of the diuretic phase followed by acquisition of one final image. The upright image was then compared to the last 5 min of the diuretic phase. Using a cutoff value of >50 % residual activity after 5 min of GAD to define obstruction helped to stratify patients with halftimes in the "indeterminate" range. *In patients with a $t_{1/2}$ washout of 10–20 min, sensitivity, specificity, and accuracy for GAD >50 % in defining obstruction*

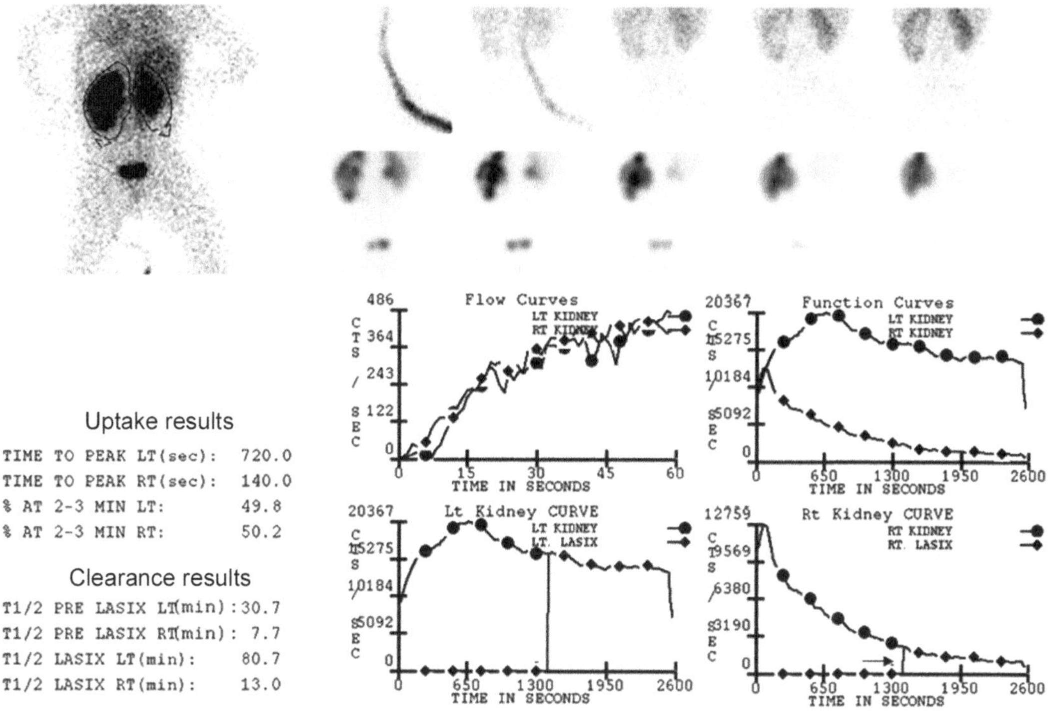

Fig. 6.7 Numeric data from the patient illustrated in Fig. 6.6. The numeric data confirm the visual impression. There is virtually no drainage from the left collecting system at any time during the test. Although the calculated $T_{1/2}$ washout from the left collecting system is 80 min, the curve is nearly flat and we would report this simply as no response to diuretic challenge, consistent with obstruction. Note also that the $T_{1/2}$ washout from the right collecting system is 13 min, which is an equivocal response to diuretic challenge. When the diuretic challenge was given (*arrow*), however, nearly all the activity already had drained from the collecting system, and consequently, this value is not meaningful. We report these situations as spontaneous drainage prior to diuretic challenge and do not report a $T_{1/2}$ washout

were 100 %, 79 %, and 83 %, respectively. In patients with $t_{1/2}$ washout >20 min, sensitivity was 88 %, specificity was 74 %, and accuracy was 84 % [63]. GAD should be a standard component in all diuresis renography studies as it can help clarify and correctly categorize some of those children with indeterminate or equivocal $t_{1/2}$ washout.

Renal Output Efficiency (OE)

Chai defined OE as the total renal output up to a time *t* expressed as a percentage of the total renal input, i.e., the amount of tracer that has left the kidney at a selected time expressed as a percentage of what the kidney has extracted from the blood [64]. OE provides an objective measure of the renal response to diuretic challenge taking into account renal function and thus may be more useful in children with reduced renal function. Images of the left ventricle are used to generate a blood clearance curve which is fitted to the rising phase of a background-corrected whole kidney time-activity curve. This represents the kidney input as a function of time. Post-diuretic background-corrected renal output is then subtracted from input and expressed as a percentage of the corrected renal input. OE can be calculated at any point during the study (time *t*); however, the input images during the first 1–2 min of the study must be used.

An OE for "normal kidneys" is defined as at least *78 % in adults* [64]. Saunders et al. compared OE to DRG in 74 young children (91 renal units) with a median age of 4 months.

Final outcomes were determined by surgical pathology and clinical follow-up. OE was calculated at 20 min post-diuretic injection and after gravity-assisted drainage. The children were initially stratified by DRG findings; obstruction on DRG was defined as at least two of the following: $t_{1/2} > 20$ min, split renal function <40 %, and by visual assessment of a flat or rising post-diuretic drainage curve. Normal OE values were obtained by assessing the non-hydronephrotic contralateral kidney. In non-hydronephrotic kidneys, the mean OE was 96 % compared to 93 % in hydronephrotic but unobstructed kidneys. The *lower limit of normal was defined as 79 %* (2 SD below the mean in hydronephrotic nonobstructed kidneys). $T_{1/2}$ washout on diuretic renography initially stratified the patients as 52 nonobstructed, 20 indeterminate, and 19 obstructed. Using a value of <79 %, OE classified 61 patients as normal and 20 as obstructed. The final diagnosis revealed true obstruction in 22 and no obstruction in 69. This resulted in an *overall diagnostic accuracy for OE of 89 %*. In the indeterminate group, OE correctly classified all cases of obstruction, and 56 % of those found not to be obstructed. Interestingly, OE performed well in a subgroup of patients with reduced differential renal function (mean DRF 32 %) detecting all true cases of obstruction and classifying ~70 % of unobstructed patients correctly. This resulted in a *sensitivity of 100 %, a specificity of 82 %, and an accuracy of 80 % in children with mild to moderate renal dysfunction* [65].

Normalized Residual Activity (NORA)

Normalized residual activity (NORA), first described by Piepsz et al. in 2000, can be thought of as complementary to OE [66]. It is the ratio between any 60-s interval of renal activity during a given time and the first 60–120 s of the study. NORA can be calculated at any point during the study regardless of whether diuretic has been given. Typical acquisition times are at the end of the renogram, the end of the furosemide test, and after voiding. In other words, while OE describes what has left the kidney, NORA describes what remains behind.

Normal values were described in *Piepsz's* study comparing NORA values to OE in 175 normal kidneys and 82 postoperative dilated but not obstructed kidneys. As expected, *NORA in normal kidneys at 20 min was almost always <1.0* because normal adequate drainage has already occurred. When NORA is plotted versus OE values obtained at 20 min, there is an excellent linear correlation ($R^2 = -0.917$), which further confirms the complementary nature of the two parameters. Of note, the choice of background correction plays a role in NORA calculations with perirenal or subrenal background ROIs making up 67 or 83 % of the value obtained without background correction. Therefore, background correction should be standardized when reporting this parameter [67]. NORA has been found to be less robust than OE in patients with diminished renal function [68]. The results of this new quantitative parameter are interesting and potentially useful, but further study is required to compare values in patients with known obstruction.

Radionuclide Cystography

Traditionally, VCUG utilizing fluoroscopy has been the standard for the initial diagnosis of vesicoureteral reflux. In an effort to minimize radiation exposure, Winter introduced direct radionuclide cystography in 1959 [69]. Because image resolution is inferior to that of VCUG and precise grading is not possible, most centers in the United States use radionuclide cystography selectively. In a survey of North American pediatric urologists, Ellison et al. reported that only 1–3 % of those polled routinely ordered radionuclide cystography for children with antenatal hydronephrosis or after a first febrile UTI compared with 97–99 % who ordered VCUG. Radionuclide cystography was, however, utilized more frequently in the setting of vesicoureteral reflux follow-up (44 %) and in sibling screening (29 %) [70].

Direct Radionuclide Cystography

Access to the bladder is made sterilely either by urethral catheter (5–8 Fr), by Foley catheter with a deflated balloon during the voiding portion of the study, or by direct percutaneous suprapubic injection [71]. ^{99m}Tc-Pertechnate is the most commonly used radiotracer, but ^{99m}Tc-sulfur colloid or ^{99m}Tc-DTPA should be used in children with augmented bladders as these compounds are not absorbed via the bowel mucosa used in the augmentation [72]. The administered dose (0.5–1.0 mCi/kg) is the same for all three tracers. The radiotracer is mixed in 250–500 mL of sterile saline and hung approximately 70–100 cm above the table. Filling is complete when the age-appropriate volume is reached or upon cessation of flow from the bottle of solution.

The gamma camera is placed under the supine patient during the filling phase, and computer images are obtained at 5 s/frame. Once filling is complete, the cooperative patient is positioned upright with the camera posterior. Computer images are obtained every 2–10 s, and analog images are taken every 30–60 s. Pre- and post-void bladder images are taken, and regions of interest are drawn around the bladder to calculate the postvoid residual.

The presence and duration of reflux, and if possible the estimated bladder volume during reflux, are reported. Grading is categorized as *mild*, tracer only in the ureter; *moderate*, tracer in a nondilated collecting system and ureter; and *severe*, tracer within a dilated collecting system and ureter (Fig. 6.8). Some authors have attempted to correlate reflux with bladder volumes and voiding with limited success [73, 74].

Acknowledged sources of error include inadequate bladder drainage in smaller caliber catheters, leakage of urine (and tracer) around the

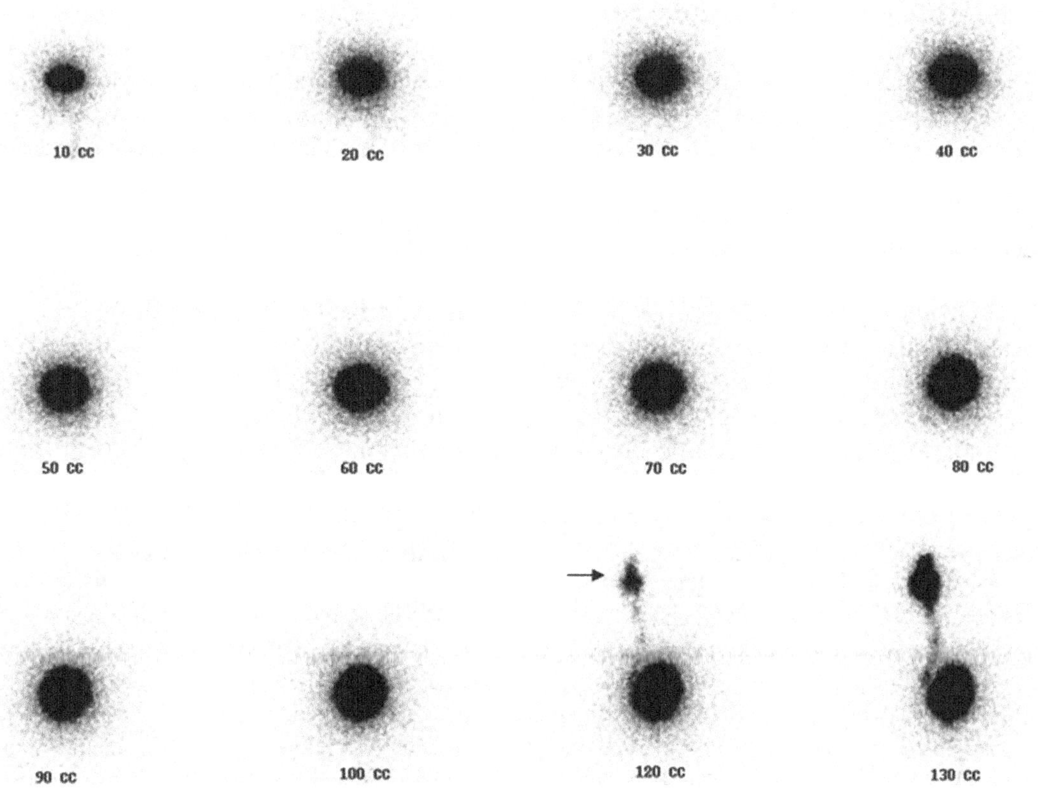

Fig. 6.8 Severe vesicoureteral reflux on direct radionuclide cystography. Activity extending into a dilated left pelvis/collecting system (*arrow*) can be appreciated when the urinary bladder volume is 120 cm^3

catheter, and skin contamination by urine. The latter two may result in false-positive exams.

Percutaneous Direct Radionuclide Cystography Technique

This technique, proposed by Wilkinson et al. in 2002, was aimed for use in older, toilet-trained children who seek to avoid the discomfort of urethral catheterization [71, 75]. EMLA or topical lidocaine is applied to the suprapubic area of puncture 45 min prior to initiation of the study. The child is encouraged to drink liquids, and bladder fullness is assessed by ultrasound. Ultrasound is also used to measure the distance between the skin and bladder, if less than 12 mm a 25 gauge needle can be used to inject the radiotracer directly into the full bladder. Larger needles may be necessary in older or more obese children.

Indirect Radionuclide Cystogram

The indirect radionuclide cystogram relies on patient cooperation to a much greater extent than direct cystography. As there is no urethral catheterization, the child must be able to voluntarily void and must remain still, or the test cannot be completed. The radiotracer of choice is ^{99m}Tc-MAG3, but ^{99m}Tc-DTPA can also be used at a dose of 0.08–0.12 mCi, administered either via venipuncture or IV catheter. Indirect cystography requires a conventional dynamic renal scan prior to the voiding phase of the study.

The child is placed supine with the camera posterior. Images are acquired at 1–4-s intervals for the first minute, followed by images at 1–5-min intervals for 30–60 min or until at least 80 % of the tracer has left the collecting system and entered the bladder. If necessary, the child can be positioned upright to aid in kidney drainage prior to voiding images. For the voiding phase, the child is asked to sit, and the camera is again placed posterior. When the child reports the urge to void, 2–10-s computer images are obtained until the end of voiding. Any patient movement during image acquisition can lead to spurious results. Of note, reflux can only be detected during the voiding phase, and if the patient cannot void, the test cannot be interpreted.

Direct Radionuclide Cystography Versus VCUG

Early studies suggest that DRC is comparable to VCUG in the detection of VUR and may be slightly more sensitive. Agreement between DRC and VCUG has been reported to be around 80 % with DRC detecting 17 % of cases missed by VCUG [76–78]. Kogan et al. report several cases of clinically significant VUR detected only on DRC and missed by VCUG in a highly selected population. They recommend supplemental DRC in those children with negative VCUG who have a clinical history of multiple febrile UTIs and/or cortical imaging suggestive of renal scarring due to occult reflux [78]. McLaren et al. found DRC to be even more sensitive than VCUG when prospectively examining infants presenting with febrile UTI. Each patient underwent both diagnostic studies yielding a sensitivity of 45 % for VCUG and 91 % for DRC. However, DRC missed half of grade 1, 20 % of grade 2, and 6 % of grade 3 VUR found on VCUG [79].

Direct Radionuclide Cystography Versus Indirect Radionuclide Cystography

Due to the nature of IRC, which relies on bladder filling after a dynamic renogram, only the voiding and postvoiding phases can be interpreted. The injected radiotracer must be cleared from the blood and excreted by the kidneys, and only after tracer has exited the collecting system and ureters can the study begin. Early reflux can potentially be masked by tracer already present in the ureter, or conversely ureteral tracer from the drainage phase could be interpreted as VUR. This significant limitation to the technique may potentially lead to false-negative or false-positive results. Early reports comparing the two tests confirm this concern. In a study of 137 patients who underwent concurrent DRC and IRC, Conway et al. reported that 21 % of cases of VUR occurred only during the filling phase and would not be detectable by IRC [80].

Despite the logistical advantages (ease of interpretation, decreased radiation dose) of DRC versus IRC, many centers in Europe and Australia prefer IRC because it avoids urethral catheterization despite decreased sensitivity and specificity versus VCUG or DRC. When compared to VCUG as the standard, sensitivities range from 41 to 82 % and specificities from 44 to 90 % [81–86].

Percutaneous Direct Radionuclide Cystography Versus IRC and VCUG

In Wilkinson's report proposing suprapubic injection of radiotracer, 94 % of injections were successful in one attempt, and approximately 82 % of patients reported the suprapubic injections caused less discomfort than the IV placement required for IRC. Detection of reflux by PDRC was approximately half that of previously reported by IRC in the same patients (28 % vs. 66 %), but 30 % of the patients studied by PDRC had previously undergone corrective surgery for their reflux. Additionally, PDRC was performed in most cases up to a year after the initial IRC, thus allowing some cases of VUR to potentially resolve [71]. Jose et al. reported slightly better results in a more carefully selected patient population with VCUG and PDRC concordant in 90 %. *Sensitivity, specificity, and accuracy compared to VCUG were 76 %, 100 %, and 92 %,* respectively. Given its feasibility and excellent patient tolerability, it seems to be a technique that warrants further study, especially in older children who seek to avoid catheterization [75].

Scrotal Scintigraphy

Differentiating testicular torsion from epididymo-orchitis relying solely on clinical judgment can be quite challenging and often results in unnecessary scrotal exploration. Scrotal scintigraphy, first introduced in 1973 by Nadel et al. [87] to evaluate acute testicular pain, for many years was used as a first-line diagnostic modality to distinguish testis ischemia from inflammatory processes. More recently, color and power Doppler ultrasonography has been shown to be a powerful and noninvasive tool for evaluating testicular blood flow that does not involve ionizing radiation. This has obviated the need for scrotal scintigraphy in most situations. Several authors advocate combined ultrasonography and scrotal scintigraphy in equivocal cases.

Scrotal Scintigraphy Technique

^{99m}Tc-Pertechnate is given intravenously at a dose of 0.1 mCi/kg, with a minimum dose of 2 mCi and a maximum dose of 15 mCi. To prevent tracer uptake by the thyroid gland, 6 mg/kg of potassium perchlorate is given orally prior to the study. The patient is placed supine and the penis is secured superiorly and the scrotum is gently elevated above the thighs. The exam is then performed in two phases, angiography and static scintigraphy.

Tracer is given IV as a rapid bolus, and a low-energy collimator is used to record one frame per second for 60 s for the flow phase. After the flow phase is completed and without moving the camera, a single static image of the scrotum is obtained for 300,000–500,000 counts. A lead apron is placed over the thighs and under the scrotum to minimize background interference, and another lead apron is placed over the suprapubic area to obscure any bladder activity. Once appropriately shielded, another anterior static image is acquired using a pinhole collimator for 150,000 counts. If necessary, a cobalt 57 line source, or lead strip, may be placed in the midline to delineate the scrotal raphe.

Interpretation of Scrotal Scintigraphy

Normally, tracer activity is rarely seen in the scrotum during the flow phase of the study due to the relatively low blood flow in the area. Instead,

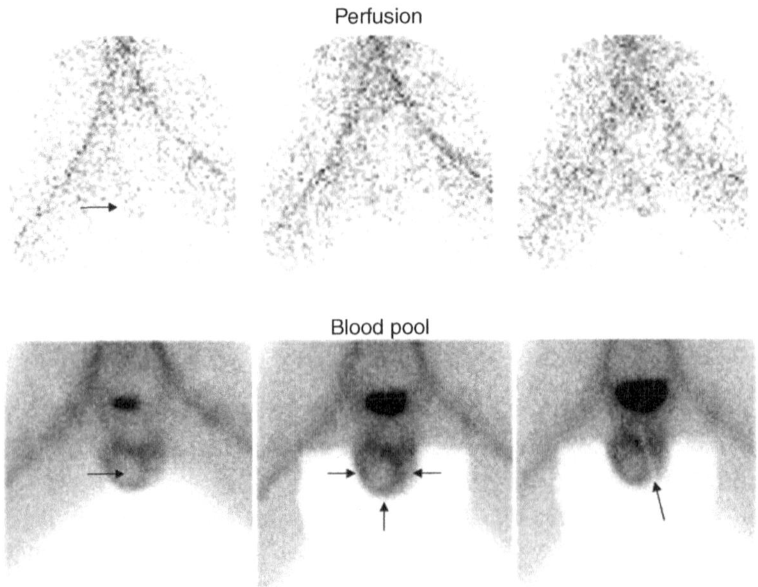

Fig. 6.9 Late testicular torsion. An 11-year-old boy presented with a 3-day history of right scrotal pain. There is mildly increased blood flow (*arrow*) to the right hemiscrotum on the perfusion (flow) phase of the study. On the blood-pool phase, in the near *left image*, there is a discrete photopenic defect (*arrow*) in the right hemiscrotum. There is a hyperemic rim (*arrows, center image*) surrounding this region. This is the typical presentation of late torsion. On the far *right image*, a lead shield has been placed on the median raphe (*arrow*), to help distinguish the right and left halves of the scrotum. A necrotic right testis was removed at surgery

tracer is more often visualized in the iliac and femoral vessels and in the soft tissue of the thighs. The static images should show symmetric uniform tracer uptake in the scrotum.

During *early acute torsion (<24 h)*, the flow phase often is normal, but on static images, there is reduced or absent uptake in the affected hemiscrotum. After a few hours of symptoms, there is sometimes a rim of increased tracer uptake surrounding the involved testicle.

In *late torsion (>24 h)*, the flow phase may show a central region of decreased or absent activity corresponding to the affected testis. There can also be a peripheral rim of increased activity. Static images also show a similar pattern of decreased or absent activity surrounded by an area of increased activity (Fig. 6.9).

In contrast to testicular torsion, *inflammatory processes such as epididymitis and orchitis* will appear as increased activity on both the flow and static images (Fig. 6.10). An abscess may have an appearance similar to that of late testicular torsion. The often irregular border of an abscess and a rim of hyperperfusion that is not always completely circumferential may help to differentiate this condition from late torsion.

Torsion of the epididymal appendage is rarely if ever demonstrated on scrotal scintigraphy as it lacks the necessary resolution. A torsed appendage can appear as normal or increased flow on the flow phase and appears as normal on the static image. However, the aim of study is to exclude testicular torsion.

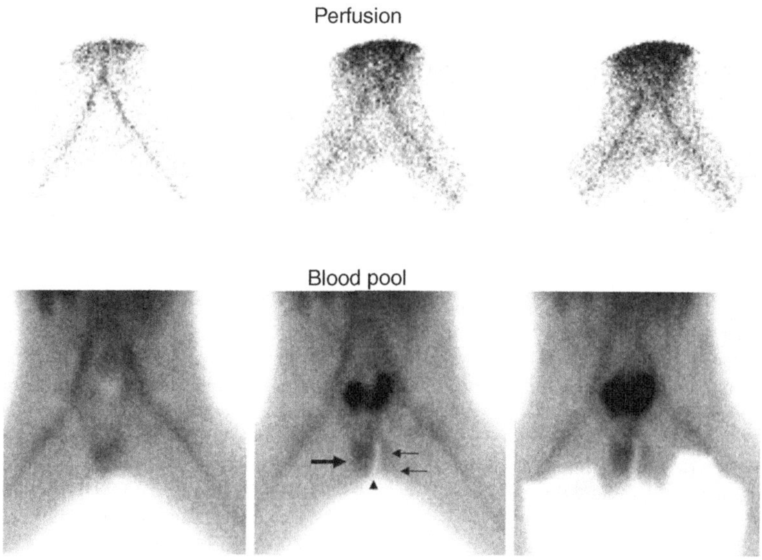

Fig. 6.10 Inflammation. A 4-year-old boy presented with a 4-day history of right scrotal pain. There is very mild hyperperfusion to the right hemiscrotum on the perfusion phase of the study. On the blood-pool images, there is diffusely increased activity throughout the right hemiscrotum (*thick arrow*). Compare with the left hemiscrotum (*arrows*). A lead strip has been placed on the median raphe (*arrowhead*)

References

1. Enlander D, Weber PM, dos Remedios LV. Renal cortical imaging in 35 patients: superior quality with 99Tc-DMSA. J Nucl Med. 1974;15:743–9.
2. Peters AM, Jones DH, Evans K, et al. Two routes for 99mTc-DMSA uptake into the renal cortical tubular cell. Eur J Nucl Med. 1988;14:555–61.
3. de Lange MJ, Piers DA, Kosterink JG, et al. Renal handling of 99mTc-DMSA: evidence for glomerular filtration. J Nucl Med. 1989;30:1219–23.
4. Kawamura J, Hosokawa S, Yoshida O, et al. Renal function studies using 99mTc-DMSA. Clin Nucl Med. 1979;4:39–46.
5. Durand E, Prigent A. Can dimercaptosuccinic acid be used to assess global renal function? Eur J Nucl Med. 2000;27(7):727–9.
6. Krill A, Cubillos J, Gitlin J, et al. Abdominopelvic ultrasound: a cost-effective way to diagnose solitary kidney. J Urol. 2012;187:2201–4.
7. Itoh K. 99mTc-MAG3: review of pharmacokinetics, clinical application to renal diseases and quantification of renal function. Ann Nucl Med. 2001;15(3):179–90.
8. Al-Nahhas AA, Jafri RA, Britton KE, et al. Clinical experience with 99mTc-MAG3, mercaptoacetyltriglycine, and a comparison with 99mTc-DTPA. Eur J Nucl Med. 1988;14:453–62.
9. Bubeck B, Brandau W, Steinbacher M, et al. Technetium-99m labeled renal function and imaging agents: II. Clinical evaluation of 99mTc-MAG3. Int J Rad App Instrum B. 1988;15:109–18.
10. Taylor A, Eshima D, Alazraki N. 99mTc-MAG3, A new renal imaging agent: preliminary results in patients. Eur J Nucl Med. 1987;12:510–14.
11. Ritchie G, Wilkinson AG, Prescott RJ. Comparison of differential renal function using 99mTc-MAG3 and 99mTc-DMSA renography in a paediatric population. Pediatr Radiol. 2008;38:857–62.
12. Gordon I, Anderson PJ, Lythgoe MF, et al. Can 99mTc-MAG3 replace 99mTc-DMSA in the exclusion of a focal renal defect? J Nucl Med. 1992;33:2090–3.
13. Bair HJ, Becker W, Schott G, et al. Is there still a need for 99mTc-DMSA renal imaging? Clin Nucl Med. 1995;20:18–21.
14. Hauser W, Atkins HL, Nelson KG, et al. 99mTc-DTPA: a new radiopharmaceutical for brain and kidney scanning. Radiology. 1970;94:679–84.
15. Klopper JF, Hauser W, Atkins HL, et al. Evaluation of 99mTc-DTPA for the measurement of GFR. J Nucl Med. 1972;13:107–10.
16. Taylor A, Nally JV. Clinical applications of renal scintigraphy. Am J Roentgenol. 1995;164:31–41.
17. Taylor A, Clark S, Ball T. Comparison of 99mTc-MAG3 and 99mTc-DTPA scintigraphy in neonates. Clin Nucl Med. 1994;19:575–80.
18. Smith T, Gordon I, Kelly JP. Comparison of radiation dose from intravenous pyelography and 99mTc-DMSA scintigraphy in children. Br J Radiol. 1998;71:314–19.
19. Stabin MG. In: Treves ST, editor. Pediatric nuclear medicine. 2nd ed. Internal Dosimetry in Pediatric Nuclear Medicine. New York: Springer; 1995. p. 556–78.

20. Ward VL, Strauss KJ, Barnewolt CE, et al. Pediatric radiation exposure and effective dose reduction during voiding cystourethrography. Radiology. 2008; 249(3):1002–9.
21. Braren V, Versage PN, Touya JJ, et al. Radioisotopic determination of glomerular filtration rate. J Urol. 1979;121:145–7.
22. Klopper JF, Hauser W, Atkins HL, et al. Evaluation of 99mTc-DTPA for the measurement of glomerular filtration rate. J Nucl Med. 1972;13:107–10.
23. Gates GF. Glomerular filtration rate: estimation from fractional renal accumulation of 99mTc-DTPA (Stannous). AJR Am J Roentgenol. 1982;138:565–70.
24. Koff SA, McDowell GC, Byard M. Diuretic radionuclide assessment of obstruction in the infant. J Urol. 1988;140:1167.
25. Gonzalez R, Chiou RK. The diagnosis of upper urinary tract obstruction in children: comparison of diuresis renography and pressure flow studies. J Urol. 1985;133:646–9.
26. Chandhoke PS, Kogan BA, Al-Dahwi A, et al. Monitoring renal function in children with urological abnormalities. J Urol. 1990;144:601–5.
27. Hansson S, Dhamey M, Sigstrom O, et al. DMSA scintigraphy instead of voiding cystourethrography for infants with urinary tract infection. J Urol. 2004;172:1071–4.
28. Pohl HG, Belman AB. The "top-down" approach to the evaluation of children with febrile UTI. Adv Urol. 2009: 1–5.
29. Prigent A, Cosgriff P, Gates G, et al. Consensus on quality control of quantitative measurements from the renogram: International Consensus Committee from the Scientific Committee of Radionuclides in Nephrourology. Semin Nucl Med. 1999;29(2):146–59.
30. Piepsz A, Blaufox MD, Gordon I, et al. Consensus on renal cortical scintigraphy in children with UTI. Semin Nucl Med. 1999;29(2):160–74.
31. Zeissman HA, Majd M. Importance of methodology on 99mTc-DMSA image quality: imaging pilot study for RIVUR multicenter investigation. J Urol. 2009;182:272–9.
32. Applegate KE, Connolly LP, Davis RT, et al. A prospective comparison of high resolution planar, pinhole and triple detector SPECT for the comparison of renal cortical defects. Clin Nucl Med. 1997; 22(10):673–8.
33. Rodriguez JL, Perera A, Fraxedas R, et al. Renal 99mTc-DMSA SPET and planar imaging: are they really the same? Nucl Med Commun. 1997;18:556.
34. Rossleigh MA, Farnsworth RH, Leighton DM, et al. 99mTc-DMSA scintigraphy studies of renal cortical scarring and length. J Nucl Med. 1998;39(7):1280–5.
35. Treves ST, Majd MM, Kuruc A, et al. Pediatric nuclear medicine. 2nd ed. Chapter 17. New York: Springer; 1995. p. 339–99.
36. Yen TC, Chen WP, Chang SL, et al. 99mTc-DMSA renal SPECT in diagnosing and monitoring pediatric acute pyelonephritis. J Nucl Med. 1996;37(8):1349–53.
37. Majd M, Rushton HG, Chandra R, et al. 99mTc-DMSA renal cortical scintigraphy to detect experimental acute pyelonephritis in piglets: comparison of planar (pinhole) and SPECT imaging. J Nucl Med. 1996;37(10):1731–4.
38. De Sadeleer C, Tondeur M, Melis K, et al. A multicenter trial on interobserver variability in reporting on 99mTc-DMSA planar scintigraphy: a Belgian survey. J Nucl Med. 2000;41(1):23–6.
39. Gacinovic S, Buscome J, Costa DC, et al. Interobserver agreement in the reporting of Tc-99m DMSA renal studies. Nucl Med Commun. 1996;17:596.
40. Craig JC, Irwig L, Ford M, et al. Reliability of DMSA for the diagnosis of renal parenchymal abnormality in children. Eur J Nucl Med. 2000;27(11):1610–16.
41. Craig JC, Wheeler DM, Irwig L, et al. How accurate is DMSA scintigraphy for the diagnosis of acute pyelonephritis? A meta-analysis of experimental studies. J Nucl Med. 2000;41(6):986–93.
42. Rushton HG, Majd M, Chandra R, et al. Evaluation of 99mTc-DMSA renal scan in experimental acute pyelonephritis in piglets. J Urol. 1998;140:1169–74.
43. Verboven M, Ingels M, Delree M, et al. 99mTc-DMSA scintigraphy in acute UTI in children. Pediatr Radiol. 1990;20:540–2.
44. Tarkington M, Fildes RD, Levin K, et al. High resolution SPECT 99mTC-DMSA renal imaging: a state of the art technique. J Urol. 1990;144:598–600.
45. Peters C, Mandell J, Treves T, et al. The "well tempered" diuretic renogram: a standard method to examine the asymptomatic neonate with hydronephrosis or hydroureteronephrosis. J Nucl Med. 1992;33(11):2047–51.
46. Mandell GA, Cooper JA, Leonard JC, et al. Procedure guidelines for diuretic renography in children. J Nucl Med. 1997;38(10):1647–9.
47. Lythgoe MF, Gordon I, Anderson PJ. The effect of renal maturation on the clearance of 99mTc-MAG3. Eur J Nucl Med. 1994;21(12):1332–7.
48. Gordon I, Piepsz A, Sixt R. Guidelines for standard and diuretic renogram in children. Eur J Nucl Med. 2011;38:1175–88.
49. Nguyen HT, Gluckman GR, Kogan BA. Changing the technique of background subtraction alters calculated renal function on pediatric MAG3 renography. J Urol. 1997;158:1252–6.
50. Ozcan Z, Anderson PJ, Gordon I. Robustness of estimation of differential renal function in infants and children with unilateral prenatal diagnosis of a hydronephrotic kidney on dynamic renography: how real is the supranormal kidney? Eur J Nucl Med Mol Imaging. 2006;33(6):738–44.
51. Oh SJ, Moon DH, Kang WC, et al. Supranormal differential renal function is real but May Be pathological: assessment by ^{99m}Technetium mercaptoacetyltriglycine renal scan of congenital unilateral hydronephrosis. J Urol. 2001;165:2300–4.
52. Capolicchio G, Jednak R, Dinh L, et al. Supranormal renographic differential function in congenital hydronephrosis: fact, not artifact. J Urol. 1999;161:1290.

53. Inanir S, Biykli N, Caliskan B, et al. Contradictory supranormal function in hydronephrotic kidneys: fact or artifact on pediatric MAG3 renal scans? Clin Nucl Med. 2005;30(2):91–6.
54. Gungor F, Anderson P, Gordon I. Effect of the size of regions of interest on the estimation of differential renal function in children with congenital hydronephrosis. Nucl Med Commun. 2002;23:147–51.
55. Piepsz A. Antenatal detection of pelviureteric junction stenosis: main controversies. Semin Nucl Med. 2011;41:11–9.
56. O'Reilly PH, Testa HJ, Lawson RS, et al. Diuresis renography in equivocal urinary tract obstruction. Br J Urol. 1978;50:76–80.
57. O'Reilly PH, Lawson RS, Shields RA, et al. Idiopathic hydronephrosis-the diuresis renogram: a New Non-invasive method of assessing equivocal pelvioureteral junction obstruction. J Urol. 1979;121:153–5.
58. Ransley PG, Dhillon HK, Gordon I, et al. The postnatal management of hydronephrosis diagnosed by prenatal ultrasound. J Urol. 1990;144:584.
59. Ulman I, Jayanthi VR, Koff SA. The long-term follow-up of newborns with severe unilateral hydronephrosis initially treated nonoperatively. J Urol. 2000;164:1101–5.
60. Ross SS, Kardos S, Krill A, et al. Observation of infants with SFU grades 3–4 hydronephrosis: worsening drainage with serial diuresis renography indicates surgical intervention and helps prevent loss of renal function. J Pediatr Urol. 2011;7:266–71.
61. Rossleigh MA, Thomas MY, Moase AL. Determination of the normal range of furosemide half-clearance times when using MAG3. Clin Nucl Med. 1994;19:880–2.
62. Rossleigh MA, Leighton DM, Farnsworth RH. Diuretic renography: the need for an additional view after gravity assisted drainage. Clin Nucl Med. 1993;18:210–13.
63. Wong DC, Rossleigh MA, Farnsworth RH. Diuretic renography with the addition of quantitative gravity-assisted drainage in infants and children. J Nucl Med. 2000;41(6):1030–6.
64. Chaiwatanarat T, Padhy AK, Bomaji JB, et al. Validation of renal output efficiency as an objective parameter in the evaluation of upper urinary tract obstruction. J Nucl Med. 1993;34(5):845–8.
65. Saunders CAB, Choong KL, Larcos G, et al. Assessment of pediatric hydronephrosis using output efficiency. J Nucl Med. 1997;38(9):1483–6.
66. Piepsz A, Tondeur M, Ham H. NORA: a simple and reliable parameter for estimating renal output with or without furosemide challenge. Nucl Med Commun. 2000;21:317–23.
67. Piepsz A, Kuyvenhoven JD, Tondeur M, et al. Normalized residual activity: usual values and robustness of the method. J Nucl Med. 2002;43(1):33–8.
68. Nimmon CC, Samal M, Britton KE. Elimination of total renal function on renal output efficiency and normalized residual activity. J Nucl Med. 2004;45(4):587–93.
69. Winter CC. A new test for vesicoureteral reflux: an external technique using radioisotopes. J Urol. 1959;81:105–11.
70. Ellison JS, Maxfield CM, Wiener JM. Voiding cystography practices of North American pediatric urologists. J Urol. 2009;182:299–305.
71. Wilkinson AG. Percutaneous direct radionuclide cystography in children: description of technique and early experience. Pediatr Radiol. 2002;32:511–17.
72. Mandell GA, Eggli DF, Gilday DL, et al. Procedure guideline for radionuclide cystography in children. J Nucl Med. 1997;38(10):1650–4.
73. McLaren CJ, Simpson ET. Direct comparison of radiology and nuclear medicine cystograms in young infants with vesico-ureteral reflux. BJU Int. 2001;87:93–7.
74. Mozley PD, Heyman S, Duckett JW, et al. Direct vesicoureteral scintigraphy: quantifying early outcome predictors in children with primary reflux. J Nucl Med. 1994;35(10):1602–8.
75. Jose TE, Mohiudheen H, Patel C, et al. Direct radionuclide cystography by suprapubic puncture: comparison with voiding cystourethrography. Nucl Med Commun. 2004;25(4):383–5.
76. Nasrallah PF, Nara S, Crawford J. Clinical applications of nuclear cystography. J Urol. 1982; 128:550–3.
77. Sukan A, Bayazit AK, Kibar M, et al. Comparison of direct radionuclide cystography and voiding direct cystography in the detection of vesicoureteral reflux. Ann Nucl Med. 2003;17(7):549–53.
78. Kogan SJ, Sigler L, Levitt SB, et al. Elusive vesicoureteral reflux in children with normal contrast cystograms. J Urol. 1986;136:325–8.
79. McLaren CJ, Simpson ET. Vesico-ureteral reflux in the young infant with follow-up direct radionuclide cystograms: the medical and surgical outcome at 5 years old. BJU Int. 2002;90:721–4.
80. Conway JJ. Kruglik. Effectiveness of direct and indirect radionuclide cystography in detecting vesicoureteral reflux. J Nucl Med. 1976;17(2):81–3.
81. Merrick MV, Uttley WS, Wild R. A comparison of Two techniques in detecting vesicoureteral reflux. Br J Radiol. 1979;50:792–5.
82. Nielsen JB, Jensen FT, Munch JT, et al. The diagnosis of VUR- radiologic and nuclear medicine methods. Scand J Urol Nephrol. 1985;19:109–12.
83. Carlsen O, Lukman B, Nathan E. Indirect radionuclide reno-cystography for determination of vesicoureteral reflux in children. Eur J Nucl Med. 1986; 12:205–10.
84. Chapman SJ, Chantler C, Haycock GB, et al. Radionuclide cystography in vesicoureteral reflux. Arch Dis Child. 1988;63:650–1.
85. Gordon I, Peters M, Morony S. Indirect radionuclide cystography: a sensitive technique for the detection of vesico-ureteral reflux. Pediatr Nephrol. 1990;4:604–6.
86. DeSadeleer C, DeBoe V, Desprechins B, et al. How good is 99mTc-MAG3 indirect cystography? Eur J Nucl Med. 1994;21(3):223–7.

87. Nadel NS, Gitter MH, Hahn LC, et al. Pre-operative diagnosis of testicular torsion. Urology. 1973;1:478.
88. Gadd R, Mountford PJ, Oxtoby JW. Effective dose to children and adolescents from radiopharmaceuticals. Nucl Med Commun. 1999;20:569.
89. Fotakis M, Athansopoulou EM, Psarrakos K, et al. Radiation doses to paediatric patients up to 5 years of age undergoing micturating cystourethrography examinations and its dependence on patient age: a Monte Carlo study. BR J Radiol. 2003;76:812.

Radiation Safety

7

Steven G. Gilbert and Richard W. Grady

Introduction

Life on earth depends on electromagnetic radiation. Plants live by converting energy through photosynthesis to grow and thrive and in turn provide food for many of the earth's animals. In our modern age, we depend on radiation-emitting devices, from the sun to our cell phones to radios, from medical imaging technologies to the electricity that powers our homes. In medicine, we derive benefits from many of these radiation-emitting devices, but there are also potential adverse health effects. To effectively explore the health effects of radiation exposure, it is necessary to examine the physics of radiation.

The electromagnetic spectrum is roughly divided into ionizing and nonionizing radiation. The distinction depends on the amount of energy carried by the radiation, which is directly related to the frequency of vibration of the electric and magnetic fields. When the frequency (and hence energy) is high enough, the radiation can separate electrons from atoms, ionizing the material it passes through.

Nonionizing radiation includes ultraviolet, visible, infrared, microwaves, radio, television, and power transmission. Ionizing radiation includes high-energy radiation such as cosmic rays, x-rays, or gamma rays generated by nuclear decay. Ionizing radiation includes several types of subatomic particles such as beta radiation (high-energy electrons) and alpha radiation (helium ions – two protons and two neutrons). Medical x-rays are an example of a common exposure to ionizing radiation used for our benefit. Nuclear radiation is used to generate electricity and cure disease, but is also an important element in military weapons. Nuclear radiation can pose significant risks regarding human exposure and environmental contamination.

History

The turn of the twentieth century marked the beginning of rapid progress in understanding and exploring the power of radiation. This period ushered in a growing appreciation of the potential adverse effects of radiation exposure. In 1903, Marie Curie and Pierre Curie, along with Henri Becquerel, were awarded the Nobel Prize

S.G. Gilbert, PhD, DABT
Institute of Neurotoxicology and Neurological Disorders, Seattle, WA, USA

Department of Environmental and Occupational Health Sciences, School of Public Health and Community Medicine, University of Washington, Seattle, WA, USA

R.W. Grady, MD (✉)
Department of Urology, The University of Washington School of Medicine, Seattle, WA, USA

Division of Pediatric Urology, Department of Surgery, Seattle Children's Hospital, 4800 Sandpoint Way NE, Seattle, WA 98105, USA
e-mail: richard.grady@seattlechildrens.org

L.S. Palmer, J.S. Palmer (eds.), *Pediatric and Adolescent Urologic Imaging*,
DOI 10.1007/978-1-4614-8654-1_7,

in physics for their contributions to understanding radioactivity, including the properties of uranium. The "curie" and the "becquerel" are still used as units of measure in radiation. In 1895, Wilhem Conrad Roentgen discovered x-rays, and in 1901 he was awarded the first Nobel Prize for physics. These discoveries lead to significant advances in medicine. However, by 1911, workers exposed to x-rays and radium (including Marie Curie) were noted to have higher rates than normal of leukemia. In addition, many of those exposed were childless or had children born with significant birth defects.

Once these associations were made, significant challenges were evident in the determination of safe or tolerable radiation dosages. Initial estimates were based on empirical observations. The construction of the Geiger-Muller counter in the 1920s helped quantify radiation intensity but did not edify health-care workers about safe levels of radiation exposure. The first safety standard was based on a measure called the erythema dose (the amount of radiation which would produce reddening of Caucasian skin). At a 1928 meeting in Stockholm, radiologists arbitrarily chose a 0.01 erythema dose per month as the upper limit of exposure. Subsequently, the Committee of Radiation Safety met with commercial manufacturers to define maximal tolerance doses. However, it was not until the United States moved into the era of nuclear weapon development and deployment with the Manhattan Project and the use of nuclear weapons on Japan that scientists were able to more fully assess the short- and long-term health effects of radiation exposure. Even today, exposure limits remain somewhat arbitrary given the low-dose exposure that we receive from naturally occurring radioactivity and cosmic rays [1, 2]. It should be remembered that we evolved with a background exposure to naturally occurring ionizing radiation and we continue to be exposed to low levels of natural background radiation. Some have estimated that 1 in 100 cancers are the result of this background exposure.

Work by Enrico Fermi and others lead to the first sustained nuclear chain reaction in a laboratory beneath the University of Chicago football stadium on December 2, 1942. Subsequently, this knowledge was used to develop the atomic bombs that were dropped on Japan in an effort to end World War II. Much of our understanding of the effects of nuclear radiation exposure has come from the victims in Japan as well as the many workers in uranium mines.

Biologic and Physical Properties

Ionizing Radiation

Ionizing radiation has sufficient energy to produce ion pairs as it passes through matter so that is it frees electrons and leaves the rest of the atoms positively charged such that there is enough energy to remove an electron from an atom. This generates free radicals that will combine with adjacent molecules. The most common free radical generated is produced from water and is a highly reactive hydroxyl radical. Similarly, the ejected free electron is left to alter the structure and activity of adjacent molecules. The energy released is enough to break bonds in DNA leading to significant cellular damage and potential cause cancer. The health effects and dose–response relationship for radiation exposure are well established from human exposures to radiation and from other research. The four main types of ionizing radiation are alpha particles, beta particles (electrons), gamma rays, and x-rays.

Alpha particles are heavyweight and relatively low-energy emissions from the nucleus of radioactive material. The transfer of energy occurs over a very short distance of about 10 cm in air. A piece of paper or layer of skin will stop an alpha particle. The primary hazard occurs in the case of internal exposure to an alpha-emitting material. Cells close to the alpha-particle-emitting material will be damaged. Typical sites of accumulation include bone, kidney, liver, lung, and spleen (see Fig. 7.1).

Beta particles, in contrast, are high-energy, high-speed positrons or electrons that emit ionizing radiation in the form of beta rays. The production of beta particles is termed beta decay. There are two forms of beta decay, β^- and β^+, which respectively give rise to the electron and the positron. Of the three common types of radiation given off by radioactive materials,

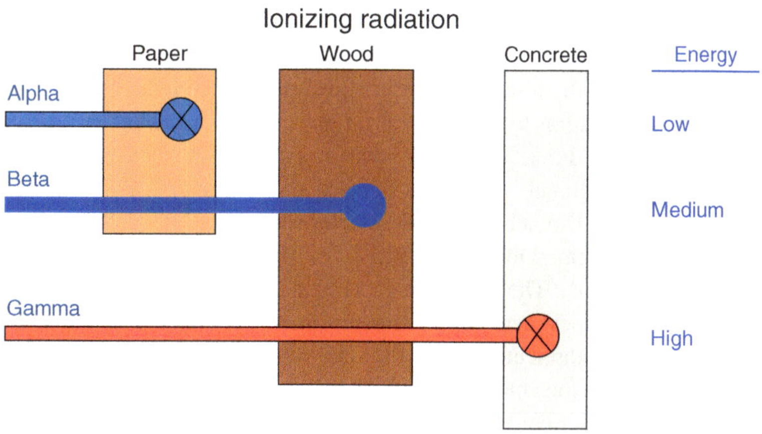

Fig. 7.1 Ionizing energy transmission associated with radiation particles (Adapted from "A Small Dose of Toxicology", with permission)

alpha (Fig. 7.1), beta, and gamma, beta has the medium penetrating power and the medium ionizing power. Although the beta particles given off by different radioactive materials vary in energy, most beta particles can be stopped by a few millimeters of metal such as aluminum or lead. Since it is composed of charged particles, beta radiation is more strongly ionizing than gamma radiation. Beta radiation is used to treat some malignancies, and beta decay is a source of positrons for PET (positron emission tomography) scans where a radiolabeled sugar (fludeoxyglucose) emits positrons that are converted to pairs of gamma rays to localize malignancies since they are typically more metabolically active than other surrounding tissues.

Gamma radiation is a high-frequency, high-energy radiation typically produced by the decay of atomic nuclei in high-energy states such as radium. Unlike alpha and beta particles, gamma rays represent a form of radiation rather than a source of radiation. Gamma rays are distinguished by x-rays by their source of origin; gamma rays are emitted by atomic nuclei, whereas x-rays are emitted by electrons [3]. Protection from gamma rays requires large amounts of mass in contrast to beta and alpha particles. Gamma radiation is used in imaging technologies such as PET scans. Other uses include technetium 99-m that emits gamma rays in the same energy range as diagnostic x-rays. During a technetium 99-m scan, a gamma camera can be used to form an image of the radioisotope's distribution by detecting the gamma radiation emitted.

X-rays are a form of electromagnetic radiation with a wavelength range of 0.01–10 nm with associated energies in the range 100 eV–100 keV. The wavelengths are shorter than those of ultraviolet radiation and typically longer than gamma radiation. X-rays are useful in imaging technology because they can penetrate tissue without significant absorption or scattering. X-ray interaction with matter for the purposes of imaging modalities occurs through photoelectric absorption.

Exposures to ionizing radiation include air travel; this increases our exposure to cosmic and solar radiation that is normally blocked by the atmosphere. Radiation intensity is greater across the poles and at higher altitudes, thus individual exposure varies depending on the route of travel. Storms on the sun can produce solar flares that can release larger amounts of radiation than normal. For the occasional traveler, this radiation exposure is well below recommended limits established by regulatory authorities. However, frequent fliers and airline workers can be exposed to levels of radiation that exceed established guidelines.

Sources of ionizing radiation or exposed populations:

- Medical x-ray devices (patients, health-care employees)
- Radioactive material producing alpha, beta, and gamma radiation (laboratory workers, health-care employees, patients)
- Cosmic rays from the sun and space (air travel)

Radiation Units

The units used to describe exposure and dose of ionizing radiation to living material are confusing, at best. First, the units have changed to an international system, SI (Systeme Internationale). The subsequent description will use the SI system. Different methods exist to measure radiation. The radiation dose that the patient experiences can be measured directly. So, while the fundamental descriptive unit of ionizing radiation is the amount energy, expressed in coulombs or joules per kilogram of air, and is the unit of exposure in air, the absorbed dose is the amount of energy absorbed by a specific material such as the human body and is described as the gray (Gy), previously the rad (radiation absorbed dose). The gray is used to assess absorbed dose in any material. One gray delivers 1 J of energy per kilogram of matter. However, the energy transfer of the different particles and gamma rays is different. A weighting factor is used to allow comparison between these different energy transfers. Further, tissues and organs have different sensitivities to radiation. As a consequence, equivalent and effective dose concepts were developed.

The unit for the equivalent dose is the sievert (Sv). The Sv is used to estimate the stochastic (see below) biologic effect of ionizing radiation on tissue and has an equivalent, effective and committed dose weighted averaging for each biologic tissue. For example, while 1 Sv = 1 J/kg = 1 Gy, the absorbed dose of 1 mGy of alpha radiation would be equal to 20 mSv because of the weighting factors of alpha radiation. A further refinement is possible that applies a weighting factor to each type of tissue. Recommended limits on radiation exposure are expressed in sieverts. Radiation imaging exposure units include milliampere-seconds (MAS).

Air kerma rate is also used to as a radiation unit. Kerma (kinetic energy released in matter) represents the kinetic energy absorbed per unit mass of a small amount of air when it is irradiated. It is associated only with indirectly ionizing radiation and is used as a replacement quantity for absorbed dose when the absorbed dose is difficult to calculate such as in fluoroscopy. Air kerma rate is the rate calculated using (u/p) value for air and is measured in Gy per unit time (Gy/h).

Several derivations on this unit exist including air kerma–area product (Pka) and air kerma at the reference point (Ka,r) [4]. Cumulative dose (CD) represents the air kerma accumulated at a specific point in space relative to the interventional reference point (typically the fluoroscope gantry). This is also referred to as cumulative air kerma. Other units include dose–area product (DAP). This measurement represents the integral of air kerma across the entire x-ray beam emission and serves as a surrogate measurement for the entire amount of energy delivered. DAP is measured in $Gy \cdot cm^2$.

Health Effects: Ionizing Radiation

Ionizing radiation is more harmful that nonionizing radiation because it has enough energy to remove an electron from an atom and thus directly damage biological material. The energy is enough to damage DNA, which can result in cell death or induce cellular neoplastic change (cancer). The study of ionizing radiation is a large area of classical toxicology, which has produced a tremendous understanding of the dose–response relationship of exposure. The primary effect of ionizing radiation resides in its effect on DNA. It can also affect the developing fetus of mothers exposed during pregnancy. Radiation exposure has a direct dose–response relationship.

Our knowledge of the effects of radiation developed gradually from experience over the last century. Early in the century, researchers such as Marie Curie died of cancer possibly related to her radiation exposure. Occupational exposure has also informed our understanding of radiation exposure risks. Young women employed to paint radium on watch dials died from bone cancer in the 1920s and 1930s [5, 6]. During this time, radium was promoted as a cure of many maladies and even recognized by the American Medical Association as a therapeutic option.

A great deal was learned from the atomic bomb survivors at Nagasaki and Hiroshima. The US military dropped the first atomic bomb on

Hiroshima, Japan, on August 6, 1945, and a second on Nagasaki, Japan, 3 days later. The bombs used two different types of radioactive material, ^{235}U in the first bomb and ^{239}PU in the second. It is estimated that 64,000 people died from the initial blasts and radiation exposure. Approximately 100,000 survivors were enrolled in follow-up studies, which confirmed an increased incidence of cancer. Ionizing radiation was also used to treat disease. From 1905 to 1960, ionizing radiation was used to treat ringworm in children and ankylosing spondylitis as well [7]. Experience with the use and misuse of ionizing radiation has demonstrated that the greater the dose, the greater the likelihood of developing cancer and that latency periods need to be measured in decades (from 10 to 60 years).

Medical Imaging

Medical imaging has become so commonplace in the United States and other resource-rich countries that the medical standard of care necessitates its use. The last two decades have seen the advancement and popularization of new imaging modalities such as magnetic resonance imaging (MRI), positron emission technology (PET) in addition to the standard use of fluoroscopy, and ultrasound technologies. It is a rare patient who has not received any imaging studies. With the widespread use of prenatal ultrasonography, most young people have experienced an imaging study even prior to birth. While ultrasound-imaging technology does not use ionizing radiation, some health concerns exist around its use. The Food and Drug Administration (FDA) has set limits on exposure at 4 T for infants less than 1 month old and 8 T for adults [8].

Nonionizing Modalities

Some modalities like ultrasonography and MRI are not associated with ionizing radiation and so are considered to have low to nonhazardous health risks to humans. The high-magnetic fields used in clinical MRI range up to 3 T. Ultrasonography employs high-frequency sound waves for visualization. The power levels used for imaging are currently believed to be below the threshold to cause short-term or long-term tissue damage.

The long-term effects due to ultrasound exposure at diagnostic intensity are still unknown, but ultrasonography as a diagnostic modality has been used in increasing frequency over the last half century [8]. The ALARA (as low as reasonably achievable) principle has been employed in this field of radiology—to minimize scanning time and power settings as low as possible while still achieving imaging goals. Nonmedical uses are discouraged under this principle as well.

Nonionizing imaging modalities are the imaging modalities of choice for children because of the recognized risks associated with ionizing radiation and cancer mortality [9]. However, ionizing radiation modalities provide diagnostic ease and clarity that cannot be reproduced by nonionizing modalities and where the risk–benefit ratio clearly rests on the side of using the study [10].

Ionizing Modalities

Radiology modalities that involve the use of ionizing radiation include diagnostic fluoroscopy, nuclear medicine imaging, and computerized tomography (CT) [11]. While the use of all these imaging modalities has increased over time, the use of CT in pediatrics has increased particularly rapidly largely because of the advent of helical CT which allows for increased accuracy in imaging over a shorter period of time [9]. This allows one to avoid the need for sedation to produce a useful study. The increase in exposure from ionizing radiation imaging modalities has increased 600 % from 1980 to 2006 (0.54–3 mSv) with medical radiation now accounting for half of the total radiation exposure in the United States. Repeated postnatal exposure of children to ionizing radiation to evaluate scoliosis is associated with increased rates of breast cancer later in life. This has raised concern for increased risk for other malignancies as well [12, 13].

Concern for increased lifetime risk for malignancies secondary to radiation exposure from these modalities was brought to attention in the late 1990s. Cancer risk estimations for children exposed to a CT (using adult radiation exposure doses) were calculated by Brenner who found a 0.18 % (abdominal) and 0.07 % (head) increased lifetime risk for cancer. These percentages were an order of magnitude higher in children than in adults based on the increased lifetime risk-dose exposure. These estimates were derived from cancer risk calculations and mortality data from atomic bomb survivors in Japan. That data demonstrated increased cancer mortality data with doses greater than 100 mSv with decreasing risk for lower radiation exposures [14–18].

Risk Assessment

Radiation risk can be considered in the following categories:

1. Stochastic risk to the individual
2. Stochastic risk to society
3. Deterministic risk to the individual
4. Pregnancy exposure-related risks

Deterministic risks represent radiation-induced tissue damage that manifests itself within days to weeks after exposure. This includes radiodermatitis and radiation-induced skin ulceration. Interventional fluoroscopic procedures represent the most common mechanism for this type of exposure. In particular, complex interventional procedures with prolonged fluoroscopy times increase deterministic risks associated with ionizing radiation exposure. Deterministic effects of tissues such as the skin, lenses of the eyes, and hair follicles are a by-product of damage to supporting tissues and sterilization of stem cells. Tissue damage occurs when the ability of the affected organ to repair itself by cellular division is overwhelmed by the cell loss due to radiation damage. Lethal levels of radiation are used to intentionally kill cancer cells. Consequently, the extent and timing of tissue damage is related to cell proliferation kinetics of the irradiated organs [19]. Deterministic risks are uncommon in general and even more uncommon in pediatrics [20, 21]. Deterministic effects occur at high doses over short exposure times and are usually seen at doses over 0.1 Gy or high-dose rates (0.1 Gy/h).

Stochastic risks represent cancer-induction risks associated with radiation exposure. They are attributable to the aftermath of DNA damage that results in malignant transformation of a cell. These risks are impacted by the tissue exposed, the severity and duration of radiation exposure, latency effects, and genetic susceptibility of the exposed individual [19]. A latency period of years to decades is taken into consideration when calculating the stochastic risks involved in radiation exposure [22]. The consensus of the nuclear industry and many government regulatory agencies is that the incidence of cancers due to ionizing radiation can be modeled linearly with an effective dose (see below) at a rate of 5.5 % per Sv [23]. Individual studies, alternate models, and earlier versions of the industry consensus have produced other risk estimates scattered around this consensus model. The BEIR VII report offers estimates of lifetime attributable to radiation exposure of specific organs [24]. This risk estimate includes cancer-related deaths that would have occurred without exposure but occurred at a younger age than anticipated as a consequence of the exposure. It is important to consider that fluoroscopic procedures do not result in whole-body irradiation so that stochastic risk estimates are better tailored for organ-specific exposures in this instance [4].

Effective dose (E) is a unit developed in an effort to quantitate the stochastic effect of a radiation dose. To calculate this dose, assumptions are made based on age, gender, and health status of the general population. In relation to fluoroscopic procedures, E is usually evaluated using Pka in addition to a procedure-specific coefficient based on Monte Carlo simulations (thermoluminescent-dosimeter measurements in phantoms) (see Fig. 7.2). This has been done for pediatric patients as well [25]. Because of the assumptions built into E calculations, the NCRP currently does not recommend using E for quantitative estimates of stochastic risk for individual patients or patient groups [4].

Consensus agreement exists that infants and children are at increased risk for the stochastic effects of ionizing radiation. As noted above,

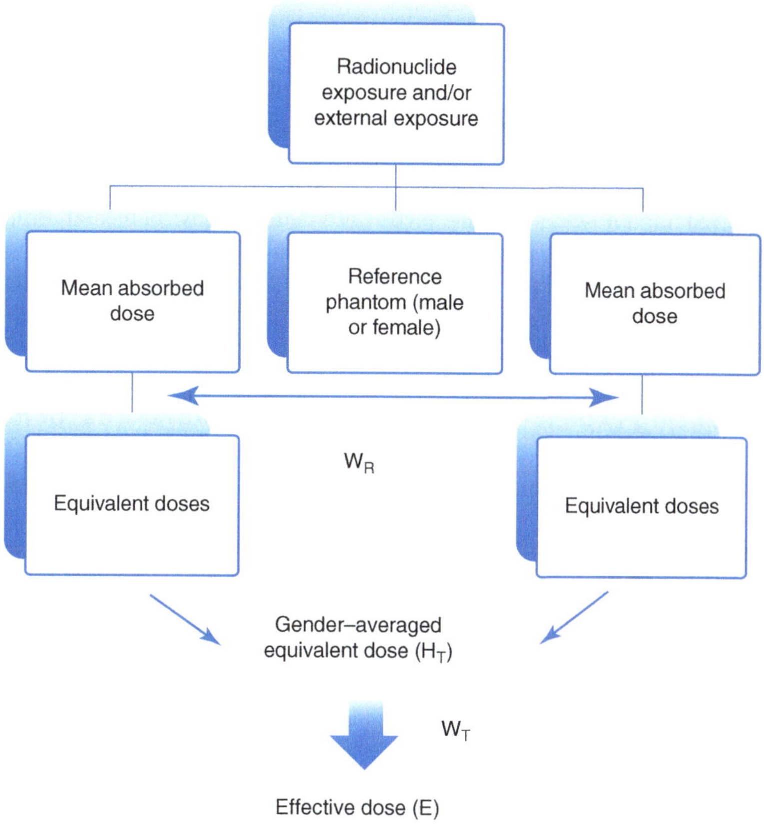

Fig. 7.2 Schematic illustration of the method used to calculate effective dose. W_R radiation weighting factor, W_T tissue weighting factor, H_T tissue weighting factor

Brenner and his colleagues raised awareness of these stochastic risks for a pediatric population by estimating the risks of inducing a fatal cancer from the ionizing radiation exposure of a computerized tomographic (CT) imaging study [9]. In this study, the authors estimated organ-dose exposures as a function of age at diagnosis for common CT examinations and then estimated lifetime cancer risks from this exposure using standard models that assumed a linear risk extrapolation. They arrived at a lifetime risk for cancer mortality for a 1-year-old exposed to a standard CT to be 0.18 % for an abdominal CT and 0.07 % for a head CT. These increased risks were attributable to an increased dose per milliampere-second and the increased lifetime risk per unit dose because of the longer latency period involved in pediatric exposures compared to adults [9].

A subsequent epidemiological study by Pearce and his colleagues of 178,064 children who received an abdominal CT or head CT between 1985 and 2002 demonstrated an increased incidence of leukemias and brain cancers that were remarkably close to the estimates of the Brenner study [26]. These studies have focused on leukemias and brain cancers because of their short latency period from radiation exposure to tumor formation. Studies of the atomic bomb survivors in Japan estimate that lifetime risk estimates for an irradiated population may need to extend 50–60 years [27].

Roughly 85 million CT scans are being performed each year in the United States, and a growing number of these are being performed on children. Several investigators have noted a high frequency of imaging studies ordered for children with an increased frequency of higher radiation exposure studies especially for diagnoses of abdominal pain, headache, and head injury [28]. The utility of imaging modalities of the CT scans due to its image quality and speed remains unsurpassed. Consequently, it is widely used in pediatric trauma situations despite the increased awareness of the long-term effects of the radiation exposure from these studies [29]. Tepper and colleagues found a mean effective ionizing radiation dose of 11.4 mSv for CT scans performed within the first 24 h for pediatric trauma patients in the North Carolina Trauma Registry [30]. In the field of pediatric urology, Page and his coworkers performed a retrospective audit of the radiation doses of patients receiving voiding cystourethrograms and nuclear medicine studies and compared them to CT scans and found the dose exposures to be comparable [31].

Reducing Exposure

In recognition of this trend and in light of increased public awareness of the stochastic risks of ionizing radiation exposure in children, pediatric imaging societies have produced new recommendations to limit ionizing radiation exposure for children from these imaging modalities. These recommendations include (1) increasing education and awareness of stochastic risks among the radiology community, (2) advocating for the use of nonionizing imaging modalities such as ultrasonography when it is an appropriate alternative, and (3) pediatric imaging protocols that reduce radiation exposure without compromising image quality [32–34]. The Image Gently campaign (http://www.pedrad.org/associations/5364/ig/) is among the best known of various efforts to reduce risk with ionizing radiation imaging sources in pediatrics. The leaders of this campaign recently published a list of goals yet to be accomplished [35]. Surveys of physicians and medical students suggest that educational gaps exist. In one survey, 25 % of physicians and 43 % of medical students were unaware that interventional procedures used ionizing radiation. The group surveyed also believed CT scans were associated with the least exposure to ionizing radiation [36].

Regulatory Standards

The first organized effort to protect people from radiation exposure began in 1915 when the British Roentgen Society adopted a resolution to protect people from x-rays.

In 1922, the United States adopted the British protection rules, and various government and nongovernmental groups were formed to protect people from radiation. In 1959, the Federal Radiation Council was formed to advise the president and recommend standards. In 1970, the US Environmental Protection Agency was formed and took over these responsibilities. Now several government agencies are responsible for protecting people from radiation-emitting devices.

Standards for Radiation Exposure

Recommended exposure limits are set by the US National Council on Radiation Protection (NCRP) and worldwide by the International Council on Radiation Protection (ICRP). The occupational exposure guidelines are 100 mSv in 5 years (average, 20 mSv per year) with a limit of 50 mSv in any single year. For the general public, the standard is 1 mSv per year. This must be put in the context of natural background radiation, which is approximately 3 mSv/year depending upon location (such as elevation) as well as other variables.

References

1. Jacob P, Stram DO. Late health effects of radiation exposure: New statistical, epidemiological, and biological approaches. Int J Radiat Biol. 2013;89(8): 673–83.
2. Cahoon EK, et al. Individual, environmental, and meteorological predictors of daily personal ultraviolet radiation exposure measurements in a United States cohort study. PLoS One. 2013;8(2):e54983.
3. Dendy PP, Heaton B. Physics for diagnostic radiology. Philadelphia: CRC Press; 1999.
4. National Council on Radiation Protection and Measurements. Radiation dose management for fluoroscopically-guided interventional medical procedures. Bethesda: NCRP Publications; 2010.
5. Evans RD. The radium standard for boneseekers–evaluation of the data on radium patients and dial painters. Health Phys. 1967;13(3):267–78.
6. Sharpe WD. The New Jersey radium dial painters: a classic in occupational carcinogenesis. Bull Hist Med. 1978;52(4):560–70.
7. Ron E, et al. Thyroid neoplasia following low-dose radiation in childhood. Radiat Res. 1989;120(3):516–31.

8. FDA. Radiation-emitting products. ultrasound imaging. Risks/Benefits; 2013. Available from: http://www.fda.gov/Radiation-EmittingProducts/RadiationEmittingProductsandProcedures/MedicalImaging/ucm115357.htm-rb
9. Brenner D, et al. Estimated risks of radiation-induced fatal cancer from pediatric CT. AJR Am J Roentgenol. 2001;176(2):289–96.
10. Coren ME, et al. The value of ultrafast computed tomography in the investigation of pediatric chest disease. Pediatr Pulmonol. 1998;26(6):389–95.
11. Linet MS, Kim KP, Rajaraman P. Children's exposure to diagnostic medical radiation and cancer risk: epidemiologic and dosimetric considerations. Pediatr Radiol. 2009;39 Suppl 1:S4–26.
12. Mettler Jr FA, et al. Medical radiation exposure in the U.S. in 2006: preliminary results. Health Phys. 2008;95(5):502–7.
13. Hoffman DA, et al. Breast cancer in women with scoliosis exposed to multiple diagnostic x rays. J Natl Cancer Inst. 1989;81(17):1307–12.
14. Pierce DA. Mechanistic models for radiation carcinogenesis and the atomic bomb survivor data. Radiat Res. 2003;160(6):718–23.
15. Pierce DA, Mendelsohn ML. A model for radiation-related cancer suggested by atomic bomb survivor data. Radiat Res. 1999;152(6):642–54.
16. Shimizu Y, et al. Studies of the mortality of A-bomb survivors. 9. Mortality, 1950–1985: part 1. Comparison of risk coefficients for site-specific cancer mortality based on the DS86 and T65DR shielded kerma and organ doses. Radiat Res. 1989; 118(3):502–24.
17. Shimizu Y, et al. Studies of the mortality of atomic bomb survivors. Report 12, part II. Noncancer mortality: 1950–1990. Radiat Res. 1999;152(4): 374–89.
18. Pierce DA, Preston DL. Radiation-related cancer risks at low doses among atomic bomb survivors. Radiat Res. 2000;154(2):178–86.
19. International Commission on Radiological Protection. Radiologic protection in medicine. IRCP, 2007. 37(6): p. publication 105.
20. Frazier TH, et al. Fluoroscopy-induced chronic radiation skin injury: a disease perhaps often overlooked. Arch Dermatol. 2007;143(5):637–40.
21. Vliestra RE, Wagner LK, Koenig T, Mettler F. Radiation burns as a severe complication of fluoroscopically guided cardiological interventions. J Interv Cardiol. 2004;17(3):1–12.
22. Hall EJ, Giaccia AJ. Radiobiology for the radiologist. 6th ed. Philadelphia: Lippincott Williams, and Wilkins; 2006.
23. ICRP. The 2007 recommendations of the International Commission on Radiological Protection. Ann ICRP. 2007;103(37):2–4.
24. National Research Council (U.S.) Committee on Health Effects of Exposure to Low Levels of Ionizing Radiations. Health risks from exposures to low levels of ionizing radiation. BEIR VII. Washington: National Academies Press; 2006.
25. Miksys N, et al. Estimating effective dose to pediatric patients undergoing interventional radiology procedures using anthropomorphic phantoms and MOSFET dosimeters. AJR Am J Roentgenol. 2010;194(5):1315–22.
26. Pearce MS, et al. Radiation exposure from CT scans in childhood and subsequent risk of leukaemia and brain tumours: a retrospective cohort study. Lancet. 2012;380(9840):499–505.
27. Hall EJ, Brenner DJ. Cancer risks from diagnostic radiology: the impact of new epidemiological data. Br J Radiol. 2012;85(1020):e1316–17.
28. Tompane T, et al. Diagnostic imaging studies performed in children over a nine-year period. Pediatrics. 2013;131(1):e45–52.
29. Kharbanda AB, et al. Analysis of radiation exposure among pediatric trauma patients at national trauma centers. J Trauma Acute Care Surg. 2013; 74(3):907–11.
30. Tepper B, Brice JH, Hobgood CD. Evaluation of radiation exposure to pediatric trauma patients. J Emerg Med. 2013;44(3):646–52.
31. Page M, et al. Paediatric urological investigations-dose comparison between urology-related and CT irradiation. Pediatr Radiol. 2013;43(7):846–50.
32. Hernanz-Schulman M, et al. Pause and pulse: ten steps that help manage radiation dose during pediatric fluoroscopy. AJR Am J Roentgenol. 2011; 197(2):475–81.
33. Goske MJ, et al. Image gently(SM): a national education and communication campaign in radiology using the science of social marketing. J Am Coll Radiol. 2008;5(12):1200–5.
34. Goske MJ, et al. Image gently: a web-based practice quality improvement program in CT safety for children. AJR Am J Roentgenol. 2010;194(5): 1177–82.
35. Goske MJ, et al. Image gently 5 years later: what goals remain to be accomplished in radiation protection for children? AJR Am J Roentgenol. 2012; 199(3):477–9.
36. Ricketts ML, et al. Perception of radiation exposure and risk among patients, medical students, and referring physicians at a tertiary care community hospital. Can Assoc Radiol J. 2013;64(3):208–12.

Part II

Clinical Imaging

8 Prenatal Imaging of the Genitourinary Tract

Carol E. Barnewolt and Marc Cendron

Introduction

Evaluation of the fetus by ultrasound goes back at least 40 years. The first report of a fetal urologic anomaly diagnosed by ultrasound was published by Garrett et al. in 1970 [1]. The overall incidence of detectable fetal anomalies has grown over the years given the improvement in technology and increased availability of prenatal screening. In the United States, 2–3 prenatal ultrasounds are performed per pregnancy [2]. Currently it is estimated that incidence of urologic anomalies detected in utero is about 1 in 500 fetuses and 50 % of these are, most commonly, in the form of dilation of the urinary tract or hydronephrosis (antenatal hydronephrosis or ANH) [3]. Recent studies have shown that the rate of hydronephrosis detected prenatally varies between 115 per 10,000 live births to 1,000/10,000 [4, 5]. With an increasing number of fetuses being diagnosed with abnormalities of the urinary tract, management has become more complex and certainly more controversial [6].

It has become clear that the prenatal diagnosis has an impact on the management of the pregnancy and has significant effect on the emotional health of both parents during the gestation [7]. Currently, in the United States, no guidelines have been set forth for the prenatal evaluation of the fetus. Prenatal ultrasound is recommended but there is no set schedule for the timing of the ultrasound. Although ultrasound is the modality of choice for fetal imaging, indication to carry out ultrasonographic evaluation of the urinary tract in the fetus is still a matter of discussion. Practice guidelines have emerged over the last 20 years. The American College of Obstetricians and Gynecology has defined three types of ultrasound examination: basic, limited, and comprehensive. In 1994 the members of the National Institute of Health Consensus Development Conference (NIHCDC) suggested that ultrasound may be beneficial and listed indications for prenatal ultrasonography [8].

Currently prenatal evaluation of the fetus by ultrasound is widely used as a screening tool in certain European countries and in Canada but has not been applied as extensively in the United States. The role of ultrasound to evaluate the fetal urinary tract can be summarized as follows: (1) to detect degrees of fetal urinary tract dilatation that may warrant monitoring during the gestation and postnatally; (2) to identify fetuses affected with such severe lesions that intervention or termination of the pregnancy might be

C.E. Barnewolt, MD
Department of Radiology, Harvard Medical School, Boston, MA, USA

Division of Ultrasound, Department of Radiology, Children's Hospital Boston, Boston, MA, USA
e-mail: carol.barnewolt@childrens.harvard.edu

M. Cendron, MD (✉)
Department of Urology, Children's Hospital Boston, Harvard Medical School, 300 Longwood Ave., Boston, MA 02115, USA
e-mail: marc.cendron@childrens.harvard.edu

L.S. Palmer, J.S. Palmer (eds.), *Pediatric and Adolescent Urologic Imaging*, DOI 10.1007/978-1-4614-8654-1_8,

considered; and (3) to provide options and management for the fetus diagnosed with urologic anomalies that will warrant postnatal evaluation and treatment [5, 9].

In general, prenatal radiologic evaluation is usually not focused on the genitourinary tract but rather on the fetus as a whole. The primary goal of sonographic screening of the fetus remains the accuracy in ascertaining a correct diagnosis [10]. As previously stated, the most common finding involving the urinary tract is dilatation of the renal collecting system otherwise known as hydronephrosis (ANH) from the Greek word for water and nephros kidney, fluid on/in the kidney. This review will go over current concepts related to fetal hydronephrosis including imaging modalities, prenatal and postnatal evaluation, and options in management.

Modalities to evaluate the genitourinary tract of the fetus include ultrasound as well as magnetic resonance imaging (MRI). Computed tomography (CT scan) is rarely if ever warranted for fear of needlessly exposing both mother and fetus to ionizing radiation. Strict indications for fetal imaging have not been established, but some relative indications include family history of genitourinary abnormalities, advanced maternal age, difficulties with the pregnancies (bleeding and/or preeclampsia), as well as concerns about fetal development or chromosomal anomalies [11]. Furthermore, standard protocols for fetal screening have not been published especially with regard to the evaluation of the genitourinary tract. Important aspects of prenatal imaging of the fetal urinary tract evaluation include, but not limited to, (1) the amount of amniotic fluid (amniotic fluid index or AFI), (2) a general fetal survey to look for any spinal abnormality as well as for pulmonary hypoplasia, and (3) a full evaluation of both kidneys, bladder, and, at a later stage of pregnancy, the genitalia.

The purpose of this chapter is to review fetal genitourinary imaging beginning with the kidneys, the ureters, and then the bladder and finally going over imaging of the genitalia [12]. A brief discussion of the use of fetal MRI will be provided.

Renal and Ureteral Imaging

The fetal kidneys will have assumed their recognizable position and shape by approximately 10–12 weeks postconception. Accurate ultrasonographic evaluation of the kidneys is usually best done after 15 weeks given the rather small size of the fetal kidneys and lack of perirenal fat which prevents clear delineation of the tissue planes. With further fetal growth, identification of the kidneys becomes much easier, and by approximately 24 weeks of gestation, a adequate evaluation of the kidney cortex as well as collecting system can be carried out. Increasing improvements in technology has allowed for better delineation of the renal cortex, collecting system, and ureters [13]. The fetal adrenal glands tend to be relatively large compared to the kidneys and can usually be identified superior to each kidneys unless the sonographic window is limited by fetal position or by maternal body habitus. It may be difficult to differentiate them from the kidneys. Kidney size measurement is an important data point in monitoring overall fetal growth. Other aspects of renal evaluation are the appearance and size of the renal collecting system. In the normal fetus, the renal collecting system is usually not clearly visualized, whereas if there is fluid either retained in the collecting system or regurgitated up the ureter, hydronephrosis will then be observed. The degree of hydronephrosis can vary widely. It is reported that approximately 10 % of all fetuses have some degree of hydronephrosis [14].

Various classification systems for hydronephrosis have been proposed. A basic classification involves grading the degree of hydronephrosis as moderate to severe based on the anteroposterior diameter of the renal pelvis [15, 16]. A more sophisticated system was proposed by the Society for Fetal Urology, but this system may be a bit cumbersome and complex [17]. Dilatation of the upper urinary tract is idiopathic in the vast majority of cases but may be associated with some type of pathological process. Given the wide variation in the degree of dilatation of the upper urinary tract seen at various stages of gestation and uncertainty regarding the etiology, managing prenatally diagnosed hydronephrosis may be difficult and is open to discussion. Mild prenatal hydronephrosis (AP diameter of less than 8 mm or SFU grades 1 through 2) is probably of no great clinical concern [18, 19] (Fig. 8.1). Studies have shown that fetuses whose renal pelvis AP diameter was <7 mm had an 80 % resolution rate of the hydronephrosis. All resolved by year one [20, 21]. However, if the dilatation is noted to be >7 mm, few or none resolved antenatally, and a number of fetus (less than 5 %), when followed postnatally, required some type of surgical procedure, most of whom having had an AP diameter of the renal pelvis >10 mm. In light of recent studies, fetal hydronephrosis was felt to be clinically significant in 5–15 % of cases usually when the renal AP diameter of the pelvis is >10 mm [22]. Other factors to consider include caliectasis, the status of the amniotic fluid volume (amniotic fluid index), as well observation of an abnormal renal parenchyma. It should be noted that dilatation of the upper urinary tract is not necessarily due to obstruction but can be due to vesicoureteral reflux (Fig. 8.2).

Ultrasound features that might be associated with some type of uropathology include pelvic AP diameter greater than 8 mm, massive dilation of the ureters and renal pelvis bilaterally, increased renal cortical echogenicity, thickened bladder wall, and reduced levels of amniotic fluid. Lee et al. in 2003 showed in a meta-analysis that moderate to severe hydronephrosis had a higher risk of pathology [23]. However, no other specific ultrasound features were found to have any predictive value [22, 24]. The differential diagnosis of fetal hydronephrosis is lengthy and includes obstructive processes such as ureteropelvic or ureterovesical obstruction as well as posterior urethral valves in boys, reflux of urine from the bladder to the renal collecting system, and more uncommon conditions such as prune-belly syndrome. Again, it is important to remember that dilatation of the upper urinary tract is not necessarily due to obstruction and that ultrasound alone is not an accurate test for obstruction as it does assess function or physiology.

The etiology of idiopathic hydronephrosis has not been determined, but the suspicion is that the ureter may have been kinked early in development as urine production starts. The kinking causes a transient obstruction to the flow of urine which will then cause back up of urine into the renal collecting system, thus, causing dilation. With differential growth of the fetus, the ureter may straighten out and the obstructive process may disappear leaving the collecting system dilated to varying degrees.

Marked dilation of the renal collecting system may be associated with high-grade obstruction (Fig. 8.3). If it is bilateral, the obstructive process may be intravesical (posterior urethral valves in males) (Fig. 8.4). As noted above, the more severe the degree of dilation of the renal collecting system, the more likely the chances of pathology [23, 25]. Vesicoureteral reflux has been mentioned as a possible etiologic factor for prenatally diagnosed hydronephrosis and is reported to be present in approximately 12 % of fetuses with ANH independent of the grade of hydronephrosis [23]. The diagnosis of reflux cannot be achieved by prenatal ultrasound but requires postnatal evaluation by VCUG (Fig. 8.5). Suspicion of vesicoureteral reflux can be raised if, while monitoring the bladder and kidneys, upper tract dilation is seen at the time of bladder contraction. This is a rather subtle and unreliable finding but has been described as a possible feature of prenatal vesicoureteral reflux [26]. Concomitant presence of both an obstructive process, as well as reflux, may also be present (Fig. 8.5).

Evaluation of the renal cortex is also an important factor in the survey of the genitourinary tract of the fetus. The echogenicity of the renal cortex should be similar to that of the fetal liver. Increased echogenicity of the renal parenchyma may be associated with renal maldevelopment otherwise known as renal dysplasia [27, 28]. Cystic renal disease of the kidney can also be identified fairly early in gestation by an increase in the echogenicity of the renal cortex (Fig. 8.6). It would be important to differentiate between congenital cystic kidney disease which is bilateral and with a genetic cause (autosomal versus dominant polycystic kidney disease ADPCKD versus ARPCKD) versus multicystic dysplastic

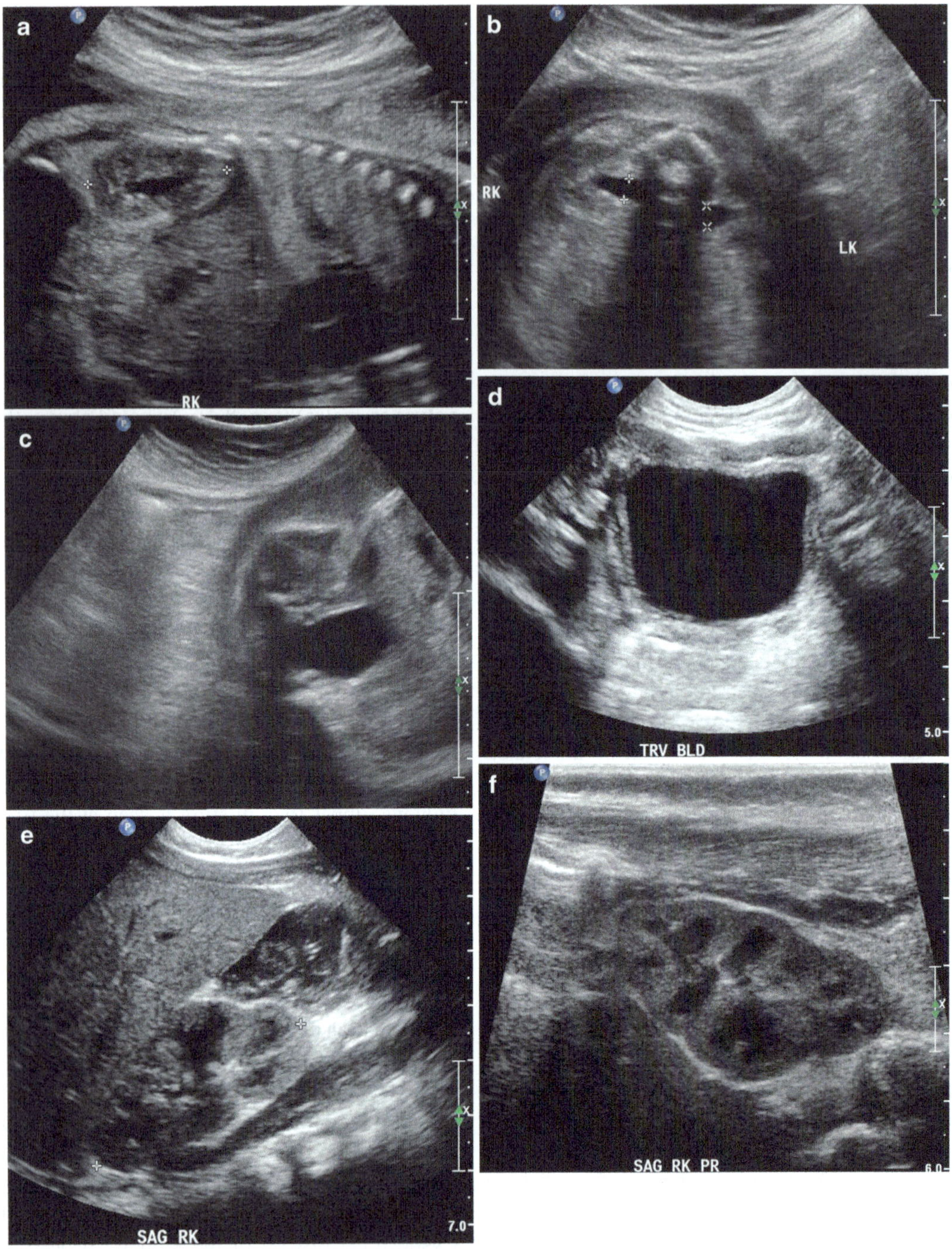

Fig. 8.1 This fetal sonogram reveals mild, bilateral hydronephrosis, in the sagittal (**a**) and transverse planes (**b**), measuring 5 mm in anterior-to-posterior dimensions, at 29 weeks gestation, with a normal, full fetal urinary bladder (**c**). After delivery, the appearance of the kidneys normalized, as is often the case. By 1 month of age, with a full urinary bladder (**d**), an 8 MHz curved probe reveals a normal appearance of the right kidney in the sagittal plane (**e**). Detail is even more apparent using a 12 MHz linear probe in the sagittal (**f**) and transverse (**g**) planes, with normal corticomedullary differentiation and no hydronephrosis

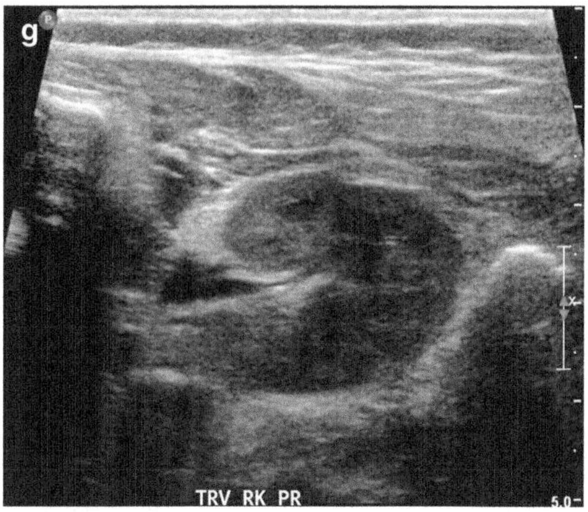

Fig. 8.1 (continued)

kidney (MCDK,) which is usually unilateral with no known genetic etiology. On fetal echography, ARPCKD displays striking features of bilateral, massively enlarged kidneys that are echogenic due to acoustic interfaces caused by the dilated tubules and cysts (Fig. 8.7). Features of multicystic dysplastic kidney as diagnosed prenatally include multiple cysts of variable sizes, no evidence of parenchyma or collecting system, and the possibility of contralateral compensatory hypertrophy (Fig. 8.8). The findings of hyperechoic kidneys in the fetus require postnatal evaluation as it may indicate some intrinsic abnormality of the renal parenchyma, although the outcomes may be quite variable [29]. Confusion may also arise with extrarenal cystic lesions which may mimic renal anomalies. For example, adrenal hemorrhage may give the appearance of an upper pole cyst. Careful, precise scanning can generally differentiate the kidney from the extrarenal lesion. Further diagnostic testing by MRI will provide additional anatomic detail (Fig. 8.9). Other abnormalities of the kidneys include anomalies of position and rotation as well as agenesis or hypoplasia, which are rare.

Any abnormalities of the renal collecting system and/or renal parenchyma should be communicated to the pediatrician who will then decide whether or not further postnatal evaluation is required. Early identification of renal or bladder anomalies warrant prenatal counseling by a pediatric urologist in order to ensure adequate postnatal evaluation and management.

Dilatation of the ureters may also be noted on prenatal ultrasound. If it is unilateral, the dilation is usually associated either with an obstructive process at the distal end of the ureter (ureterovesical junction obstruction or megaureter) or with reflux. Unilateral dilatation of the renal collecting system and ureter does not usually warrant any further intervention during pregnancy but will require postnatal evaluation. Bilateral dilatation of the ureters, on the other hand, warrants careful evaluation of the bladder to look for intravesical obstruction. Other anomalies associated with bilateral dilatation of the renal collecting system and ureters include prune-belly syndrome as well as high-grade vesicoureteral reflux.

Duplication anomalies of the kidneys can be identified later in gestation when the renal parenchyma may be seen to have a band of tissue separating the renal collecting system one or both showing some degree of dilatation (Fig. 8.10). Duplication anomalies diagnosed prenatally should raise the suspicion for vesicoureteral reflux (usually to the lower pole), ureterocele, and ectopic ureters and warrant postnatal evaluation.

Absence of a one or both of the kidneys can be observed prenatally. It is important to ensure that the apparently absent kidney is not ectopic (usually in the lower abdomen or bony pelvis) before making a diagnosis of renal agenesis. Bilateral renal agenesis is rare and occurs in 1–4,800 to 1 in 10,000 births [30]. Unilateral renal agenesis occurs in 1 in 1,100 births. There is usually a male predominance (75 %). There may be an autosomal recessive inheritance associated with this condition. Unilateral renal agenesis should be confirmed postnatally. Bilateral renal agenesis is thought to be incompatible with survival of the fetus and is associated with gradual or sudden drop in amniotic fluid leading to anhydramnios low or inexistent levels of amniotic fluid as the pregnancy progresses leading to fetal crowding and profound lung hypoplasia (Potter's syndrome) [31].

Renal and suprarenal masses will, occasionally, may be identified prenatally. These include mesoblastic nephroma which is a benign lesion of the kidney. Adrenal hemorrhage may be also

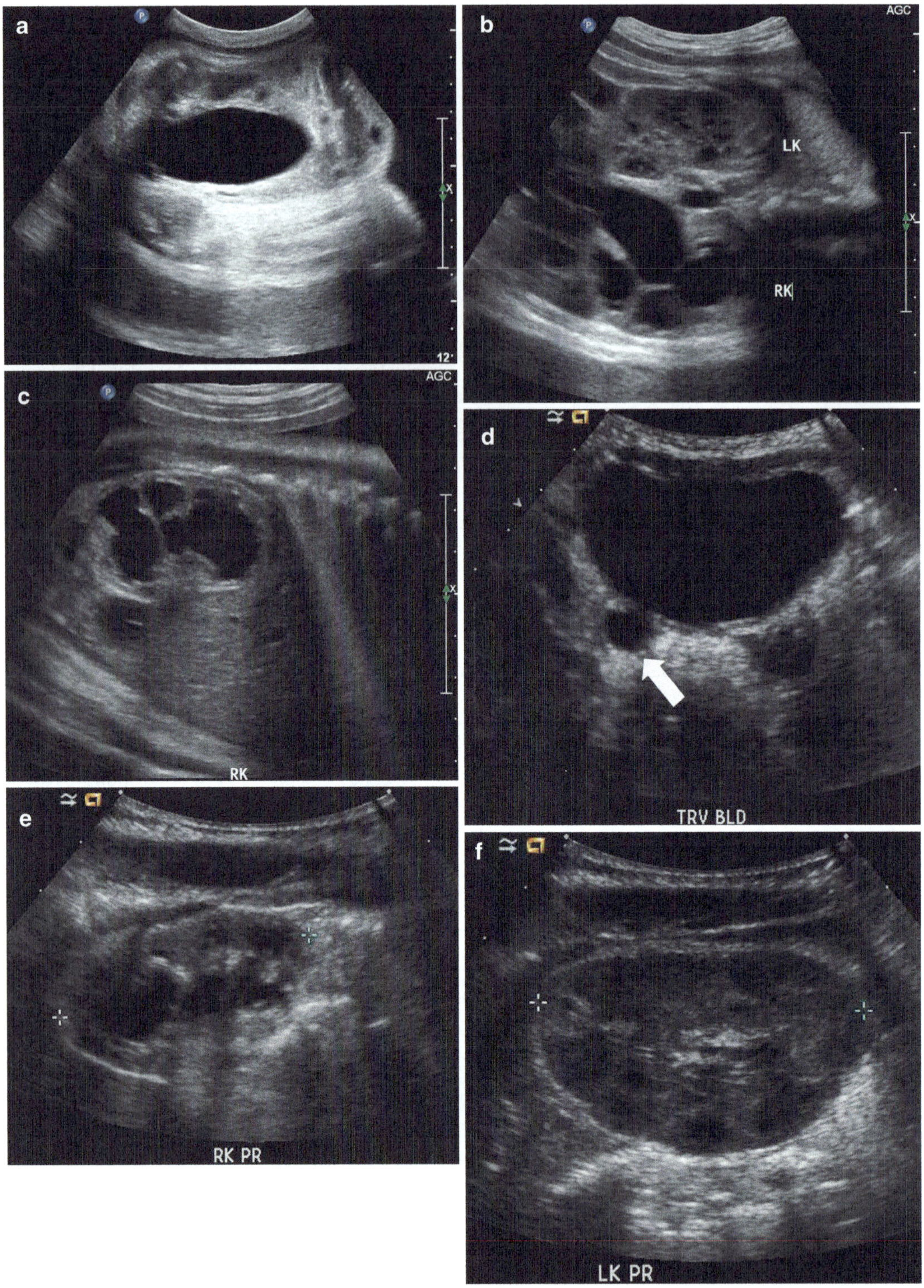

Fig. 8.2 This sonogram of a 33-week male fetus demonstrates a rather full but not thick-walled bladder (**a**) and moderate to severe right hydroureteronephrosis (**b** and **c**). Sonography at 4 weeks old confirms the presence of moderate to severe right hydroureteronephrosis (**d** and **e**, *arrow*=right distal ureter), some evidence for right-sided renal cortical loss (**e**), and a normal-appearing left kidney (**f**). VCUG on the same day proves that the dilatation is due to high-grade, right-sided reflux (**g**) that drains well (**h**), with no evidence for posterior urethra valves on voiding (**i**). Renal scintigraphy was performed at age 3 months, and this posterior view reveals evidence for diffuse cortical loss on the right (**j**)

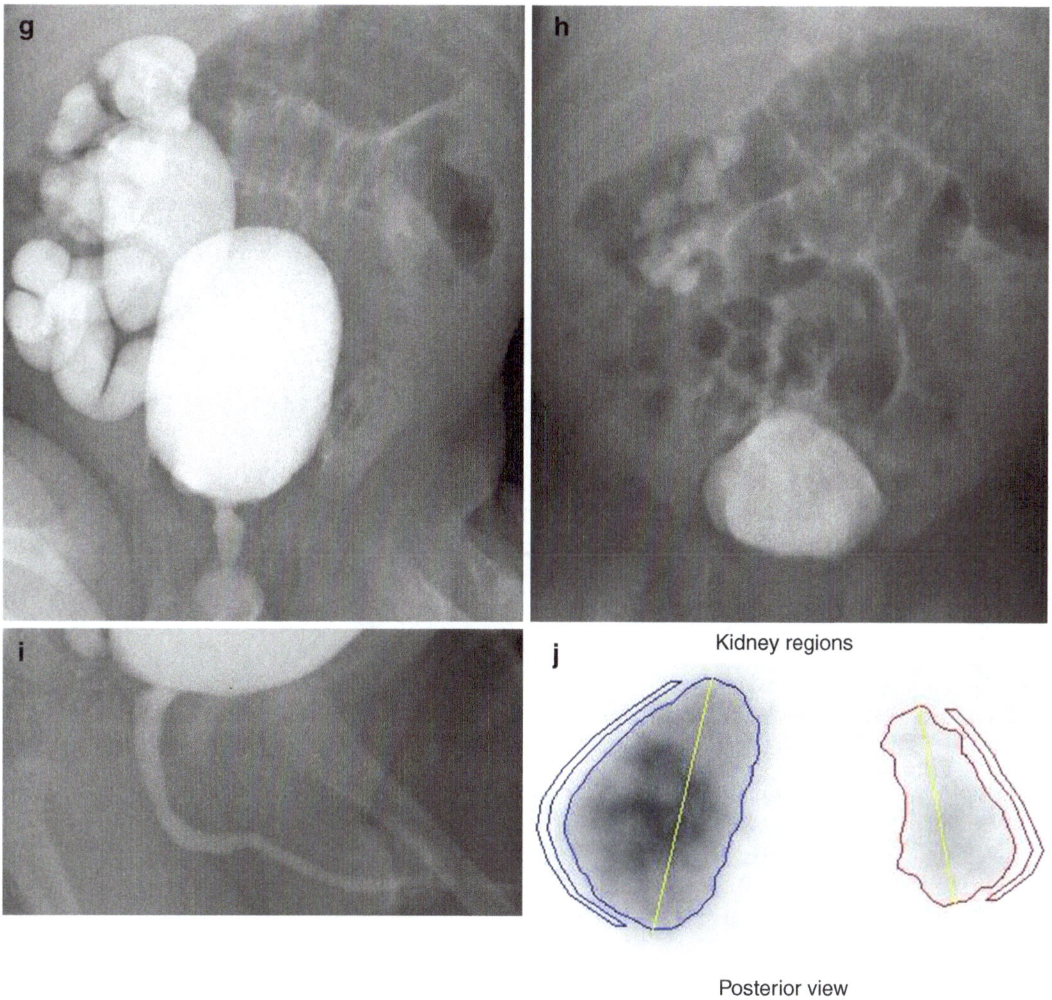

Fig. 8.2 (continued)

identified as a large hypo- or hyperechoic mass above the kidney (Fig. 8.9). Neuroblastoma can also be diagnosed prenatally typically in a suprarenal position but can occasionally be seen in the abdomen or the retroperitoneum.

Postnatal evaluation is dictated by the prenatal findings. No guidelines have been set up for postnatal evaluation of patients diagnosed with hydronephrosis. However, currently it would be reasonable to suggest that any child whose AP diameter of the renal pelvis is <7 mm, probably does not require any follow-up postnatally. A postnatal ultrasound certainly is not an unreasonable approach for patients with an AP diameter of 8 mm or greater. The timing of the first postnatal ultrasound is a matter of debate. An early evaluation (within the first days of life) may allow for early identification of those fetuses who may require follow-up. It is important to realize, however, that sonography during the first 24 h of life may significantly underestimate the degree of hydronephrosis because of physiologic oliguria, so most authorities recommend evaluation after the first few days of life, or later, unless a serious abnormality, requiring urgent treatment, is suspected. Evaluation for vesicoureteral reflux or posterior urethral valves would be in the form of a voiding cystourethrogram (VCUG); for an obstructive process, a MAG 3 radioisotope study would be indicated.

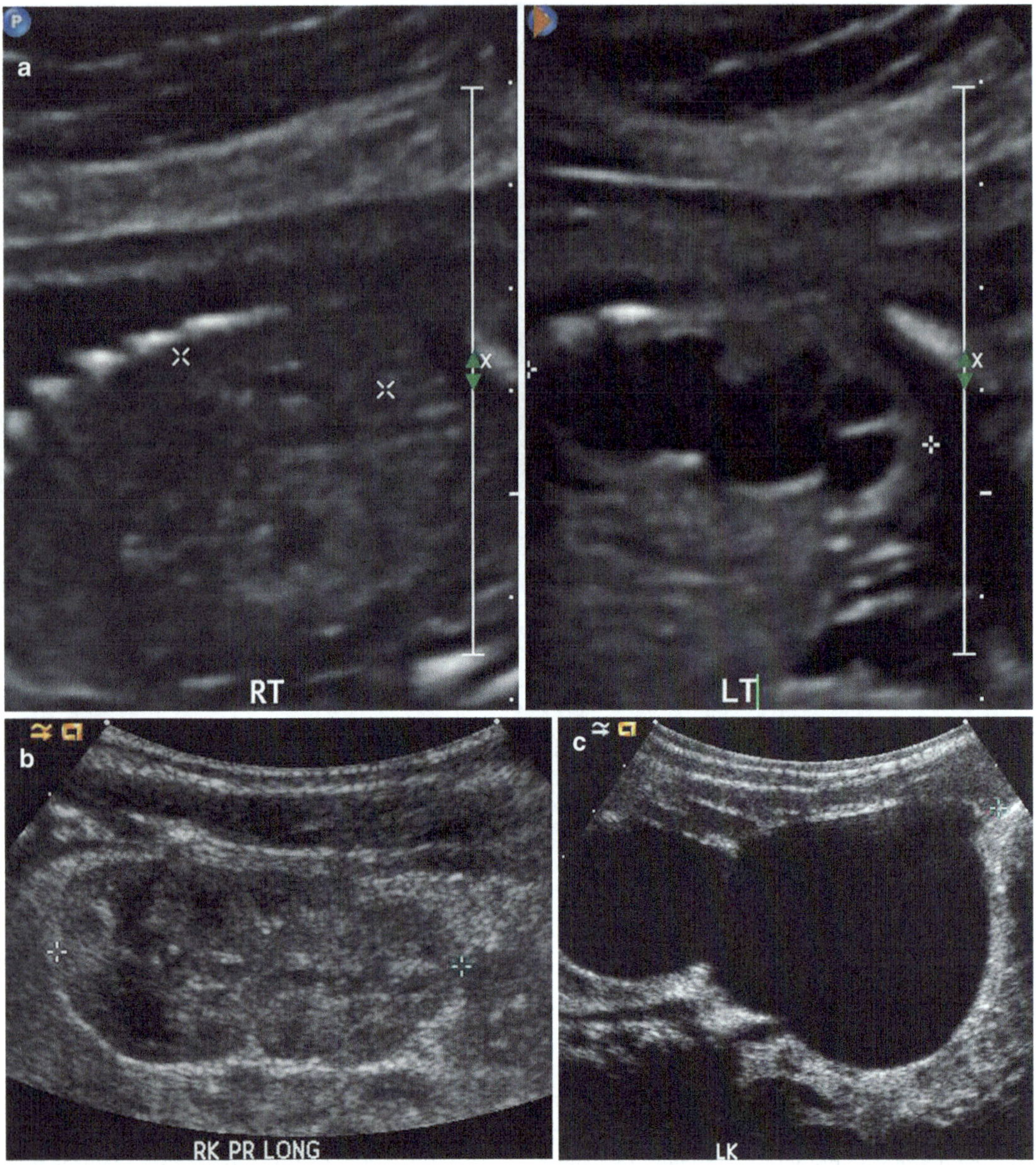

Fig. 8.3 At 21 weeks gestation, fetal sonography reveals moderate to severe left hydronephrosis, without hydroureter, and a normal-appearing right kidney (**a**). At age 4 weeks, postnatal renal sonography confirms this suspicion, and the degree of left hydronephrosis is even worse, with very little visible cortex, with a still normal-appearing right kidney (**b** and **c**). Diuretic nuclear renography (not shown) demonstrates a clearly obstructive pattern of excretion, indicating that the fetal hydronephrosis was due to isolated ureteropelvic junction obstruction

The Fetal Bladder

Evaluation of the bladder carried out during a fetal sonogram is an integral part of the fetal survey. The bladder is usually seen as a hypoechoic ovoid structure in the lower portion of the abdomen extending from the fetal pelvis. It can be detected as early as 11–12 weeks of gestation as urine production begins [32]. Variability in the size of the bladder is explained by the rhythmic filling and emptying of the fetal bladder. Incomplete fetal bladder emptying is usually the

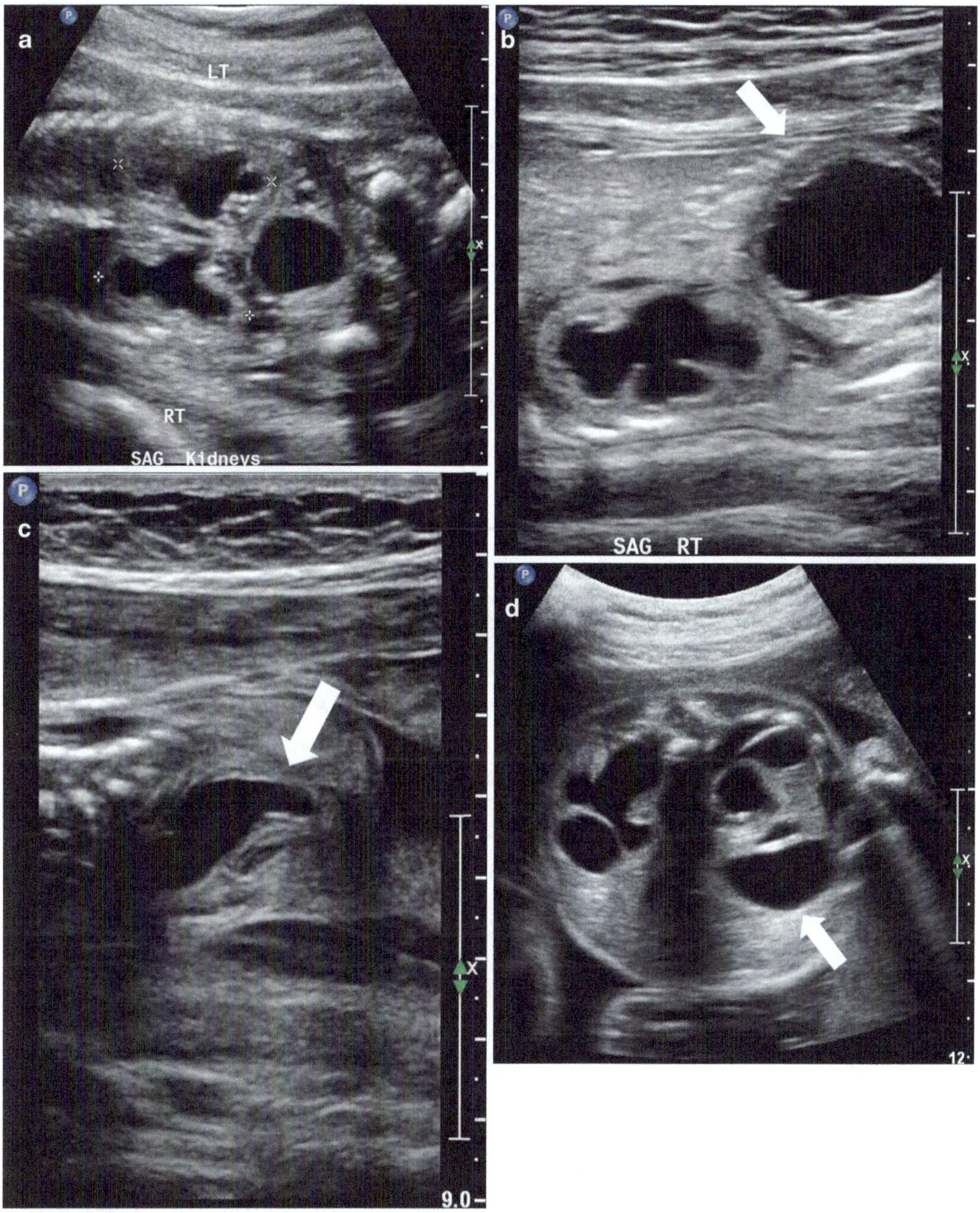

Fig. 8.4 This figure demonstrates four different examples of fetuses with posterior urethral valves. The first presents at 20 weeks gestation with anhydramnios, bilateral hydronephrosis (**a**), a dilated, thick-walled urinary bladder (**b**, *arrow*), and dilated posterior urethra (**c**, *arrow*). The second example is one of the diamniotic-dichorionic twins (**d**, **e**, and **f**), presenting at 26 weeks gestation, with bilateral hydronephrosis, perinephric urinomas (**d**, *arrow*, **e**), and compression of the abnormally echogenic renal cortex by the urinoma (**f**, *arrow*). The third example is revealed by both sonography (**g**) and MRI (**h**), with oligohydramnios, a dilated urinary bladder, and dilated posterior urethra (*arrow*). Finally, the fourth example presents at 24 weeks with a dilated, thick-walled urinary bladder (**i** and **j**), asymmetric hydronephrosis (**k**), and a dilated posterior urethra by sonography (**l**, *arrow*). After delivery, a voiding cystourethrogram proves the presence of posterior urethra valves (**m**, *arrow*) and high-grade, right-sided vesicoureteric reflux, with multiple bladder diverticula (**n**). Postnatal sonography reveals diffuse, right-sided renal cortical thinning, but no hydronephrosis (**o**), while the left renal cortex is normal, but there is both hydronephrosis (**p** and **q**) and hydroureter. All but the fourth example died shortly after delivery as a result of pulmonary hypoplasia

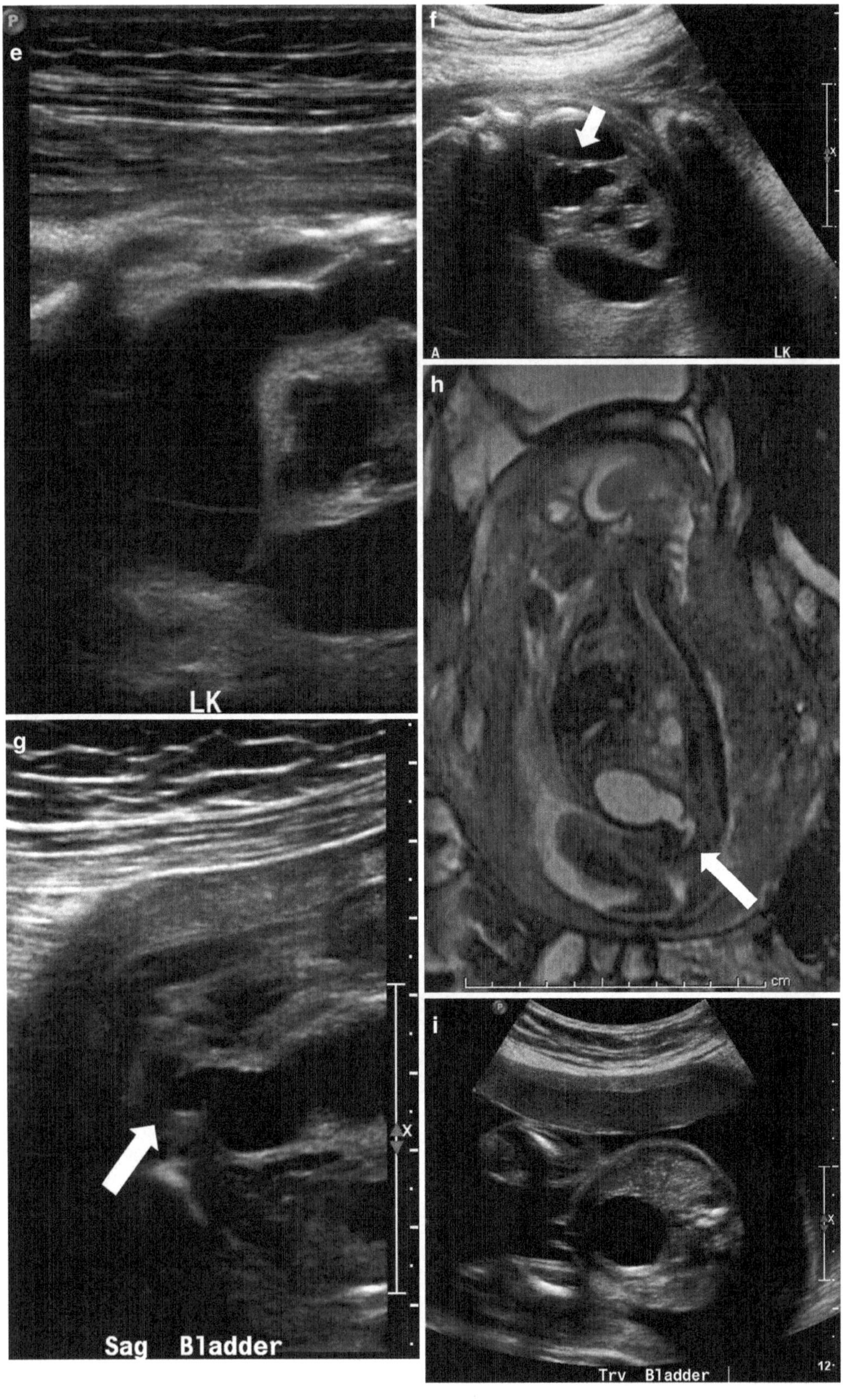

Fig. 8.4 (continued)

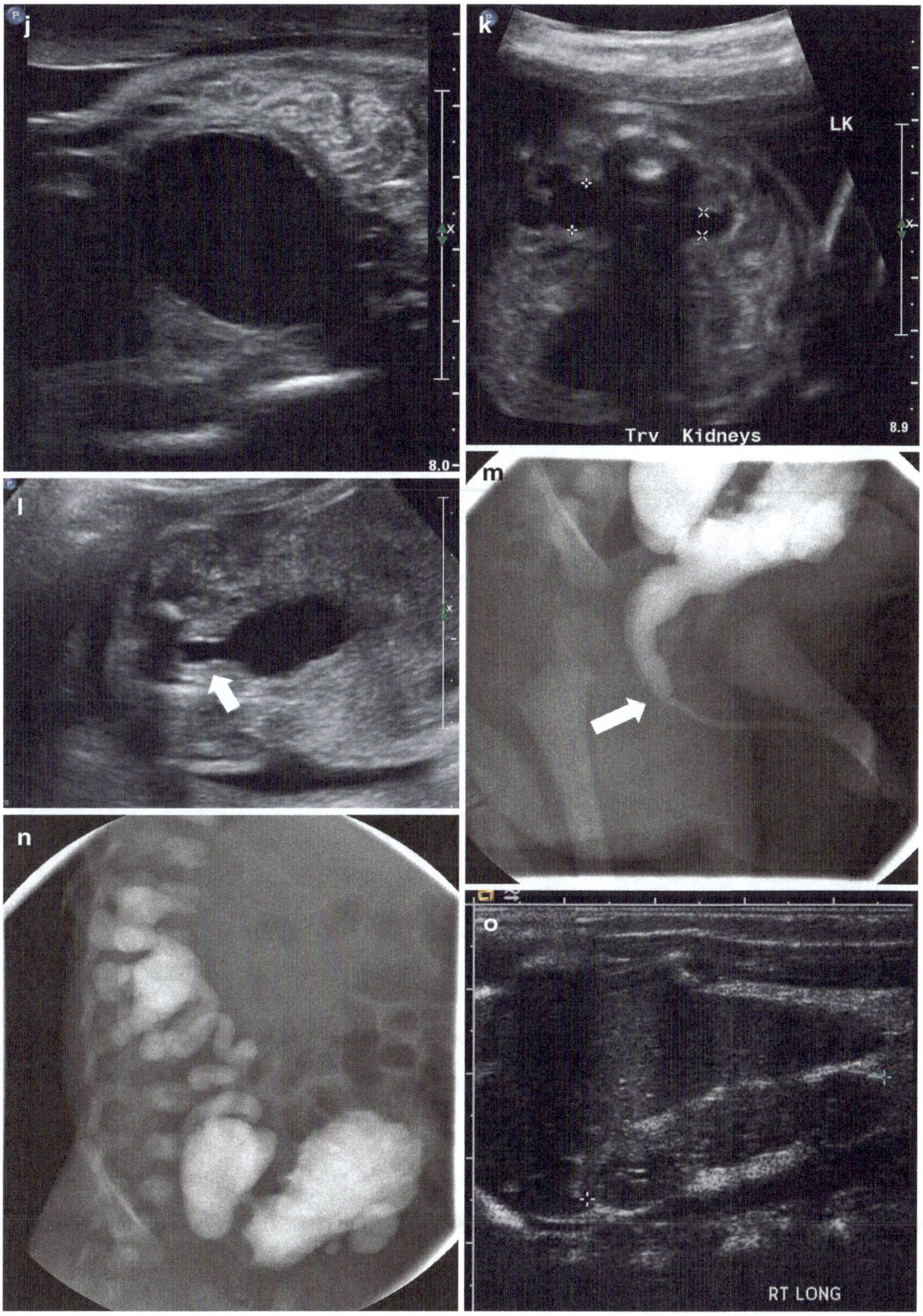

Fig. 8.4 (continued)

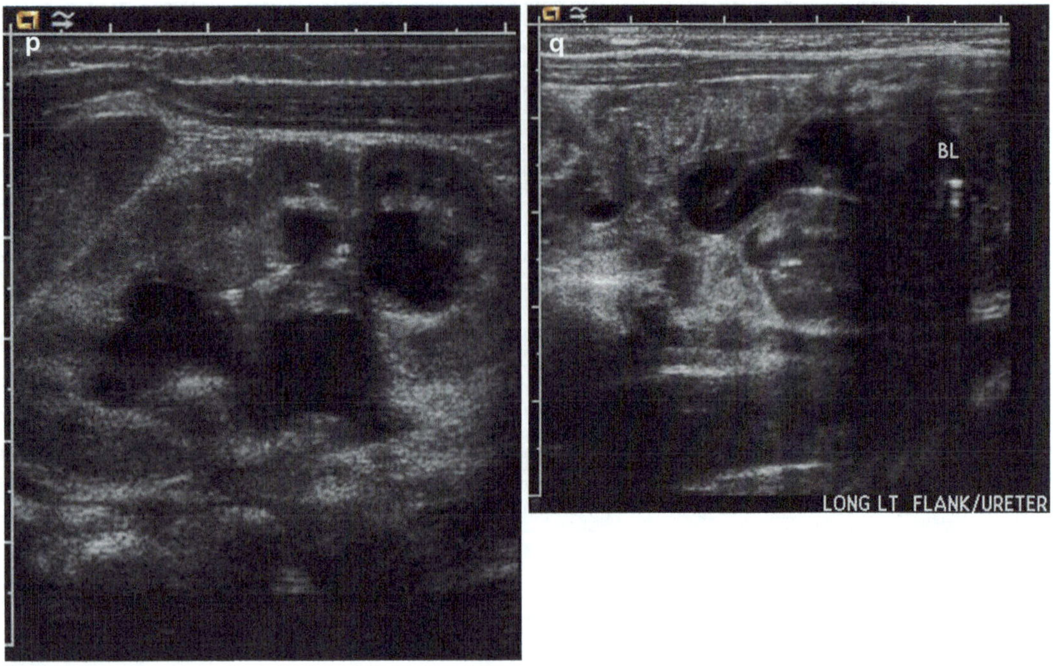

Fig. 8.4 (continued)

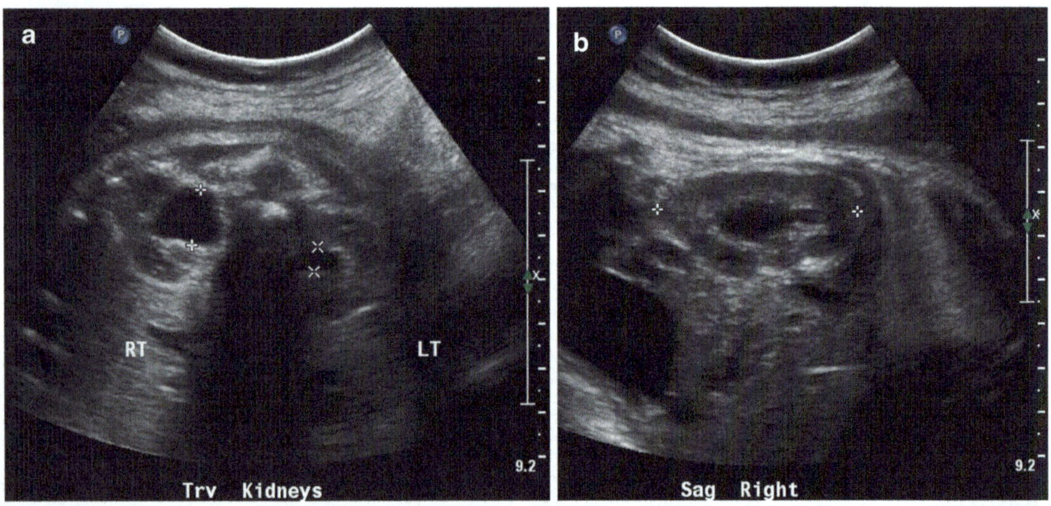

Fig. 8.5 On this 34-week fetal sonogram, we see moderate right and mild left fetal hydronephrosis in the transverse plane (**a**) and in the sagittal plane on the right (**b**). Postnatal sonography is fairly similar, with moderate right hydronephrosis, and very minimal residual pelviectasis on the left side (**c** and **d**). Voiding cystourethrography reveals bilateral, high-grade vesicoureteric reflux (**e**) and delay in drainage of refluxed contrast after voiding (**f**), suggesting the presence of a degree of concomitant, right-sided ureteropelvic junction obstruction. It is important to note that the left-sided fetal hydronephrosis was minor, but the documented, left-sided reflux was considerable on postnatal VCUG, indicating the poor sensitivity of sonography for identification of reflux

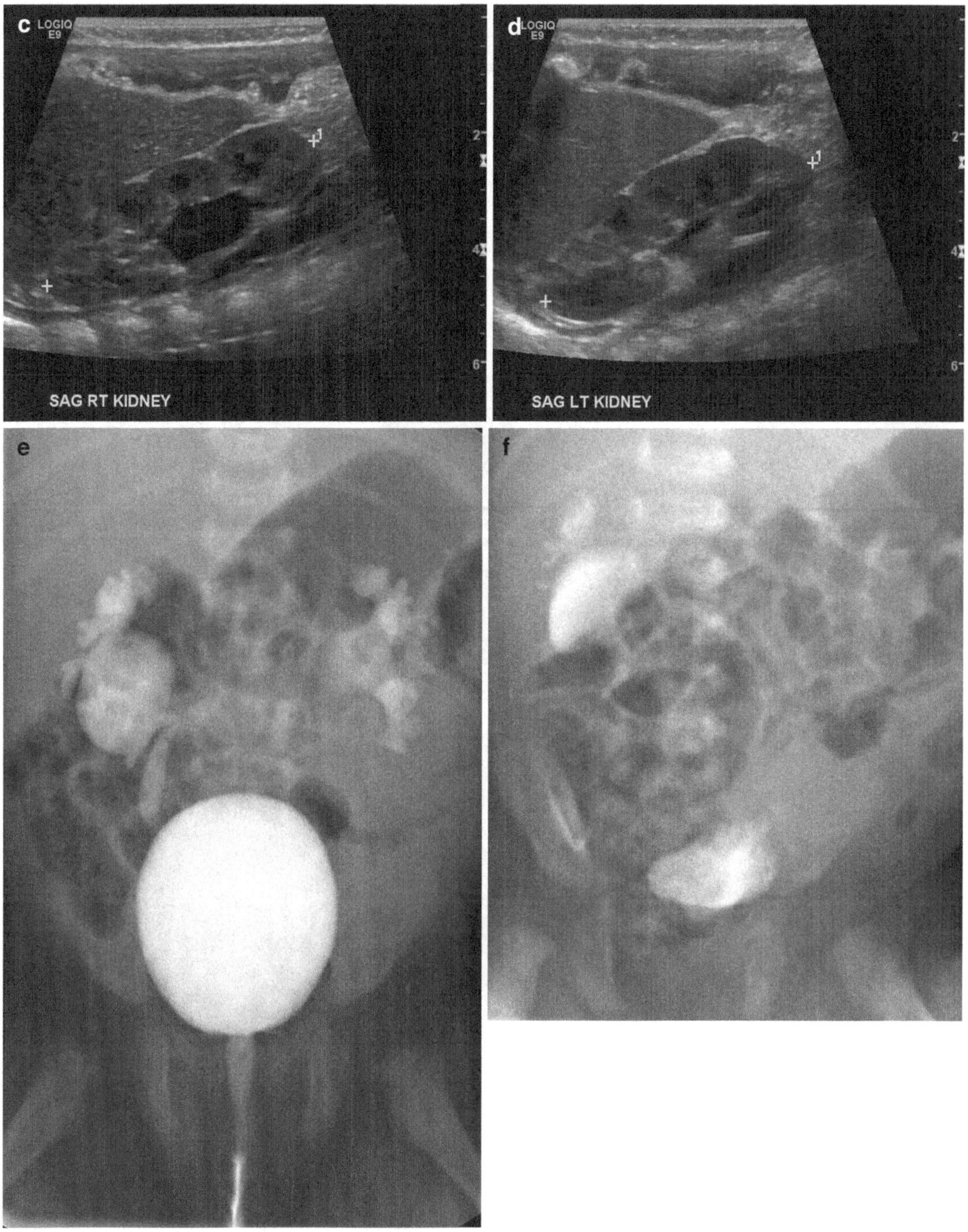

Fig. 8.5 (continued)

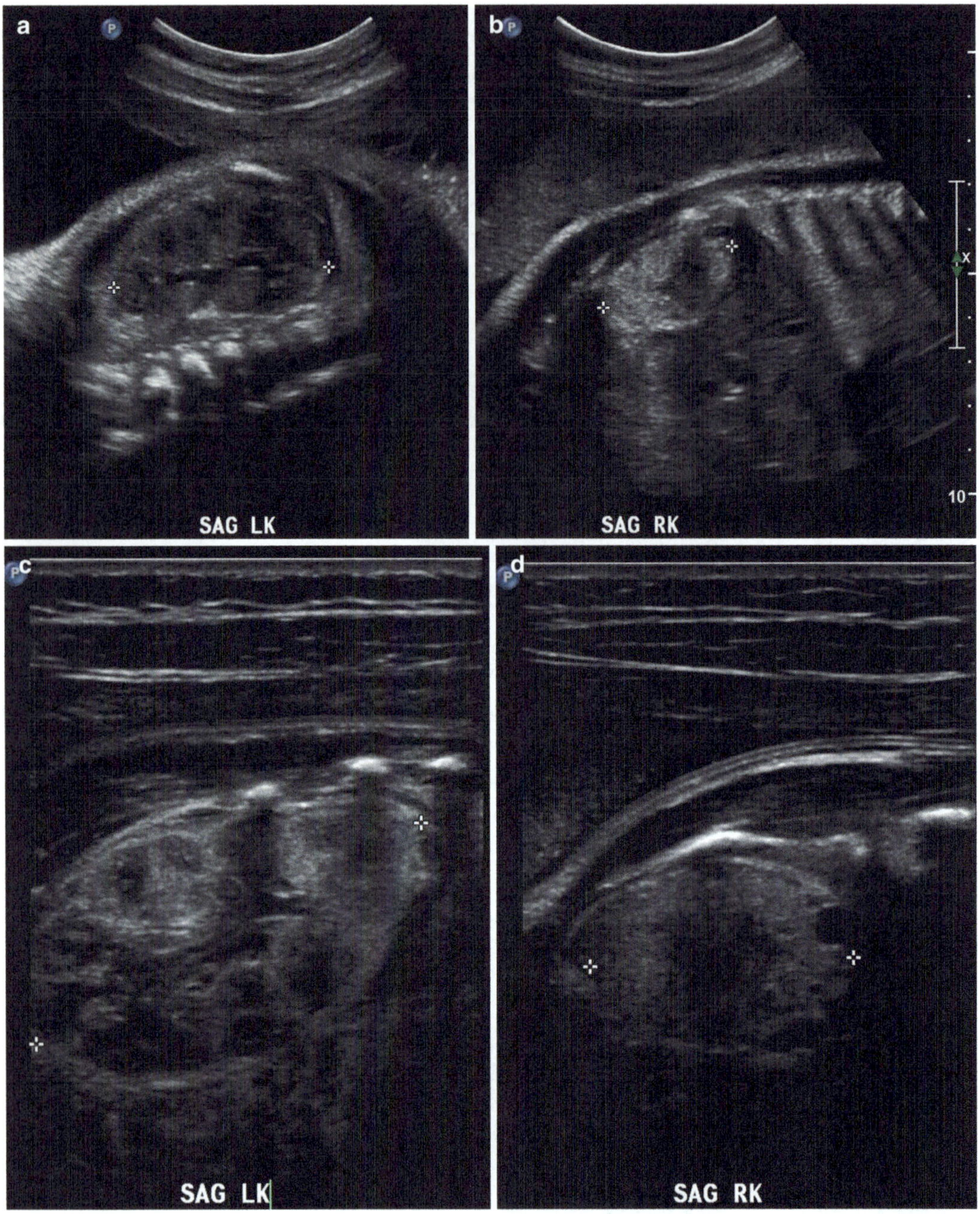

Fig. 8.6 This fetus was followed by sonography with a small, echogenic, dysplastic right kidney and a normal, compensatory hypertrophy of the left kidney. Sonography at 32 weeks shows the striking difference between the kidneys using a curved transducer (**a** and **b**) and linear probe views obtained on the same day show even greater detail (**c** and **d**), with at least one discernible cortical cyst on the right. Findings are confirmed after birth, at 1 month of age (**e** and **f**)

Fig. 8.7 At 32 weeks gestation, this fetus was shown to have bilaterally enlarged kidneys, with a brightly echogenic renal cortex (**a**). The linear probe shows that the kidney is so large that it reaches well below the level of the aortic bifurcation (**b**). Additional views of the fetal left upper quadrant reveal a single, simple cyst in the fetal spleen (**c**, *arrow*). This fetus proved to have autosomal recessive polycystic kidney disease (*ARPKD*)

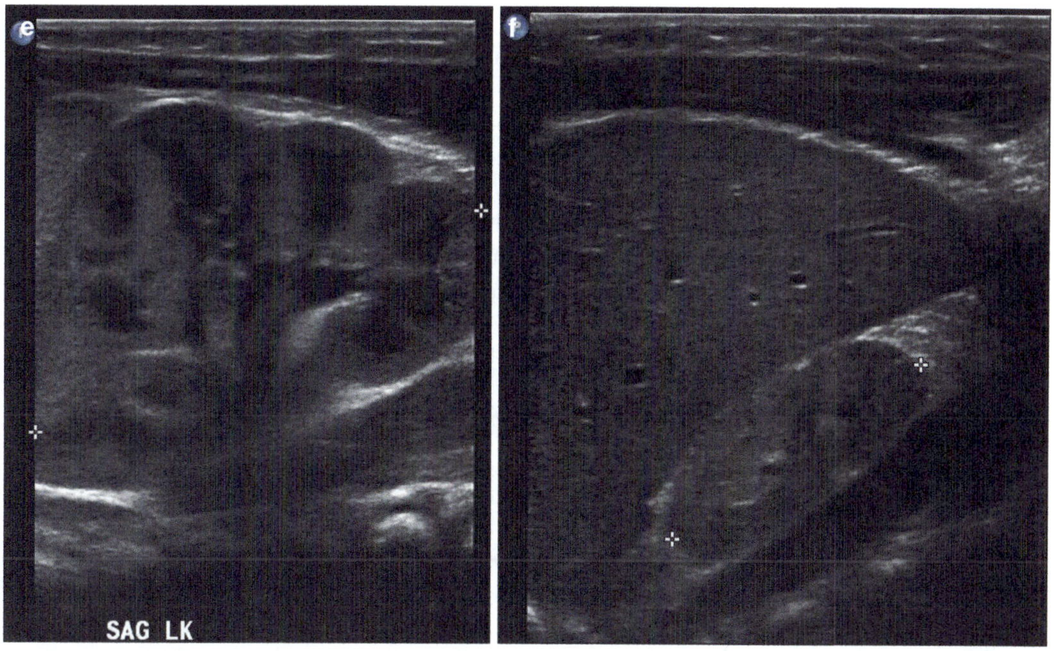

Fig. 8.6 (continued)

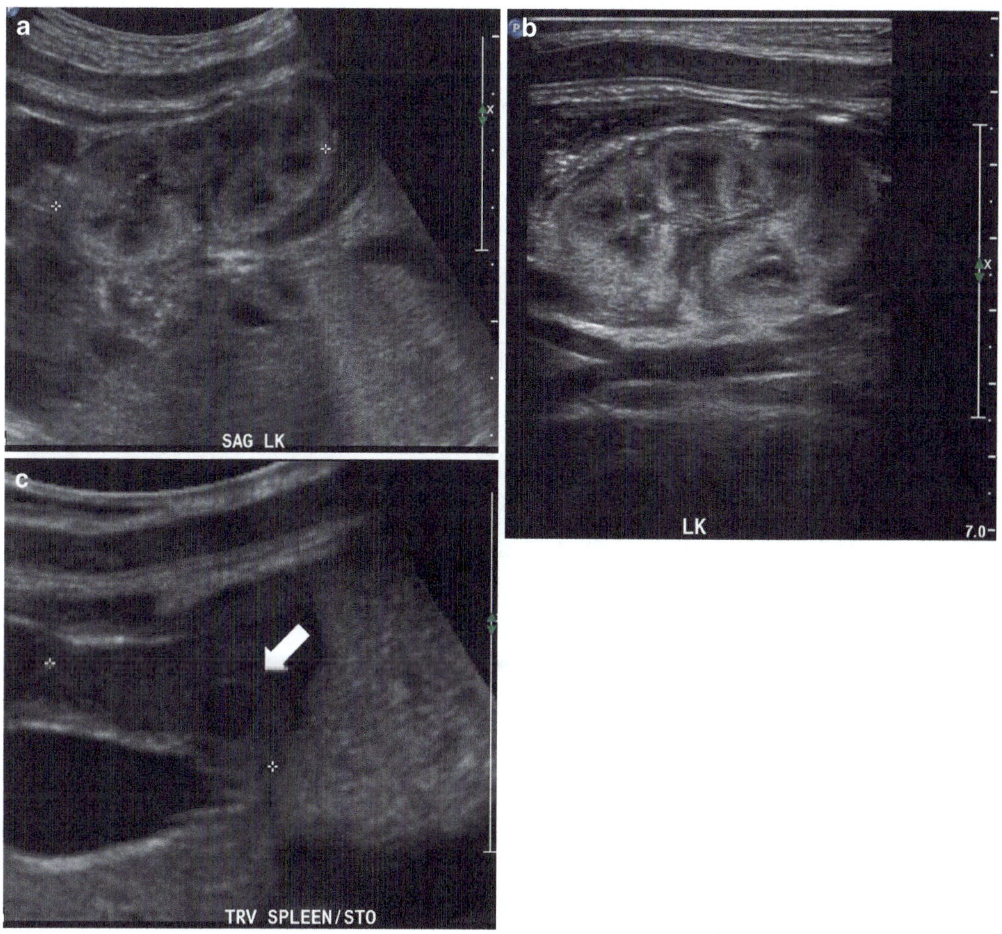

norm. However, a persistently dilated bladder with a thickened wall may correlate with infravesical obstruction. It is referred to as megacystis and may be found in 1 out 1,831 pregnancies [33], although more than half resolve spontaneously [34]. While fetal bladder diameter will increase over time, it will always be less than 10 % of the crown-rump length. In general patients with bladder diameter greater than 17 mm in the first trimester will be found to have some form of obstruction [35]. The cause of bladder outlet obstruction in the male is usually posterior urethral valves which should be confirmed by postnatal evaluation using a VCUG. Very rarely will urethral atresia or anterior urethral cause bladder outlet in males. The diagnosis of posterior urethral valves should be considered if there is decreased amniotic fluid

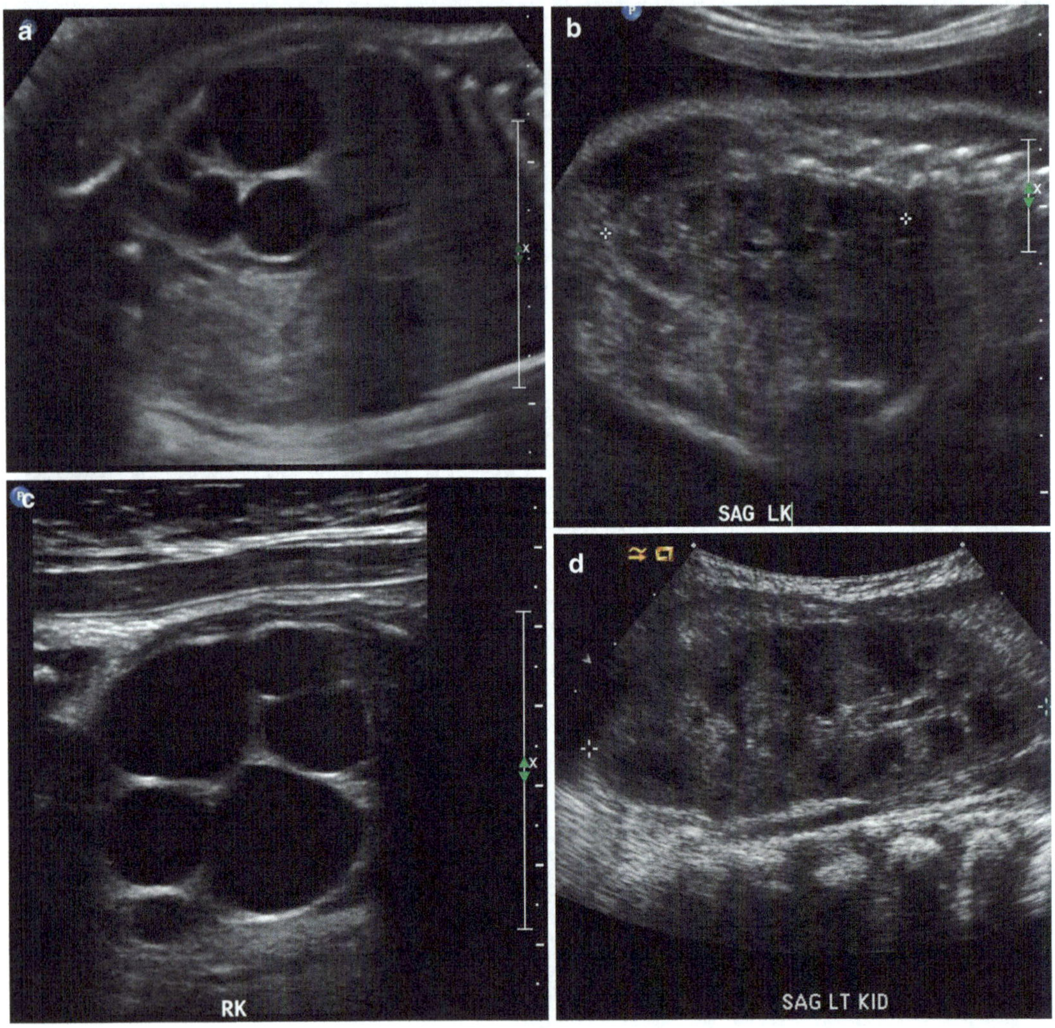

Fig. 8.8 Fetal sonography at 32 weeks gestation reveals a large conglomerate of cysts in the right renal fossa and a normal-appearing left fetal kidney, using a curved probe (**a** and **b**). With a high-resolution linear probe, further detail is revealed (**c**). This is the classic appearance of a multicystic dysplastic kidney. Sonography was performed 6 weeks after delivery, revealing the expected compensatory hypertrophy of the left kidney (**d**) and some interval involution in the cysts on the right side, as is typical (**e**). In a different fetus at 25 weeks gestation, we see another minor variation in the fetal appearance of multicystic dysplastic kidneys. This kidney is even larger than the first example, with some visible intervening echogenic, dysplastic renal parenchyma, and multiple scattered cysts (**f**). By 2 months of age, there had been considerable interval involution of this nonfunctioning dysplastic kidney (**g**)

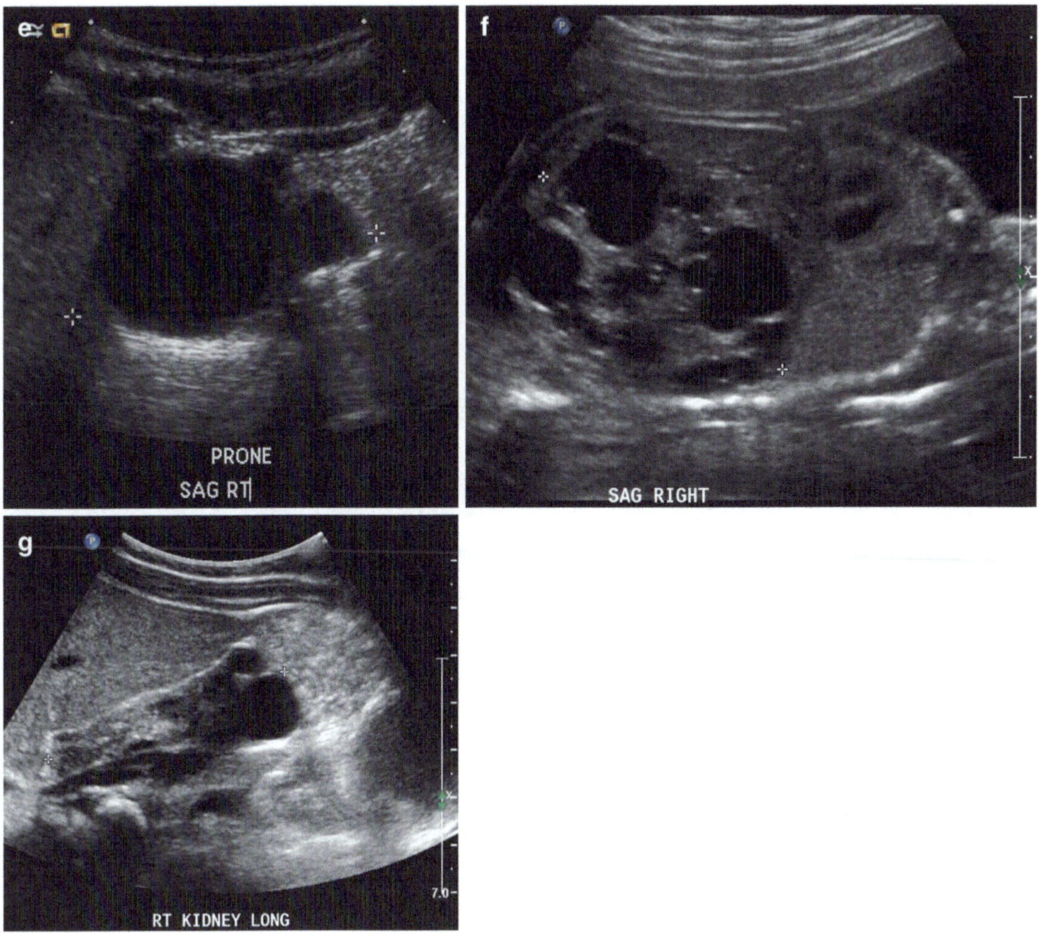

Fig. 8.8 (continued)

volume (oligohydramnios) or if there is significant dilation of the bladder, both ureters and upper urinary tract. The prostatic urethra may also appear dilated assuming the shape of a keyhole (Fig. 8.4). In the female, bladder outlet obstruction is exceedingly rare and is usually seen in cases of prolapsing ureterocele where the ureterocele will ball valve down into the urethra and may cause intermittent bladder outlet obstruction.

Another identifiable lesion in the bladder is a ureterocele which represents cystic dilation of the distal ureter within the bladder lumen (Fig. 8.10). Ureteroceles may be associated with duplication of the kidney and, if so, are virtually always associated with the upper pole. When ureteroceles occur in association with the upper pole of a duplex kidney, there may be also dilation of one or both ureters, more commonly the upper pole ureter which may, itself, be quite dilated up to the renal collecting system. The upper pole of the kidney may vary in size and may show evidence of hyperechogenicity indicative of dysplasia. Ureteroceles tend to vary in size and appearance and are best imaged prenatally when the fetal bladder is partially full. This congenital lesion may be associated with vesicoureteral reflux classically to the lower pole moiety of the duplex kidney.

Anomalies of the bladder such as exstrophy may also be diagnosed prenatally although the diagnosis is not always unequivocal (Fig. 8.11) [36, 37]. Lack of visualization of the bladder, despite repeated attempts with protrusion of the

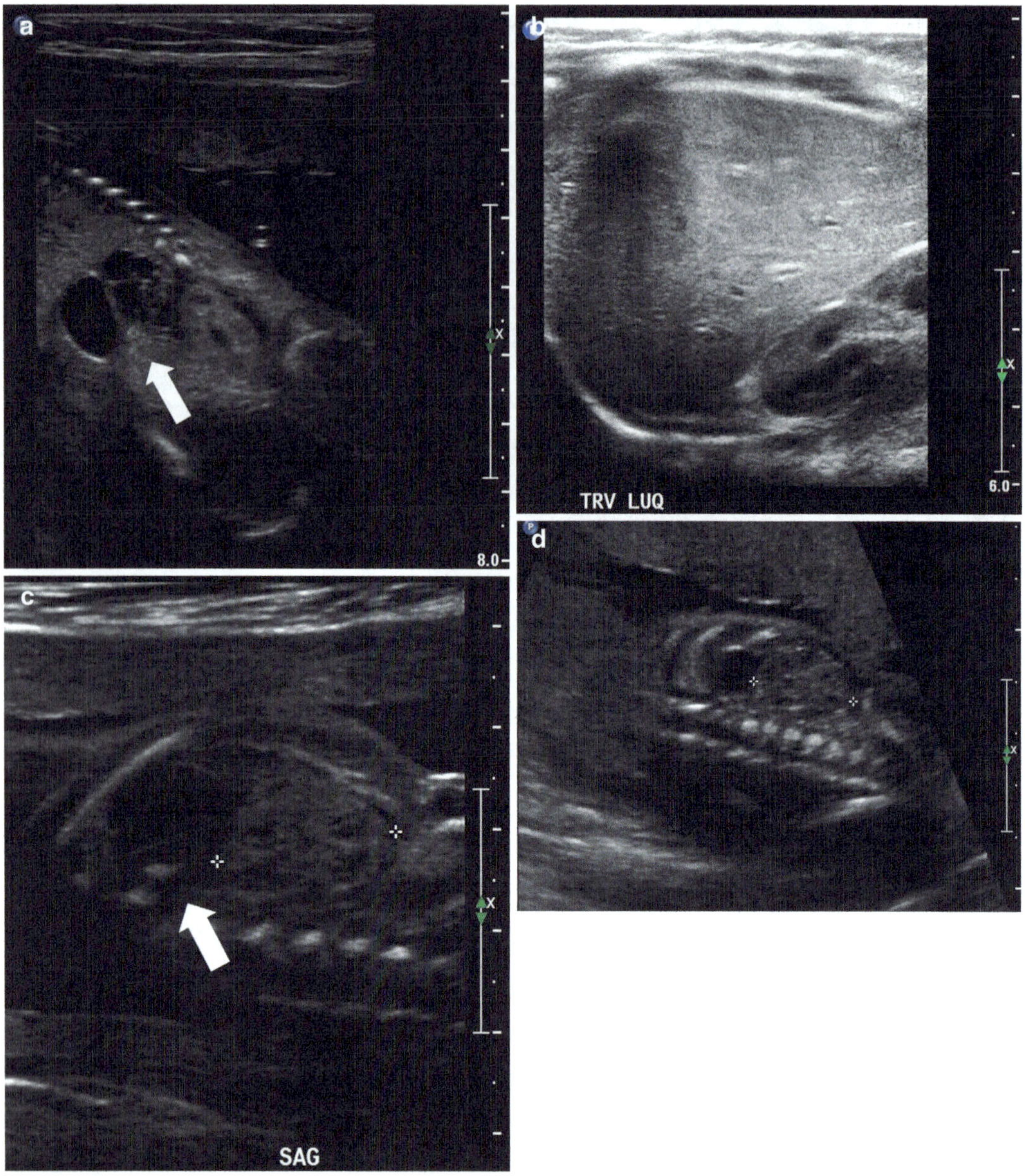

Fig. 8.9 This fetus was referred at 19 weeks gestation with the working diagnosis of left upper pole renal cysts. However, upon our assessment, it was clear that the kidney and the cystic conglomerate moved separately from one another on real-time sonography (*arrow*), suggesting that this was a cystic adrenal mass, likely evolving hemorrhage (**a**). On postnatal sonography, this had resolved entirely by 6 weeks of age (**b**). In another pregnancy, also at 19 weeks gestation, similar, bilateral cystic adrenal masses were also observed (*arrow*, **c** and **d**). It is interesting to note that this patient had also been referred with the erroneous diagnosis of upper pole renal cysts. Single-shot FSE T2 images in the coronal (**e**, *arrow*) and sagittal (**f**) planes reveal complex, bilateral adrenal masses with both T2 bright and T2 dark material, suggesting the presence of hemorrhage. This is proved on the axial gradient echo sequence, with marking, the so-called blooming artifact of Fe products (*arrow*, **g**)

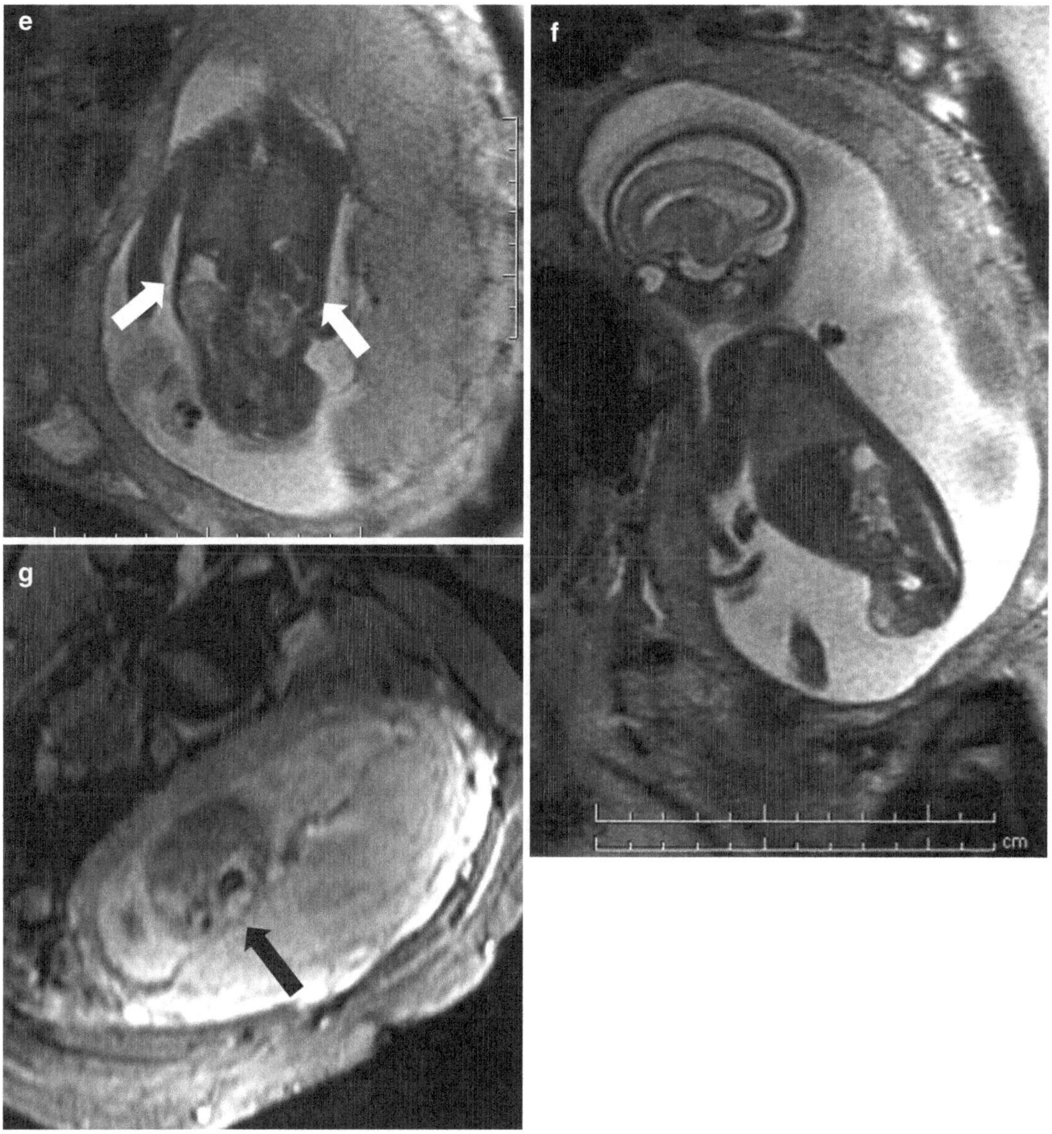

Fig. 8.9 (continued)

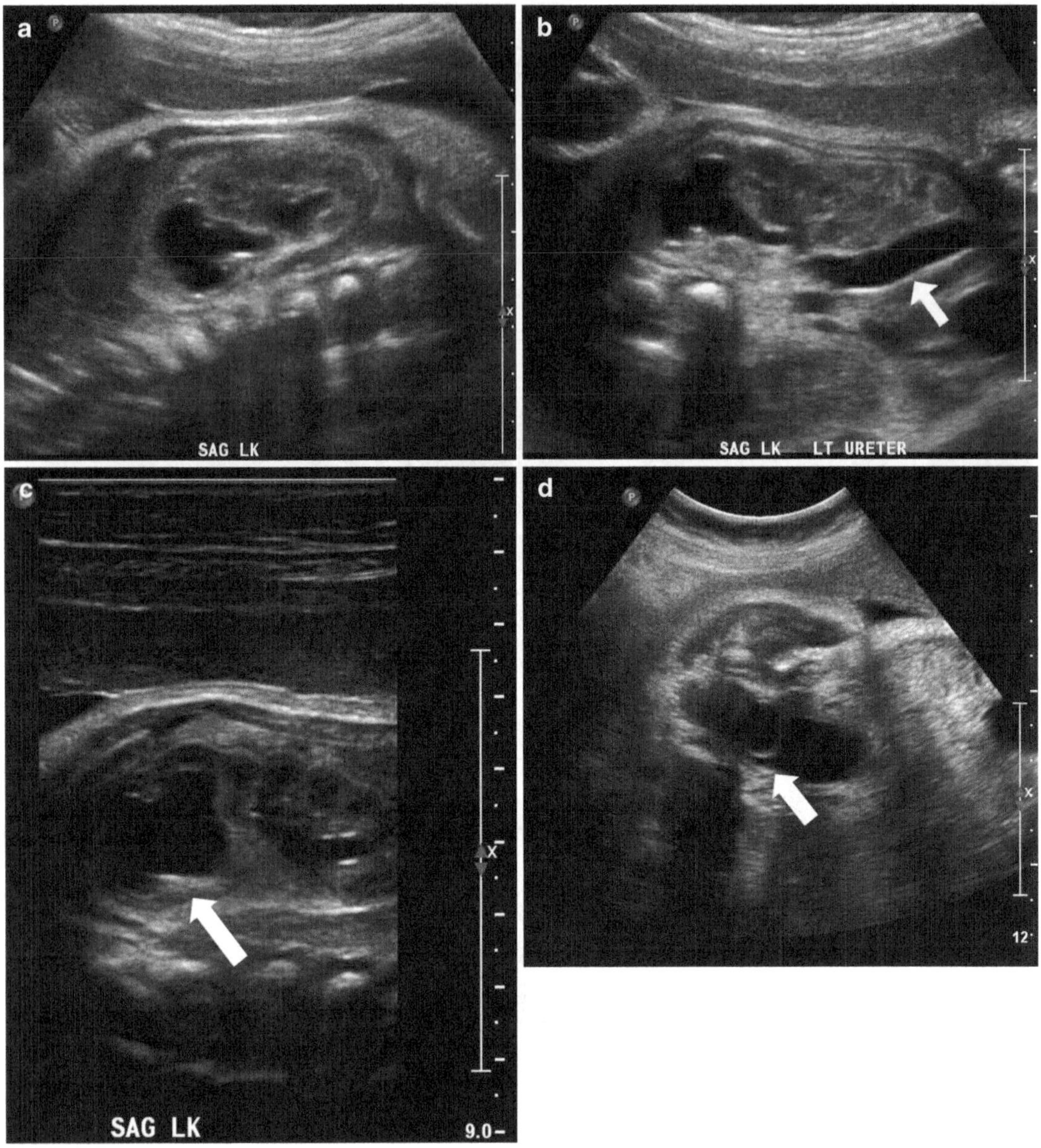

Fig. 8.10 At 33 weeks gestation, this fetal sonogram reveals a duplex left kidney, with both upper and lower pole hydronephrosis (**a**), as well as upper pole hydroureter (**b**, *arrow*). A 12 MHz linear probe can be used to obtain additional detail in this fetus as the mother is slender, so less depth of penetration is required (**c**), showing disproportionate distention of the upper pole pelvis (*arrow*). With careful attention to the moderately full fetal bladder, a ureterocele is visible (**d**, *arrow*). After delivery, initial evaluation with sonography (**e**, **f**, **g**) and voiding cystourethrography (**h**) confirms the presence of a duplex kidney with disproportionate upper pole hydroureteronephrosis (**e**, **f**, **g**, *arrow*), associated with an obstructed ureterocele (**h**, *arrow*), but no vesicoureteric reflux. Scintigraphy was performed at 2 months, and posterior views of the left (**i**) and right kidneys (**j**) reveal clearly diminished function of the left upper pole cortex

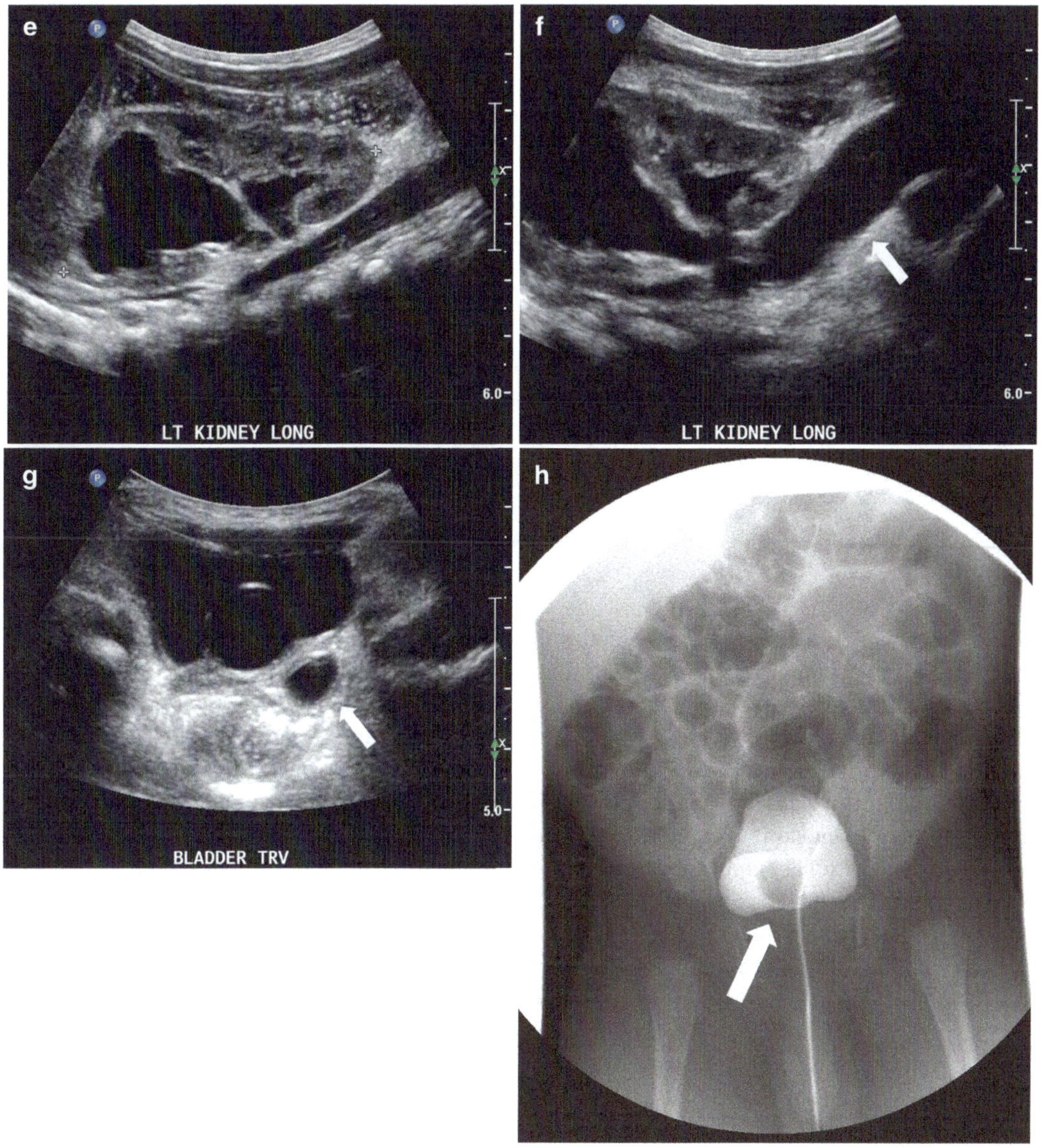

Fig. 8.10 (continued)

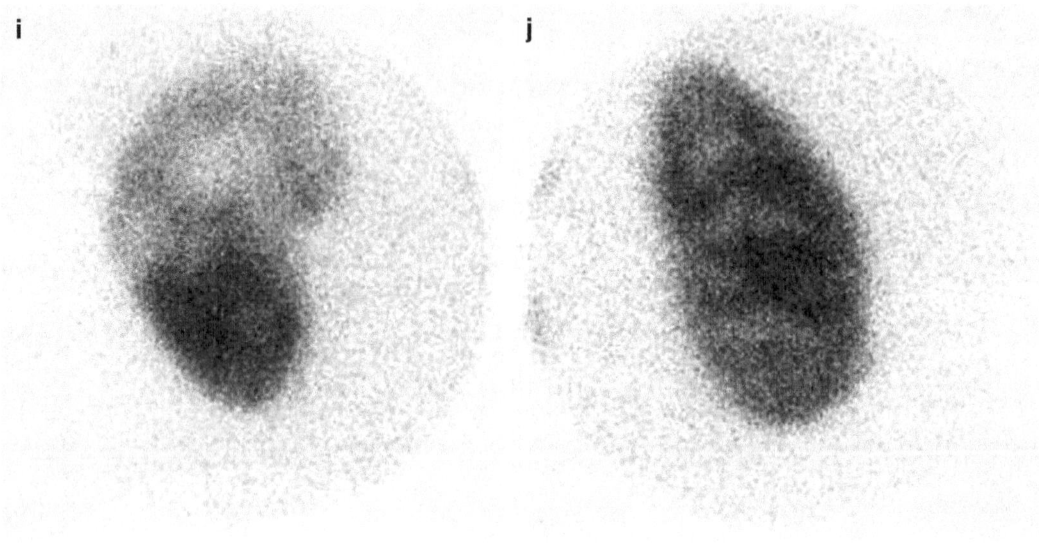

Fig. 8.10 (continued)

lower abdominal wall may be consistent with bladder exstrophy and warrant require further evaluation and monitoring in addition to prenatal counseling. It is important to distinguish bladder exstrophy from the more extensive anomaly of cloacal exstrophy, which is associated with protrusion of bowel beyond the anterior abdominal wall, anomalies of renal number and position, as well as complex vertebral and spinal cord abnormalities. More rare abnormalities such as genitourinary sinus and the cloacal malformation may also be suspected prenatally, typically due to the presence of a fluid-filled pelvic structure in a female fetus representing a distended vagina which may extend into the abdomen.

Fetal Imaging of the Genitalia

Assessment by prenatal ultrasound has been used primarily to determine fetal gender for expectant parents and their families should they wish to know the sex of the child [38]. Gender assignment had significant clinical implication for fetuses at risks of either x-linked disease or gender-specific conditions such as posterior urethral valves. Abnormal genital findings may occur as isolated events or can be associated with other syndromes [39, 40]. Fetal gender assignment and antenatal diagnosis of genital anomalies may be provided to the parents and should be part of prenatal counseling. Care should be given to ensure that the parents understand that the radiologic findings are not always accurate and that the diagnosis may remain elusive until the child is born. A recent study showed no advantage of multiplanar 3-dimensional ultrasonography in predicting fetal sex but may provide better measurement of the genitalia [41]. However, the prenatal findings may provide important information for postnatal management. Late in gestation the diagnosis of hypospadias can be made. Features include ventral curvature, shortening of the penis, and occasionally an unusual relationship between the penis and scrotum (penoscrotal transposition) (Fig. 8.12). However, this finding should have no significance with regard to the prenatal management of the fetus. Megalourethra can also be diagnosed in the later part of gestation as seen with a marked dilation of the penile urethra. In general, bladder and renal anomalies are seen concomitantly. Other abnormalities involving the genitalia have also been reported. Scrotal anomalies can also be seen such as hydroceles, but these should have no impact on the fetus's health.

Patients with a family history of congenital adrenal hyperplasia should have a careful evaluation looking for the presence of ambiguous genitalia.

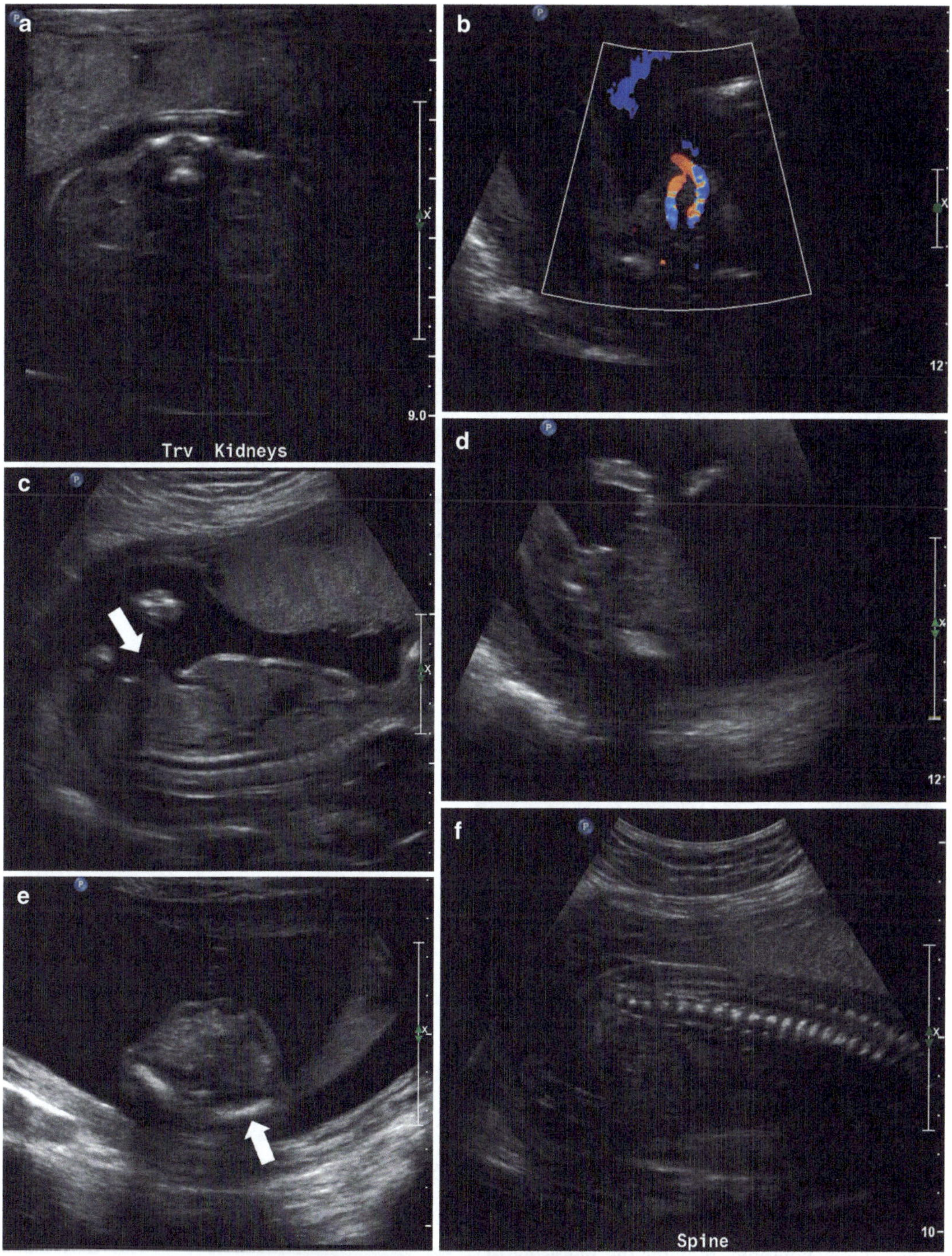

Fig. 8.11 At 21 weeks gestation, this fetus has normal appearing kidneys on sonography in the transverse plane (**a**), but no visible urinary bladder (**b**). We know that we are in the region of the bladder because both umbilical arteries are documented with color Doppler. The umbilical cord inserts in an unusually low position, and there is a subtle bulge seen just inferior to the cord in the sagittal (**c**, *arrow*) and transverse planes (**d**). The iliac wings project in a so-called open book configuration (*arrow*, **e**), and the spinal cord and vertebrae are normal in appearance (**f**). All features suggest a diagnosis of classic bladder exstrophy. This is also apparent by fetal MRI, with sagittal (**g**) and transverse (**h**) T2 images, also showing the low anterior abdominal wall bulge and the contour of the scrotum (**h**, *arrow*). The low anterior abdominal wall bulge is also visible on this axial FIESTA sequence (*arrow*, **i**)

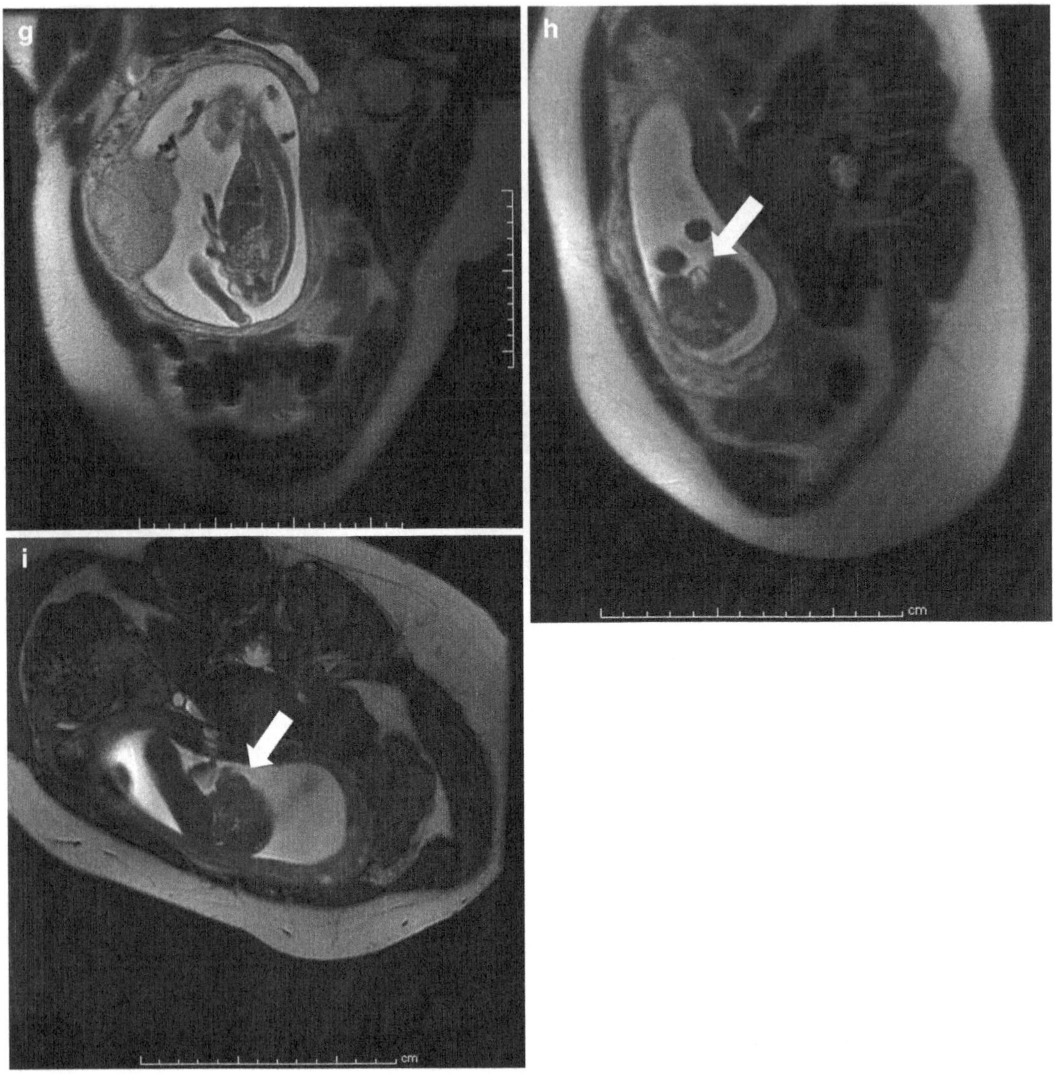

Fig. 8.11 (continued)

Should the diagnosis be confirmed, prenatal treatment with corticosteroids may be considered [42].

MRI Evaluation of the Fetus

While ultrasonography remains the mainstay of fetal imaging, MRI has also been a helpful adjunct to the evaluation of fetuses with complex genitourinary anomalies when the findings on ultrasound do not provide satisfactory information or if technical factors such as oligohydramnios, unfavorable fetal position, or maternal body habitus [43]. MRI has been shown to be safe in the fetus [44]. Widespread use of MRI has not been encouraged given the complexity and cost of the modality. However, in patients with complex anomalies such as the cloacal malformation or urogenital anomalies, MRI may help further delineate precise fetal anatomy [45] (Fig. 8.13).

Prenatal Intervention and Postnatal Evaluation

While fetal imaging has provided an insight into possible fetal pathology, ultrasound of the fetus is limited by (1) variability in maternal body

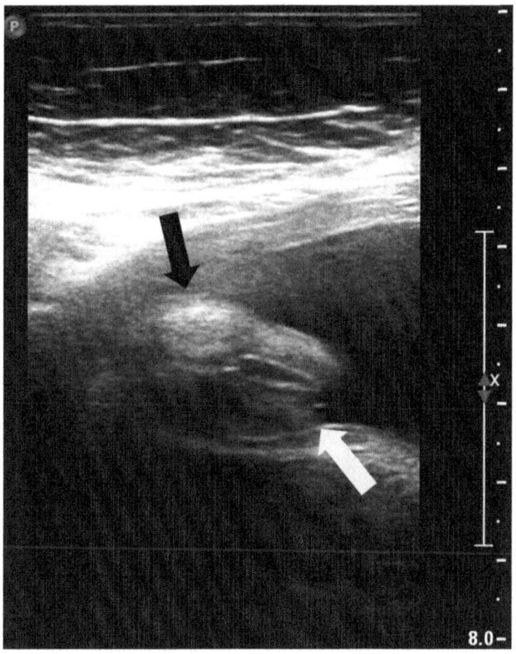

Fig. 8.12 This fetal sonogram was performed at 29 weeks gestation and reveals penoscrotal transposition in a confirmed XY male, with the phallus (*black arrow*) positioned inferior and posterior to the labioscrotal folds (*white arrow*)

habitus, (2) variability in the timing of presentation, and (3) variability in the experience of the ultrasound operator. In addition, variability in the technology may also be a confounding factor. Finally, there is a lack of consistency in follow-up and management protocols for patients who are diagnosed with conditions such as hydronephrosis [6]. Use of prophylactic antibiotics has not been studied well enough to justify use in all patients. Lack of communication between subspecialties with the obstetricians carrying out the evaluation, the pediatrician having to deal with the patient postnatally, and finally the subspecialists being called in after the child is born may lead to inconsistent patient follow-up.

Important prenatal predictors of significant pathology include the amniotic fluid volume which, as mentioned above, is an indirect indicator of renal function, the severity of the dilatation of the renal collecting system and ureters, the appearance of the renal cortex, and the possible association with other abnormalities of the urinary tract such as bladder outlet obstruction or abnormalities of the spine such as spina bifida. The indisputable advantage of fetal imaging for the urinary tract is the opportunity to provide parents with counseling and to map out the postnatal evaluation of the child who is diagnosed with any genitourinary anomaly. Once it has been determined that postnatal evaluation is warranted, follow-up should at the least include a renal and bladder ultrasound. Timing of the initial postnatal ultrasound depends on the severity of the lesion(s) noted prenatally. In general, a delay of 24–48 h for the first ultrasound may minimize the rate of false negative scans except in cases of severe bilateral hydronephrosis [46]. Subsequent radiologic evaluation should be tailored to the findings of the postnatal ultrasound.

In very select cases, prenatal intervention can be offered. Since 1984, when Harrison proposed the first surgical intervention to alleviate bladder outlet obstruction, several studies have documented the feasibility of treating prenatally diagnosed uropathy but have also demonstrated the difficulties in ascertaining an accurate diagnosis [47–49]. The rationale for fetal intervention in urology includes preservation of renal function and preservation of pulmonary function [50, 51]. Preservation of renal function can be achieved by relieving the obstructive process that may lead to renal maldevelopment (dysplasia). In turn, with alleviation of the obstructive process, normal amniotic fluid production is restored, promoting normal development of both the kidneys and lungs, which require adequate amniotic fluid for normal maturation [52].

Options for prenatal intervention include open fetal surgery, early delivery, and elective termination [53]. Several options for fetal surgical intervention have been investigated: vesicoamniotic shunting, vesicocentesis, and renal pelvis aspiration as well as restoration of amniotic fluid [54]. To date, antenatal intervention is and should only be carried out in specialized centers. It is reserved for patients felt to have severe bladder outlet obstruction. Unfortunately, studies that have followed these children have not shown a significant improvement in survival or in preservation of renal function [49]. Furthermore, fetal intervention has been associated with significant maternal and fetal risks [55, 56].

Conclusion

Prenatal imaging of the genitourinary tract has opened a new diagnostic window. Improved technology in ultrasonography and MRI provide two- and three-dimensional views which may help clinicians diagnose and manage a variety of congenital lesions involving the kidneys, ureters, bladder, and genitalia. Most of the more severe conditions will be treated after delivery of the child. Prenatal counseling will help expectant parents prepare for the postnatal evaluation. Prenatal intervention remains experimental. Whether prenatal diagnosis has improved postnatal long-term outcomes remains to be determined.

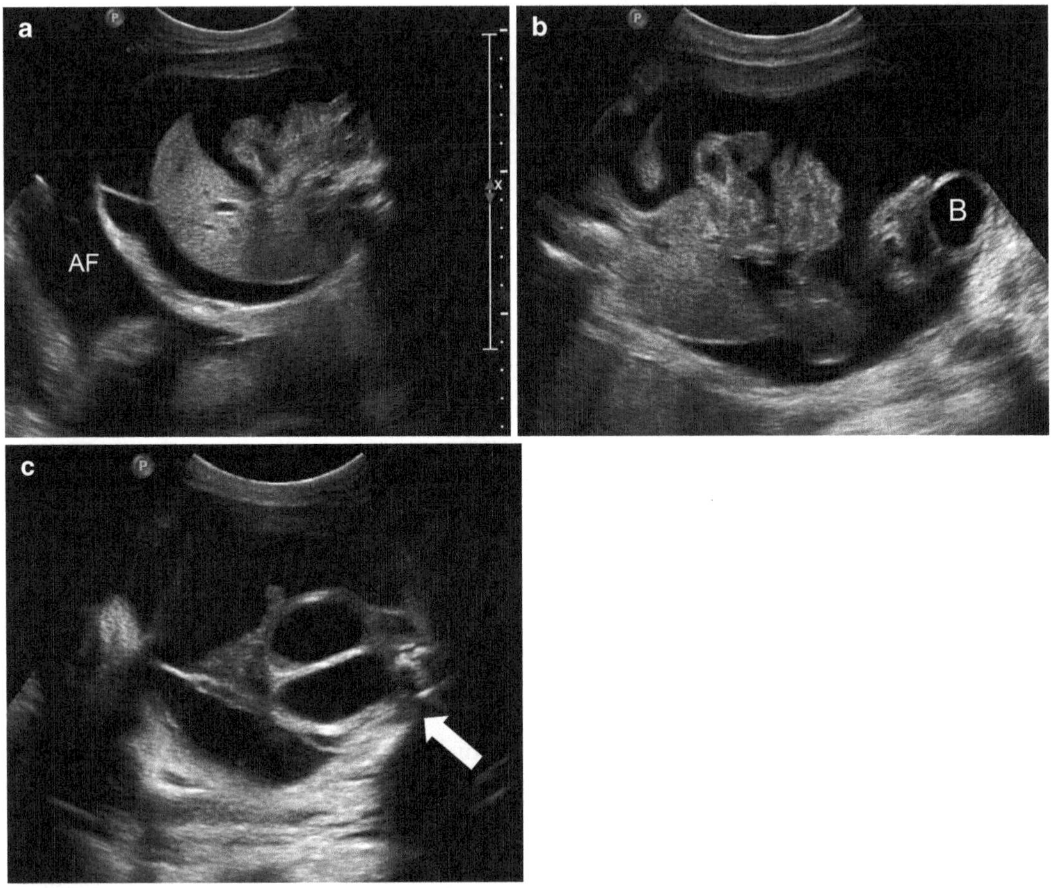

Fig. 8.13 This female fetus presented to care with massive ascites at 30 weeks gestation on sonography. On this axial view of the fetal abdomen, amniotic fluid (*AF*) is seen around the margins of the fluid-filled abdomen, with visualization of the falciform ligament within the ascites (**a**). On a coronal view (**b**), ascites surrounds bowel and a fluid-filled bladder (*B*) is seen. On an axial view of the pelvis (**c**), two ovoid structures were identified (*arrow*). MRI was performed for further evaluation on the same day. Serial coronal views (**d** and **e**) and serial sagittal views (**f**, **g**, and **h**) document the ascites and hydronephrosis. They also prove that the paired ovoid structures seen on sonography represent dilated, fluid-filled hemivaginas (*arrows*), in contiguity with small, decompressed hemiuteri in a patient with the cloacal malformation. A cloacagram performed at age 3 months by opacifying the common cloaca in a retrograde manner, prior to surgical correction (**j**), fills both the paired hemivaginas with contrast (*open arrow*) as well as the distal rectum (*closed arrow*), that is in direct communication with the distal vaginas at the point of the common cloaca. The correlation with coronal views obtained on MRI at 30 weeks gestation (**j** and **k**, *open arrow*=hemivaginas, *closed arrow*=distal rectum) is striking

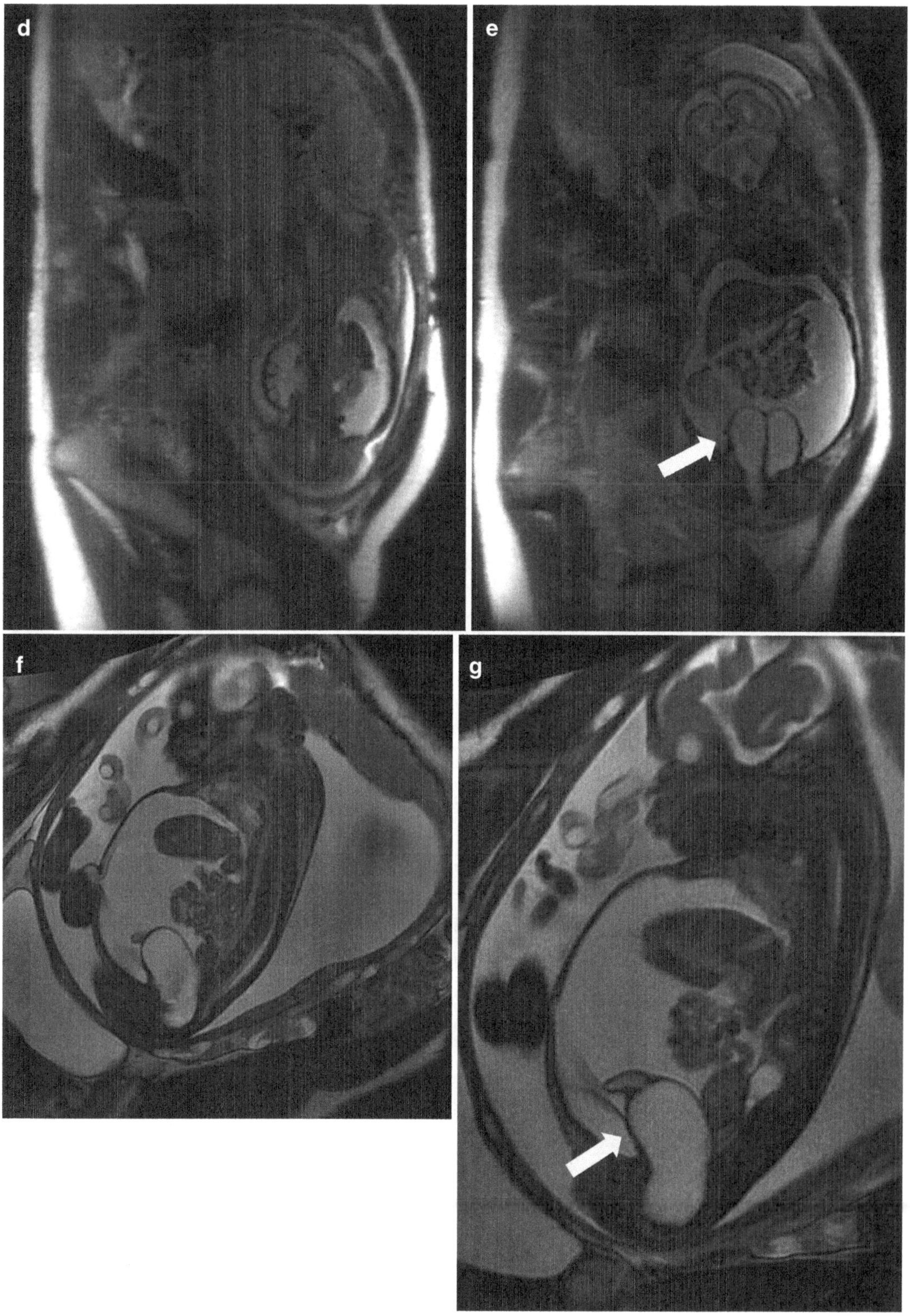

Fig. 8.13 (continued)

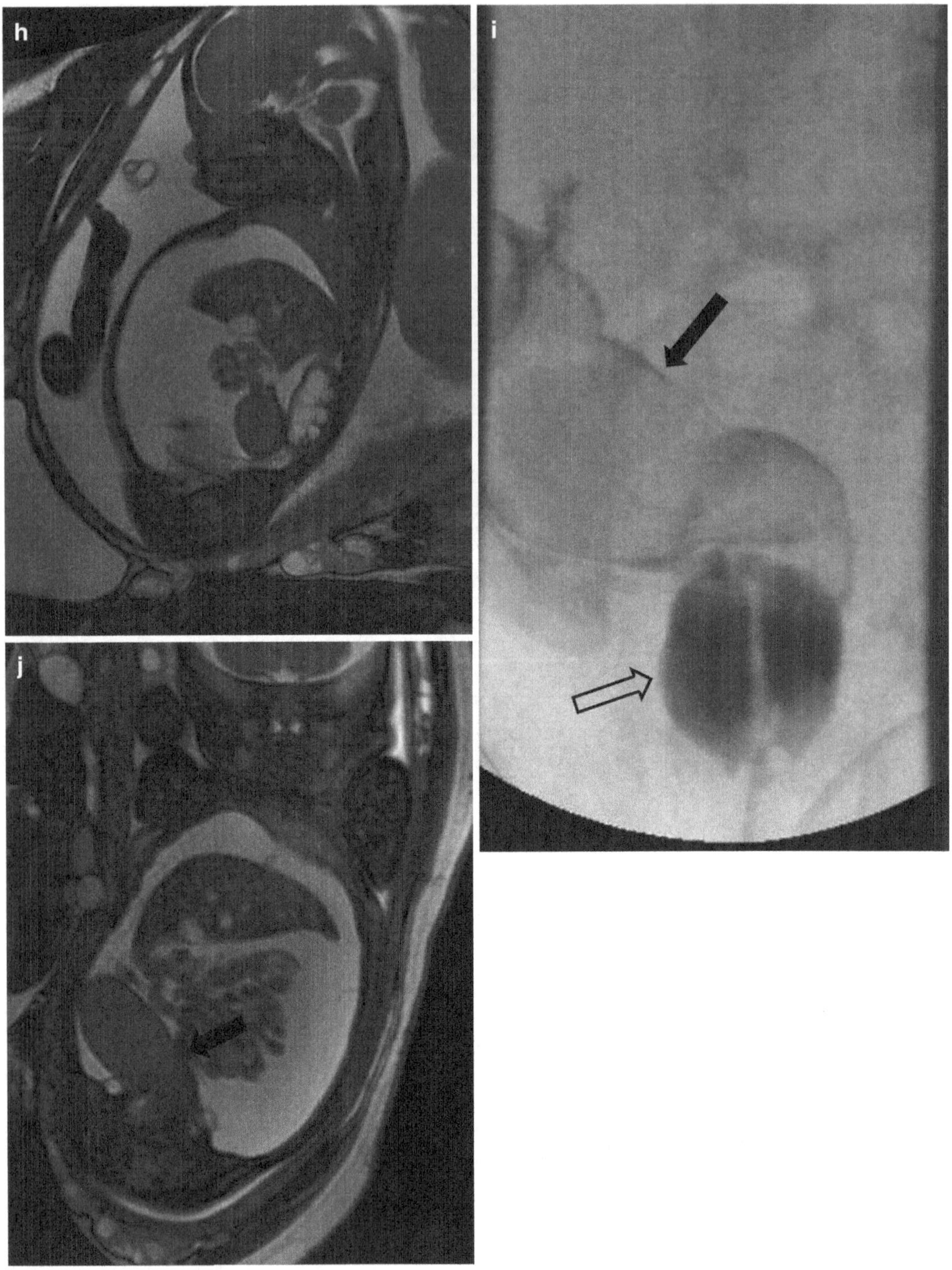

Fig. 8.13 (continued)

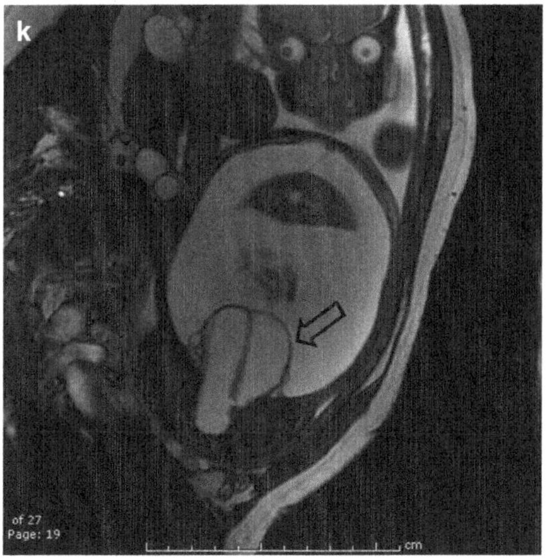

Fig. 8.13 (continued)

References

1. Garrett WJ, Grunwald G, Robinson DE. Prenatal diagnosis of fetal polycystic kidney by ultrasound. Aust N Z J Obstet Gynecol. 1970;10:7–9.
2. Siddique J, Lauderdale DS, VanderWeele TJ, Lantos JD. Trends in prenatal ultrasound use in the United States: 1995 to 2006. Med Care. 2009;47:1129–35.
3. Grandjean H, Larroque D, Levi S. The performance of routine ultrasonographic screening of pregnancies in the Eurofetus Study. Am J Obstet Gynecol. 1999;181:446–54.
4. Garne E, Loane M, Wellesley D, Barisic I, Eurocat Working Group. Congenital hydronephrosis: prenatal diagnosis and epidemiology in Europe. J Pediatr Urol. 2009;5:47–52.
5. Hsieh MH, Lai J, Saigal CS. Urologic diseases in America Project. J Pediatr Urol. 2009;5:490–4.
6. Zanetta VC, Rosman BM, Bromley B, Shipp TD, et al. Variations in management of mild prenatal hydronephrosis among maternal-fetal medicine obstetricians and pediatric urologists and radiologists. J Urol. 2012;188:1935–9.
7. Skari H, Bjornland K, Egeland T, Haugen G, Skreden M, Dalholt Bjork M, Bjornstad Ostensen A, Emblem R. Prenatal diagnosis of congenital malformations and parental psychological distress- a prospective longitudinal cohort study. Prenat Diagn. 2006;26:1001–9.
8. American College of Obstetricians and Gynecologists. ACOG practice bulletin no. 101: ultrasonography in pregnancy. Obstet Gynecol. 2009;113:451–61.
9. Cromie WJ, Lee K, Houde K, Holmes L. Implications of prenatal ultrasound screening in the incidence of major genitourinary malformations. J Urol. 2001;165:1677–80.
10. Isaksen CV, Eik-Nes SH, Blaas HG, Torp SH. Fetuses and infants with congenital urinary system anomalies: correlation between prenatal ultrasound and postmortem findings. Ultrasound Obstet Gynecol. 2000;15:177–85.
11. Garmel SH, D'Alton ME. Fetal ultrasonography. West J Med. 1993;159:273–85.
12. Chapman T. Fetal genitourinary imaging. Pediatr Radiol. 2012;42 Suppl 1:S115–23.
13. Lawson TL, Foley WD, Berland LL, Clark KE. Ultrasonic evaluation of fetal kidneys. Radiology. 1981;138:153–6.
14. Ek S, Lidefeldt KJ, Varricio L. Fetal hydronephrosis; prevalence, natural history and postnatal consequences in an unselected population. Acta Obstet Gynecol Scand. 2007;86:1463–6.
15. Corteville JE, Gray DL, Crane JP. Congenital hydronephrosis: correlation of fetal ultrasonographic findings with infant outcome. Am J Obstet Gynecol. 1991;165:384–8.
16. Pereira AK, Reis ZS, Bouzada MC, de Oliveira EA, Osanan G, Cabral AC. Antenatal ultrasonographic anteroposterior renal pelvis diameter measurement: is it a reliable way of defining fetal hydronephrosis? Obstet Gynecol Int. 2011;2011:861–5.
17. Fernbach SK, Maizels M, Conway JJ. Ultrasound grading of hydronephrosis: introduction to the system used by the Society for Fetal Urology. Pediatr Radiol. 1993;23:478–80.
18. Morin L, Cendron M, Crombleholme TM, Garmel SH, Klauber GT, D'Alton ME. Minimal hydronephrosis in the fetus: clinical significance and implications for management. J Urol. 1996;155:2047–9.
19. Harding LJ, Malone PS, Wellesley DG. Antenatal minimal hydronephrosis: is its follow-up an unnecessary cause of concern? Prenat Diagn. 1999;19:701–5.
20. Sairam S, Al-Habib A, Sasson S, Thilaganathan B. Natural history of fetal hydronephrosis diagnosed on mid-trimester ultrasound. Ultrasound Obstet Gynecol. 2001;17:191–6.
21. Wollenberg A, Neuhaus TJ, Willi UV, Wisser J. Outcome of fetal renal pelvic dilatation diagnosed during the third trimester. Ultrasound Obstet Gynecol. 2005;25:483–8.
22. Passerotti CC, Kalish LA, Chow J, Passerotti AM, Recabal P, Cendron M, et al. The predictive value of the first postnatal ultrasound in children with antenatal hydronephrosis. J Pediatr Urol. 2011;7:128–36.
23. Lee RS, Cendron M, Kinnamon DD, Nguyen HT. Antenatal hydronephrosis as predictor of postnatal outcome: a meta-analysis. Pediatrics. 2006;118:586–93.
24. Longpre M, Nguan A, Macneily AE, Afshar K. Prediction of the outcome of antenatally diagnosed

hydronephrosis: a multivariable analysis. J Pediatr Urol. 2012;8:135–9.
25. Ulrike J, Kahler C, Schulz S, Mentzel HJ, Vogt S, Misselwitz J. The impact of fetal renal pelvic diameter on postnatal outcome. Prenat Diagn. 2004;24:591–5.
26. Blane CE, DiPietro MA, Zerin JM, Sedman AB, Bloom DA. Renal sonography is not a reliable screening examination for vesicoureteral reflux. J Urol. 1993;150:752–5.
27. Woolf A. Perspectives on human perinatal renal tract disease. Semin Fetal Neonatal Med. 2008;13:196–201.
28. Cendron M. Reflux nephropathy. J Pediatr Urol. 2008;4:414–21.
29. Tsatsaris V, Gagnadoux MF, Aubry MC, Gubler MC, Dumez Y, Dommerques M. Prenatal diagnosis of bilateral isolated fetal hyperechogenic kidneys. Is it possible to predict the long-term outcome? BJOG. 2002;109:1388–93.
30. Latini JM, Curtis MR, Cendron M, Crow HC, Baker E, Marin-Padilla M. Prenatal failure to visualize kidneys: a spectrum of disease. Urology. 1998;52:306–11.
31. Potter EL. Bilateral absence of ureters and kidneys: a report of 50 cases. Obstet Gynecol. 1965;25:3–12.
32. Rosati P, Guariglia L. Transvaginal sonographic assessment of the fetal urinary tract in early pregnancy. Ultrasound Obstet Gynecol. 1996;7:95–100.
33. Sepulveda W. Megacystis in the first trimester. Prenat Diagn. 2004;24:144–9.
34. Sebire NJ, Von Kaisenberg C, Rubio C, Snijders RJ, Nicolaides KH. Fetal megacystis at 10-14 weeks of gestation. Ultrasound Obstet Gynecol. 1996;8:387–90.
35. Yiee J, Wilcox D. Abnormalities of the fetal bladder. Semin Fetal Neonatal Med. 2008;13:164–70.
36. Gearhardt JP, Ben-Chaim J, Jeffs RD, Sanders RC. Criteria for the prenatal diagnosis of classic bladder exstrophy. Obstet Gynecol. 1995;85:961–4.
37. Goyal A, Fishwick J, Hurrell R, Cervellione RM, Dickson AP. Antenatal diagnosis of bladder/cloacal exstrophy: challenges and possible solutions. J Pediatr Urol. 2012;8:140–4.
38. Odeh M, Granin V, Kais M, et al. Sonographic fetal sex determination. Obstet Gynecol Surv. 2009;64:50–7.
39. Smith PD, Felker RE, Noe N, Emerson DS, Mercer B. Prenatal diagnosis of genital anomalies. Urology. 1996;47:114–19.
40. Shapiro E. The sonographic appearance of normal and abnormal fetal genitalia. J Urol. 1999;162:530–3.
41. Hackett LK, Tarsa M, Wolfson TJ, et al. Use of multiplanar 3-dimensional ultrasonography for prenatal sex identification. J Ultrasound Med. 2010;29:195–202.
42. Lajic S, Nordenstrom A, Ritzen EM, Wedell A. Prenatal treatment of congenital adrenal hyperplasia. Eur J Endocrinol. 2004;151:1163–9.
43. Quinn T, Hubbard A, Adzick SN. Prenatal magnetic resonance imaging enhances fetal diagnosis. J Pediatr Surg. 1998;33:55308.
44. Myers C, Duncan K, Gowland P, et al. Failure to detect intrauterine growth retardation restriction following in utero exposure to MRI. Br J Radiol. 1998;71:549–51.
45. Barseghyan K, Jackson HA, Chmait R, et al. Complementary roles of sonography and magnetic resonance imaging in the assessment of fetal urinary tract anomalies. AJR Am J Roentgenol. 2004;182(3):689–95.
46. Docima SG, Silver RI. Renal ultrasonography in newborns with prenatally detected hydronephrosis: why wait? J Urol. 1997;19:642–8.
47. Hoosley HT, Harrison MR. Fetal urinary tract abnormalities. Natural history, pathophysiology, and treatment. Urol Clin North Am. 1998;25:63–73.
48. Crmbleholme TM, Harrison MR, Golbus MS, et al. Fetal intervention in obstructive uropathy; prognostic indicators and efficacy of intervention. Am J Obstet Gynecol. 1994;170:1770–6.
49. Freedman AL, Johnson MP, Smith CA, et al. Long-term outcome in children after antenatal intervention for obstructive uropathies. Lancet. 1999;354:374–7.
50. Harrison MR, Nakayam DK, Noall R, deLorimer AA. Correction of congenital hydronephrosis in utero II: decompression reverses the effects of obstruction on the fetal lung and urinary tract. J Pediatr Surg. 1982;17:965–74.
51. Peters CA, Reid LM, Docimo SG, et al. The role of the kidney in lung growth and maturation in the setting of obstructive uropathy and oligohydramnios. J Urol. 1991;146:597–600.
52. Chevalier RL. Prenatal obstructive uropathy. Semin Perinatol. 2004;28:124–31.
53. Herndon CDA, Ferrer FA, Freedman FA, McKenna PH. Consensus on the prenatal management of antenatally detected urological abnormalities. J Urol. 2000;354:374–6.
54. Chevalier RL, Klahr S. Therapeutic approaches in obstructive uropathy. Semin Nephrol. 1998;18:652–8.
55. Golan A, Lin G, Evron S, et al. Oligohydramnios; maternal complications and fetal outcomes in 145 cases. Gynecol Obstet Invest. 1994;37:91–5.
56. Robichaux III AG, Green MJ, Green MF, et al. Fetal abdominal wall defect: a new complication of vesicoamniotic shunting. Fetal Diagn Ther. 1991;6:11–3.

9 Renal Imaging: Congenital Anomalies of the Kidney and Urinary Tract

Bruce J. Schlomer, Ronald A. Cohen, and Laurence S. Baskin

Introduction

Congenital anomalies of the kidney and urinary tract (CAKUT) account for up to 30 % of all congenital anomalies diagnosed [1]. These anomalies are often prenatal diagnoses by screening prenatal ultrasound, but can present in childhood or adolescence with a urinary tract infection (UTI) and less commonly with pain. CAKUT diseases are responsible for around 50 % of end-stage renal disease (ESRD) in children in North America [2]. In this chapter we will discuss the relevant embryology, the scope of congenital anomalies of the kidney and urinary tract (CAKUT), the approach to prenatal diagnosis and imaging of fetuses with CAKUT, and the approach to postnatal diagnosis and imaging of children with CAKUT. More time will be allotted to the more common congenital anomalies.

B.J. Schlomer, MD • L.S. Baskin, MD (✉)
Department of Urology, University of California, 400 Parnassus Ave., A633, San Francisco, CA 94143, USA
e-mail: bruce.schlomer@ucsf.edu; lbaskin@urology.ucsf.edu

R.A. Cohen, MD
Diagnostic Imaging, Children's Hospital and Research Center, 747 52nd St., Oakland, CA 94609, USA
e-mail: rcohen@mail.cho.org

Embryology of Normal Kidney and Bladder Development

To help understand congenital anomalies of the kidney and urinary tract, an understanding of embryologic development is needed.

Kidney Development

In humans, three kidneys develop in the course of gestation with the first two regressing in utero and the third becoming the definitive kidney. All of the three kidneys develop from the intermediate mesoderm. The first kidney, the pronephros, develops near the beginning of the fourth week of gestation and is a nonfunctional system composed of 5–7 paired segments located in the region of the future head and neck. The pronephros develops cranial to caudal and degenerates by the end of the fourth week of gestation.

The mesonephros is the next rudimentary kidney that develops in the fifth week of development. It also develops cranial to caudal and is composed of 40–42 pairs of tubules. The mesonephros does produce a small amount of urine starting around 10 weeks of gestation, and the mesonephric duct contributes to development of the bladder and male genital ducts. By the end of 12 weeks of gestation, most of the mesonephros has degenerated except for the mesonephric duct, which in males develops into the vas deferens, seminal vesicles, epididymis, and ejaculatory ducts, and some cranial tubules that develop into the efferent ductules

L.S. Palmer, J.S. Palmer (eds.), *Pediatric and Adolescent Urologic Imaging*, DOI 10.1007/978-1-4614-8654-1_9, © Springer Science+Business Media New York 2014

of the testis. In females, the cranial and caudal portions of the mesonephric duct form the vestigial structures epoophoron and paroophoron. Parts of the mesonephric duct form the ureter and part of the bladder as discussed in the next section.

The final stage in kidney development involves development of the metanephros which begins around 5–6 weeks of gestation. The metanephros is composed of the metanephric mesenchyme derived from the intermediate mesoderm in the pelvis and the ureteric bud derived from the distal part of the mesonephric duct. Complex interactions between the metanephric mesenchyme and the ureteric bud induce nephron development in the metanephric mesenchyme and collecting duct development from ureteric bud branching [1]. The metanephric mesenchyme develops into the glomeruli, proximal tubules, loops of Henle, and distal tubules, while the ureteric bud branching develops into the collecting ducts, calyces, renal pelvis, and ureters. The developing kidney migrates from the pelvis to its final position in the lumbar region by the eighth week and begins making urine by the ninth week. During renal ascent, the kidney rotates so the pelvis, which starts oriented anteriorly, is medially oriented when it completes ascent. Kidney maturation continues after birth in humans, but nephron formation is complete in utero.

Ureter and Bladder Development

Around the fifth week of gestation, the mesonephric duct that gives rise to the ureteric bud elongates and dilates and fuses with the endoderm-lined cloaca. After the mesonephric duct fuses with the cloaca, the urogenital septum divides the cloaca into the urogenital sinus and the anorectal canal with the mesonephric duct fused with the urogenital sinus. The urogenital sinus develops into the bladder and urethra in both sexes. Part of the mesonephric duct that fused with the urogenital sinus is incorporated in a caudal to cranio-lateral direction. The bladder trigone forms from the fusion and incorporation of the mesonephric ducts. The location of the ureteral orifice in the bladder is related to the location of the ureteric bud on the mesonephric duct; the more caudal the ureteric bud on the mesonephric duct, the more cranial and lateral the ureteral orifice is in the bladder [3].

The ureter develops from the non-branching part of the ureteric bud closest to the mesonephric duct. The ureter is a simple cuboidal epithelial-lined tube with a lumen by 4 weeks of gestation. It is thought that the lumen of the ureter closes briefly and then reopens by week 7 when urine production ensues. The ureter attains its mature transitional epithelium by 14 weeks, and muscle fibers are seen by 12 weeks.

The bladder is composed of two parts that arise from different structures embryologically, the trigone and the bladder body. The trigone is derived from the incorporation and fusion of the distal part of the mesonephric duct into the urogenital sinus. The bladder body is formed from the endoderm-lined urogenital sinus and the surrounding mesenchyme. The bladder apex is the urachus which connects to the allantois. The urachus degenerates by week 12 of gestation into the median umbilical ligament. Similar to the ureter, the bladder has primitive cuboidal epithelium around week 7 and transitional-appearing epithelium by 14 weeks. The bladder wall muscle also develops during this time and may be dependent upon fetal urine production for a change from a low-compliance system to a high-compliance system [4].

Normal Kidney and Collecting System Anatomy

Normal Kidney Anatomy

The mature kidney is located in the retroperitoneum, anterior to the psoas muscle, with the upper pole at T12 to L1 spinal column level and lower pole at L3 level. The left kidney is slightly higher than the right kidney usually. Adult kidneys are around 10–12 cm cranial to caudal, 5–7 cm wide, and 3–4 cm anterior to posterior.

The kidney is divided into the cortex and medulla. The medulla is made up of pyramid-shaped areas called medullary pyramids. The cortex contains glomeruli and nephron tubules, while the medullary pyramids contain the collecting ducts. The collecting ducts drain urine into the renal calyx in areas called renal papilla. The calyceal system generally contains 7–9 renal papilla, but can range from 4 to 18 [5]. The upper pole of the kidney generally contained 3–4 calyces, the middle pole 1–2,

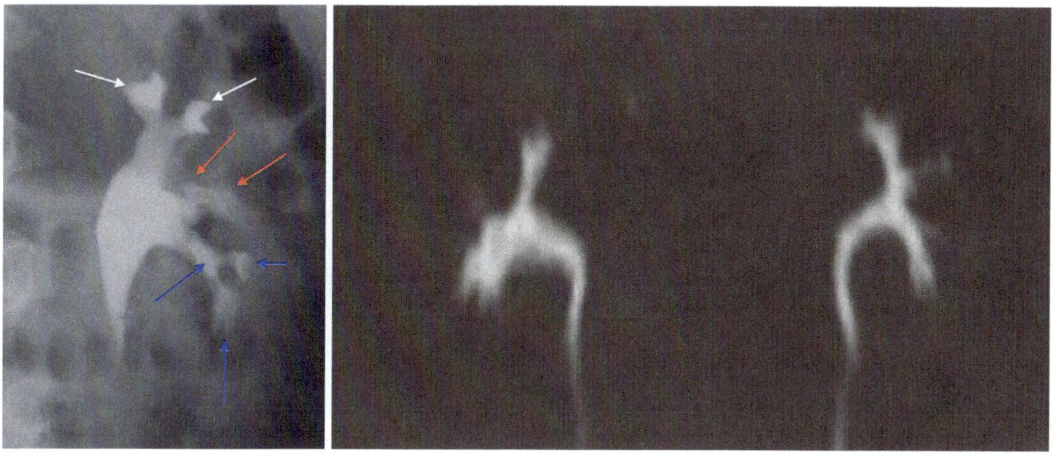

Fig. 9.1 *Left image*: Intravenous pyelogram demonstrating normal configuration of a left kidney with upper-pole (*white arrows*), mid-pole (*red arrows*), and lower-pole (*blue arrows*) calyces. *Right image*: MR urogram of normal kidneys with distinguishable upper, mid, and lower poles

and the lower pole 3–4 calyces. Compound calyces occur when 2 renal papilla fuse, which tends to occur more frequently in the upper and lower poles. Each minor calyx narrows to an infundibulum and then combines with 2–3 other infundibulum to form the major calyces, of which there are generally 2–3 (Fig. 9.1). The major calyces drain into the renal pelvis which can vary in size from small and nondilated intrarenal pelvis to a large, dilated extrarenal pelvis. There is a wide range of normal configurations for the renal pelvicalyceal collecting system. The number and size of the minor and major calyces can vary, the renal pelvis can be bifid, and the collecting system may be completely bifid with two separate ureters draining into the bladder.

Renal vasculature is highly variable with up to 40 % of kidneys not having the classic renal blood supply with one renal vein and one renal artery. The renal artery branches into 4–5 segmental arteries which are end arteries supplying a distinct area of the kidney with no collateral arterial blood flow. The segmental arteries branch into lobar arteries which branch into the interlobar arteries which give rise to the arcuate arteries. The arcuate arteries run along the corticomedullary junction and branch into the interlobular arteries which give rise to the afferent arterioles that supply the glomerulus. From the glomerulus, the efferent arterioles give rise to the vasa recta. The venous drainage parallels the arterial supply with the major difference that there is collateral venous drainage. The main renal vein is generally anterior to the renal artery.

Normal Kidney Imaging

Antenatally and early in life, the kidneys show corticomedullary differentiation on renal ultrasound which can be confused with hydronephrosis of the calyces (Fig. 9.2). In addition, fetal lobulation of the kidney is seen at birth and generally disappears by 1 year of age but may persist (Fig. 9.3). Generally, the pelvicalyceal anatomy is not seen well on ultrasound unless there is significant hydronephrosis (Fig. 9.4). A normal kidney on ultrasound is slightly less echogenic than the liver with the difference in echogenicity generally increasing with age (Fig. 9.5).

The normal kidney on the noncontrast phase of a CT scan should have a radiodensity measured in Hounsfield units of around 30. The renal cortex, medulla, and calyces are generally not distinguishable on a noncontrast phase. After infusion of intravenous contrast, the cortex is able to be distinguished from the medulla on an early nephrogram phase. On a later nephrogram phase, the cortex and medulla may be less distinguishable, and the contrast enhancement should be symmetric between the two kidneys. On the excretory phase, the renal calyces should be crisp and not dilated (Fig. 9.6).

In a normal kidney imaged by T1-weighted MRI, the cortex has a higher signal intensity than the medulla and therefore appears brighter than the medulla allowing the cortex and medulla to be differentiated (Fig. 9.7). On T2-weighted MRI, the medulla has a higher signal intensity and appears

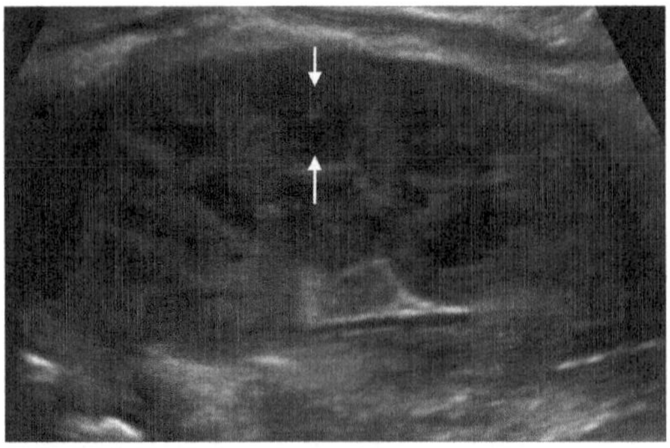

Fig. 9.2 Ultrasound of the left kidney in a 1-week-old infant demonstrating corticomedullary differentiation. The hypoechoic areas are the renal pyramids (one pyramid identified by *white arrows*)

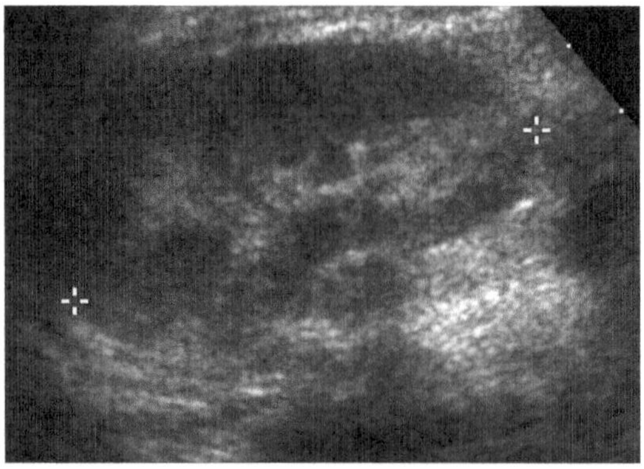

Fig. 9.4 Normal renal ultrasound of the left kidney in a 1-year-old demonstrating inability to discern pelvicalyceal anatomy (*asterisk* denote renal polar length)

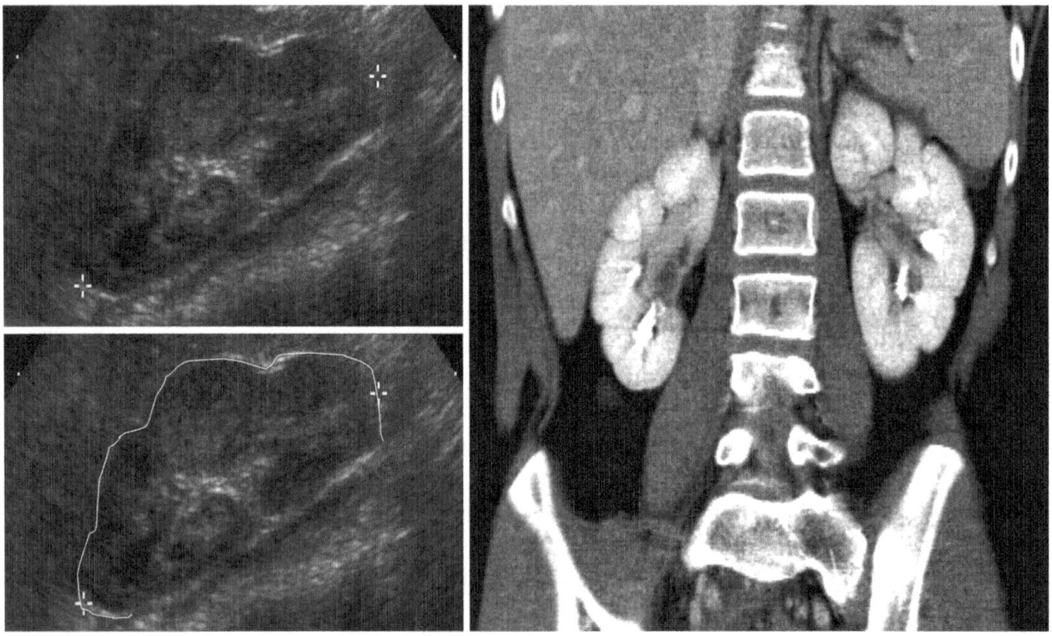

Fig. 9.3 Renal ultrasound of the right kidney in a 1-year-old demonstrating fetal lobulations (*left images*) with the renal contour highlighted in the lower image. CT scan with IV contrast in a 10-year-old demonstrating persistence of fetal lobulations into childhood (*right*)

brighter than the cortex. In addition, the collecting system has a higher signal intensity on T2-weighted MRI and can be somewhat visualized. Visualization of the collecting system and vascular supply can be improved with the addition of intravenous contrast such as gadolinium (Fig. 9.7).

The normal kidneys on radionuclide scans should uptake radiotracer symmetrically and homogeneously throughout the kidneys (Fig. 9.8). In the case of a MAG3 renal scan, the radiotracer should begin excretion into the collecting system within 10 min and should wash out promptly if furosemide is given. A time for half of the radiotracer to wash out (T ½) under 10–15 min is considered unobstructed. The differential function on a MAG3 renal scan is determined by the amount of radiotracer taken up by the kidneys within the first 2–3 min after radiotracer infusion.

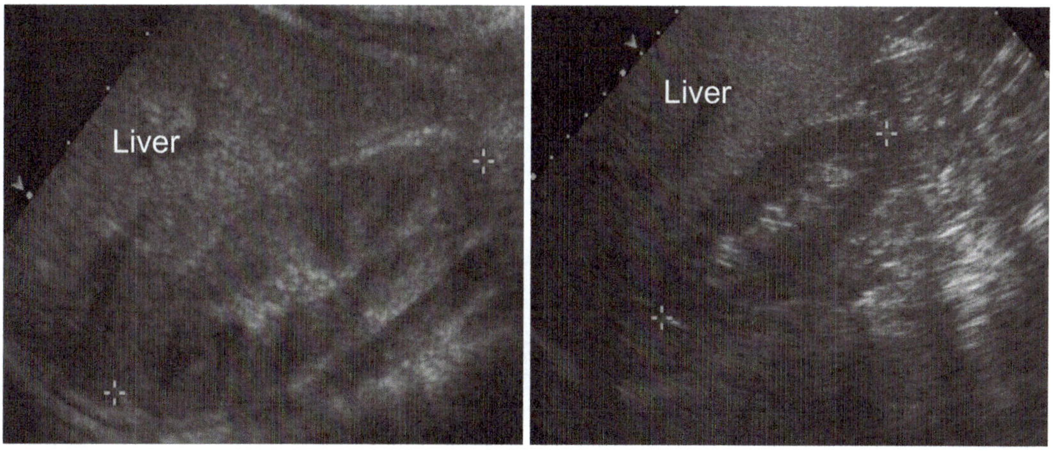

Fig. 9.5 Normal renal ultrasound of the right kidney in a 1-year-old demonstrating normal echogenicity compared to the liver (*left*). Normal renal ultrasound of the right kidney in a 10-year-old demonstrating that difference in echogenicity generally becomes more pronounced (*right*)

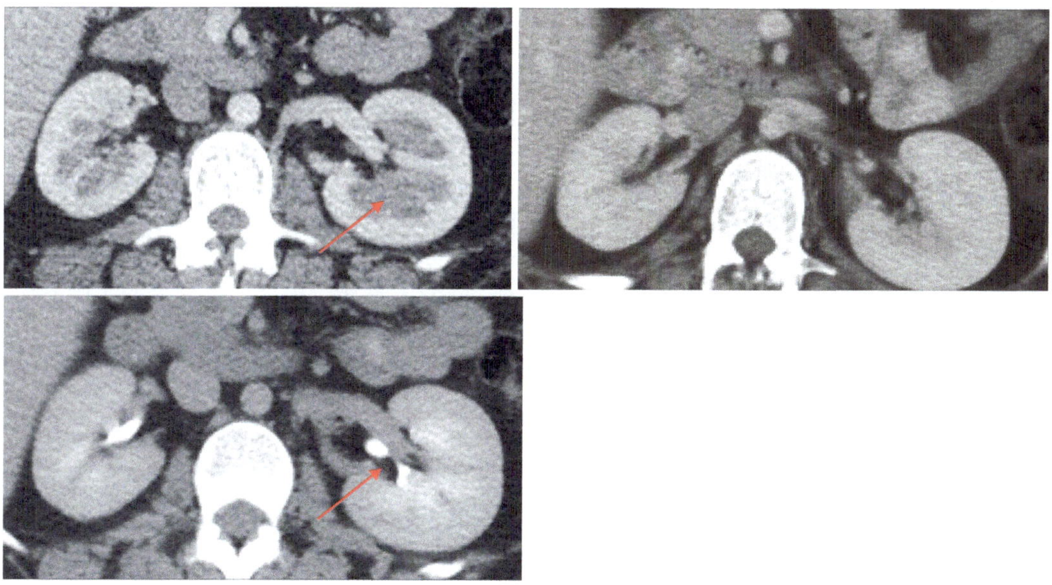

Fig. 9.6 Axial CT scan of the kidneys with intravenous contrast. The *upper left image* shows an early nephrogram phase, note how the medulla of the kidney has yet to fully enhance with contrast and is distinguishable from the cortex (*arrow*). The *upper right image* shows a later nephrogram phase of the same patient at another time where the contrast has now reached the medulla. The *lower image* shows the excretory or urogram phase with contrast easily visible within the renal collecting systems (*arrow*)

Normal Ureter Anatomy

The renal pelvis drains to the ureter whose origin is normally posterior to the renal artery. The ureter courses caudally and anterior to the psoas muscle toward the pelvis. The ureter crosses the iliac vessels close to its bifurcation. Once in the pelvis, the ureter passes posteroinferiorly along the lateral walls of the pelvis and then courses anteromedially to come into contact with the bladder. The ureter travels 2–3 cm within the bladder wall before the ureteral orifice. There are three points of anatomical narrowing in the ureter that are common sites of ureteral nephrolithiasis: the ureteropelvic junction, the iliac vessels, and the ureterovesical junction. The normal ureter size in adults is 1.8 mm (SD 0.9 mm) with 96 % of ureters less than 3 mm [6]. The blood supply

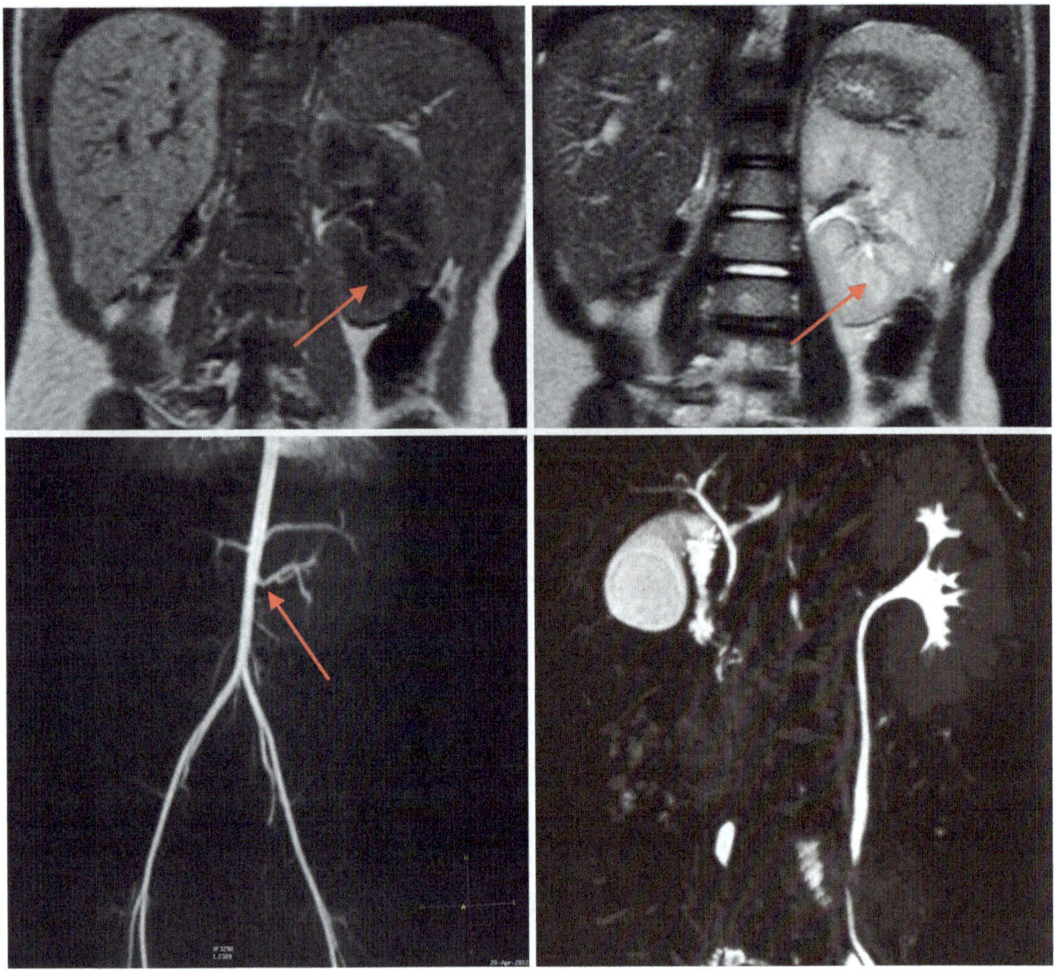

Fig. 9.7 MRI of a 4-year-old with solitary left kidney. *Upper left image* is a T1-weighted MRI image, note the cortex has a higher signal intensity than the medulla (*arrow*). On the T2-weighted MRI image in the *upper right*, the medulla (*arrow*) has a higher signal intensity than the cortex, and the collecting system is somewhat discernable. The *lower left image* is a three-dimensional reconstruction of an arterial phase demonstrating MR angiography; the arrow denotes the renal artery. The *lower right image* is a three-dimensional reconstruction of the excretory phase after addition of intravenous contrast demonstrating the collecting pelvicalyceal collecting system

of the upper ureter comes medially from the aorta, and the blood supply of the lower ureter comes laterally from the iliac vessels.

Normal Ureter Imaging

Most ureters are not able to be visualized their entire length by ultrasonography unless there is hydroureter. Normal ureters can be visualized on CT and MRI, and their visualization is enhanced on the delayed excretory phase of a contrast-enhanced study (Fig. 9.9). A retrograde pyelogram can also be used to study the ureters but requires cystoscopy and anesthesia (Fig. 9.10).

Normal Bladder Anatomy

The bladder is a retroperitoneal pelvic organ. The superior surface is covered with peritoneum, and the urachus attaches the bladder to the anterior abdominal wall. When full, the bladder is an ovoid shape.

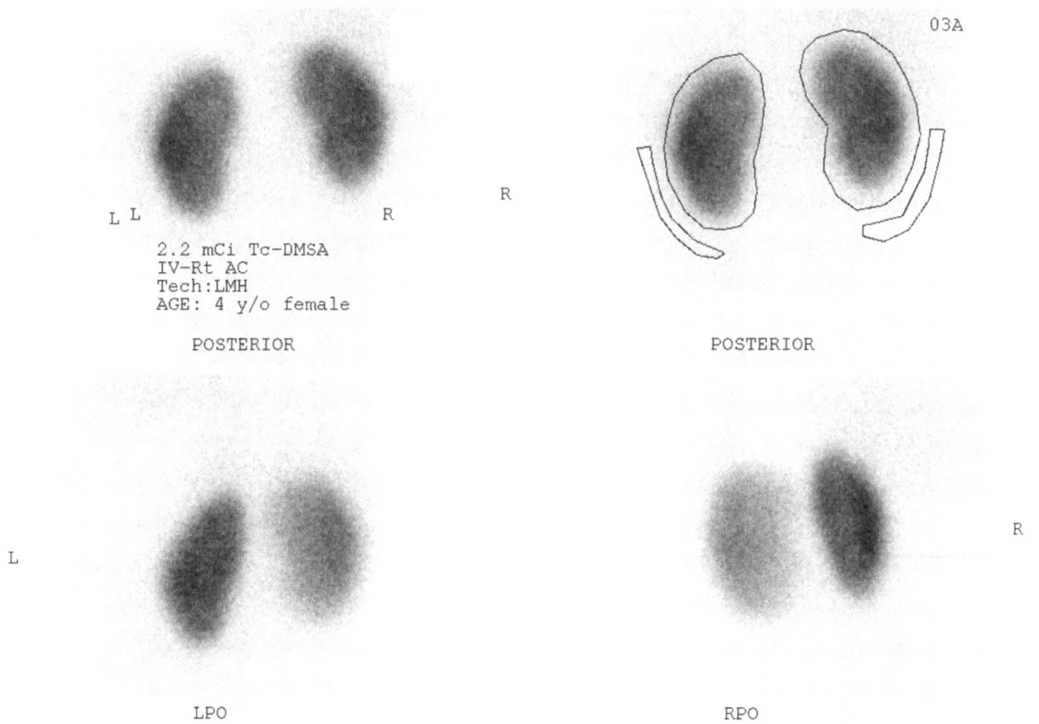

TECH LMH	COUNTS/TOTAL VOL	%DIFF/TOTAL VOL	COUNTS/UNIT VOL	%DIFF/UNIT VOL
Left Kidney - BKG	129410	48.897	41.16	51.911
Right Kidney - BKG	135251	51.103	38.13	48.089

Fig. 9.8 Normal DMSA scan of a 4 year old female with vesicoureteral reflux. The kidneys uptake the radiotracer symmetrically and homogeneously on the posterior images (*upper images*). Posterior oblique images (*lower images*) give an asymmetrical appearance

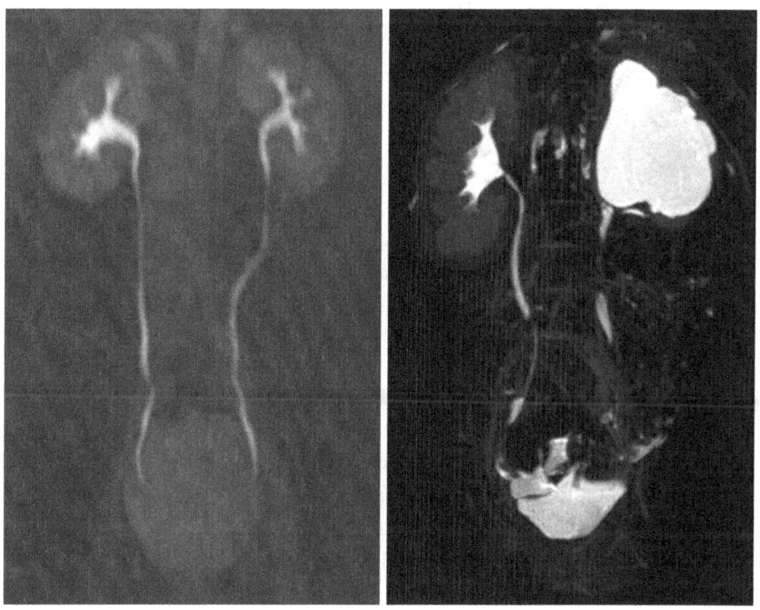

Fig. 9.9 Normal ureters on excretory phase of MRI (*left image*). It is normal for the entire ureter not to be visualized on the excretory phase as some parts of the ureter may be undergoing peristalsis. The *right image* shows a normal left kidney and a right kidney with hydronephrosis and thin parenchyma on excretory phase of MRI

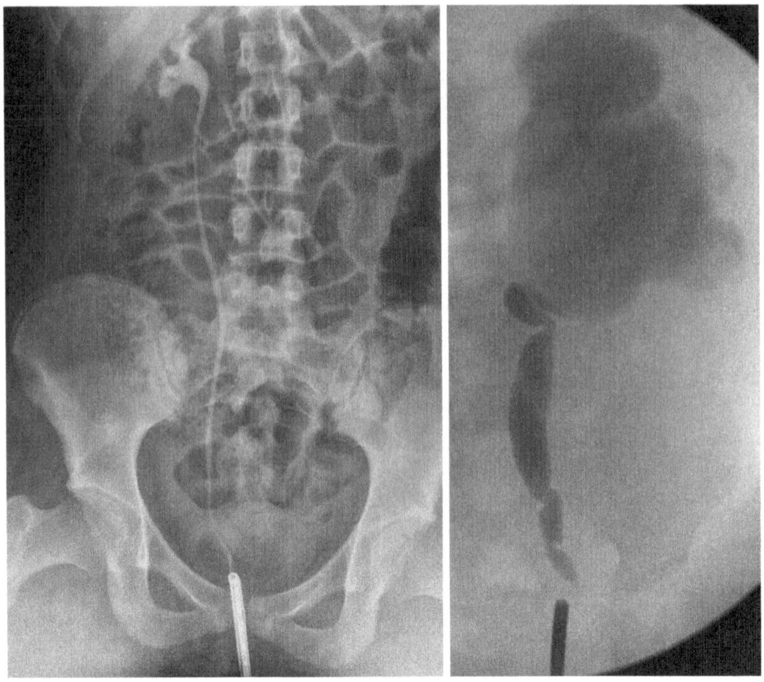

Fig. 9.10 Normal right ureter on retrograde pyelogram in a 10-year-old (*left image*). Left kidney with UPJ obstruction in a 1-year-old (*right image*), the ureter has evidence of fetal folds which are a normal variant in young children

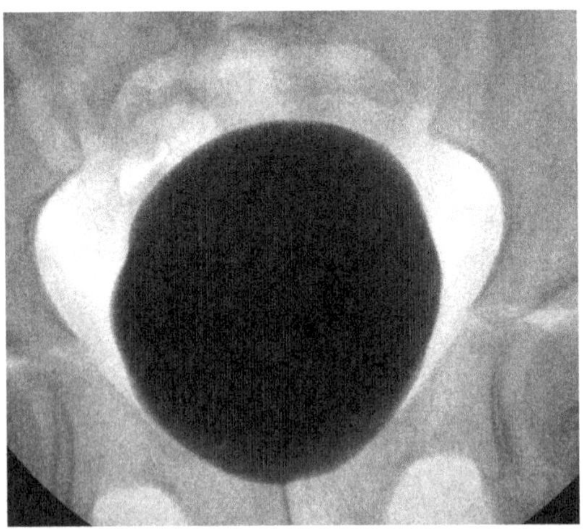

Fig. 9.11 Normal appearance of the bladder on VCUG with no trabeculations and a smooth, *ovoid shape*

Normal Bladder Imaging

The bladder can be visualized by ultrasound, and the volume of urine can be estimated. The normal bladder wall thickness in adults is around 3 mm [7]. In school-age children, the normal bladder wall thickness is 1–2 mm [8]. Another study found that the normal bladder wall thickness for all ages of children from newborn to teenager was around 2 mm [9]. A VCUG can demonstrate the size of a bladder as well as its contour. The bladder contour should be smooth and ovoid shaped without trabeculations and diverticulum (Fig. 9.11).

Congenital Anomalies of the Kidney and Urinary Tract

CAKUT represents a wide variety of malformations and disorders that result from abnormal development of the kidney and collecting system. They can be divided in to three major categories:

1. Anomalies of renal parenchyma development
2. Anomalies of embryonic renal migration and fusion
3. Anomalies of collecting system development

Anomalies of Renal Parenchyma Development

Anomalies of renal parenchyma development result in renal dysplasia. Renal dysplasia is

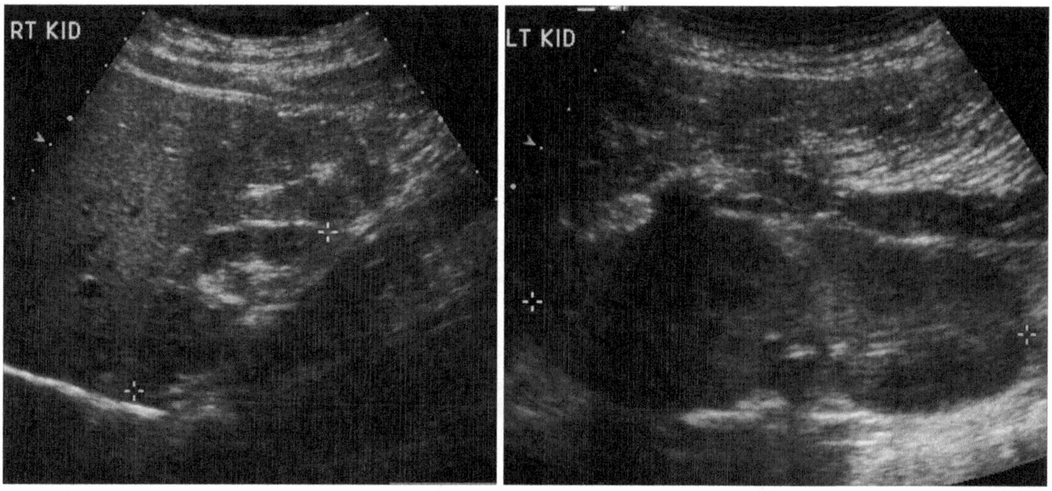

Fig. 9.12 Renal ultrasound of a 13-year-old with right renal hypoplasia. The right kidney (*left image*) is 2 standard deviations smaller than the mean size for age, and the left kidney demonstrates compensatory hypertrophy

characterized by abnormal nephron and collecting system development that leads to malformed kidney tissue with pathologic findings such as primitive-appearing tubules, fibrosis or scarring, and metaplastic tissue such as cartilage being present. This process can lead to several different clinical diagnoses such as renal hypoplasia, renal dysplasia or hypodysplasia, multicystic dysplastic kidney, polycystic kidney disease, or renal agenesis. The genes associated with renal dysplasia are often genes expressed during kidney development [10]. Exposure to angiotensin converting enzyme inhibitors in utero has been associated with renal dysplasia and is an example of an environmental exposure associated with renal dysplasia [11].

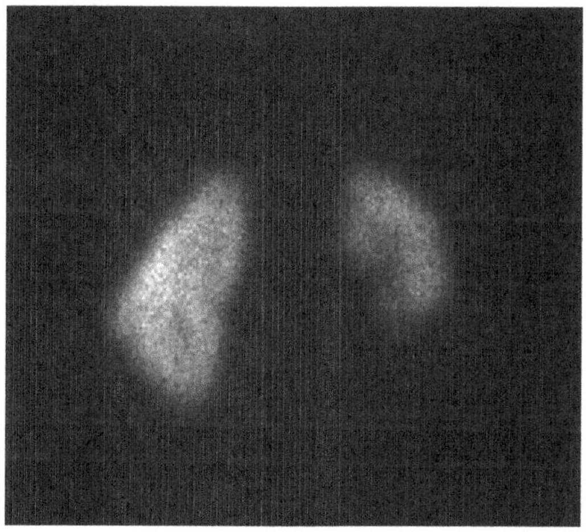

Fig. 9.13 DMSA radionuclide renal scan of a 13-year-old from Fig. 9.12 with right renal hypoplasia with absence of renal scarring. The right kidney contributes 30 % of overall renal function

Renal Hypoplasia

Renal hypoplasia is a rare entity that results in congenitally small kidneys with normal architecture but reduced number of nephrons. Renal hypoplasia may be unilateral with contralateral compensatory hypertrophy. Bilateral renal hypodysplasia can be part of genetic syndromes such as branchio-oto-renal syndrome and renal-coloboma syndrome [12, 13]. When bilateral, renal hypoplasia often results in end-stage renal disease (ESRD) with pathology consistent with focal segmental glomerular sclerosis and interstitial fibrosis presumably from hyperfiltration injury of the reduced number of nephrons [14].

The diagnosis of renal hypoplasia is a clinical diagnosis when an imaging study, typically renal ultrasonography, demonstrates a kidney smaller than 2 standard deviations of the mean kidney size by age (Fig. 9.12) [15]. Absence of renal scarring on a 99mTc-dimercaptosuccinic acid (DMSA) radionuclide scan is expected (Fig. 9.13).

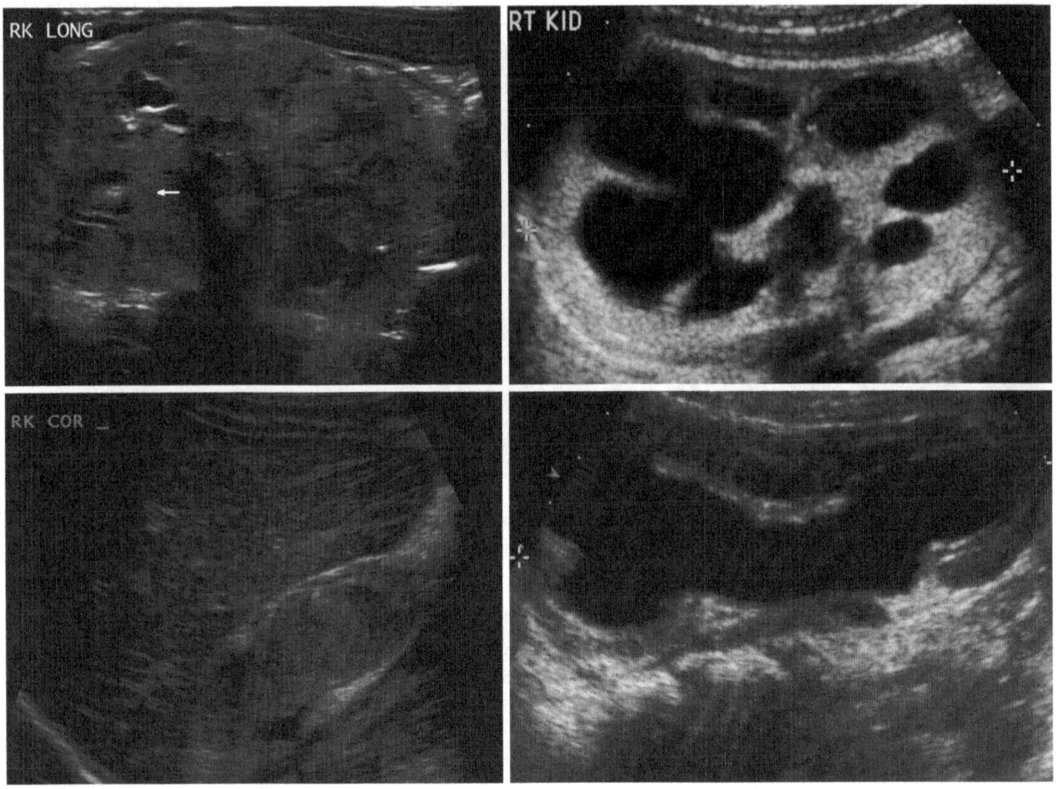

Fig. 9.14 Renal dysplasia can have many different appearances on renal ultrasound. An 8-day-old with areas of cystic renal dysplasia (*Top left*). A 4-year-old with echogenic renal cortex and hydronephrosis (*Top right*). A 2-year-old with renal hypodysplasia with cystic areas (*bottom left*). A 6-month-old with thin renal parenchyma and hydronephrosis (*bottom right*)

Renal Dysplasia

Renal dysplasia is more common than renal hypoplasia and is characterized by a kidney that is often smaller than normal depending on the size of associated cysts. Renal dysplasia occurs in about 3 of every 1,000 births and can be bilateral or unilateral with males affected 30–90 % more frequently than females [16]. Collecting system anomalies such as VUR, megaureter, ureteral atresia, and duplicated ureters occur at an increased incidence in kidneys with dysplasia [17–19]. Therefore, a voiding cystourethrogram (VCUG) is often obtained along with a renal ultrasound. As with renal hypoplasia, unilateral renal dysplasia is often associated with contralateral renal hypertrophy, and bilateral renal dysplasia is often associated with ESRD.

In children, ultrasonography is often the first imaging modality to evaluate renal dysplasia. Cystic areas, echogenic renal parenchyma, small kidneys, and hydronephrosis with thin renal parenchyma are examples of ultrasound findings with dysplasia but findings can be quite variable (Fig. 9.14). Findings on CT scan for renal dysplasia can also be quite variable (Fig. 9.15). A static renal scan such as a DMSA scan will show heterogenous, decreased uptake of radionuclide and possibly a small kidney representing poor renal function compared to a normal contralateral kidney (Fig. 9.16). As stated above, a VCUG is often obtained to evaluate for VUR which is often associated with renal dysplasia.

Multicystic Dysplastic Kidney

A multicystic dysplastic kidney (MCDK) is a very severe form of renal dysplasia characterized by a kidney that is non-reniform in shape, composed of noncommunicating cysts, lacking functional renal tissue, and has an absent or atretic ureter [20]. Most

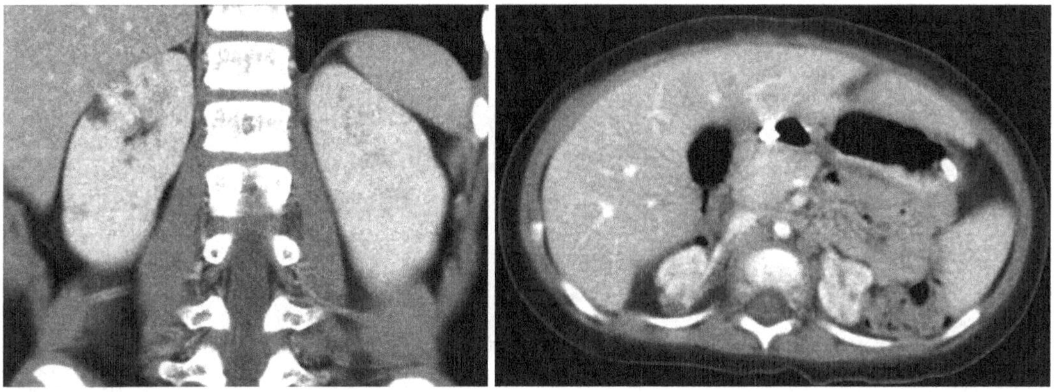

Fig. 9.15 Small areas of cystic renal dysplasia (*left image*). Bilateral renal dysplasia with hypoplastic kidneys demonstrating heterogeneous uptake of contrast and cystic areas (*right image*)

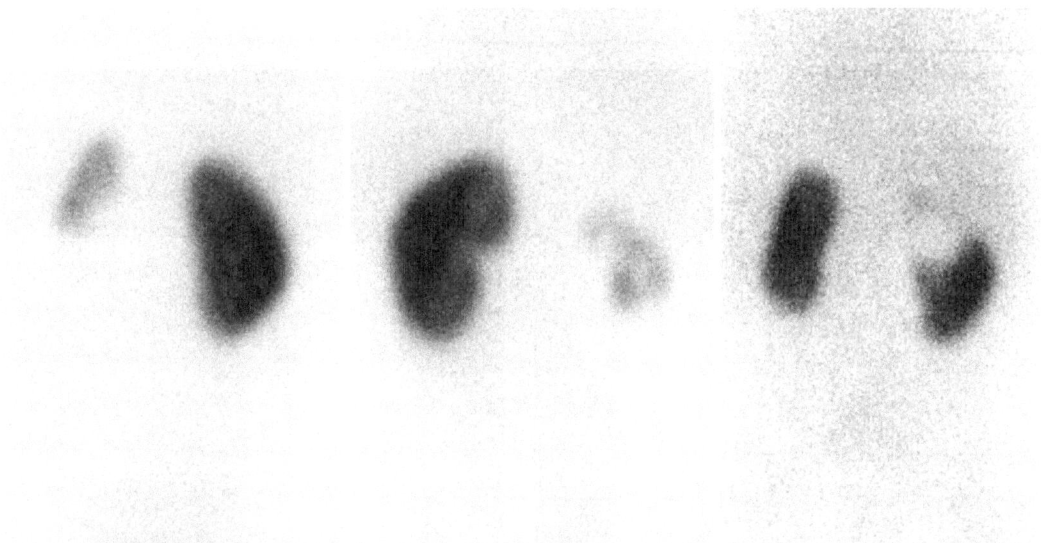

Fig. 9.16 DMSA scans demonstrating heterogeneous uptake of radiotracer with renal dysplasia. *Left image* is a 4-year-old with small congenitally dysplastic left kidney associated with vesicoureteral reflux. The *middle image* is a 7-year-old with dysplastic and hydronephrotic right kidney associated with ectopic ureter. The *right image* is a 4-month-old with a duplex right kidney with the upper pole associated with an ectopic ureter

cases of MCDK are detected antenatally by ultrasound and are found between 0.3 and 1 in 1,000 live births [21]. As with other forms of renal dysplasia, if the contralateral kidney is normal, it often shows compensatory hypertrophy. Children with unilateral MCDK have a low risk of any significant sequelae such as hypertension, proteinuria, significant renal impairment, or contralateral abnormalities such as VUR or ureteropelvic junction obstruction (UPJO) that require surgical correction [22, 23]. Historical concerns about an increased risk of malignancy in children with unilateral MCDK are not supported by current literature [24, 25].

On ultrasound, a MCDK generally appears as a collection of noncommunicating cystic structures of variable size. MCDK can be quite large in neonates and may even be palpable, but the majority of children with unilateral MCDK show involution of the MCDK over the first few years of childhood (Fig. 9.17). Cross-sectional imaging with CT scan will demonstrate similar findings as ultrasound as well as contralateral compensatory

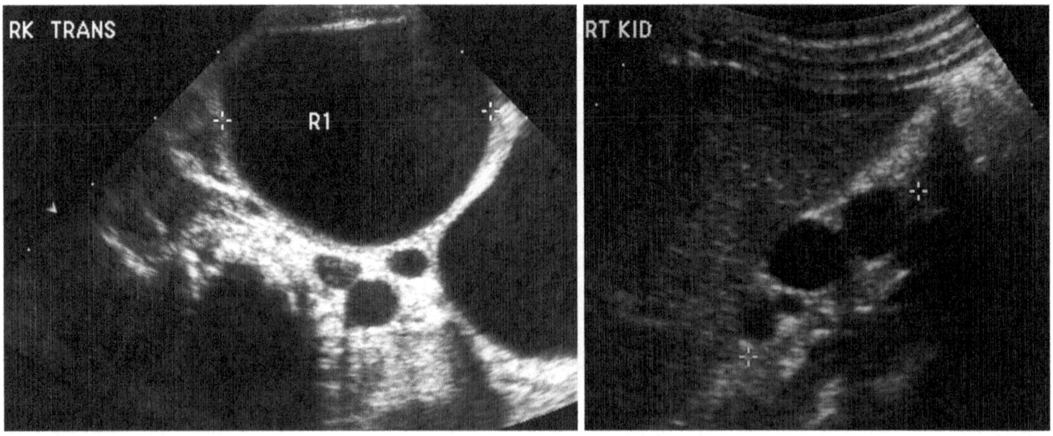

Fig. 9.17 A large multicystic dysplastic kidney in a newborn infant (*left*). Note the multiple noncommunicating cysts of varying size. The same child at age 2 with involuting MCDK (*right*)

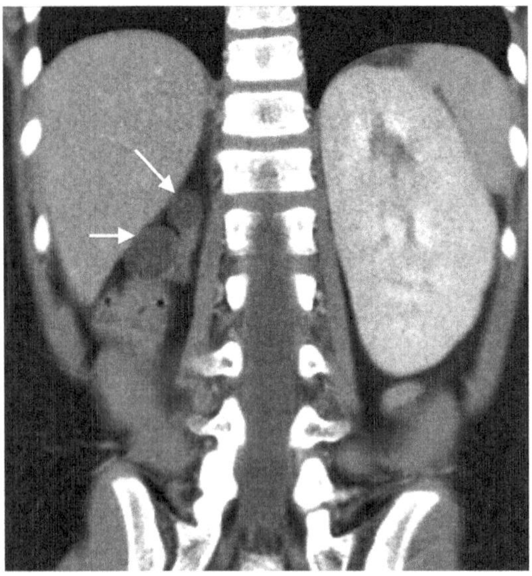

Fig. 9.18 CT scan with right MCDK (*arrows*) and compensatory renal hypertrophy on *left*

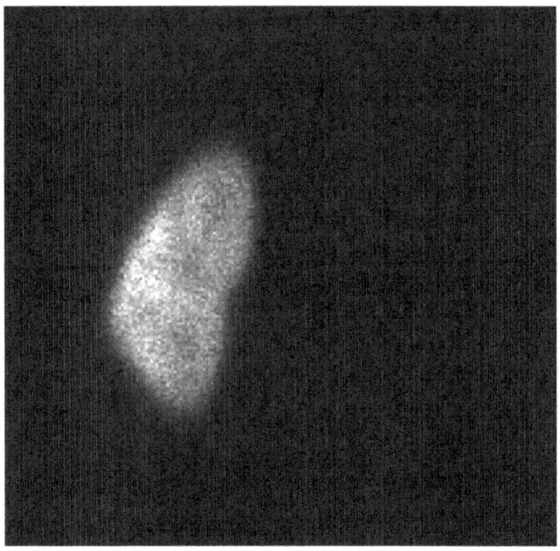

Fig. 9.19 DMSA scan of a 9-year-old child with right MCDK and normal left kidney

hypertrophy (Fig. 9.18). DMSA radionuclide scan demonstrates no significant update to the MCDK (Fig. 9.19). Grossly, a MCDK does not have the typical reniform shape, contains multiple cysts, and the ureter may be atretic (Fig. 9.20).

Autosomal Recessive Polycystic Kidney Disease

Autosomal recessive polycystic kidney disease (ARPKD), previously called infantile polycystic kidney disease, has an estimated incidence of 1 per 10,000–40,000 births [26, 27]. Mutations in the PKHD1 gene on chromosome 6p12 that encodes for the protein fibrocystin are responsible for ARPKD with over 200 mutations identified [28]. The kidneys are increased in size and are filled with small cysts (<3 mm) arising from the collecting ducts that appear to radiate from the medulla to the cortex. The liver is also affected in ARPKD with evidence of congenital fibrosis due to malformation of the biliary system

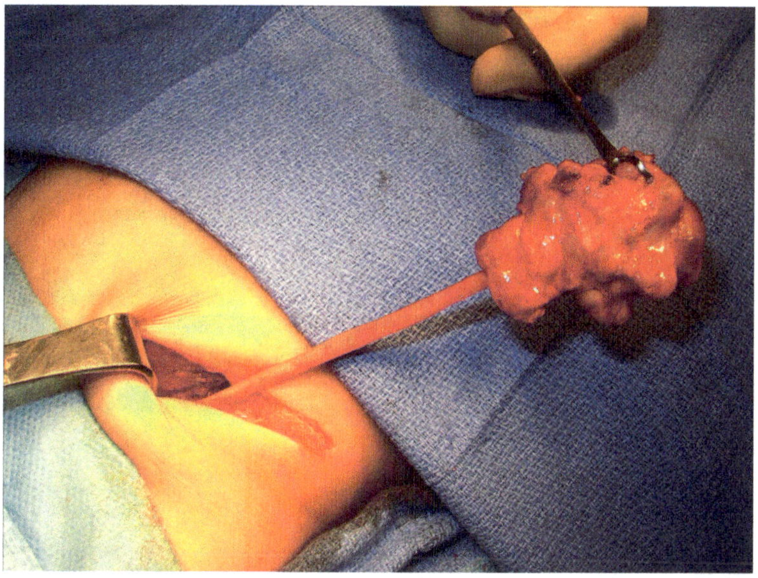

Fig. 9.20 Gross image of MCDK at time of removal. This particular example has a well-defined ureter, but the ureter may also be atretic

and may show hepatomegaly, increased echogenicity, and dilation of bile ducts on ultrasonography [29]. The clinical spectrum of ARPKD varies widely from death in utero or in infancy due to complications of oligohydramnios, to bilateral nephrectomies at birth with dialysis, and to delayed diagnosis into early adulthood with only signs of hepatic fibrosis [30]. In general, the earlier the diagnosis is discovered, the more severe the renal impairment will be. Most severe cases of ARPKD are detected by prenatal ultrasound.

On ultrasound, the kidneys are large most commonly have a reniform shape but will be filled with multiple small cysts causing the echotexture to be hyperechoic (Fig. 9.21). Cross-sectional imaging can demonstrate the cysts that arise in the cortex and radiate from the medulla to the cortex (Fig. 9.22). A newborn with severe ARPKD will have oligohydramnios, and the kidneys can be quite large and may need to be removed for any potential for survival with dialysis (Fig. 9.23).

Autosomal Dominant Polycystic Kidney Disease

Autosomal dominant polycystic kidney disease (ADPKD), previously adult polycystic kidney disease, may present in childhood. ADPKD is much more common than ARPKD with 1 case occurring every 400–1,000 live births. The mutation for ADPKD occurs in the PKD1 or PKD2 gene with PKD1 mutations accounting for 85 % of the cases [31]. The PKD1 and PKD2 genes encode the polycystin-1 and polycystin-2 proteins, respectively. Pathologically, the kidneys develop cysts of variable size in all parts of the nephron. Since the number of cysts generally increases with age, children may only have a few cysts. The natural history of ADPKD is a progressive increase in the number and size of cysts with corresponding deterioration of renal function resulting in renal replacement in middle age to late adulthood. Most children with ADPKD are asymptomatic, but occasionally complications associated with the later stages of ADPKD such as ESRD, hypertension, pain, hematuria, or cyst infection can occur [32]. Other significant organ involvement occurs including hepatic, pancreatic, or splenic cysts; cerebral aneurysms in up to 10 % of patients; and increased left ventricular size [33, 34].

Renal ultrasound in children with ADPKD can be normal, have a small number of cysts, or demonstrate kidneys that are filled with cysts (Fig. 9.24). The cysts on cross-sectional imaging often have varying signal intensity due to hemorrhage or infection history (Fig. 9.24).

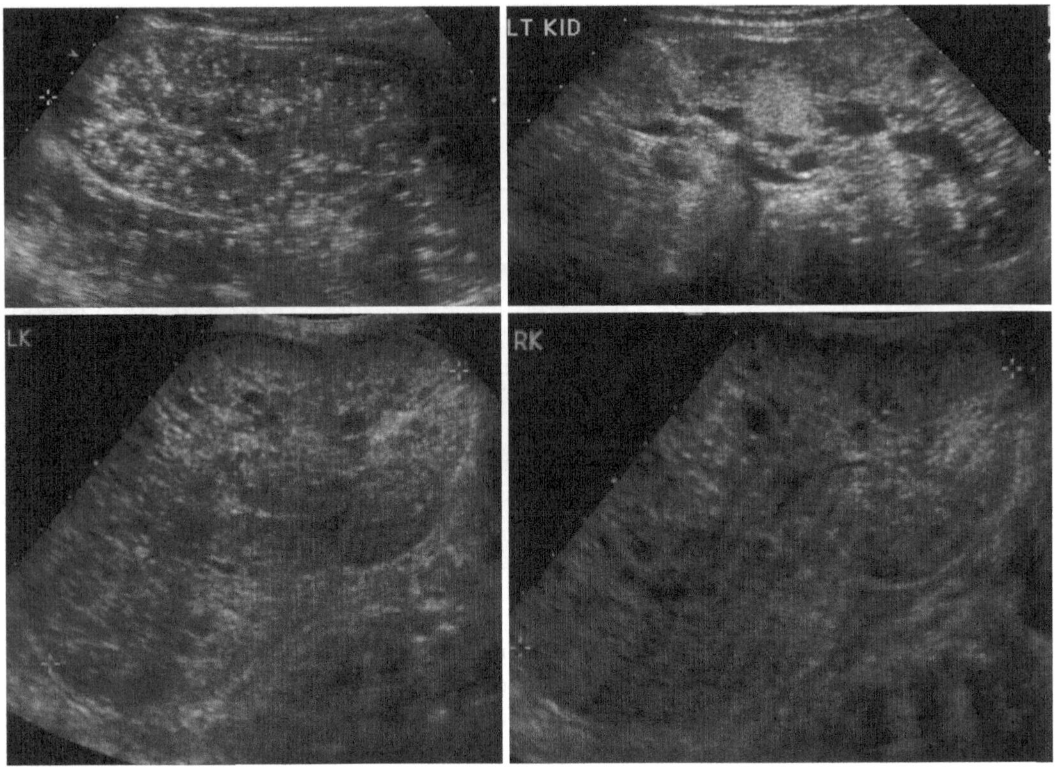

Fig. 9.21 Ultrasound examples of a newborn with ARPKD. Multiple small cysts in a reniform-shaped kidney that are both over 11 cm in length. The kidney also has increased echogenicity

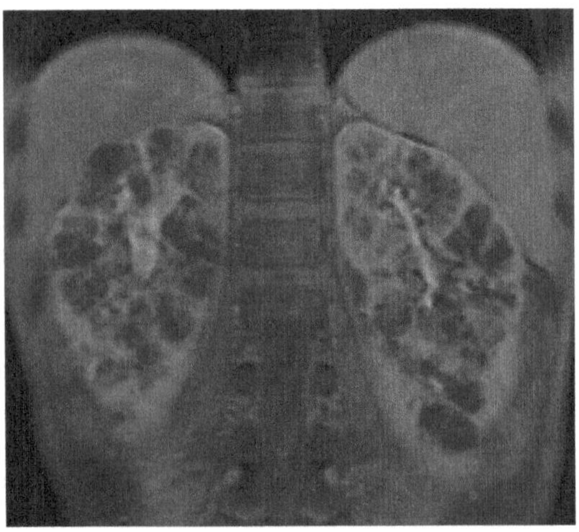

Fig. 9.22 MRI image of ARPKD in a 7-year-old. The kidneys retain a reniform shape, and multiple small cysts are seen radiating from the medulla to the cortex

Isolated Renal Cysts

Isolated renal cysts are common incidental findings with the prevalence increasing with increasing age. Given how common isolated renal cysts are and the concern about risk of malignancy with complex renal cysts, the Bosniak classification system was created in which cysts are classified into one of five categories based upon morphologic and enhancement characteristics with CT scanning [35].

- Category I: Benign simple cysts with thin wall and without septations, calcifications, or solid components. It has the density of water and does not enhance with contrast (Fig. 9.25).
- Category II: Benign cystic lesions that may have a few thin septa, fine calcifications, or a short segment of thickened calcification. No contrast enhancement. Also includes lesions less than 3 cm in size with higher attenuation than water but without enhancement.
- Category IIF: More complicated cystic lesions than category II but without contrast enhancement. Multiple thin septa may be present as well as thick calcifications. Also includes lesions greater than 3 cm in size with higher

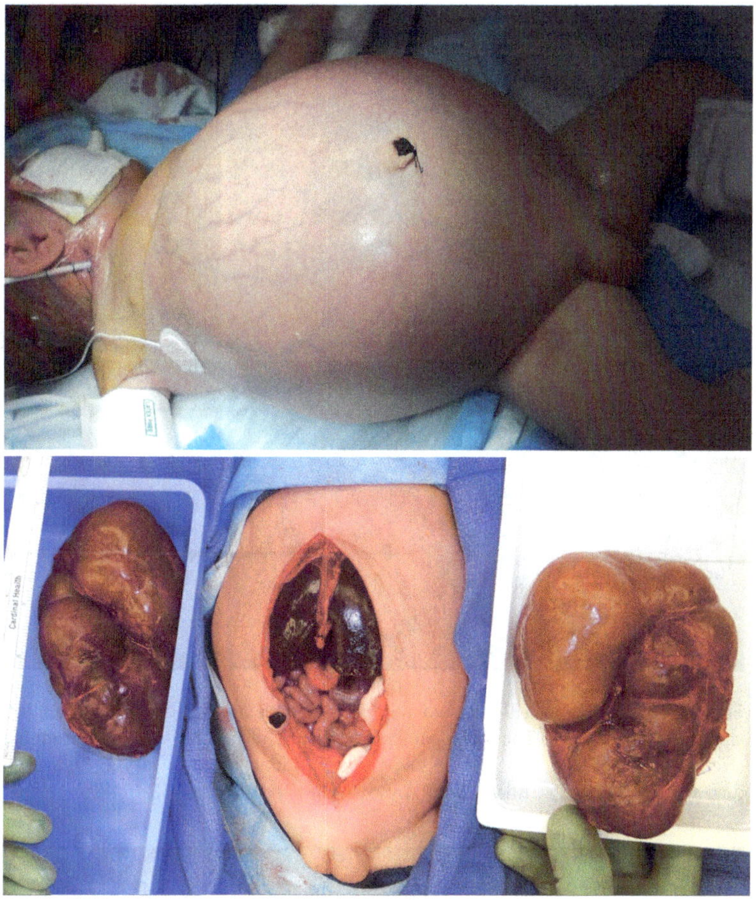

Fig. 9.23 Newborn female with ARPKD, oligohydramnios, renal failure, and pulmonary insufficiency (ultrasound shown in Fig. 9.20). Gross images after bilateral native nephrectomy

attenuation than water but without enhancement. Considered nonmalignant but follow-up required.

- Category III: Cystic lesions that can be complex with measurable contrast enhancement. Approximately 50 % are malignant with low-grade renal cell carcinoma as the most common diagnosis (Fig. 9.26) [36].
- Category IV: These lesions are similar to category III lesions, and they contain contrast-enhancing soft tissue components. Greater than 75 % chance of malignancy with category IV lesions.

The Bosniak classification system has been evaluated on a limited scale in children with complex renal cysts. In one study, 5 of 39 children with complex renal cysts underwent resection; three had a benign cyst (Category IIF in 2, Category III in 1), and two had renal cell carcinoma (Category III in 1 and Category IV in 1) [37]. In another study of 22 children, all lesions classified as Category I or II were benign, and all malignant lesions were classified as Category III or IV [38].

The most common type of isolated renal cyst seen in children and adults is the simple renal cyst. Among adults, the prevalence of simple renal cysts increases from approximately 5 % in the fourth decade of life to over 30 % in the eighth decade of life [39]. The prevalence among people age 15–30 years old is less than 1 % [40]. One study evaluated over 16,000 renal ultrasounds of children from birth to age 18 found that the prevalence of simple renal cysts was 0.22 %, which was relatively stable across all age groups [41]. The average cyst size was 1 cm (range 0.3–7 cm), and of the 23 cysts followed, only 2 were slightly larger and only 1 cyst required treatment with percutaneous drainage [41].

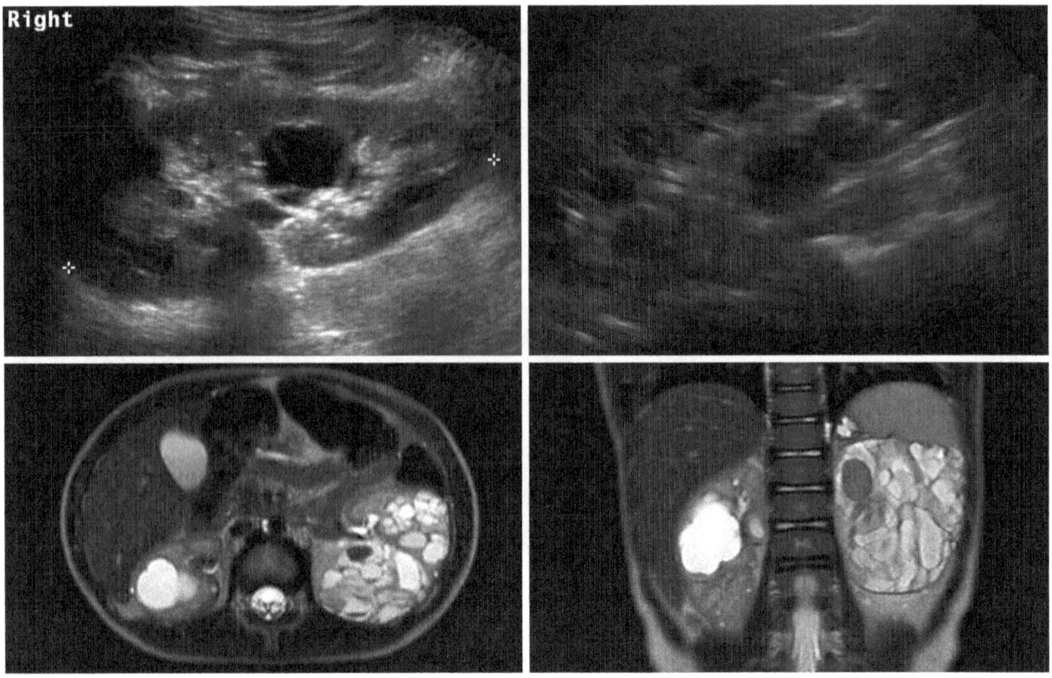

Fig. 9.24 ADPKD in a 9-year-old (*left image*) with a small number of cysts. The same patient at 20 years old (*right image*) showing progression and the right kidney now almost entirely filled with cysts. The lower T2-weighted MRI images of a 4-year-old demonstrate that ADPKD in children can be quite severe. The cysts have varying signal intensity likely due to hemorrhage

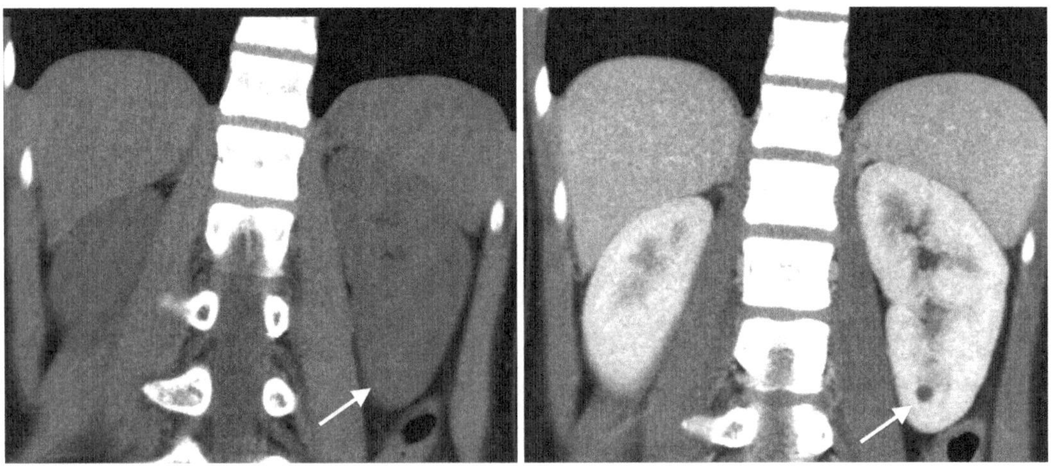

Fig. 9.25 CT scan images of a category I simple renal cyst (*arrows*). They cyst is smooth and round without any calcifications or solid components. The fluid within cyst is homogenous with a density similar to water (Hounsfield units less than 20). No contrast enhancement exists

Ultrasound is used most commonly in children to evaluate simple renal cysts, and a CT scan is not needed if a cyst meets ultrasound criteria for a simple cyst. On ultrasound a simple renal cyst is defined as being round and sharply demarcated with smooth walls, no internal echoes within the cyst, and there is a posterior wall echo with enhanced transmission beyond the cyst (Fig. 9.27) [42]. Rarely, a large simple cyst will cause pain and will require treatment such as laparoscopic cyst decortication or percutaneous drainage (Fig. 9.28).

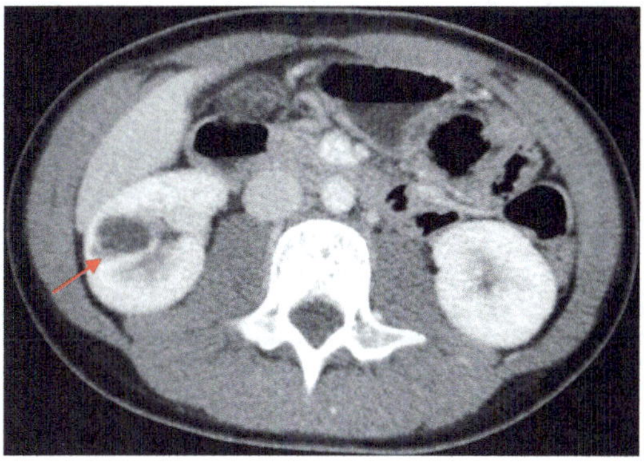

Fig. 9.26 CT scan image showing category III renal cystic lesion (*red arrow*) in a 13-year-old. Note the presence of septations with measurable contrast enhancement. Contrast enhancement of septations (Bosniak III) and soft tissue components (Bosniak IV) are the main distinguishing factors for renal cysts considered to have a high risk of malignancy

Renal Agenesis

The congenital absence of renal parenchymal tissue, renal agenesis, results from an early disruption of metanephric development and occurs approximately every 1 per 3,000–5,000 births [1, 43]. Renal agenesis is thought to be due to a failure of ureteral bud induction or development of the mesonephric duct [1]. Most patients are asymptomatic and are diagnosed during screening antenatal ultrasound or for imaging performed for other reasons showing an absent renal fossa and contralateral compensatory renal hypertrophy. A postnatal ultrasound and radionuclide scan confirm the diagnosis. Other congenital anomalies such as VUR, UPJO, and ureterovesical junction obstruction (UVJO) are more common in the remaining kidney [44, 45]. Unilateral renal agenesis in males can be associated with abnormalities or absence of structures derived from the mesonephric duct such as the seminal vesicles, vas deferens, and epididymis

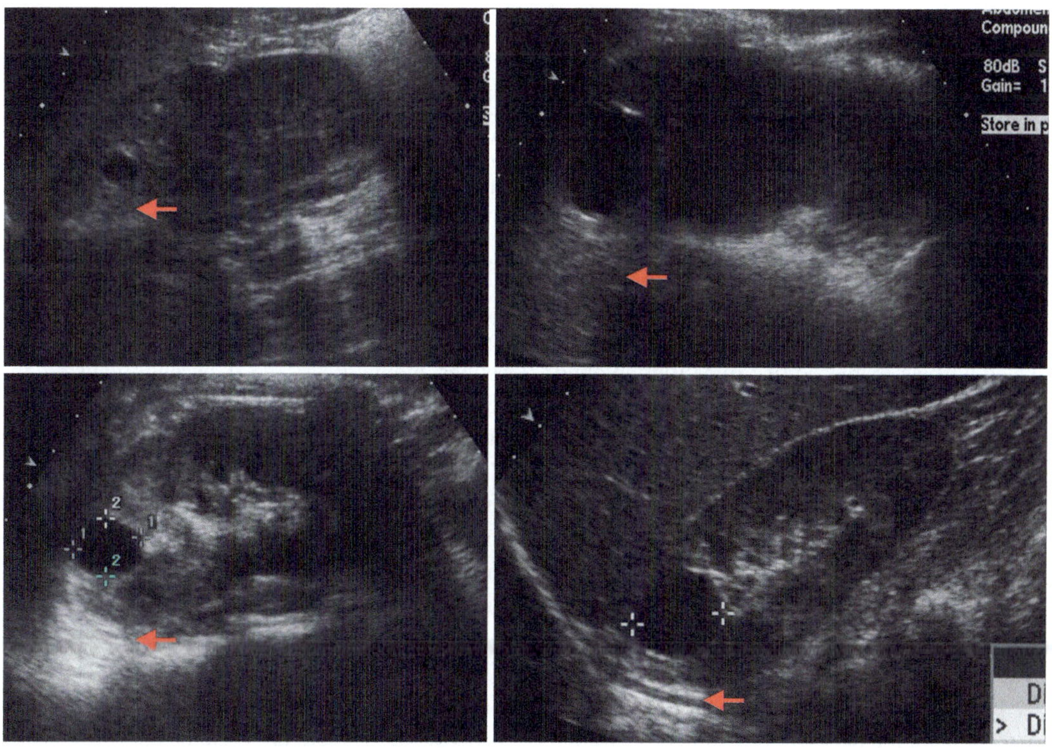

Fig. 9.27 Examples of ultrasound images of simple cysts in four different children. The cysts are round with smooth walls, there are no internal echoes, and there is a posterior wall echo with enhanced transmission beyond the cyst (*arrows* showing enhanced transmission)

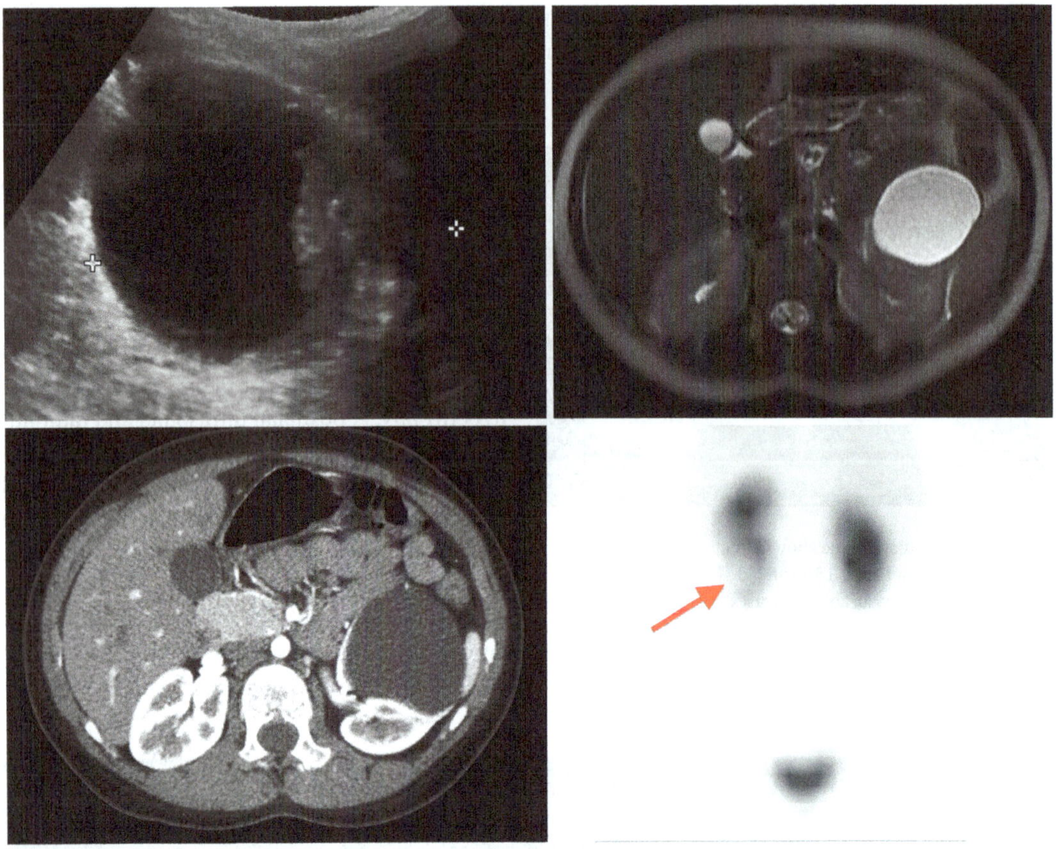

Fig. 9.28 Preoperative evaluation prior to laparoscopic decortication of a symptomatic left lower-pole renal cyst. The renal ultrasound shows a large lower-pole cystic structure with questionable thick walls (*upper left*). The MRI (*upper right*) and CT scan (*lower left*) demonstrate a non-enhancing simple cyst. The MAG3 renal scan demonstrated a left kidney that functions well but had an area in the lower pole with lack of contrast uptake (*arrow*) that corresponded to the cyst (*lower right*)

[46]. Unilateral renal agenesis in females is associated with an increased risk of Mullerian abnormalities such as uterine didelphys, duplicated vagina, and obstructed hemivagina [47].

Anomalies of Renal Migration and Fusion

Renal migration and fusion anomalies result in renal ectopia and renal fusion anomalies, respectively. The kidney normally ascends during development from the pelvis to the lumbar position by week 8 of gestation. As the kidney ascends, the kidney obtains its blood supply from nearby vessels. As a result, ectopic kidneys have an anomalous blood supply. The kidney also normally rotates medially 90° as it ascends causing the renal hilum to be oriented medially. Fusion anomalies occur when the developing kidneys fuse abnormally prior to ascent. All forms of ectopic or fused kidneys are associated with an increased risk of ipsilateral and contralateral renal abnormalities such as VUR, UPJO, hydronephrosis, kidney stones, and urinary tract infections [48].

Renal Ectopia

The most common position for an ectopic kidney is below the ipsilateral pelvic brim. These pelvic kidneys are found in 1 in 500–1,200 births [46]. Pelvic kidneys also fail to rotate properly and tend to have an anteriorly directed blood supply

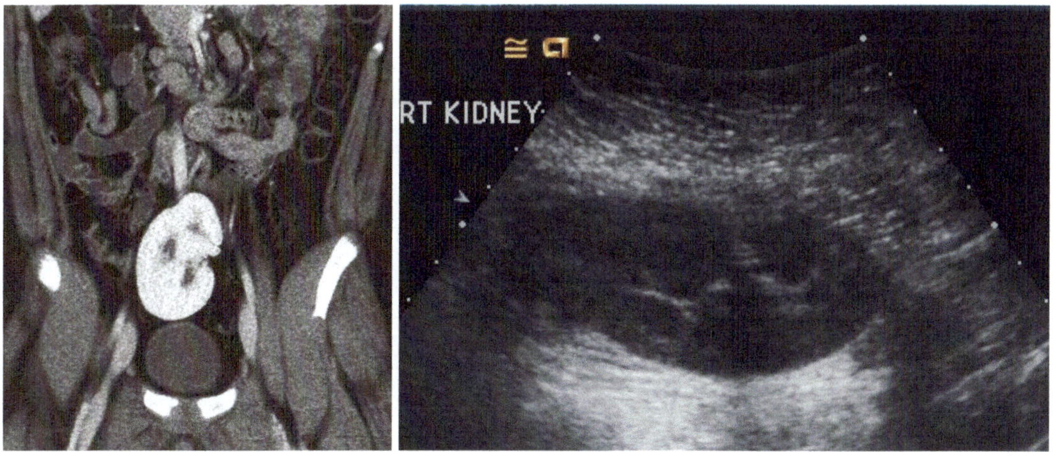

Fig. 9.29 CT and ultrasound images of a 10-year-old with right ectopic kidney (pelvic kidney)

and renal pelvis. The blood supply is variable and can come from a one or a combination of the internal iliac, external iliac, common iliac, or aorta. Rarely, an ectopic kidney can be located in the thoracic region [49]. There is an increased incidence of other urologic abnormalities in the ectopic kidney as well as the contralateral kidney with vesicoureteral reflux to the ectopic kidney being the most common [48]. In females, Mullerian abnormalities have been associated with ectopic kidneys such as Mayer-Rokitansky-Kuster-Hauser syndrome or ipsilateral uterine agenesis [50, 51].

Simple renal ectopia is often evaluated with ultrasonography or cross-sectional imaging (Fig. 9.29). A DMSA scan can be obtained to evaluate function of the ectopic kidney (Fig. 9.30). A VCUG is commonly obtained to evaluate for VUR in the ectopic or contralateral kidney.

Crossed Renal Ectopia

Crossed renal ectopia occurs in 1 in 1,000–2,000 births and is associated with some fusion to the other kidney 90–95 % of the time [46, 52]. Most commonly, the fusion is between the upper pole of the crossed ectopic kidney and the lower pole of the kidney on the appropriate side. The ureter of the crossed ectopic kidney generally crosses back to the other side and inserts into the bladder trigone. Other rare forms of crossed renal ectopic include crossed unfused renal ectopia and bilateral crossed renal ectopia.

Crossed renal ectopia can also be detected with ultrasonography and cross-sectional imaging, and an excretory phase can be obtained to further characterize the anatomy if needed (Fig. 9.31). Radionuclide scans are also helpful in determining the anatomy and relative function of the kidneys (Fig. 9.32).

Horseshoe Kidney

Horseshoe kidneys are the most common renal fusion abnormality occurring in 1 in 600 individuals [53]. The horseshoe kidney occurs when the lower poles of the developing kidneys fuse prior to renal ascent. The part of the horseshoe kidney that connects the two sides is called the isthmus and can contain functional renal tissue or just be a fibrous band depending on how early the fusion event occurred. The fused kidneys are not able to rotate properly, and ascent is limited by the isthmus coming into contact with the inferior mesenteric artery. As a result, a horseshoe kidney has its distinct horseshoe shape, is located more caudal than normal kidneys, has an anteriorly directly renal pelvis, and has a highly variable blood supply from the aorta and iliac vessels [54, 55]. The presence of a horseshoe kidney is often asymptomatic but is associated with an increased risk of VUR, hydronephrosis, UPJO, kidney stones, and UTIs [21].

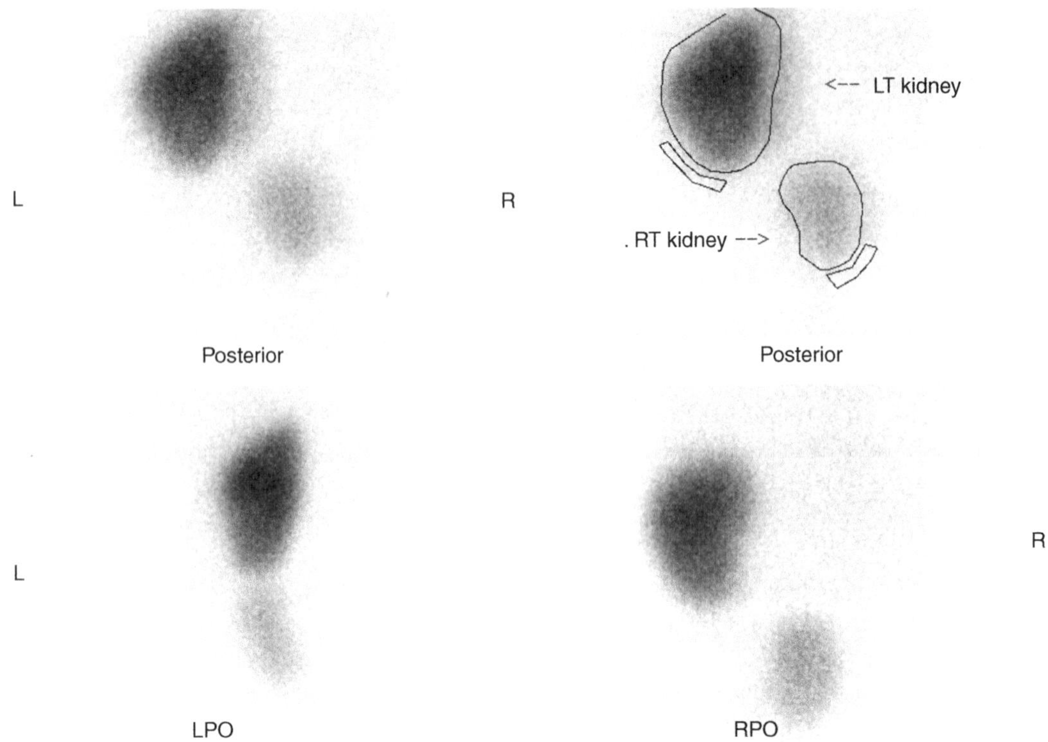

TECH CAN	Counts/total vol	%Diff/total vol	Counts/unit vol	%Diff/unit vol
LT KIDNEY - BKG	145,791	83.614	44.46	70.106
RT KIDNEY - BKG	28,571	16.386	18.96	29.894

Fig. 9.30 DMSA scan of the right pelvic kidney. Note the decreased function that is typical of ectopic kidneys with the right pelvic kidney contributing 16 % of total renal function

Ultrasonography can usually detect the isthmus of a horseshoe kidney (Fig. 9.33), but sometimes cross-sectional imaging is needed (Fig. 9.34). In addition, studies such as a VCUG or MAG3 furosemide renal scan are obtained if there is the presence of hydronephrosis and/or urinary tract infections (Fig. 9.35).

Anomalies of Collecting System Development

Anomalies of collecting system development constitute some of the more common CAKUT diseases. Anomalies of the renal pelvis include congenital hydronephrosis, congenital UPJ obstruction, and megacalycosis. Anomalies of the ureter include primary megaureter, ectopic ureter, duplicated ureter, ureteroceles, and vesicoureteral reflux. Anomalies of the bladder and urethra include bladder exstrophy and epispadias complex, prune-belly syndrome, posterior urethral valves, bladder diverticulum, duplicated urethra, and urethral atresia.

Congenital Hydronephrosis

Antenatal hydronephrosis is found in approximately 1–2 % of all fetuses screened by prenatal ultrasound and seems to be more common in male fetuses [56, 57]. Clinical outcomes are related to severity of hydronephrosis, and two main grading systems are used. The Society for Fetal Urology (SFU) criteria grade antenatal hydronephrosis and postnatal hydronephrosis based upon the degree and location of hydronephrosis as well as presence of thinned renal parenchyma [58].

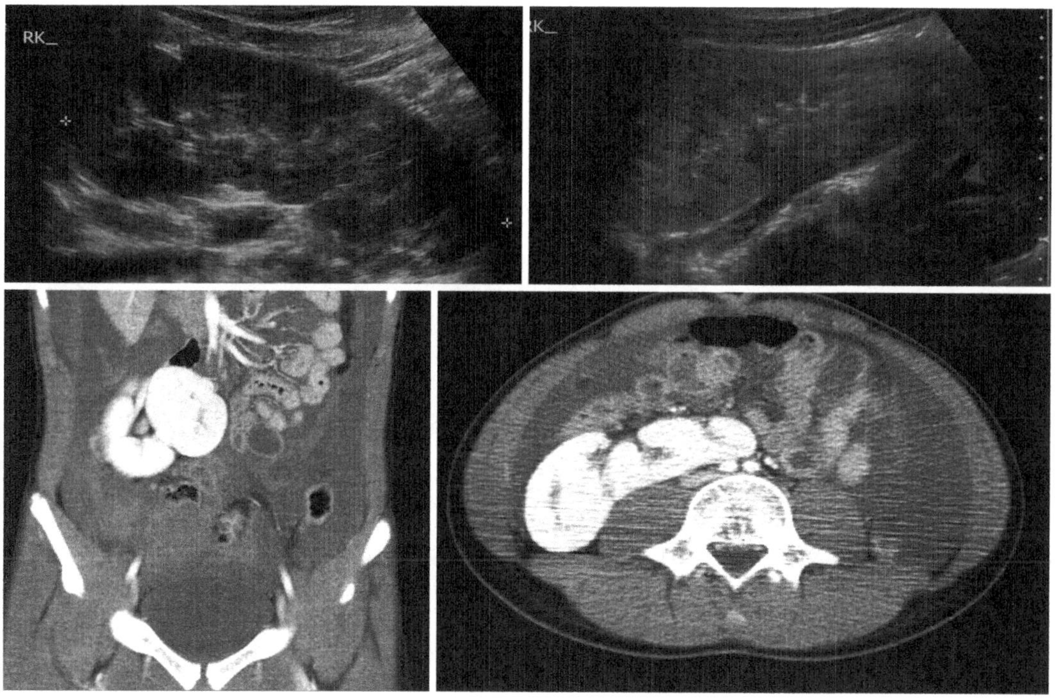

Fig. 9.31 Ultrasound and CT imaging of crossed fused ectopia found incidentally after trauma (note free fluid on CT images). The ectopic kidney has anteriorly facing renal pelvis

- Grade 0: Normal examination with no dilatation of the renal pelvis
- Grade 1: Mild dilatation of renal pelvis only (Fig. 9.36)
- Grade 2: Moderate dilatation of the renal pelvis including a few calyces (Fig. 9.36)
- Grade 3: Dilatation of the renal pelvis with visualization of all the calyces, which are uniformly dilated, and normal renal parenchyma (Fig. 9.36)
- Grade 4: Similar appearance of the renal pelvis and calyces as Grade 3 plus thinning of the renal parenchyma (Fig. 9.36)

The other method of grading antenatal hydronephrosis is measurement of the anterior-posterior renal pelvis diameter (RPD). Several studies have found an association with increasing RPD and increasing risk of postnatal UTI, diagnosis of a significant CAKUT, and undergoing surgery [59–64]. A RPD of >4 mm and <10 mm is generally considered mild renal pelvis dilatation, and >15 mm is considered severe (Fig. 9.37). For mild renal pelvis dilatation, over 75 % of the cases are likely to resolve spontaneously [64]. Mild renal pelvis dilatation is the most commonly seen type of antenatal hydronephrosis, so the etiology is transient hydronephrosis accounts for around 50 % of all cases. The next most common causes of congenital hydronephrosis are physiologic hydronephrosis without obstruction (15 %), UPJO (11 %), and VUR (9 %) [65].

Ureteropelvic Junction Obstruction (UPJO)

As mentioned in the previous section, UPJO is the most common diagnosis given for children with antenatal hydronephrosis. Congenital UPJO is caused by an anatomical or functional intrinsic stenosis of the UPJ or less commonly by an extrinsic compression of the UPJ usually by a lower-pole renal artery. The exact mechanism of intrinsic stenosis of the UPJ is not known. The reported incidence of UPJO is 1 in 500–1,500 births [66]. UPJO can be bilateral in a minority of cases, and boys are more frequently affected [66].

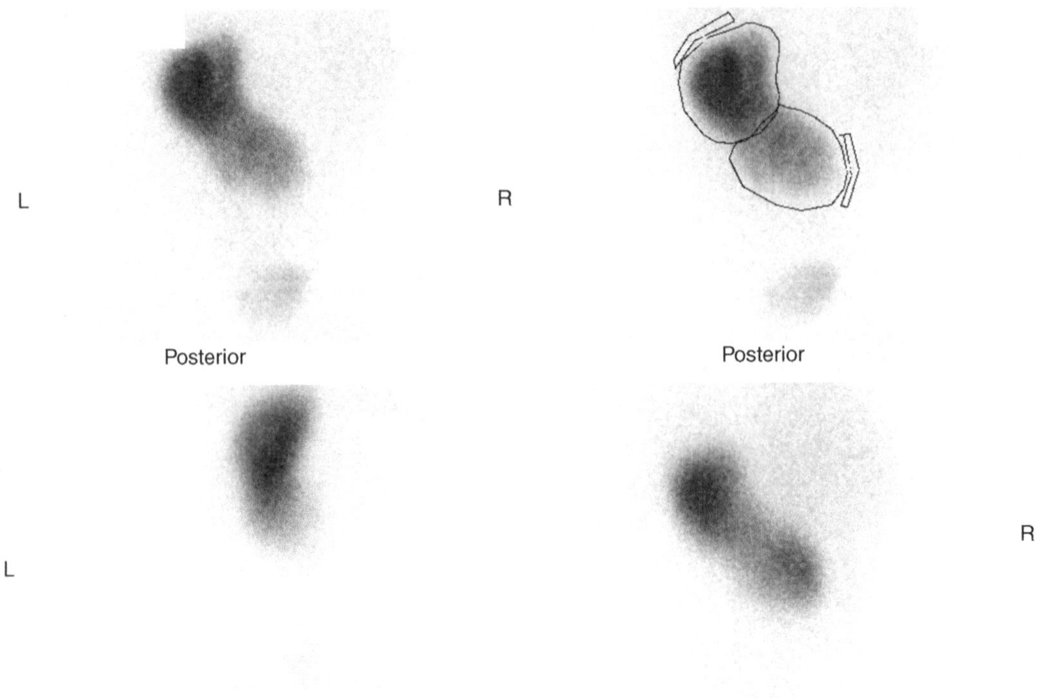

	LPO		RPO	
TECH BKS	Counts/total vol	%Diff/total vol	Counts/unit vol	%Diff/unit vol
LT KID - BKG	116,164	67.034	55.90	65.109
RT KID - BKG	57,127	32.966	29.96	34.891

Fig. 9.32 DMSA scan of crossed fused renal ectopia. The ectopic kidney has decreased function compared to the non-ectopic kidney

Most congenital UPJO cases are detected by prenatal ultrasound. The diagnosis is supported by the presence of hydronephrosis, but that is not sufficient (Fig. 9.38). The diagnosis is confirmed by diuretic renography, such as a MAG3 diuretic renal scan, that demonstrates delayed washout of radiotracer from the renal pelvis (Fig. 9.39). The washout time of interest is the number of minutes it takes for the amount of radiotracer in the renal pelvis to decrease in half. A washout time of <15 min is considered unobstructed, and a washout time of >20 is considered consistent with obstruction. A washout time between 15 and 20 min is considered intermediate. Another important piece of information obtained from diuretic renography is the split function of the two kidneys. If the split function is equal in a patient with a unilateral kidney with a washout time consistent with obstruction, that kidney can often be observed conservatively and surgery avoided [67]. However, an initial split renal function <40 % and severe hydronephrosis are associated with increased risk of undergoing surgery [67].

Ureteral Fibroepithelial Polyps

Fibroepithelial polyps are rare causes of UPJ obstruction in children. They are benign tumors that can occur anywhere in the urinary tract, but the most common locations are the UPJ, upper ureter, and posterior urethra [68]. While seen rarely, these lesions are often encountered unexpectedly at time of UPJ repair (Fig. 9.40).

The diagnosis of a fibroepithelial polyp prior to surgery requires an index of suspicion. Often the ultrasound will have the appearance of a typical UPJ obstruction with hydronephrosis without hydroureter, and the diagnosis is not suspected. One study reported that subtle finding of a

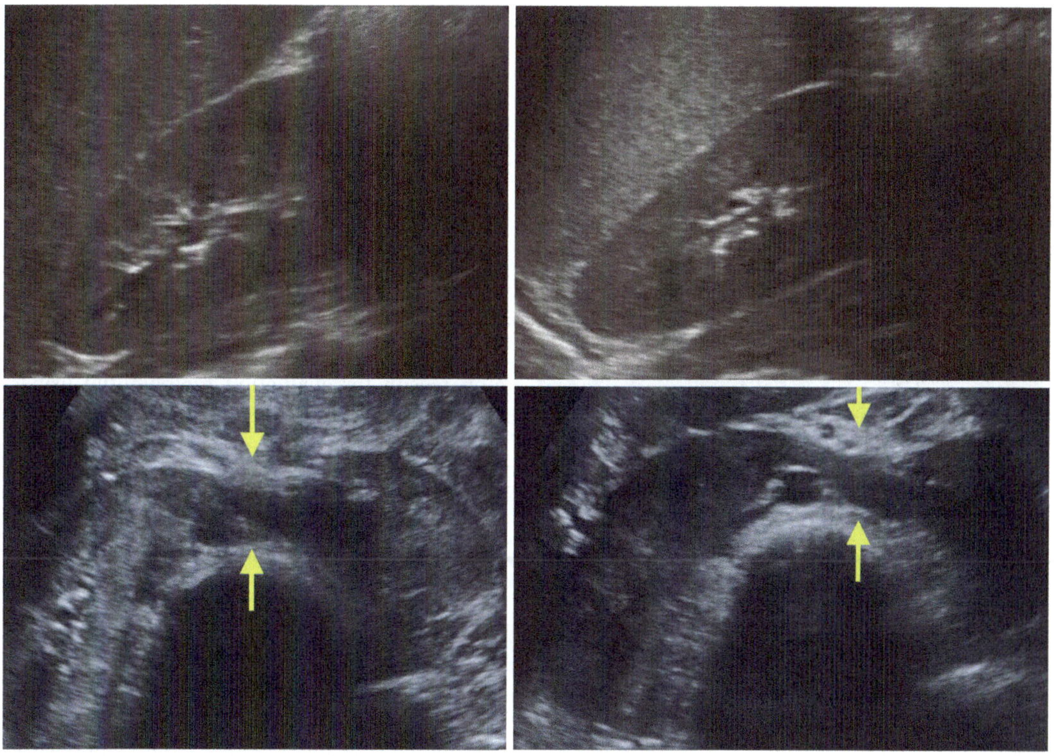

Fig. 9.33 Ultrasound images of a 7 year old with a horseshoe kidney. Right kidney (*upper left*), left kidney (*upper right*), and isthmus indicated by *arrows* (*bottom images*)

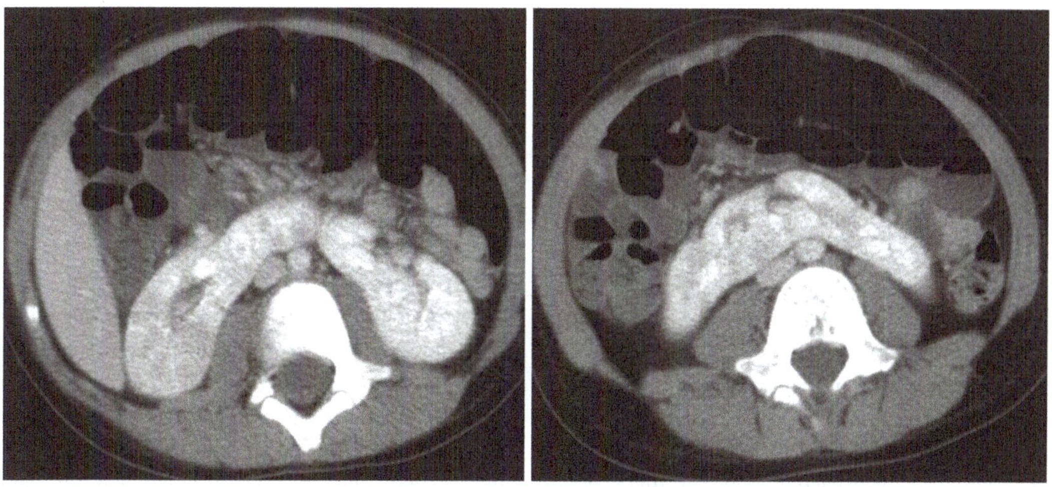

Fig. 9.34 CT images of horseshoe kidney demonstrating prominent isthmus in a 10-year-old

fibroepithelial polyp was detected by ultrasound preoperatively in 62 % of 35 children undergoing UPJ repair [68]. The authors report that blood flow was detected in all polyps that were suspected prior to surgery. Retrospective analysis of preoperative imaging of the child in Fig. 9.40 demonstrates blood flow to a polyp in the region of the UPJ (Fig. 9.40).

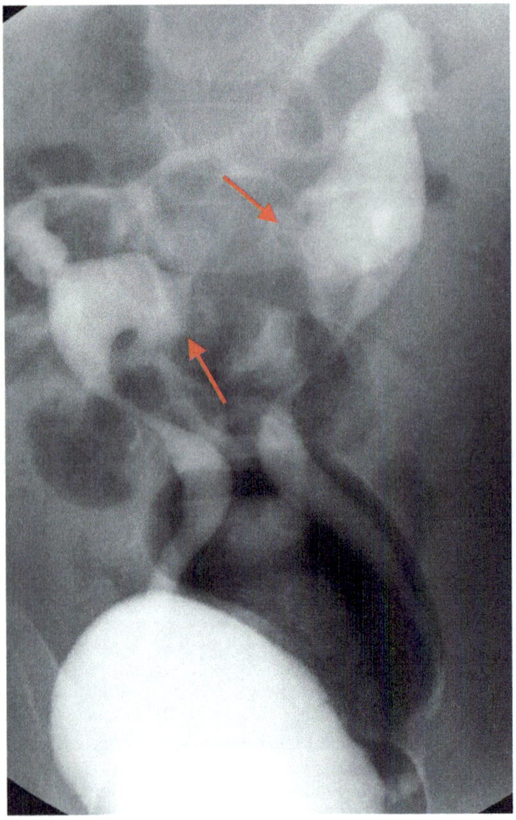

Fig. 9.35 VCUG demonstrating bilateral vesicoureteral reflux into a horseshoe kidney. Note the medially directed calyces (*red arrows*) typical of a horseshoe kidney

Primary Megaureter

A megaureter is a descriptive term given to a ureter >7 mm in diameter in children <12 years old and neonates greater than 30 weeks gestation (Fig. 9.41) [69]. There are four types of megaureter based upon the presence or absence of obstruction and reflux [70].

- Refluxing, non-obstructed megaureter: this is a common type of megaureter caused by high-grade vesicoureteral reflux that leads to a dilated ureter.
- Refluxing, obstructed megaureter: this is generally associated with an ectopic ureter that inserts into the external sphincter and is relatively rare.
- Nonrefluxing, non-obstructed megaureter: this is a common variant of megaureter and is also called primary dilated megaureter.
- Nonrefluxing, obstructed megaureter: this type of primary megaureter is relatively rare and often leads to a decrease in renal function, infection, or pain.

The refluxing, non-obstructed megaureter will be discussed in the section on vesicoureteral reflux, and the refluxing, obstructed megaureter will be discussed in the section on ectopic ureters. This section focuses on nonrefluxing, primary megaureter where the pathology is due to an intrinsic abnormality of the ureter and not bladder outlet obstruction or high intravesical pressures.

Nonrefluxing primary megaureter is a common reason for evaluation for potential urinary tract obstruction. Boys are affected more frequently than girls, the left side is more common, bilateral cases occur in 25 %, and the contralateral kidney can be absent or dysplastic in 10–15 % of cases [71]. The cause of primary megaureter is thought to be a defect in the muscle and collagen development in the distal ureter resulting in an aperistaltic segment near the ureterovesical junction which can lead to obstruction (Fig. 9.42) [71]. The main question with primary megaureter is whether there is significant obstruction and risk of renal deterioration. As in evaluation for UPJO, primary megaureter is evaluated with diuretic renography with the area of interest including the ureter (Fig. 9.43). If the split function is equal and UTIs are not a significant problem, primary megaureters are often observed even if the washout time is greater than 20 min. A high percentage of primary megaureters does not lead to renal deterioration and resolves spontaneously (Fig. 9.44) [72–75].

Ectopic Ureter

An ectopic ureter drains to an abnormal location. In males, the ureteral orifice of an ectopic ureter is always proximal to the external urethral sphincter and can be located distal to the trigone, in the posterior urethra, seminal vesicle, vas deferens, ejaculatory duct, and epididymis. The reason for these locations is explained embryologically (see above). Given the association of duplex kidneys and upper-pole ectopic ureters, ultrasonography often reveals a duplex kidney with upper-pole hydronephrosis (Fig. 9.45). There can be significant dysplasia associated with ectopic ureters, and the associated kidneys or upper-pole segments are

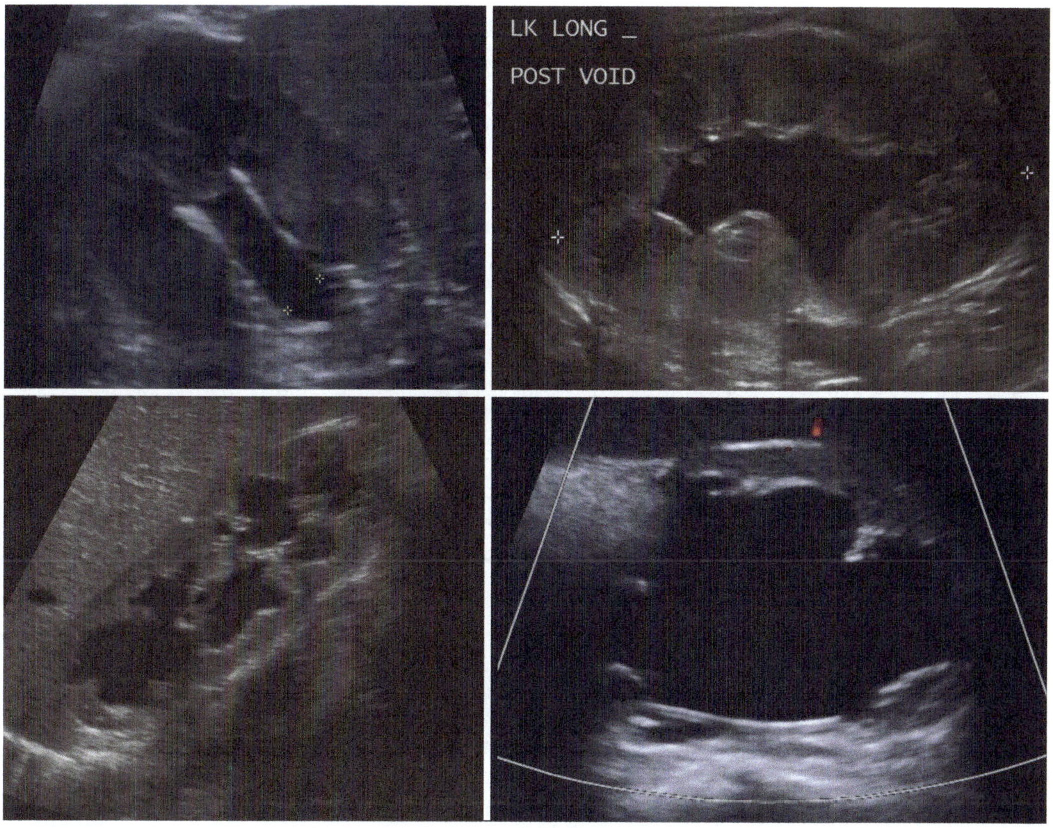

Fig. 9.36 Hydronephrosis grades. Grade 1 (*upper left*), grade 2 (*upper right*), grade 3 (*lower left*), and grade 4 (*lower right*). The distinction between grade 3 and 4 is the presence of thinning of the renal parenchyma in grade 4

often poorly functioning (Fig. 9.46). The location of the ectopic ureter insertion is often not able to be determined by ultrasonography. If the ectopic ureteral orifice is in the external urethral sphincter, a unique situation can occur where an obstructed, refluxing megaureter is found. The reflux in these ureters is usually seen only during the voiding phase when the external sphincter is relaxed (Fig. 9.47).

Ureterocele

A cystic dilation of the distal ureter where it inserts into the bladder or urethra is called a ureterocele (Fig. 9.48). Ureteroceles are most commonly associated with the upper pole in a duplex kidney and occur more frequently in females [76]. The reported incidence of ureteroceles is 1 in every 1,000 births [77]. The risk of UTI in children with ureteroceles may be as high as 50 % [78]. Ureteroceles are classified as intravesical if they are entirely within the bladder or ectopic if part of the ureterocele extends into the urethra. The exact embryologic explanation for ureteroceles is unknown, but one popular theory is that there is a membrane between the mesonephric duct and the ureteric bud that does not completely break down and leads to a stenotic ureteral orifice and obstruction [79].

Ureteroceles can be detected antenatally by screening ultrasound (Fig. 9.49) or postnatally after a urinary tract infection. Most ureteroceles are diagnosed by ultrasonography that demonstrates a cystic mass within the bladder and potentially hydroureteronephrosis (Fig. 9.50). A VCUG is generally performed as well because of the increased incidence of ipsilateral lower-pole reflux in duplex systems. Early images of the bladder with the VCUG will often demonstrate

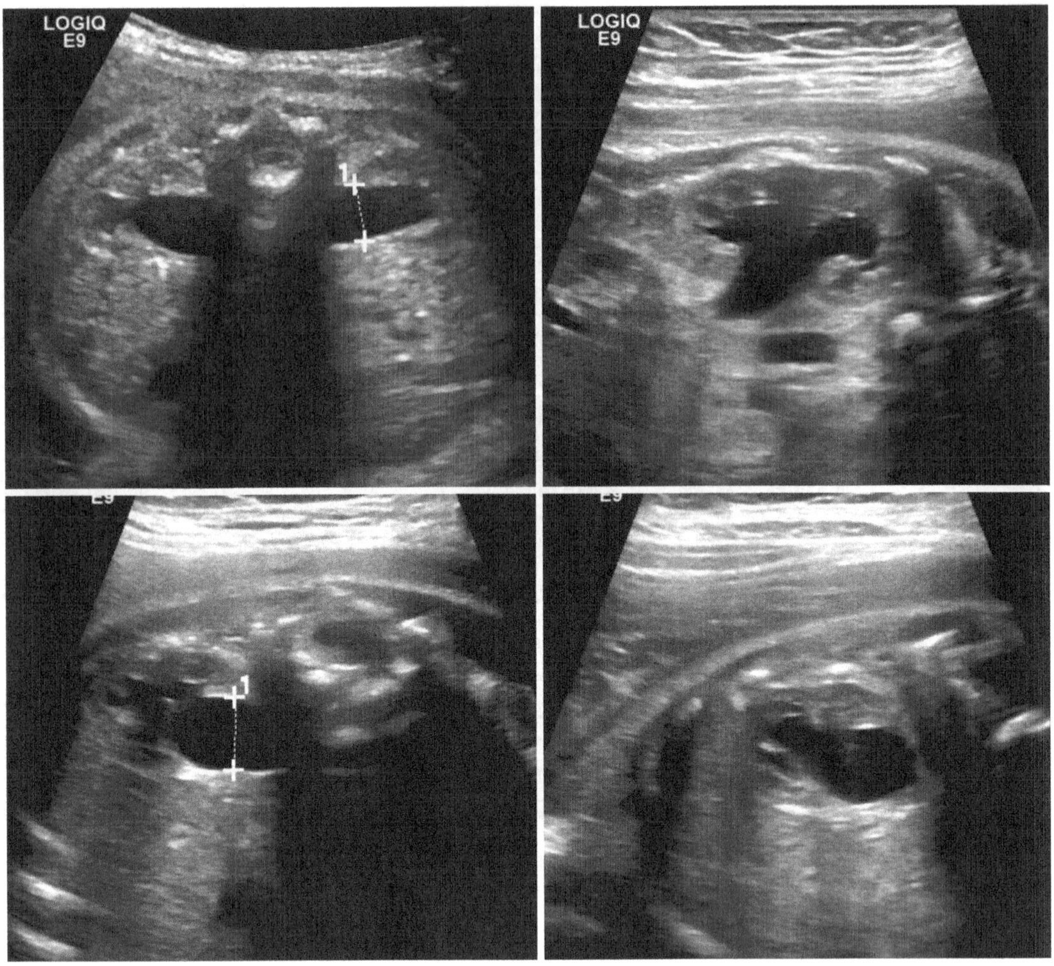

Fig. 9.37 Prenatal ultrasound of a 32-week-old fetus with bilateral grade 3 hydronephrosis. The left kidney has an anterior-posterior diameter of 10 mm (*upper left image*) with no parenchymal thinning (*upper right image*). The right kidney has an anterior-posterior diameter of 11 mm (*lower left image*) with no parenchymal thinning (*lower right image*)

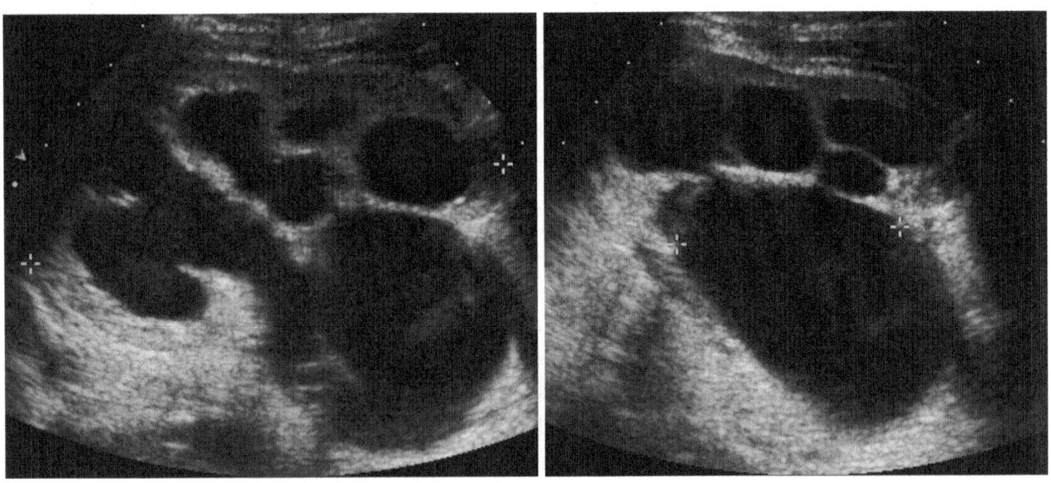

Fig. 9.38 Ultrasound images of a 10-month-old with left ureteropelvic junction obstruction with grade 4 hydronephrosis. No hydroureter was seen (images not shown). The presence of hydronephrosis suggests obstruction, but is not diagnostic

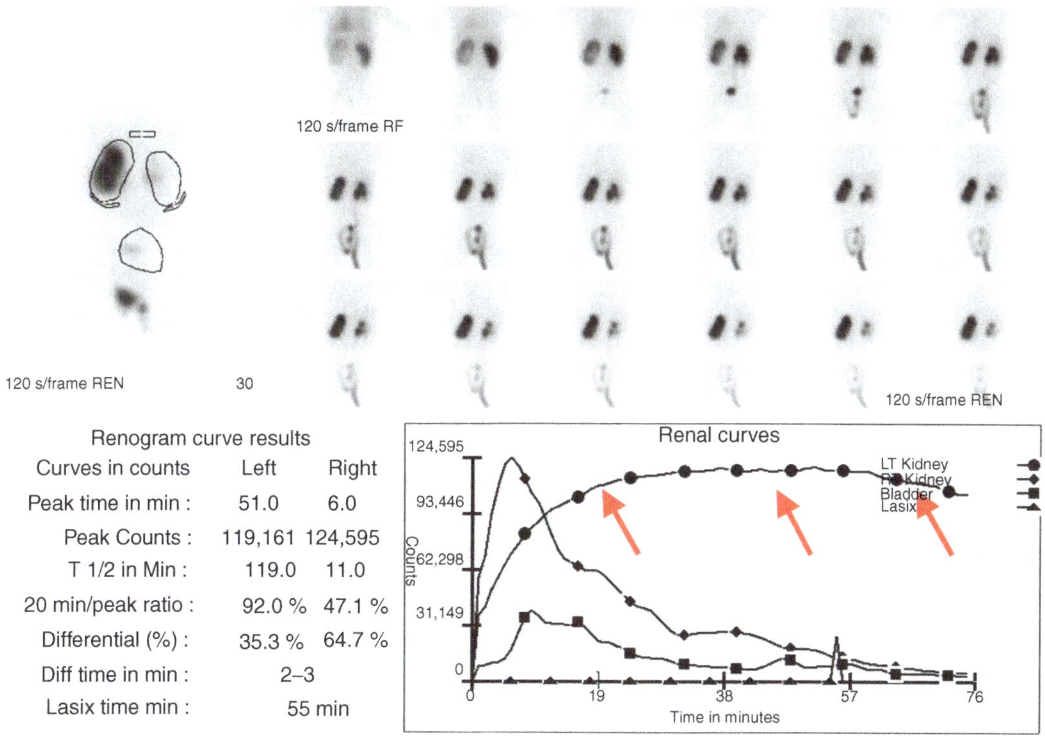

Fig. 9.39 MAG3 diuretic renal scan demonstrating left ureteropelvic junction obstruction in a 10-month-old. The left kidney has decreased relative function at 35 % and a very prolonged T ½ washout time (*arrows*) even after diuretic was given at 55 min. No radiotracer is seen along the course of the left ureter

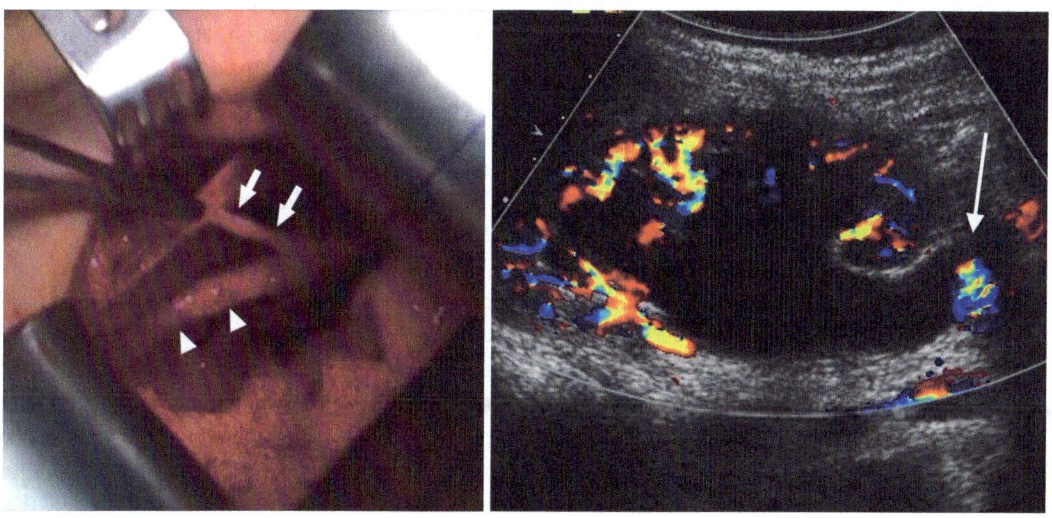

Fig. 9.40 Gross image: benign fibroepithelial polyp (*arrows*) in the proximal ureter (*arrowheads*) seen at time of UPJ repair in a child. Ultrasound image: the presence of the polyp was not known prior to surgery, but a polyp with blood flow was retrospectively appreciated on preoperative ultrasound

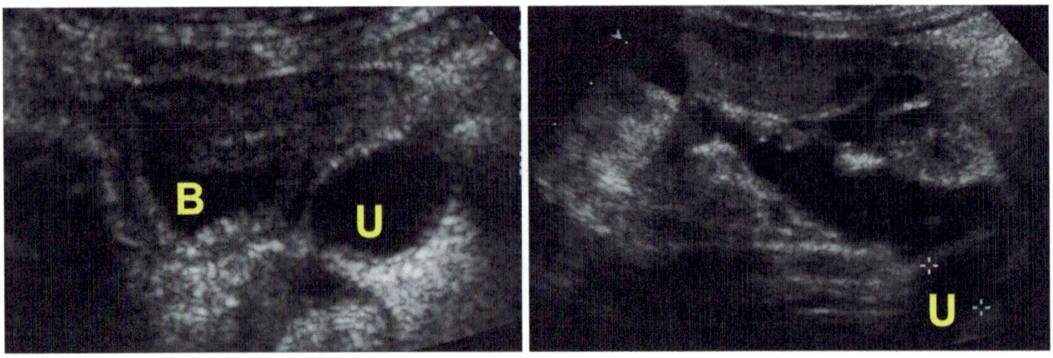

Fig. 9.41 : Megaureter in a 10-month-old. The ureter (*U*) is dilated distally near the bladder (*B*) on the left image and proximally near the kidney on the right image

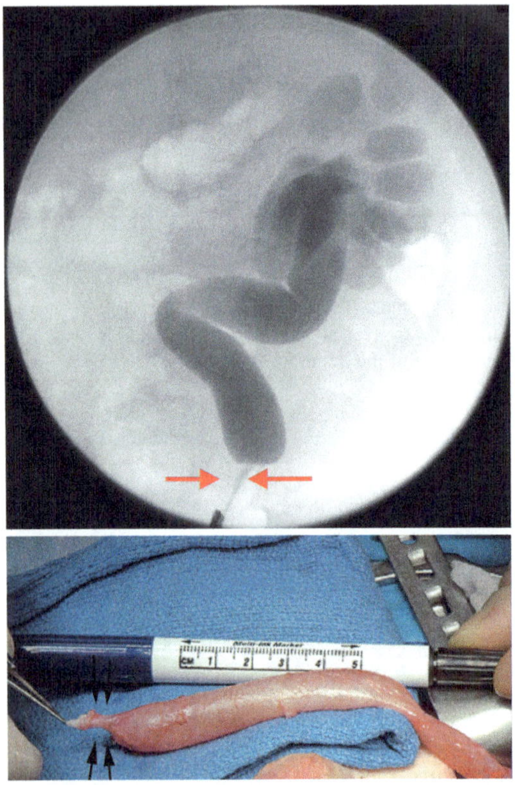

Fig. 9.42 Retrograde pyelogram of left megaureter demonstrating distal aperistaltic segment (*red arrows*) (*upper image*). Gross appearance of distal aperistaltic segment (*black arrows*) at time of ureter reimplantation for nonrefluxing, obstructed megaureter (*lower image*)

the ureterocele (Fig. 9.50). As with ectopic ureters associated with duplex kidneys, renal scans are also used clinically in determining the relative function of the different poles in a duplex kidney.

Duplex Kidney

The most common congenital anomaly of the urinary tract is complete or partial duplication of the collecting system with an estimated incidence of 1–5 % [80]. Partial duplication is more common than complete duplication. In collecting systems that have complete duplication, separate ureters drain the upper and lower poles of the duplex kidney. As mentioned in prior sections, the upper-pole ureteric bud arises higher on the mesonephric duct and may lead to an ectopic ureter or ureterocele, while the lower-pole ureteric bud arises lower on the mesonephric duct and can lead to VUR and a more craniolateral insertion into the bladder. In addition, the lower pole in a duplex kidney can develop a UPJ obstruction. However most completely duplicated systems do not lead to ectopic ureters, ureteroceles, UPJ obstructions, or VUR. The upper-pole ureter simply inserts medial and caudal to the lower-pole ureter. This relationship is referred to the Weigert-Meyer rule, but rare exceptions exist [81, 82].

Duplicated collecting systems are often detected by ultrasonography (Fig. 9.51) or incidentally on cross-sectional imaging (Fig. 9.51). In cases of UTI in children, a VCUG will often demonstrate lower-pole VUR (Fig. 9.52) or an upper-pole ectopic ureter or ureterocele discussed in the previous sections. Renal scans for kidneys with complete duplication can have the area of interest drawn around the upper and lower poles of a kidney to obtain the relative function of each.

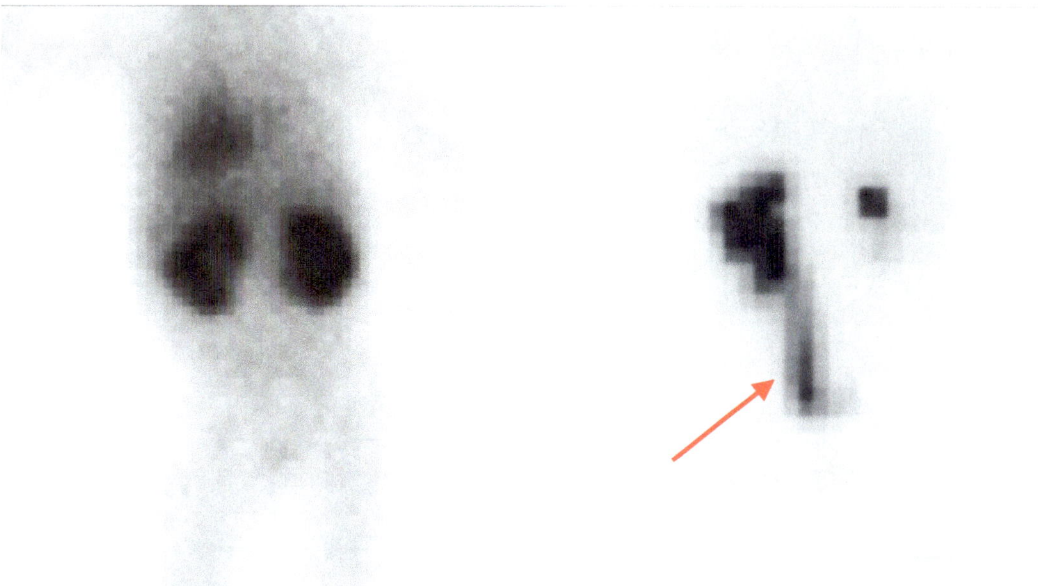

Fig. 9.43 MAG3 diuretic renal scan images of nonrefluxing, non-obstructed megaureter. The left and right kidney have symmetrical uptake of radiotracer with approximately equal split function (*left image*). The left kidney has a megaureter (*arrow*) with delayed drainage, but no obstruction

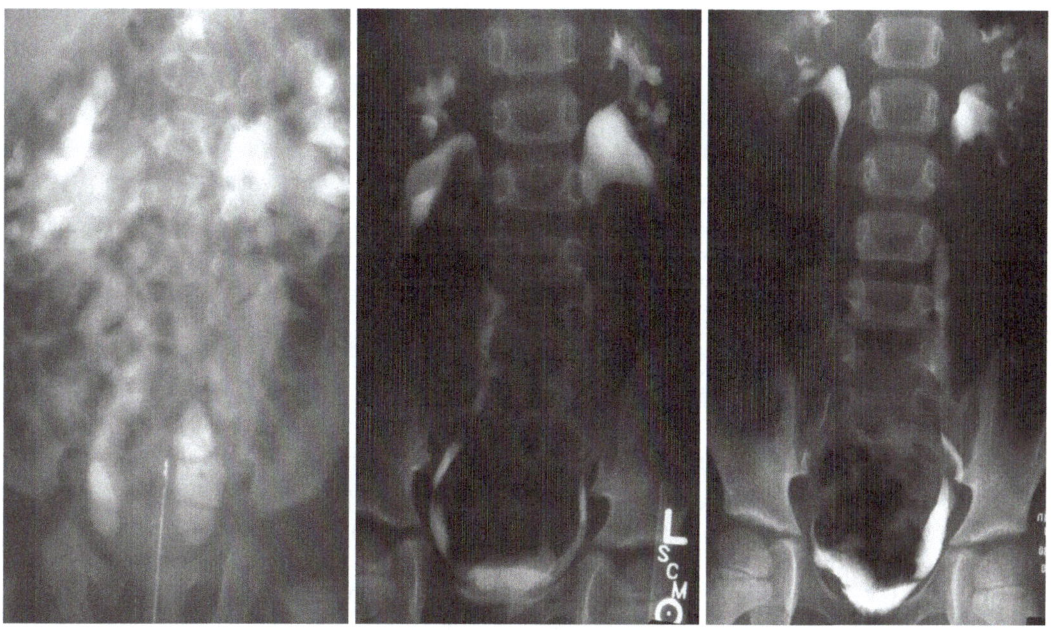

Fig. 9.44 Natural history of megaureters by intravenous pyelogram. The *right image* shows an infant with bilateral non-refluxing, non-obstructed megaureters. The *middle image* is at 5 years old and *right image* is at 8 years old demonstrating marked improvement on the *left side* and resolution on the *right*

Vesicoureteral Reflux

Vesicoureteral reflux (VUR) is the flow of urine retrograde from the bladder to the ureters. The two most common presentations for VUR are a neonate with a history of antenatal hydronephrosis or a young child with a febrile UTI.

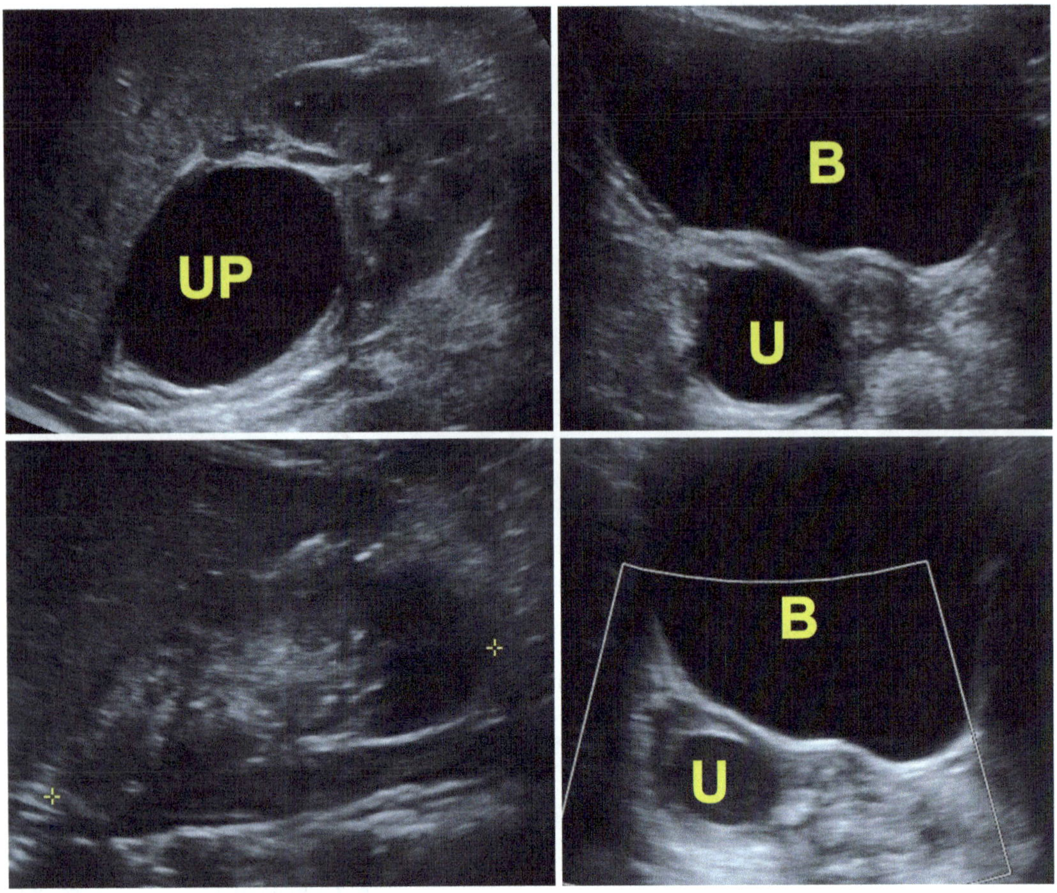

Fig. 9.45 Upper pole (*UP*) of duplex kidney with ectopic ureter (*upper left image*) and distal ureter (*U*) behind the bladder (*B*) (*upper right*) in a 4-month-old. The same patient at 14 months old after laparoscopic upper-pole heminephrectomy demonstrating removal of upper pole (*lower left image*) and persistence of some distal hydroureter behind the bladder (*lower right image*)

VUR is found in approximately 1 % of newborns and 30–45 % of children with a febrile UTI [83]. Caucasians and females are at increased risk of being diagnosed with VUR. VUR is divided into primary and secondary. Primary VUR is the most common form of VUR and is thought to occur because the ureterovesical junction (UVJ) is incompetent or the intravesical tunnel of the ureter is too short to allow closure with voiding. Secondary VUR occurs in the setting of high bladder pressures often associated with bladder outlet obstruction or neurogenic bladder.

The diagnosis of VUR is most commonly confirmed by a voiding cystourethrogram (VCUG) or a radionuclide cystogram (RNC). A VCUG is performed by placing a catheter into the bladder and filling the bladder retrograde with contrast. Images of the bladder are obtained during the filling and voiding phase. The International Reflux Study Group developed a 5-level grading method for VUR detected by VCUG [84].

Fig. 9.47 Example of refluxing, obstructed megaureter in a duplex kidney of a male child. The reflux is seen as the child starts to void (*left image*) and does not drain after completion of voiding (*right image*). Some prostatic ducts (*arrows*) are seen suggesting the ectopic ureter inserts near ejaculatory duct in the prostate

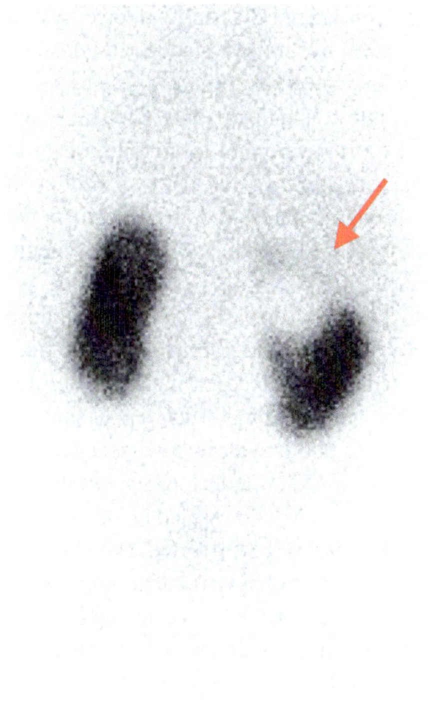

Fig. 9.46 DMSA scan demonstrating dysplasia and lack of function of the upper pole (*arrow*) of the right kidney that is often associated with an ectopic ureter

- Grade 1: Reflux into ureter only without dilation (Fig. 9.53).
- Grade 2: Reflux into ureter and renal collecting system without dilation (Fig. 9.53).
- Grade 3: Reflux fills and mildly dilates the ureter and renal collecting system with mild blunting of the calyces (Fig. 9.53).
- Grade 4: Reflux fills and grossly dilates the ureter and renal collecting system with blunting of the calyces. The ureter is also somewhat tortuous (Fig. 9.53).
- Grade 5: Reflux massively dilates the ureter and renal collecting system with blunted calyces. The ureter is significantly tortuous (Fig. 9.53).

The International Reflux Study Group also developed a grading method for RNC [85].

- Mild VUR – reflux into ureter only without dilation (Fig. 9.54)
- Moderate VUR – reflux into ureter and renal collecting systems with or without mild dilation and blunting of calyces (Fig. 9.54)
- Severe VUR – reflux that grossly dilates the ureter and renal colleting system with tortuosity in the ureter (Fig. 9.54)

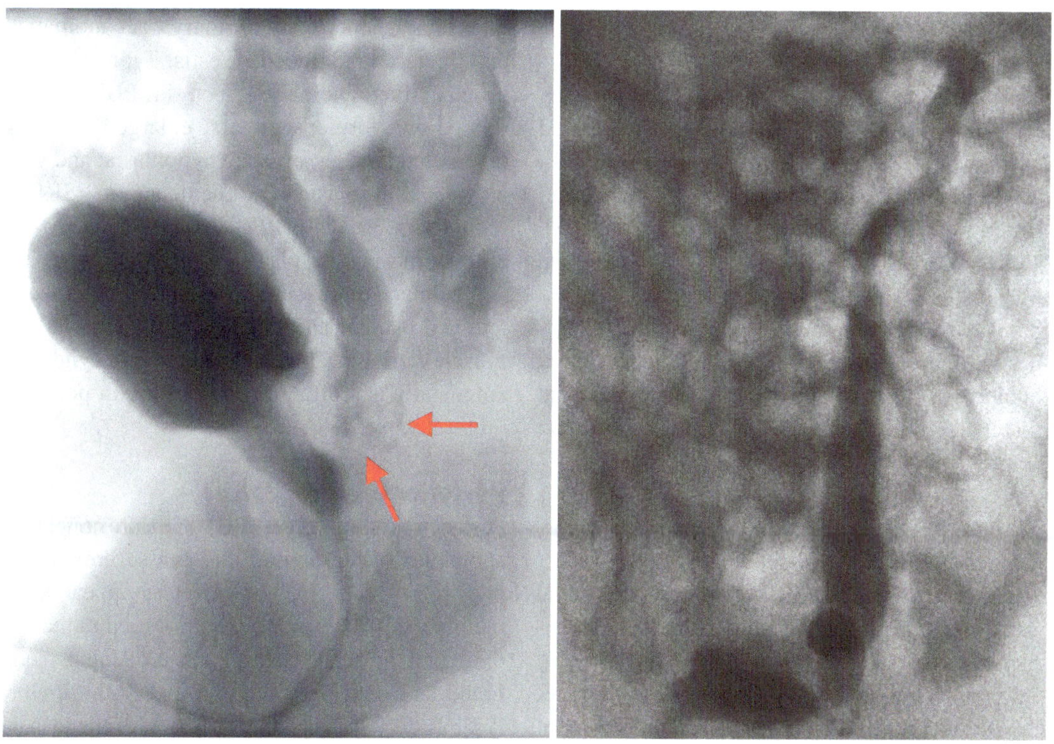

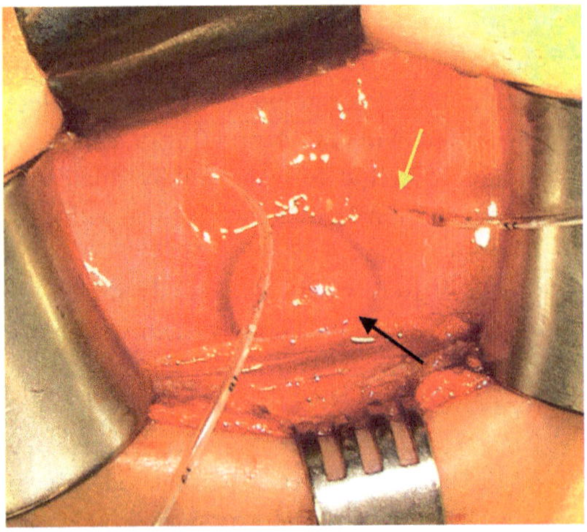

Fig. 9.48 Gross image of ureterocele in a bladder at time of surgery. The left kidney is a duplex kidney with a ureteral stent in the lower-pole ureter (*yellow arrow*) and upper pole associated with a ureterocele (*black arrow*)

The VCUG is the most widespread test used to diagnose VUR but has the disadvantage of more radiation exposure than the RNC. In RNC, one possible disadvantage is decreased anatomical detail. Several groups have attempted to use ultrasonography to diagnose VUR using ultrasound contrast media, but its use is not widespread [86].

Megacalycosis

Megacalycosis is a very rare entity characterized by an increased number of renal calyces [12–20], caliectasis in the absence of obstruction, and hypoplasia of the medullary pyramids [87]. The cause of megacalycosis is not known. Megacalycosis can present as prenatal hydronephrosis, and the diagnosis is confirmed by postnatal ultrasonography which shows the increased number of renal calyces with caliectasis and diuretic renography without obstruction (Fig. 9.55).

Bladder Exstrophy and Epispadias Complex (BEEC)

BEEC composes rare and complex congenital anomalies including epispadias, bladder exstrophy, and cloacal exstrophy. Epispadias is defined by an open urethra dorsally on the penis in males or a bifid clitoris in females. Isolated cases of epispadias can occur. Classic bladder exstrophy is characterized by an open bladder and posterior urethra in the lower abdomen, diastasis of the symphysis pubis, and epispadias. Cloacal exstrophy is the most severe and least common of the BEEC diseases and involves an open bladder and hindgut through a large abdominal wall defect, anal atresia, omphalocele, and genital anomalies.

BEEC complex diseases can be diagnosed antenatally by ultrasonography. Classic bladder exstrophy can be detected prenatally with ultrasonography with findings such as absence of bladder filling, pubic symphysis diastasis, small genitalia in males, and low-set umbilicus. However, prenatal MRI may also be useful in the diagnosis (Fig. 9.56) [88]. Around 3 % of bladder exstrophy patients will have renal anomalies such as duplex kidney, UPJO, pelvic kidney, and MCDK that are usually diagnosed by renal ultrasonography [89].

Prune Belly

Prune-belly or Eagle-Barrett syndrome (PBS) is a rare congenital syndrome of unknown etiology characterized by a triad of findings: abdominal muscle deficiency, genitourinary tract anomalies, and bilateral undescended testis. Typical genitourinary tract anomalies seen in PBS include dilated and tortuous ureters, enlarged but non-obstructed bladder, prostate hypoplasia, and variable renal dysplasia. The incidence of ESRD is around 25–30 % in PBS and is related to the amount of renal dysplasia [90, 91].

Antenatal ultrasound may show dilated ureters and bladder and the lack of abdominal wall muscle. The appearance of prune-belly syndrome antenatally can often be confused with posterior urethral valves.

Posterior Urethral Valves

Posterior urethral valves (PUV) are rare congenital anomalies of the urethra that can severely affect the urinary tract. PUV themselves appear to be membranous folds in the posterior urethra that are the result of persistence of the urogenital membrane and deficient cannulization of the urethra [92]. The PUV leads to obstruction of the urinary

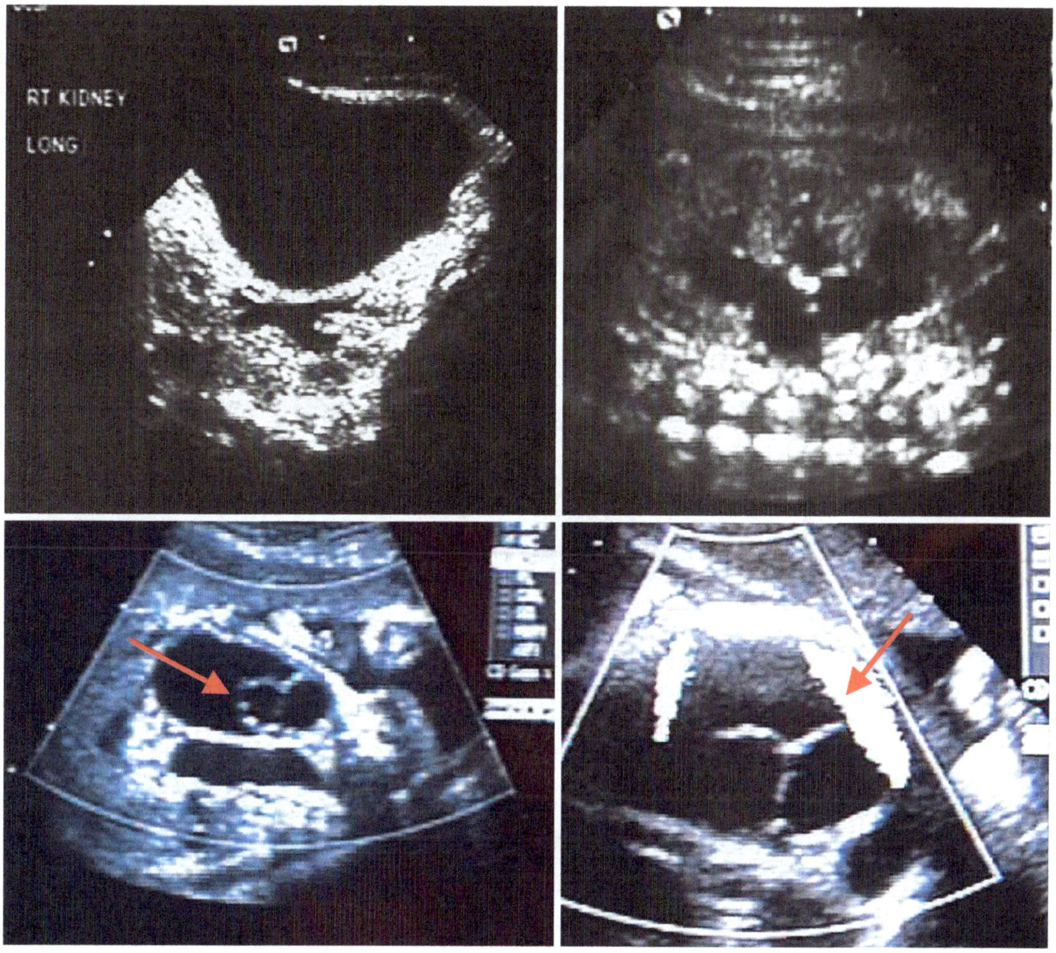

Fig. 9.49 Prenatal diagnosis of bilateral ureteroceles. The right kidney is a duplex kidney (*upper left*) with an upper-pole segment associated with a ureterocele (*bottom left*). The left kidney is a single system (*upper right*) associated with a ureterocele (*lower right*). The ureteroceles within the bladder are highlighted by *arrows*; there are clearly two cystic structures in this case of bilateral ureteroceles

tract with resulting collecting system anomalies including abnormal bladder function, hydroureteronephrosis, VUR, renal dysplasia, and ESRD.

The majority of PUV cases are detected by prenatal ultrasound that may show unilateral or bilateral hydroureteronephrosis and dilated bladder and posterior urethra (Fig. 9.57). Postnatally, PUV cases are evaluated with a VCUG, which shows the characteristic dilated posterior urethra during the voiding phase and often trabeculated bladder (Fig. 9.58). VUR is present in up to 50 % of all patients with PUV [93]. Renal dysplasia and differential renal function can be evaluated by radionuclide scans such as the DMSA scan.

Antenatal and Postnatal CAKUT Evaluation

Antenatal Evaluation

The majority of clinically significant CAKUT diseases are detected by fetal ultrasonography. The most common time to obtain a screening antenatal ultrasound is between 16 and 20 weeks of gestation. At this time there is good visualization of urinary tract anatomy with a high sensitivity for detecting CAKUT diseases. In addition, it is early enough in the gestation where other prenatal testing such as karyotype can be performed as well as termination of the pregnancy.

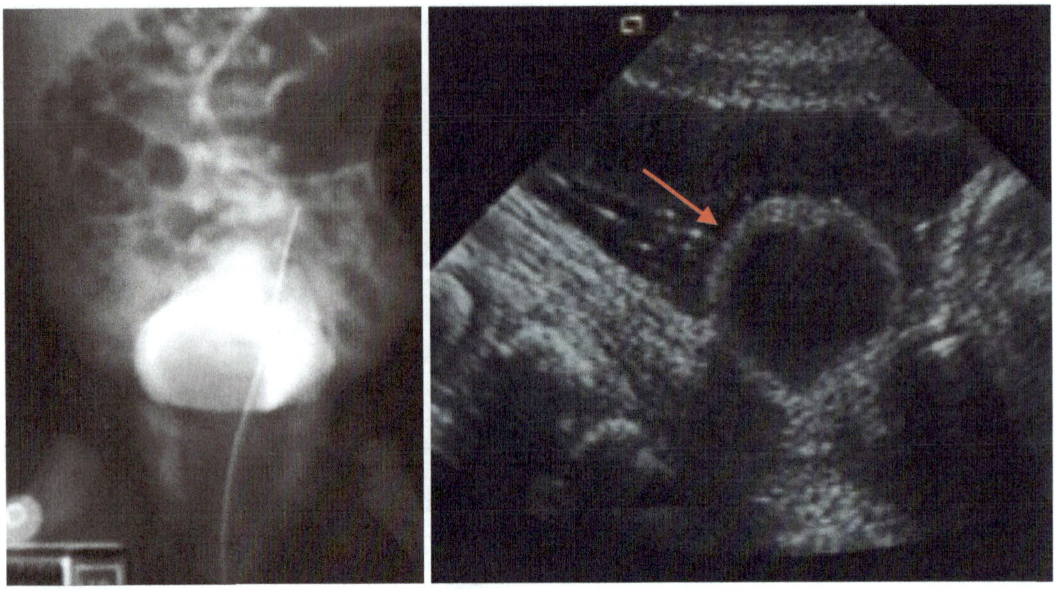

Fig. 9.50 Right-sided ureterocele. On early filling images of VCUG, the ureterocele is visible as a filling defect (*left image*). Ultrasound demonstrates a cystic structure within the bladder (*red arrow*) (*right image*)

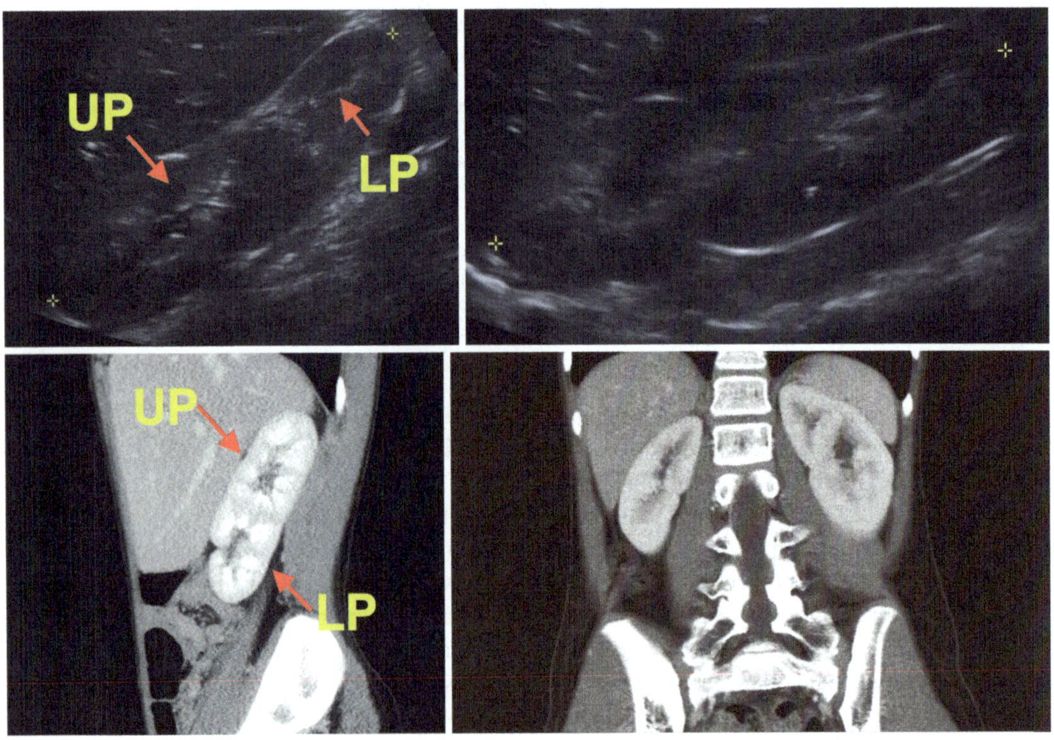

Fig. 9.51 Ultrasound of a 10-month-old with duplex right kidney without hydronephrosis (*Top images*). The duplex kidney is longer than a normal kidney, and a strip of kidney parenchyma can be seen that divides the poles. CT scan of an 11-year-old with right duplex kidney (*lower left*) and CT scan of a 10-year-old with left duplex kidney (*lower right*). The upper pole (*UP*) and lower pole (*LP*) of the duplex kidneys are highlighted in two of the images

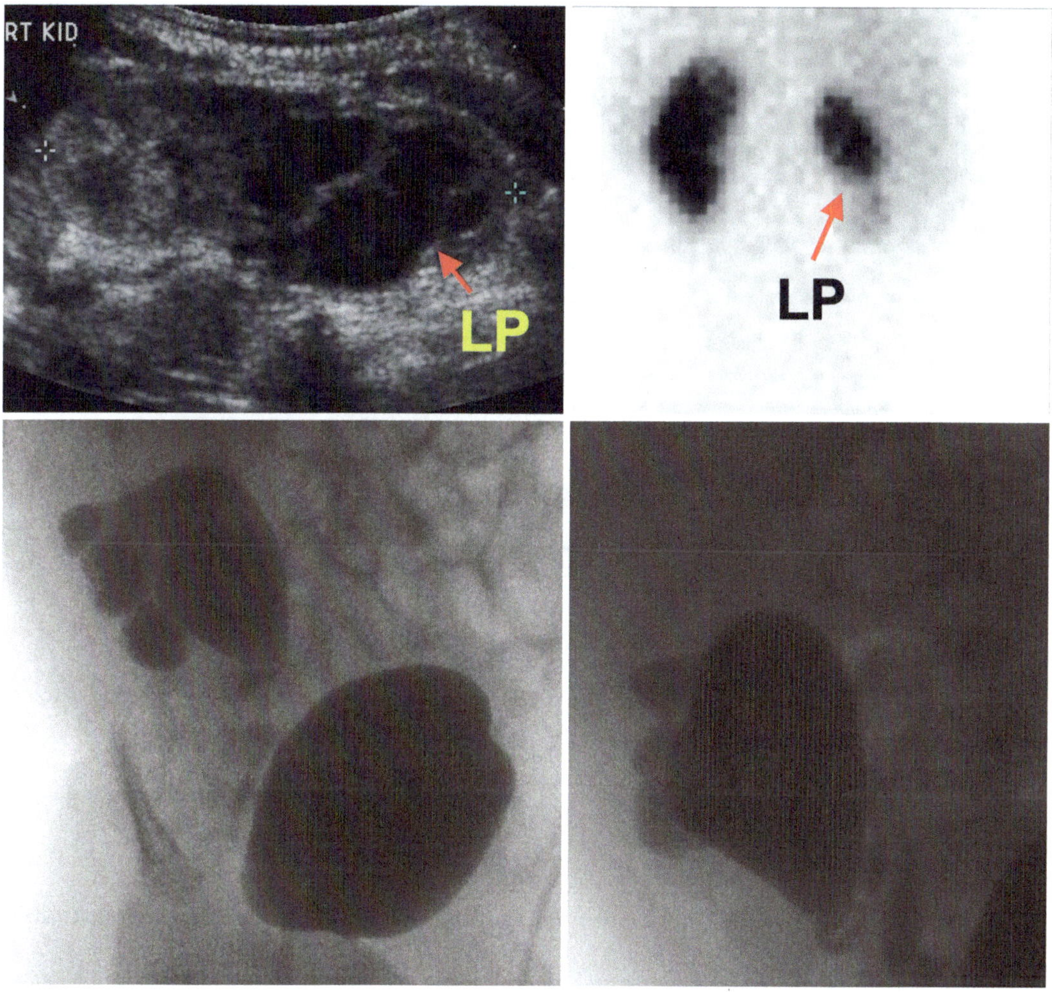

Fig. 9.52 Duplex kidney with lower-pole (*LP*) reflux. Note the grade 4 hydronephrosis in the lower pole on ultrasound (*upper left*) and the decreased function seen on MAG3 renal scan of the lower pole (*upper right*). The reflux is grades 4–5 and the drooping lily appearance of the lower-pole calyces is demonstrated (*lower images*)

The fetal kidneys and bladder can be detected by the 15th week of gestation [94, 95]. The fetal ureters are normally not seen on prenatal ultrasound. The amount of hydronephrosis, if present, can be graded by SFU grade or the RPD measured. The bladder wall should be thin. The decrease in the volume of amniotic fluid (oligohydramnios) is a sensitive marker for abnormal fetal renal function because by 20 weeks gestation fetal urine accounts for the majority of amniotic fluid volume [96, 97]. There are several methods for assessing amniotic fluid volume by prenatal ultrasound with the single deepest pocket (SDP) measurement and amniotic fluid index (AFI) being the most common. The SDP measurement is obtained by measuring the vertical length of the largest pocked of amniotic fluid measured at a right angle to the uterus. The SDP can be interpreted accordingly: 0–2 cm, oligohydramnios; 2.1–8 cm, normal; and greater than 8 cm, polyhydramnios [98]. The AFI is a slightly more complicated measurement that is obtained by dividing the uterus into four quadrants and then obtaining the vertical length of the largest amniotic fluid pocket in each quadrant then summing the four measurements. The AFI can be interpreted accordingly: 0 to less than 4 cm,

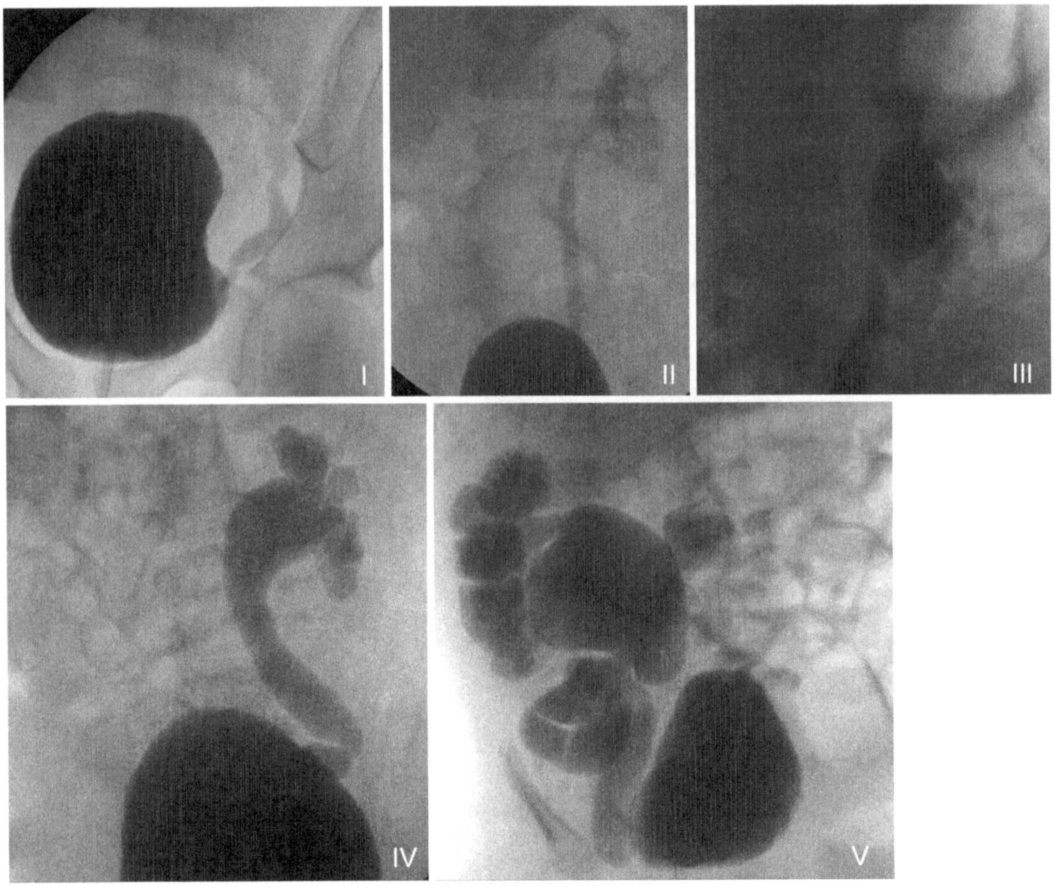

Fig. 9.53 Reflux grades on VCUG. Grade I (*upper left*). Grade II (*upper middle*). Grade III (*upper right*). Grade IV (*lower left*). Grade V (*lower right*)

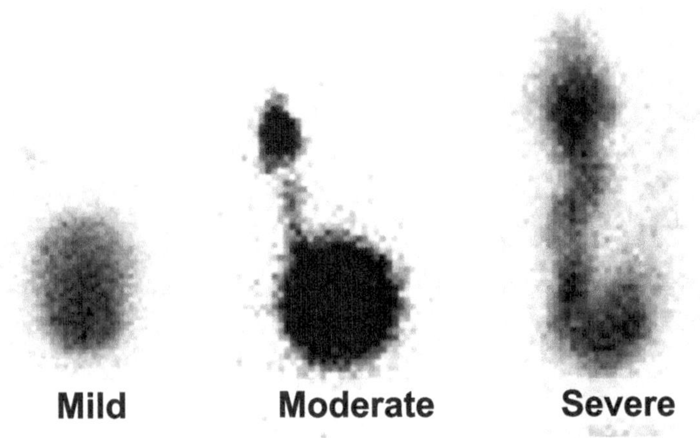

Fig. 9.54 Reflux grades on RNC. Mild VUR (*left*). Moderate VUR (*middle*). Severe VUR (*left*)

oligohydramnios; 5–25 cm, normal; and greater than 25 cm, polyhydramnios [99]. A Cochrane Collaboration meta-analysis comparing the SDP and AFI found that no method was superior in prevention of poor peripartum outcomes. However, the AFI diagnosed oligohydramnios

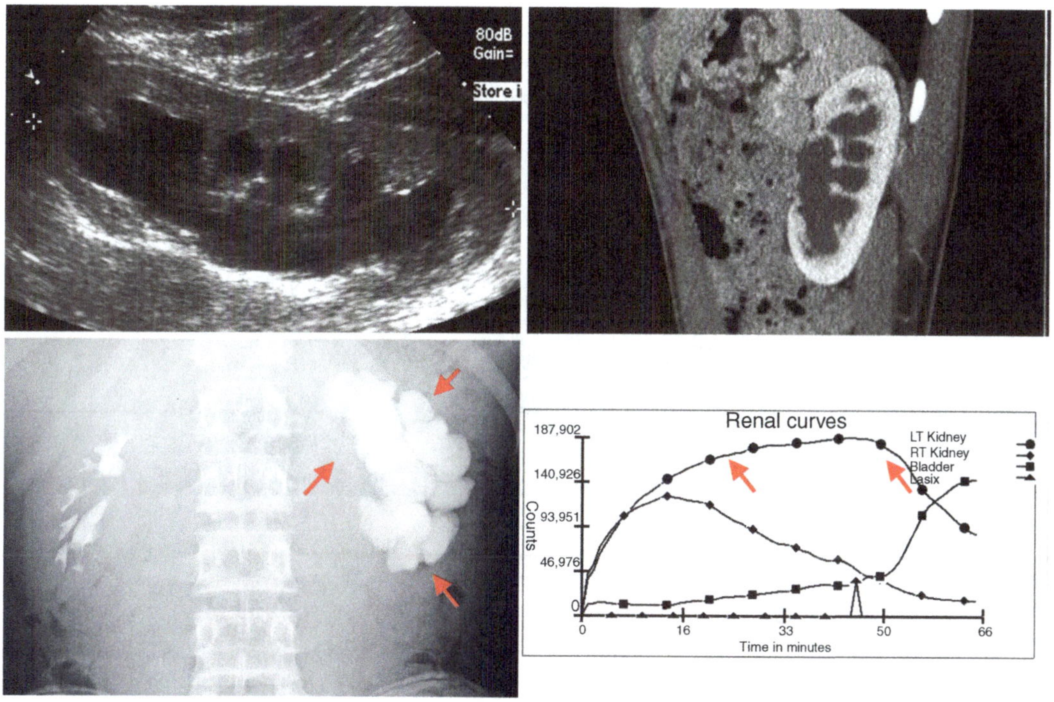

Fig. 9.55 Megacalycosis in a 15-year-old. Ultrasonography of megacalycosis (*upper left image*) will show an increased number of calyces as well as CT (*upper right image*). Perhaps the best demonstration of the increased number of calyces (*arrows*) is a plain film obtained during excretory phase of CT scan (*lower left image*). In megacalycosis, diuretic renography typically demonstrates lack of obstruction with radiotracer washout (*arrows*) after diuretic administration (*lower right image*)

more frequently, which led to more labor inductions and cesarean section deliveries. Therefore, the SDP was recommended [100].

Fetal MRI is increasing in use in the evaluation of CAKUT diseases [101, 102]. In one report, 35 women with 37 fetuses underwent fetal MRI with a gestational age range of 17–35 weeks. Fetal MRI was able to evaluate the kidneys and bladder in all infants and the perineum in 27 of the 35 pregnancies. In four cases of renal agenesis, the fetal MRI was able to detect the kidneys. Fetal MRI was able to distinguish between PUV and PBS by detecting the dilated posterior urethra in all cases of PUV and no posterior urethral dilation in the PBS cases. The authors suggest that fetal MRI has advantages in pregnancies with significant oligohydramnios and cases where evaluation of the perineum is important [102]. MRI can be a useful adjunct to ultrasound when the diagnosis is inconclusive on ultrasound [103].

Postnatal Evaluation

The postnatal evaluation strategy varies by the severity of antenatal findings and presumed diagnosis. A detailed pregnancy and maternal history should be performed as well as a physical examination of the newborn for all infants with a CAKUT finding prenatally. In infants with severe oligohydramnios, the infant's pulmonary function and efforts toward pulmonary resuscitation will be most important. Some CAKUT diseases will be obvious such as prune-belly syndrome or BEEC syndromes.

Postnatal radiologic evaluation of CAKUT diseases usually begins with abdominal ultrasonography. In infants with severe prenatal findings, oligohydramnios, an abnormal solitary kidney, or bilateral disease an ultrasound within the first 24 h of life is appropriate. In infants with only unilateral involvement, it is recommended to perform ultrasonography after 48 h but within the first week of life. The reason to wait 48 h is

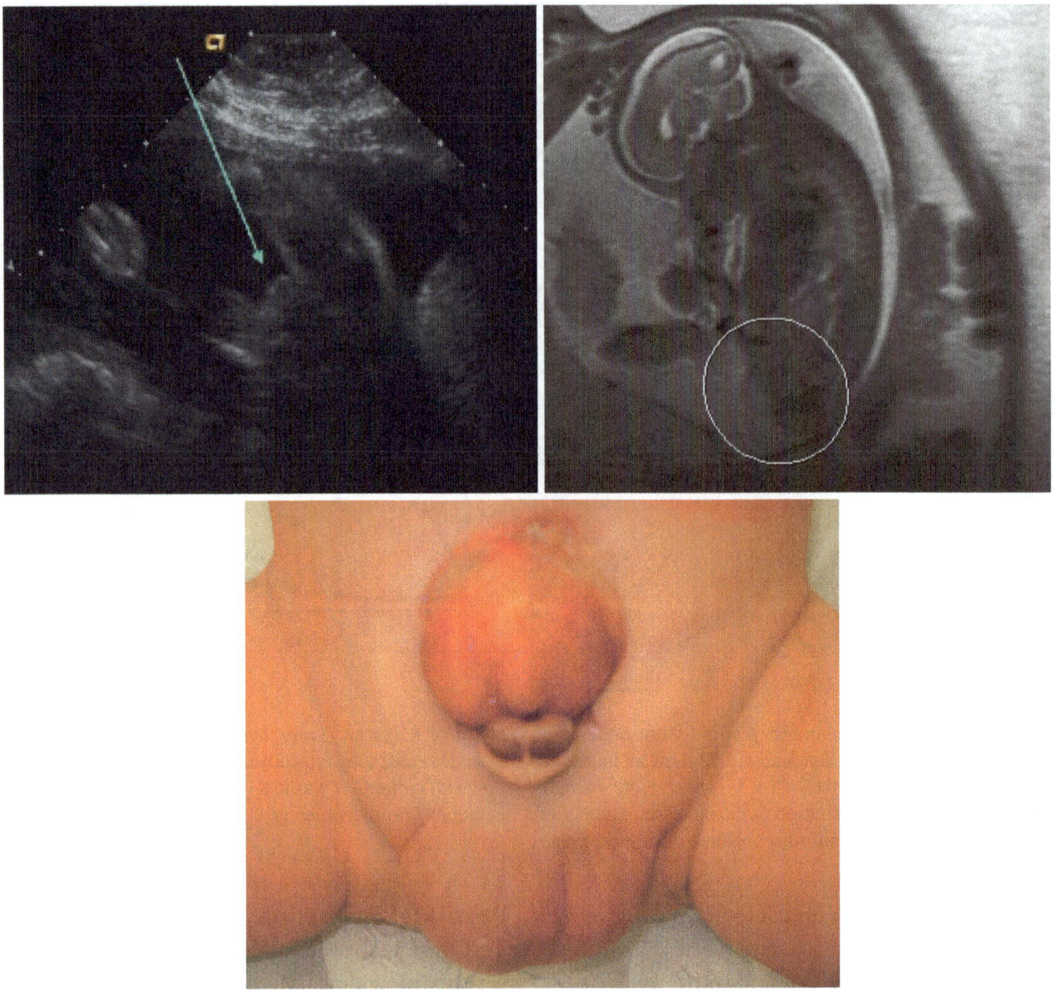

Fig. 9.56 Classic bladder exstrophy. The findings on prenatal ultrasound done at 20 weeks included a small penis (*arrow*) with no bladder visualized (*upper left image*). A prenatal MRI performed at 21 weeks visualized the abdominal wall defect with the herniated bladder (*circle*) typical of classic bladder exstrophy (*upper right image*). The bottom image shows the appearance just prior to surgical reconstruction at 3 weeks of age with a small, wide penis with epispadias and abdominal wall defect with open bladder

that infants are relatively dehydrated, and severity of findings such as hydronephrosis may be underestimated earlier. A VCUG is often performed within the first week of life in infants with severe findings, oligohydramnios, an abnormal solitary kidney, or those with severe disease. However, it is controversial whether a VCUG should be performed in infants with bilateral or unilateral low-grade hydronephrosis. If there is severe hydronephrosis or megaureter, a MAG3 diuretic renal scan is often performed within the first weeks of life to assess for obstruction. A static renal scan such as a DMSA scan can also be performed within the first few weeks of life to evaluate for severity of dysplasia and differential function. In many cases of mild hydronephrosis, only serial ultrasounds are performed as the hydronephrosis is very likely to resolve spontaneously [61].

Other imaging modalities such as MRI or CT are performed occasionally to evaluate complex CAKUT malformations. However, ultrasonography,

VCUG, and radionuclide renal scans remain the main imaging modalities for postnatal evaluation of CAKUT diseases.

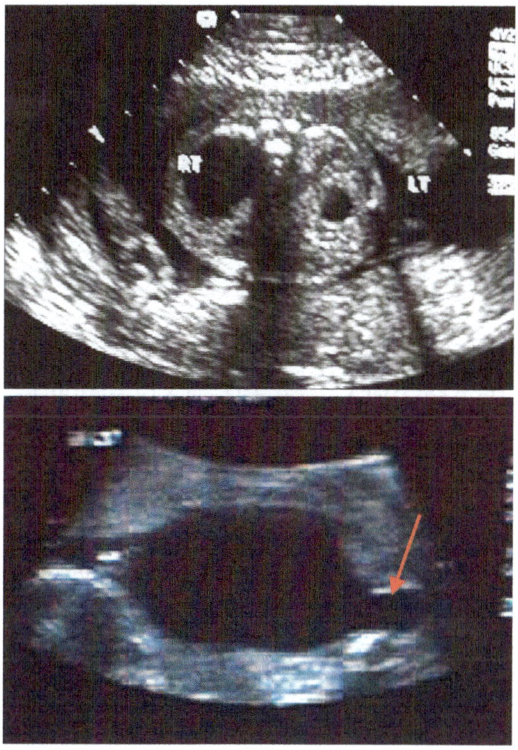

Fig. 9.57 Antenatal ultrasound of posterior urethral valves. This fetus had bilateral hydroureteronephrosis (*upper image*); however, unilateral or no hydroureteronephrosis is also possible with posterior urethral valves. The bladder (*lower image*) had the typical appearance of posterior urethral valves with a dilated posterior urethra (*arrow*) known as the keyhole sign

Diagnosis of CAKUT Diseases in Childhood or Adolescence

Ureteropelvic Junction Obstruction

The most common presentations of a UPJO in childhood or adolescence are episodes of pain called Dietl's crises, after evaluation for UTI, after trauma, or incidentally. Usually, the first test obtained is a renal ultrasound which shows dilation of the renal pelvis and calyces, but not hydroureter as mentioned in previous sections. A MAG3 diuretic renal scan is then obtained to evaluate the kidneys for differential function and obstruction. In older children, the concern for a crossing lower-pole renal vessel is higher than in infants, so occasionally CT or MR angiography is sometimes obtained to look for lower-pole crossing vessels (Fig. 9.59).

Vesicoureteral Reflux

Vesicoureteral reflux (VUR) is commonly found after a VCUG is performed in a child with a febrile UTI. Approximately 30–45 % of children with a febrile UTI will be found to have VUR [83]. VUR in childhood is more common in females and Caucasians [104]. Most cases of VUR resolve spontaneously with lower-grade VUR resolves at a higher rate than high-grade VUR [105]. VUR can be associated with renal scarring or dysplasia with higher grades of VUR having a higher risk of abnormalities seen on DMSA scan (Fig. 9.60).

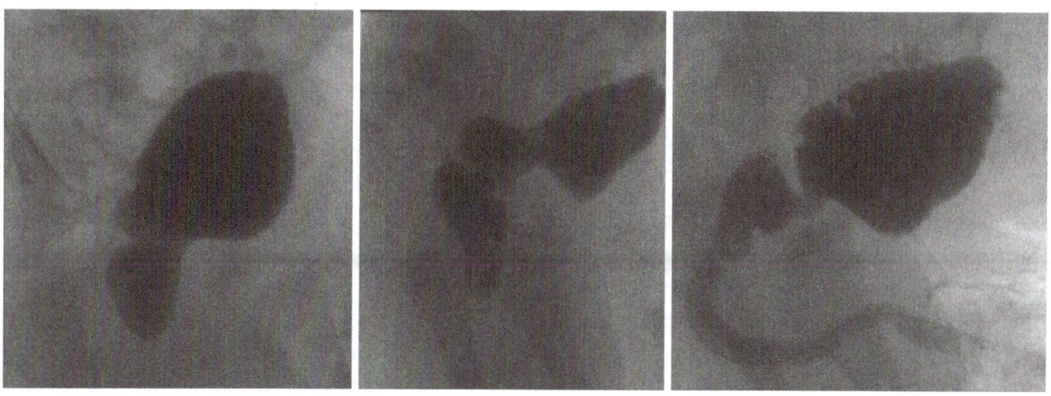

Fig. 9.58 Postnatal VCUG of three different infants with posterior urethral valves. Vesicoureteral reflux is also a common finding on VCUG

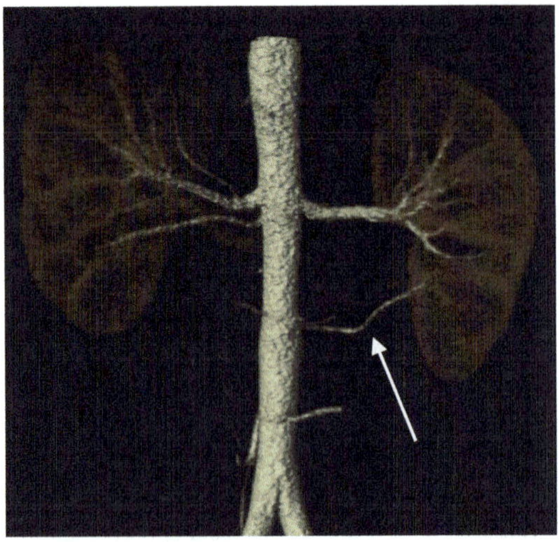

Fig. 9.59 Three-dimensional reconstruction of CT angiography images showing vascular supply to kidneys in a child with a history consistent with left UPJ obstruction. A lower-pole crossing vessel was detected on the left (*arrow*)

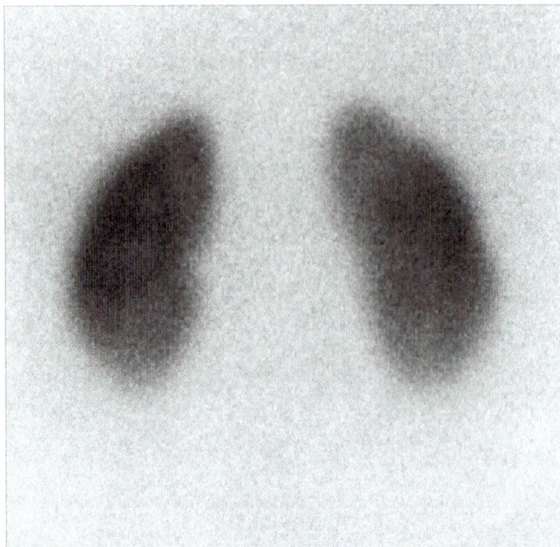

Fig. 9.60 DMSA scan of child with bilateral VUR demonstrating renal scarring in upper and lower poles of right kidney and scarring in the lower pole of the left kidney

Congenital Renal Vein Thrombosis

Congenital (neonatal) renal vein thrombosis (RVT) is a rare entity occurring in 2–3 infants per 100,000 live births [106]. The exact etiology is often unclear, but perinatal dehydration and/or asphyxia are thought to be risk factors as well as hereditary prothrombotic states such as lupus anticoagulant, prothrombin gene mutations, factor V Leiden mutation, and others. Hereditary prothrombotic states are found in around 50 % of cases of RVT [107]. The classic presentation includes the triad of gross hematuria, palpable abdominal mass, and thrombocytopenia although a minority of patients present with the classic triad of findings [108]. There is no consensus on the optimal management of neonates with RVT [107].

Ultrasound is a common method for diagnosing congenital RVT [107]. The kidneys affected by RVT are enlarged and with increased echogenicity and loss of corticomedullary differentiation. In addition, a renal vein thrombus may be able to be seen on ultrasound. Blood flow in the main renal vein may still be present in kidneys with RVT, but an increased resistance to flow may be seen in the renal arteries. Given the propensity for renal scarring with RVT, radionuclide scans are often used to assess the kidneys in follow-up.

Key Points to Remember

- Congenital anomalies of the kidney and urinary tract are the most common causes of end-stage renal disease in childhood.
- Understanding the embryology of kidney development helps understand the pathology seen in CAKUT diseases.
- Anomalies in renal parenchymal development can result in renal dysplasia, renal hypoplasia, and cystic renal diseases including multicystic dysplastic kidney.
- Anomalies in renal fusion or ascent during development can result in ectopic kidneys, horseshoe kidneys, and crossed fused ectopic kidneys.
- Anomalies in collecting system development can result in ectopic ureter, vesicoureteral reflux, ureteropelvic junction obstruction, ureterocele, megaureter, and other collecting system anomalies.
- Anomalies in collecting system development are commonly associated with renal dysplasia.

- Anomalies in renal fusion or ascent are commonly associated with renal dysplasia and anomalies in collecting system development.
- Many CAKUT diseases are diagnosed prenatally by ultrasonography.
- Renal ultrasonography is the first imaging modality for most CAKUT diseases with radionuclide scanning and voiding cystourethrograms utilized frequently. MRI is increasing in use for CAKUT diseases.

References

1. Schedl A. Renal abnormalities and their developmental origin. Nat Rev Genet. 2007;8(10):791–802.
2. Harambat J, van Stralen KJ, Kim JJ, Tizard EJ. Epidemiology of chronic kidney disease in children. Pediatr Nephrol. 2012;27(3):363–73.
3. Pope JC, Brock 3rd JW, Adams MC, Stephens FD, Ichikawa I. How they begin and how they end: classic and new theories for the development and deterioration of congenital anomalies of the kidney and urinary tract, CAKUT. J Am Soc Nephrol. 1999;10(9):2018–28.
4. Baskin L, Meaney D, Landsman A, Zderic SA, Macarak E. Bovine bladder compliance increases with normal fetal development. J Urol. 1994;152(2 Pt 2):692–5; discussion 696–7.
5. Anderson JK, Kabalin JN, Cadeddu JA. Chapter 1: Surgical Anatomy of the Retroperitoneum, Adrenals, Kidneys, and Ureters. Campbell-Walsh Urology. 9th ed. Philadelphia: Saunders Elsevier; 2007.
6. Zelenko N, Coll D, Rosenfeld AT, Smith RC. Normal ureter size on unenhanced helical CT. AJR Am J Roentgenol. 2004;182(4):1039–41.
7. Hakenberg OW, Linne C, Manseck A, Wirth MP. Bladder wall thickness in normal adults and men with mild lower urinary tract symptoms and benign prostatic enlargement. Neurourol Urodyn. 2000; 19(5):585–93.
8. Uluocak N, Erdemir F, Parlaktas BS, Caglar MK, Hasiloglu Z, Etikan I. Bladder wall thickness in healthy school-aged children. Urology. 2007; 69(4):763–6; discussion 766.
9. Jequier S, Rousseau O. Sonographic measurements of the normal bladder wall in children. AJR Am J Roentgenol. 1987;149(3):563–6.
10. Weber S, Moriniere V, Knuppel T, Charbit M, Dusek J, Ghiggeri GM, et al. Prevalence of mutations in renal developmental genes in children with renal hypodysplasia: results of the ESCAPE study. J Am Soc Nephrol. 2006;17(10):2864–70.
11. Cooper WO, Hernandez-Diaz S, Arbogast PG, Dudley JA, Dyer S, Gideon PS, et al. Major congenital malformations after first-trimester exposure to ACE inhibitors. N Engl J Med. 2006;354(23): 2443–51.
12. Weaver RG, Cashwell LF, Lorentz W, Whiteman D, Geisinger KR, Ball M. Optic nerve coloboma associated with renal disease. Am J Med Genet. 1988; 29(3):597–605.
13. Fraser FC, Ling D, Clogg D, Nogrady B. Genetic aspects of the BOR syndrome–branchial fistulas, ear pits, hearing loss, and renal anomalies. Am J Med Genet. 1978;2(3):241–52.
14. Broyer M, Soto B, Gagnadoux MF, Adi M, Rica C, Gubler MC. Oligomeganephronic renal hypoplasia. Adv Nephrol Necker Hosp. 1997;26:47–63.
15. Sanna-Cherchi S, Caridi G, Weng PL, Scolari F, Perfumo F, Gharavi AG, et al. Genetic approaches to human renal agenesis/hypoplasia and dysplasia. Pediatr Nephrol. 2007;22(10):1675–84.
16. Harris J, Robert E, Kallen B. Epidemiologic characteristics of kidney malformations. Eur J Epidemiol. 2000;16(11):985–92.
17. Murawski IJ, Gupta IR. Vesicoureteric reflux and renal malformations: a developmental problem. Clin Genet. 2006;69(2):105–17.
18. Mackie GG, Stephens FD. Duplex kidneys: a correlation of renal dysplasia with position of the ureteral orifice. J Urol. 1975;114(2):274–80.
19. Risdon RA. Renal dysplasia. I. A clinico-pathological study of 76 cases. J Clin Pathol. 1971;24(1):57–71.
20. Ismaili K, Avni FE, Alexander M, Schulman C, Collier F, Hall M. Routine voiding cystourethrography is of no value in neonates with unilateral multicystic dysplastic kidney. J Pediatr. 2005;146(6):759–63.
21. Eckoldt F, Woderich R, Smith RD, Heling KS. Antenatal diagnostic aspects of unilateral multicystic kidney dysplasia–sensitivity, specificity, predictive values, differential diagnoses, associated malformations and consequences. Fetal Diagn Ther. 2004; 19(2):163–9.
22. Aslam M, Watson AR. Unilateral multicystic dysplastic kidney: long term outcomes. Arch Dis Child. 2006;91(10):820–3.
23. Kuwertz-Broeking E, Brinkmann OA, Von Lengerke HJ, Sciuk J, Fruend S, Bulla M, et al. Unilateral multicystic dysplastic kidney: experience in children. BJU Int. 2004;93(3):388–92.
24. Narchi H. Risk of Wilms' tumour with multicystic kidney disease: a systematic review. Arch Dis Child. 2005;90(2):147–9.
25. Beckwith JB. Should asymptomatic unilateral multicystic dysplastic kidneys be removed because of the future risk of neoplasia? Pediatr Nephrol. 1992; 6(6):511.
26. Shaikewitz ST, Chapman A. Autosomal recessive polycystic kidney disease: issues regarding the variability of clinical presentation. J Am Soc Nephrol. 1993;3(12):1858–62.
27. Zerres K, Hansmann M, Mallmann R, Gembruch U. Autosomal recessive polycystic kidney disease. Problems of prenatal diagnosis. Prenat Diagn. 1988;8(3):215–29.

28. Bergmann C, Kupper F, Dornia C, Schneider F, Senderek J, Zerres K. Algorithm for efficient PKHD1 mutation screening in autosomal recessive polycystic kidney disease (ARPKD). Hum Mutat. 2005;25(3):225–31.
29. Wen J. Congenital hepatic fibrosis in autosomal recessive polycystic kidney disease. Clin Transl Sci. 2001;4(6):460–5.
30. Adeva M, El-Youssef M, Rossetti S, Kamath PS, Kubly V, Consugar MB, et al. Clinical and molecular characterization defines a broadened spectrum of autosomal recessive polycystic kidney disease (ARPKD). Medicine (Baltimore). 2006;85(1):1–21.
31. Peters DJ, Spruit L, Saris JJ, Ravine D, Sandkuijl LA, Fossdal R, et al. Chromosome 4 localization of a second gene for autosomal dominant polycystic kidney disease. Nat Genet. 1993;5(4):359–62.
32. Mekahli D, Woolf AS, Bockenhauer D. Similar renal outcomes in children with ADPKD diagnosed by screening or presenting with symptoms. Pediatr Nephrol. 2010;25(11):2275–82.
33. Belz MM, Hughes RL, Kaehny WD, Johnson AM, Fick-Brosnahan GM, Earnest MP, et al. Familial clustering of ruptured intracranial aneurysms in autosomal dominant polycystic kidney disease. Am J Kidney Dis. 2001;38(4):770–6.
34. Cadnapaphornchai MA, McFann K, Strain JD, Masoumi A, Schrier RW. Increased left ventricular mass in children with autosomal dominant polycystic kidney disease and borderline hypertension. Kidney Int. 2008;74(9):1192–6.
35. Israel GM, Bosniak MA. An update of the Bosniak renal cyst classification system. Urology. 2005;66(3):484–8.
36. Harisinghani MG, Maher MM, Gervais DA, McGovern F, Hahn P, Jhaveri K, et al. Incidence of malignancy in complex cystic renal masses (Bosniak category III): should imaging-guided biopsy precede surgery? AJR Am J Roentgenol. 2003;180(3):755–8.
37. Wallis MC, Lorenzo AJ, Farhat WA, Bagli DJ, Khoury AE, Pippi Salle JL. Risk assessment of incidentally detected complex renal cysts in children: potential role for a modification of the Bosniak classification. J Urol. 2008;180(1):317–21.
38. Peng Y, Jia L, Sun N, Li J, Fu L, Zeng J, et al. Assessment of cystic renal masses in children: comparison of multislice computed tomography and ultrasound imaging using the Bosniak classification system. Eur J Radiol. 2010;75(3):287–92.
39. Terada N, Ichioka K, Matsuta Y, Okubo K, Yoshimura K, Arai Y. The natural history of simple renal cysts. J Urol. 2002;167(1):21–3.
40. Ravine D, Gibson RN, Donlan J, Sheffield LJ. An ultrasound renal cyst prevalence survey: specificity data for inherited renal cystic diseases. Am J Kidney Dis. 1993;22(6):803–7.
41. McHugh K, Stringer DA, Hebert D, Babiak CA. Simple renal cysts in children: diagnosis and follow-up with US. Radiology. 1991;178(2):383–5.
42. Curry NS. Small renal masses (lesions smaller than 3 cm): imaging evaluation and management. AJR Am J Roentgenol. 1995;164(2):355–62.
43. Parikh CR, McCall D, Engelman C, Schrier RW. Congenital renal agenesis: case-control analysis of birth characteristics. Am J Kidney Dis. 2002;39(4):689–94.
44. Song JT, Ritchey ML, Zerin JM, Bloom DA. Incidence of vesicoureteral reflux in children with unilateral renal agenesis. J Urol. 1995;153(4):1249–51.
45. Kaneyama K, Yamataka A, Satake S, Yanai T, Lane GJ, Kaneko K, et al. Associated urologic anomalies in children with solitary kidney. J Pediatr Surg. 2004;39(1):85–7.
46. Singer A, Simmons MZ, Maldjian PD. Spectrum of congenital renal anomalies presenting in adulthood. Clin Imaging. 2008;32(3):183–91.
47. Smith NA, Laufer MR. Obstructed hemivagina and ipsilateral renal anomaly (OHVIRA) syndrome: management and follow-up. Fertil Steril. 2007;87(4):918–22.
48. Guarino N, Tadini B, Camardi P, Silvestro L, Lace R, Bianchi M. The incidence of associated urological abnormalities in children with renal ectopia. J Urol. 2004;172(4 Pt 2):1757–9; discussion 1759.
49. Murphy JJ, Altit G, Zerhouni S. The intrathoracic kidney: should we fix it? J Pediatr Surg. 2012;47(5):970–3.
50. D'Alberton A, Reschini E, Ferrari N, Candiani P. Prevalence of urinary tract abnormalities in a large series of patients with uterovaginal atresia. J Urol. 1981;126(5):623–4.
51. Fedele L, Bianchi S, Agnoli B, Tozzi L, Vignali M. Urinary tract anomalies associated with unicornuate uterus. J Urol. 1996;155(3):847–8.
52. McDonald JH, McClellan DS. Crossed renal ectopia. Am J Surg. 1957;93(6):995–1002.
53. Weizer AZ, Silverstein AD, Auge BK, Delvecchio FC, Raj G, Albala DM, et al. Determining the incidence of horseshoe kidney from radiographic data at a single institution. J Urol. 2003;170(5):1722–6.
54. O'Brien J, Buckley O, Doody O, Ward E, Persaud T, Torreggiani W. Imaging of horseshoe kidneys and their complications. J Med Imaging Radiat Oncol. 2008;52(3):216–26.
55. Boatman DL, Cornell SH, Kolln CP. The arterial supply of horseshoe kidneys. Am J Roentgenol Radium Ther Nucl Med. 1971;113(3):447–51.
56. Ek S, Lidefeldt KJ, Varricio L. Fetal hydronephrosis; prevalence, natural history and postnatal consequences in an unselected population. Acta Obstet Gynecol Scand. 2007;86(12):1463–6.
57. Sairam S, Al-Habib A, Sasson S, Thilaganathan B. Natural history of fetal hydronephrosis diagnosed on mid-trimester ultrasound. Ultrasound Obstet Gynecol. 2001;17(3):191–6.
58. Fernbach SK, Maizels M, Conway JJ. Ultrasound grading of hydronephrosis: introduction to the system used by the Society for Fetal Urology. Pediatr Radiol. 1993;23(6):478–80.

59. Tombesi MM, Alconcher LF. Short-term outcome of mild isolated antenatal hydronephrosis conservatively managed. J Pediatr Urol. 2011;8(2):129–33.
60. de Kort EH, Bambang Oetomo S, Zegers SH. The long-term outcome of antenatal hydronephrosis up to 15 millimetres justifies a noninvasive postnatal follow-up. Acta Paediatr. 2008;97(6):708–13.
61. Coelho GM, Bouzada MC, Pereira AK, Figueiredo BF, Leite MR, Oliveira DS, et al. Outcome of isolated antenatal hydronephrosis: a prospective cohort study. Pediatr Nephrol. 2007;22(10):1727–34.
62. Coelho GM, Bouzada MC, Lemos GS, Pereira AK, Lima BP, Oliveira EA. Risk factors for urinary tract infection in children with prenatal renal pelvic dilatation. J Urol. 2008;179(1):284–9.
63. Wollenberg A, Neuhaus TJ, Willi UV, Wisser J. Outcome of fetal renal pelvic dilatation diagnosed during the third trimester. Ultrasound Obstet Gynecol. 2005;25(5):483–8.
64. Lee RS, Cendron M, Kinnamon DD, Nguyen HT. Antenatal hydronephrosis as a predictor of postnatal outcome: a meta-analysis. Pediatrics. 2006;118(2):586–93.
65. Woodward M, Frank D. Postnatal management of antenatal hydronephrosis. BJU Int. 2002;89(2):149–56.
66. Liang CC, Cheng PJ, Lin CJ, Chen HW, Chao AS, Chang SD. Outcome of prenatally diagnosed fetal hydronephrosis. J Reprod Med. 2002;47(1):27–32.
67. Chertin B, Pollack A, Koulikov D, Rabinowitz R, Hain D, Hadas-Halpren I, et al. Conservative treatment of ureteropelvic junction obstruction in children with antenatal diagnosis of hydronephrosis: lessons learned after 16 years of follow-up. Eur Urol. 2006;49(4):734–8.
68. Wang XM, Jia LQ, Wang Y, Wang N. Utilizing ultrasonography in the diagnosis of pediatric fibroepithelial polyps causing ureteropelvic junction obstruction. Pediatr Radiol. 2012;42(9):1107–11.
69. Cussen LJ. Dimensions of the normal ureter in infancy and childhood. Invest Urol. 1967;5(2): 164–78.
70. Report of working party to establish an international nomenclature for the large ureter. Birth Defects Orig Artic Ser. 1977;13(5):3–8.
71. Hodges SJ, Werle D, McLorie G, Atala A. Megaureter. ScientificWorldJournal. 2010;10:603–12.
72. Arena F, Baldari S, Proietto F, Centorrino A, Scalfari G, Romeo G. Conservative treatment in primary neonatal megaureter. Eur J Pediatr Surg. 1998;8(6):347–51.
73. Liu HY, Dhillon HK, Yeung CK, Diamond DA, Duffy PG, Ransley PG. Clinical outcome and management of prenatally diagnosed primary megaureters. J Urol. 1994;152(2 Pt 2):614–17.
74. Baskin LS, Zderic SA, Snyder HM, Duckett JW. Primary dilated megaureter: long-term followup. J Urol. 1994;152(2 Pt 2):618–21.
75. Shukla AR, Cooper J, Patel RP, Carr MC, Canning DA, Zderic SA, et al. Prenatally detected primary megaureter: a role for extended followup. J Urol. 2005;173(4):1353–6.
76. Shokeir AA, Nijman RJ. Ureterocele: an ongoing challenge in infancy and childhood. BJU Int. 2002;90(8):777–83.
77. Jelen Z. The value of ultrasonography as a screening procedure of the neonatal urinary tract: a survey of 1021 infants. Int Urol Nephrol. 1993;25(1): 3–10.
78. Besson R, Ngoc BT, Laboure S, Debeugny P. Incidence of urinary tract infection in neonates with antenatally diagnosed ureteroceles. Eur J Pediatr Surg. 2000;10(2):111–13.
79. Coplen DE, Duckett JW. The modern approach to ureteroceles. J Urol. 1995;153(1):166–71.
80. Decter RM. Renal duplication and fusion anomalies. Pediatr Clin North Am. 1997;44(5):1323–41.
81. Zamani R, Martinez R, Reddy MP. Duplicated collecting system: not following Weigert-Meyer rule as a result of renal stone obstructing the lower ureteropelvic junction. Clin Nucl Med. 2004;29(6): 386–7.
82. Jain P, Parelkar S, Shah H, Sanghavi B, Mishra P. Uncrossed complete ureteral duplication with dysplastic lower moiety: a violation of the Weigert-Meyer law. J Pediatr Urol. 2008;4(5):404–6.
83. Hoberman A, Charron M, Hickey RW, Baskin M, Kearney DH, Wald ER. Imaging studies after a first febrile urinary tract infection in young children. N Engl J Med. 2003;348(3):195–202.
84. Medical versus surgical treatment of primary vesicoureteral reflux: report of the International Reflux Study Committee. Pediatrics. 1981;67(3): 392–400.
85. Willi U, Treves S. Radionuclide voiding cystography. Urol Radiol. 1983;5(3):161–73, 175.
86. Darge K. Diagnosis of vesicoureteral reflux with ultrasonography. Pediatr Nephrol. 2002;17(1): 52–60.
87. Pieretti-Vanmarcke R, Pieretti A, Pieretti RV. Megacalycosis: a rare condition. Pediatr Nephrol. 2009;24(5):1077–9.
88. Gearhart JP, Ben-Chaim J, Jeffs RD, Sanders RC. Criteria for the prenatal diagnosis of classic bladder exstrophy. Obstet Gynecol. 1995;85(6):961–4.
89. Stec AA, Baradaran N, Gearhart JP. Congenital renal anomalies in patients with classic bladder exstrophy. Urology. 2012;79(1):207–9.
90. Noh PH, Cooper CS, Winkler AC, Zderic SA, Snyder 3rd HM, Canning DA. Prognostic factors for long-term renal function in boys with the prune-belly syndrome. J Urol. 1999;162(4):1399–401.
91. Reinberg Y, Manivel JC, Pettinato G, Gonzalez R. Development of renal failure in children with the prune belly syndrome. J Urol. 1991;145(5): 1017–19.
92. Krishnan A, de Souza A, Konijeti R, Baskin LS. The anatomy and embryology of posterior urethral valves. J Urol. 2006;175(4):1214–20.
93. DeFoor W, Clark C, Jackson E, Reddy P, Minevich E, Sheldon C. Risk factors for end stage renal disease in children with posterior urethral valves. J Urol. 2008;180(4 Suppl):1705–8; discussion 1708.
94. Dugoff L. Ultrasound diagnosis of structural abnormalities in the first trimester. Prenat Diagn. 2002; 22(4):316–20.

95. Cohen HL, Kravets F, Zucconi W, Ratani R, Shah S, Dougherty D. Congenital abnormalities of the genitourinary system. Semin Roentgenol. 2004;39(2):282–303.
96. Vanderheyden T, Kumar S, Fisk NM. Fetal renal impairment. Semin Neonatol. 2003;8(4):279–89.
97. Leibovitch L, Kuint J, Rosenfeld E, Schushan-Eisen I, Weissmann-Brenner A, Maayan-Metzger A. Short-term outcome among term singleton infants with intrapartum oligohydramnios. Acta Paediatr. 2012;101(7):727–30.
98. Chamberlain PF, Manning FA, Morrison I, Harman CR, Lange IR. Ultrasound evaluation of amniotic fluid volume. I. The relationship of marginal and decreased amniotic fluid volumes to perinatal outcome. Am J Obstet Gynecol. 1984;150(3):245–9.
99. Rutherford SE, Phelan JP, Smith CV, Jacobs N. The four-quadrant assessment of amniotic fluid volume: an adjunct to antepartum fetal heart rate testing. Obstet Gynecol. 1987;70(3 Pt 1):353–6.
100. Nabhan AF, Abdelmoula YA. Amniotic fluid index versus single deepest vertical pocket as a screening test for preventing adverse pregnancy outcome. Cochrane Database Syst Rev. 2008;3:CD006593.
101. Chauvin NA, Epelman M, Victoria T, Johnson AM. Complex genitourinary abnormalities on fetal MRI: imaging findings and approach to diagnosis. AJR Am J Roentgenol. 2012;199(2):W222–31.
102. Caire JT, Ramus RM, Magee KP, Fullington BK, Ewalt DH, Twickler DM. MRI of fetal genitourinary anomalies. AJR Am J Roentgenol. 2003;181(5):1381–5.
103. Alamo L, Laswad T, Schnyder P, Meuli R, Vial Y, Osterheld MC, et al. Fetal MRI as complement to US in the diagnosis and characterization of anomalies of the genito-urinary tract. Eur J Radiol. 2010;76(2):258–64.
104. Vates TS, Shull MJ, Underberg-Davis SJ, Fleisher MH. Complications of voiding cystourethrography in the evaluation of infants with prenatally detected hydronephrosis. J Urol. 1999;162(3 Pt 2):1221–3.
105. Estrada Jr CR, Passerotti CC, Graham DA, Peters CA, Bauer SB, Diamond DA, et al. Nomograms for predicting annual resolution rate of primary vesicoureteral reflux: results from 2,462 children. J Urol. 2009;182(4):1535–41.
106. Bokenkamp A, von Kries R, Nowak-Gottl U, Gobel U, Hoyer PF. Neonatal renal venous thrombosis in Germany between 1992 and 1994: epidemiology, treatment and outcome. Eur J Pediatr. 2000;159(1–2):44–8.
107. Lau KK, Stoffman JM, Williams S, McCusker P, Brandao L, Patel S, et al. Neonatal renal vein thrombosis: review of the English-language literature between 1992 and 2006. Pediatrics. 2007;120(5):e1278–84.
108. Winyard PJ, Bharucha T, De Bruyn R, Dillon MJ, Van't Hoff W, Trompeter RS, et al. Perinatal renal venous thrombosis: presenting renal length predicts outcome. Arch Dis Child Fetal Neonatal Ed. 2006;91(4):F273–8.

Renal Imaging: Hydronephrosis and Renal Obstruction

10

Liza M. Aguiar, Kathleen McCarten, and Anthony A. Caldamone

Introduction

Obstructive uropathy is defined as a structural or functional restriction of urinary flow, which if left uncorrected will lead to impairment of renal function. There are numerous radiologic signs that suggest and help define genitourinary obstruction. This chapter aims to describe the imaging modalities and findings used to characterize and diagnose genitourinary obstruction in specific pathologic entities.

Imaging Modalities

Ultrasound

Ultrasound is the mainstay of urinary tract evaluation in children. It is noninvasive, easily performed, relatively low in cost, and readily repeated as needed. A renal bladder ultrasound should be performed in routine fashion evaluating size, echo architecture, corticomedullary differentiation, collecting system appearance, and bladder characteristics. The highest-frequency transducer for the child's size should be used, and subsequent focused imaging of regions of concern with an even higher-frequency linear array transducer may demonstrate a specific abnormality in better detail. In the setting of obstruction, specific areas require more detailed evaluation. If there is hydronephrosis present, the calyceal configuration is important as to whether they are delicately configured or blunted and rounded. Attention should be paid to the ureteropelvic junction as to whether it can be followed into a dilated upper ureter or has an abrupt termination. In the setting of an extrarenal pelvis, there is dilation of the renal pelvis with no extension into the calyceal system.

Ideally, the urinary bladder should be well distended before starting the study. Having the child well hydrated will facilitate adequate visualization. In the case of infants and toddlers who are not potty trained, it is helpful to image the bladder first in the exam so that the chance is not lost to image optimal distention. If the bladder is not distended at the beginning of the exam, it can then be reevaluated later in the exam after good hydration has refilled it. Distal ureters are much better seen with a full bladder, and the ureterovesical junction can be most optimally scrutinized for an underlying abnormality. Normal nondilated ureters are not visualized, but it is essential to identify any dilated distal ureter to

L.M. Aguiar, MD • A.A. Caldamone, MD (✉)
Department of Urology,
The Warren Alpert Medical School of Brown University, Hasbro Children's Hospital,
2 Dudley Street, Suite 175,
Providence, RI 02905, USA
e-mail: lizaaguiar@gmail.com;
acaldamone@lifespan.org

K. McCarten, MD
Department of Pediatric Radiology,
The Warren Alpert Medical School of Brown University, Hasbro Children's Hospital,
593 Eddy Street, Providence, RI, USA
e-mail: kmccarten@lifespan.org

L.S. Palmer, J.S. Palmer (eds.), *Pediatric and Adolescent Urologic Imaging*,
DOI 10.1007/978-1-4614-8654-1_10, © Springer Science+Business Media New York 2014

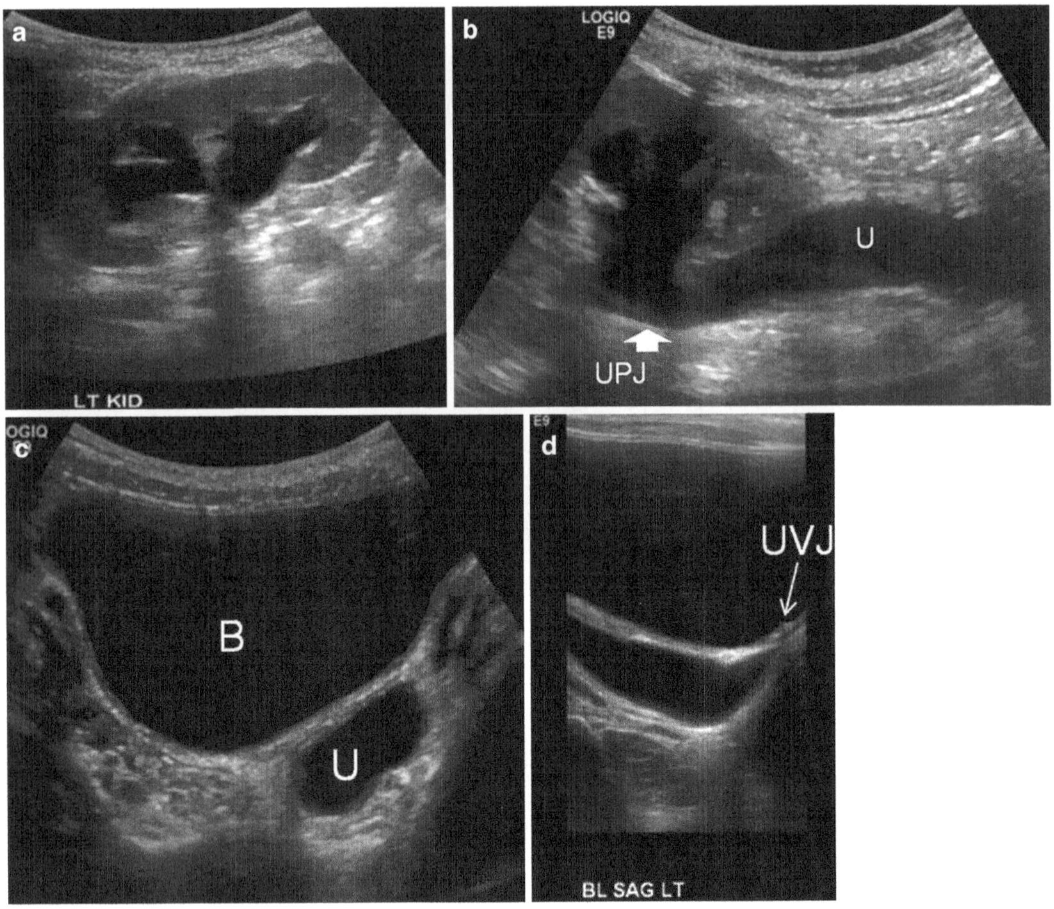

Fig. 10.1 Optimal evaluation by ultrasound requires identification of the calyceal system, renal pelvis (**a**), the ureteropelvic junction, and as much of the upper ureter as possible (**b**). Transverse images of the bladder with the relationship of the distal ureter (**c**) and the ureterovesical junction (**d**) are shown. *U* ureter, *B* bladder, *UVJ* ureterovesical junction, *UPJ* ureteropelvic junction

help to determine the level of obstruction. The region from the renal pelvis to the bladder is the most difficult to image due to overlying bowel gas. The optimal method to visualize this area is imaging in the coronal plane from the flank often using the iliopsoas muscle as a window to avoid the bowel gas (Fig. 10.1).

Prenatal Ultrasound

Perinatal urology has changed significantly since the advances of prenatal ultrasound. Prenatal ultrasound is a noninvasive tool that can determine gestational age, fetal number, viability, placental location, and some fetal anomalies. Although prenatal ultrasound screening may detect congenital abnormalities, the benefit of this knowledge in measured postnatal outcomes is unproven. The a priori deduction that early diagnosis can prevent future complications is controversial, as in many cases, early diagnosis may lead to unnecessary interventions. Additionally, it can lead to significant parental anxiety.

Although the use of prenatal ultrasound in diagnosing genitourinary abnormalities has not been proven to change postnatal outcome relative to renal function, more women are undergoing routine prenatal counseling and screening ultrasound [1].

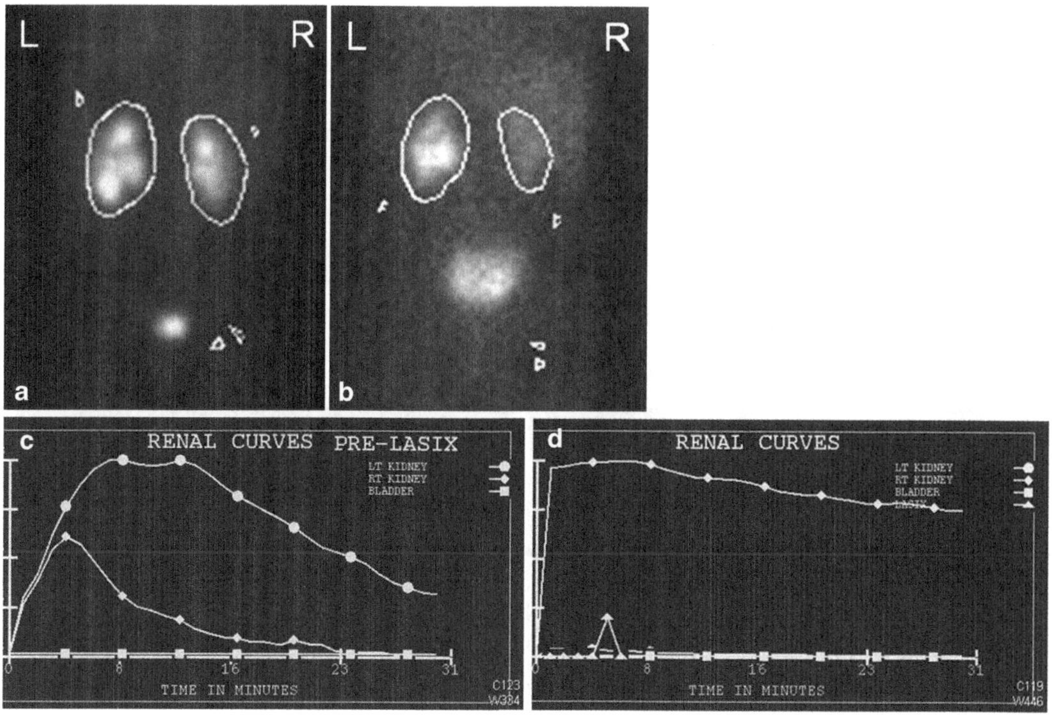

Fig. 10.2 This Tc-99m Mag3 diuretic renogram demonstrates delayed emptying of the left renal pelvis on the pre diuretic urogram (**a**) and flow curve (**b**) but with improved excretion post diuretic (**c** and **d**)

Diuretic Renogram

In addition to anatomic detail, it is important to determine the degree of obstruction and the relative function of the kidneys. The purpose of a diuretic renogram is to distinguish between non-obstructive hydronephrosis and mechanically obstructed hydronephrosis (Figs. 10.2 and 10.3). Historically, the intravenous urogram was the study of choice, often requiring delayed images with dilute contrast in an attempt to identify the level of abnormality. The IVU has been replaced primarily by nuclear medicine as the functional modality of choice. Technetium-99m is the ideal agent because of availability, short half-life, low-energy photopeak (140 keV), and ability to bind to agents such as MAG3 (mertiatide). Appropriate gamma camera and collimator are necessary. Because radioactive isotope is excreted into the bladder, care should be taken that the bladder is emptied by continuous bladder drainage or as soon as possible after the exam, especially in females where the ovaries are adjacent. This is aided by appropriate hydration. Because time is required to acquire images, swaddling of infants or sedation if the child cannot cooperate may be necessary.

Magnetic Resonance Urography

Magnetic resonance urography (MRU) is a more recently developed modality for evaluation of the genitourinary tract, particularly with obstruction. Magnetic resonance imaging was first introduced in 1986 [2]. MRU later came along and has been used to not only assess differential function and drainage as with a diuretic renogram but also to provide anatomic detail of the kidneys and collecting system. MRU also avoids exposure to radiation and iodine contrast. Volumetric differential renal function (DRF) is calculated by comparing the volume of enhancing renal parenchyma of each kidney prior to

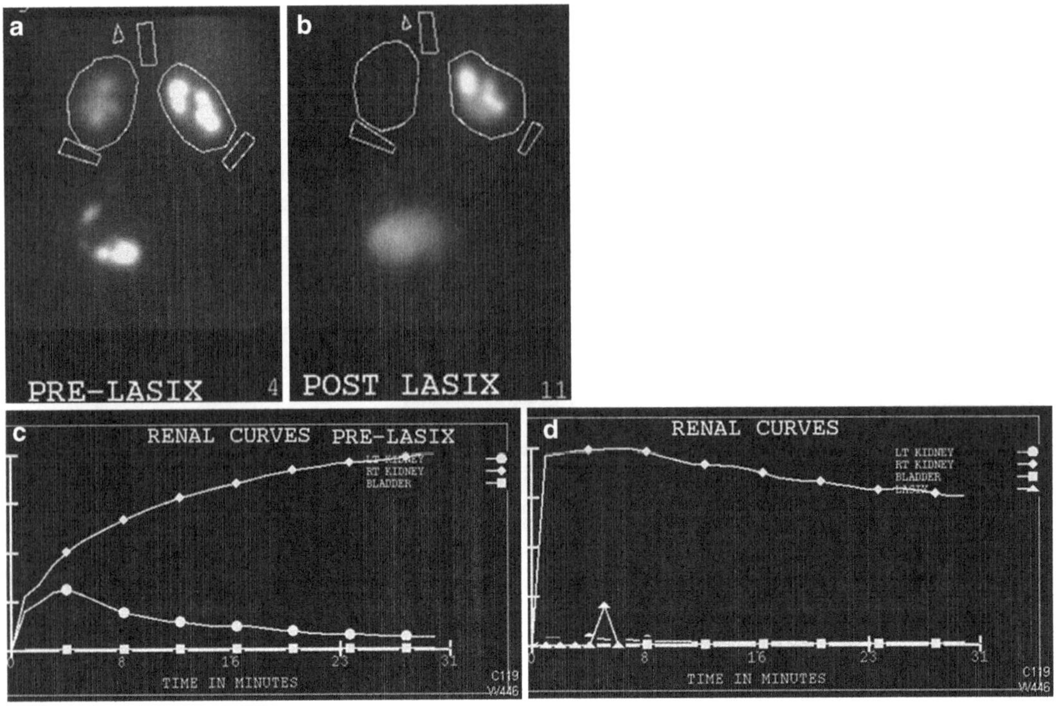

Fig. 10.3 If the degree of obstruction at the UPJ is significant, there will not be appreciable excretion of the isotope before or after diuretic administration. Here, the post diuretic images (**c**) and flow chart (**d**) show little change from pre diuretic (**a** and **b**)

contrast excretion in the kidneys. Gadolinium-diethylenetriaminepentaacetate dimeglumine (Gd-DTPA) is the contrast used. Sequential imaging allows for evaluation of contrast parenchymal concentration, excretion, and drainage [3]. The anatomic detail of MRU is considered its main advantage. With a variety of technical sequences, exquisite anatomic detail is possible. With administration of MR contrast agents, such as gadolinium, functional information is possible as well. With the addition of diuretics, dynamic information is obtained as with renal scintigraphy but with the additional benefit of superior contrast, spatial, and temporal resolution. The major disadvantages are cost, access, and time required for imaging acquisition, necessitating sedation in younger or certain disabled patients.

Computed Tomography

Computed tomography is a modality that provides excellent anatomic detail. With intravenous contrast, it also performs the additional role of a functional modality. Non-contrast CT has become the modality of choice for the detection of calculi in adults. Contrast CT can demonstrate a delayed nephrogram, as was seen with intravenous urography, or, with delayed images, can illustrate the detail of the etiology of the obstruction such as mass, stricture, or congenital abnormality. Radiation exposure to children from CT scans can be quite high, and evaluation by alternative imaging procedures when possible is the recommended approach to evaluation.

Fluoroscopy/Voiding Cystourethrogram

The voiding cystourethrogram remains the best imaging modality to diagnose bladder outlet obstruction because it defines the anatomy of the bladder, bladder neck, and urethra. Imaging of the urethra is best obtained during the voiding phase of the VCUG.

It can, however, result in significant radiation exposure. Advances in equipment development now allow varying degrees of pulsed fluoroscopy in which the X-ray beam is functioning only intermittently rather than continuously. In addition, "fluoro store" is a function where the image on the monitor screen can be stored without requiring additional spot film exposures.

Use of Imaging Modalities in Specific Pathologic Entities

Prenatal Hydronephrosis

Prenatal hydronephrosis, or dilation of renal collecting system, is the most common abnormality detected on prenatal ultrasound. It is estimated that antenatal hydronephrosis is detected in 1–5 % of all pregnancies [4]. There are many etiologies of prenatal hydronephrosis, including transient and non-transient hydronephrosis, upper tract and lower tract obstruction, and vesicoureteral reflux (VUR) (Table 10.1).

The Society for Fetal Urology (SFU) categorizes antenatal hydronephrosis in the second and third trimester based on the pelvic anterior-posterior diameter (APD), which is obtained in the axial plane (Table 10.2). Factors that influence APD are maternal hydration, gestational age, and degree of bladder distension [5–8]. The degree of hydronephrosis has been shown to correlate with an increasing risk of certain postnatal pathology, such as ureteropelvic junction obstruction and posterior urethral valves (Table 10.3).

Table 10.1 The etiology of ANH

Etiology	Incidence (%)
Transient hydronephrosis	41–88
UPJ obstruction	10–30
VUR	10–20
UVJ obstruction/megaureters	5–10
Multicystic dysplastic kidney	4–6
PUV/urethral atresia	1–2
Ureterocele/ectopic ureter/duplex system	5–7
Others: prune belly syndrome, cystic kidney disease, congenital ureteric strictures, and megalourethra	Uncommon

Modified from Nguyen et al. [4]

Table 10.2 Definition of ANH by APD

Degree of ANH	Second trimester (mm)	Third trimester (mm)
Mild	4 to <7	4 to <9
Moderate	7 to ≤10	9 to ≤15
Severe	>10	>15

Modified from Nguyen et al. [4]

Table 10.3 Risk of specific postnatal pathologic conditions by the degree of ANH

	% ANH [95 % CI]		
	Mild	Moderate	Severe
UPJ	4.9 [2.0–11.9]	17.0 [7.6–33.9]	54.3 [21.7–83.6]
VUR	4.4 [1.5–12.1]	14.0 [7.1–25.9]	8.5 [4.7–15.0]
PUV	0.2[0.0–1.4]	0.9[0.2–2.9]	5.3[1.2–21.0]
Ureteral obstruction	1.2 [0.2–8.0]	9.8 [6.3–14.9]	5.3 [1.4–18.2]
Other	1.2 [0.3–4.0]	3.4 [0.5–19.4]	14.9 [3.6–44.9]

Other: prune belly syndrome, VATER syndrome, solitary kidney, renal mass, and unclassified
Modified from Nguyen et al. [4]

In assessing the genitourinary system of a fetus on prenatal ultrasound, it is important to not only identify the presence of hydronephrosis but also to further characterize the kidneys, ureters, bladder, and urethra (Fig. 10.4). In examining the kidney, one should note their size, single or duplex collecting system, echogenicity of the renal parenchyma, presence of hydronephrosis, and presence of cystic structures. All of this information can suggest specific diagnoses.

The echogenicity of a fetal kidney should be less than that of the liver and spleen. The medullary pyramids should be lucent. Increased echogenicity can suggest dysplasia or high-grade obstruction and is commonly seen in multicystic dysplastic kidney (MCDK) and in autosomal recessive polycystic kidney disease (ARPKD). Hydronephrosis can be due to transient or non-transient physiologic hydronephrosis, obstruction, or vesicoureteral reflux (VUR). Cystic structures in the renal parenchyma may be

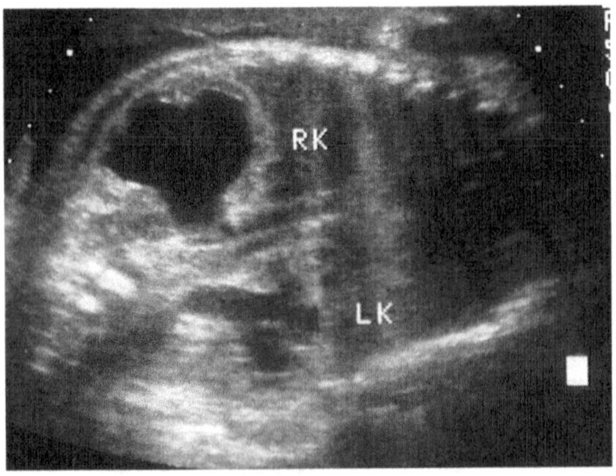

Fig. 10.4 A coronal image of a fetus demonstrates significant hydronephrosis of the right with cortical thinning (*RK*) and moderate hydronephrosis on the left with more substantial cortex (*LK*)

confused for hydronephrosis. Cysts, however, do not communicate with one another and can be a sign of MCDK or autosomal dominant polycystic kidney disease (ADPKD).

Normal ureters are not seen on prenatal ultrasound. The presence of a dilated structure between the kidneys and the bladder or the presence of cystic structures posterior to the bladder on transverse imaging suggests dilated ureters. Dilated ureters can be seen with VUR, various types of megaureters, duplication anomalies including ureterocele, and bladder outlet obstruction.

It is also important to evaluate the bladder on prenatal ultrasound. Increase in size or the presence of a thick bladder wall can indicate bladder outlet obstruction. In the case of posterior urethral valves, the posterior urethra as well as the bladder is distended giving a "keyhole" configuration.

Postnatally, the voiding cystourethrogram is the best imaging modality to diagnose bladder outlet obstruction because it defines the anatomy of the bladder, bladder neck, and urethra during its voiding phase. In bladder outlet obstruction, the bladder wall is usually thickened, and a VCUG can demonstrate a trabeculated appearance to the bladder wall or bladder diverticula. Fluoroscopy can also help determine whether hydroureteronephrosis is secondary to obstruction or due to vesicoureteral reflux. A dilated, thick-walled bladder or severely enlarged bladder is highly suggestive of bladder outlet obstruction, including posterior urethral valves, urethral atresia, congenital urethral stricture, or urethral polyp. It can also be the result of extrinsic compression of the bladder outlet as with hindgut duplication anomalies or pelvic masses. The presence of a cystic structure within the bladder can be a sign of a ureterocele, which is most commonly associated with duplication and can cause obstructive uropathy and hydronephrosis.

Although the use of prenatal ultrasound in diagnosing genitourinary abnormalities has not been proven to change postnatal renal function, prenatal ultrasound imaging can be viewed as a way of preparing for the postnatal diagnosis and management. The 2010 Society for Fetal Urology guidelines recommend a follow-up postnatal ultrasound within the first week of life or earlier in cases of bilateral hydronephrosis, hydronephrosis in a solitary kidney, or suspected bladder outlet obstruction [4].

Upper Tract Obstruction: Ureteropelvic Junction and Obstructed Megaureter

Ureteropelvic junction obstruction is the most common cause of hydronephrosis. These patients are commonly diagnosed with prenatal hydronephrosis. Although increasing size of the AP diameter correlates with the risk of obstruction, the presence of hydronephrosis does not definitively diagnose obstruction. However, the presence of hydronephrosis without ureteral dilation can be suggestive of ureteropelvic junction obstruction (Fig. 10.5).

Megaureter is a term to describe a dilated ureter measuring >7 mm regardless of the etiology. The dilation does not necessarily mean there is an obstruction, as megaureters are classically categorized as obstructive, refluxing, obstructive and refluxing, and nonobstructive and nonrefluxing. Primary obstructed megaureters are thought to be caused by an aperistaltic distal segment of the ureter that prevents urine from flowing at a normal rate. Secondary obstructed megaureters can

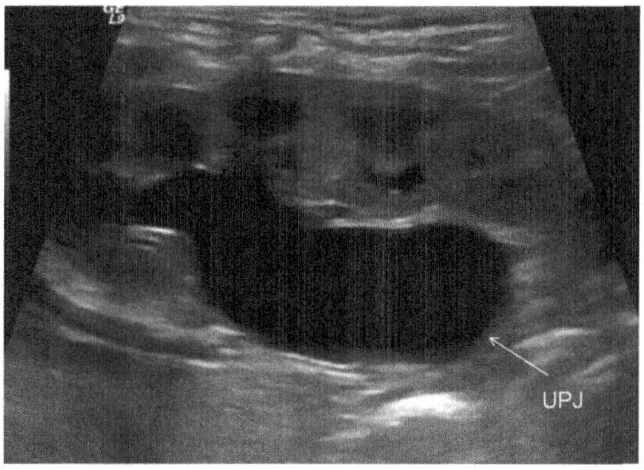

Fig. 10.5 With upper tract dilation, all attempts should be made to identify whether there is an abrupt termination of the dilation at the ureteropelvic junction, as in this case (*arrow*), or whether there is extension into a dilated ureter. *UPJ* ureteropelvic junction

be due to elevated intravesical pressures in the setting of bladder outlet obstruction or bladder dysfunction.

Ultrasound is a noninvasive tool to image the kidneys and the bladder, and it is usually the initial study in any child with a suspected genitourinary abnormality. Although ultrasound may not image normal-sized ureters well, it can easily identify dilated ureters, especially posterior to a fluid-filled bladder. It is commonly the primary means of diagnosing megaureter.

Ultrasound has not been considered a dependable way to assess for obstruction because it does not evaluate function or drainage of the kidney, as other modalities such as diuretic urography. In order to improve the predictive value of ultrasound in the diagnosis of obstruction, Cost et al. compared the renal parenchymal and pelvicaliceal area measurements to diuretic renography and found that a ratio of less than 1.6 correlates with obstruction [9].

Resistive index (RI), defined as the highest systolic velocity minus the lowest diastolic velocity divided by the peak systolic velocity, is also an objective measurement on ultrasound that may be indicative of obstruction. An RI of $\geq$0.75 suggests obstruction [10, 11]. An advantage to using RI in diagnosing obstruction is its noninvasive nature. However, resistive indices can be elevated in the setting of dehydration, medical renal disease, and decreased absolute blood flow, as in the case of young children or in chronic high-grade obstruction.

The Whitaker test is a pressure-flow study involving percutaneous insertion of a catheter into the renal pelvis with infusion of fluid at 10 mL/s into the kidney. The high flow rate is easily tolerated in a nonobstructed system. In obstructed systems, however, the pressure will rise above 12 cm H_2O. This test, however, is invasive and not widely used except in equivocal situations [12, 13].

Intravenous urography was once commonly used to diagnose UPJ obstruction with retained contrast in the collecting system on delayed imaging indicating obstruction. This, however, was replaced by radionuclide diuretic renography, which can assess differential renal function and presence of obstruction by evaluating the ability of the pelvis and ureter to drain in response to a diuresis. The results of diuretic renograms are influenced by multiple patient factors, including hydration status, renal function and its ability to respond to the diuretic, and state of bladder fullness. In addition, there is variability in the procedure between institutions, making it difficult to compare results. Effort has been made to standardize the technique. The Society for Fetal Urology and the Pediatric Nuclear Medicine Council described the "well-tempered" diuretic renogram, which included patient prehydration, placement of a bladder catheter for decompression, and the use of weight-based dose of technetium-99m mercaptoacetyltriglycine (MAG3) and furosemide [14]. Furosemide is administered after the renogram phase (20–30 min) or when the entire collecting system is full. Static images at 5-min intervals are then taken. The time-activity curve is plotted out and pelvic T1/2 clearance time is calculated. A washout T1/2 of <10 min suggests a nonobstructed renal unit, T1/2 10–20 min is indeterminate, and >20 min suggests the system is obstructed.

Ureteral strictures and fetal folds, commonly associated with hydronephrosis, can be seen on MRU, eliminating the need for a retrograde pyelogram performed in the operating room. Also, other ureteral abnormalities such as ecto-

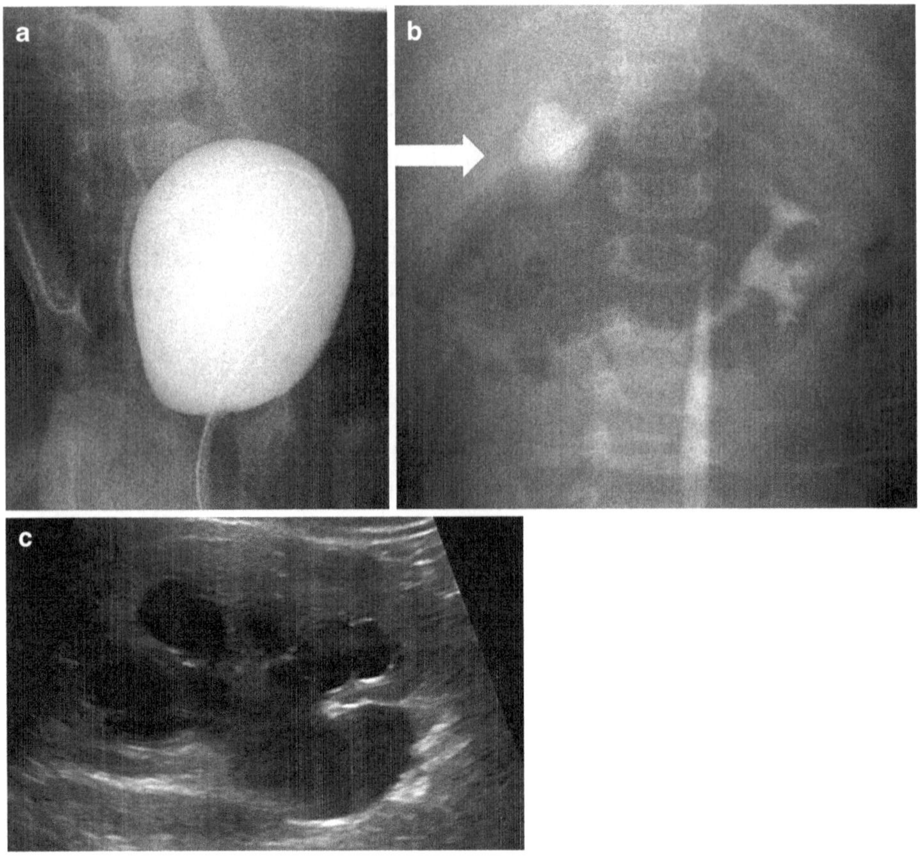

Fig. 10.6 VCUG images demonstrating reflux into bilateral ureters (**a**) with contrast in a hydronephrotic renal pelvis on the right (**b**, *arrow*). Image (**c**) demonstrating a dilated renal pelvis, suspicious for a UPJ obstruction

pia and duplication can be very well characterized on MRU, especially on delayed contrast imaging or T2-weighted imaging. Megaureter is easily diagnosed, as fluid-filled structures are well defined on T2-weighted imaging. T1-weighted imaging can define more subtle findings such as small diverticula and small ureteroceles. Renal transit time (RTT) is defined as the time of contrast passage from the cortex into the ureter below the renal pelvis. A normal RTT is ≤245 s, equivocal is 245–490 s, and obstructive is >490 s [15]. Disadvantages of MRU are the need for sedation in children of preschool age and younger; possible, although rare, adverse reaction to gadolinium; inability to perform with metallic foreign bodies/implants; and its significant cost.

Although the voiding cystourethrogram (VCUG) is viewed as the primary imaging modality for diagnosing vesicoureteral reflux and characterizing the anatomy of the urethra, certain findings on a VCUG can suggest presence of a ureteropelvic junction obstruction. There are often normal caliber ureter and dilution of contrast in an obstructed hydronephrotic renal pelvis or retained contrast in the renal pelvis on the postvoid images (Fig. 10.6).

Duplicated Collecting Systems

In the absence of hydronephrosis, a duplicated collecting system may be difficult to diagnose. A total renal length greater than the opposite kidney or longer than would be expected by age or body size may give a clue. Renal tissue separating perisinus fat or minimal amounts of collecting system fluid may be another. If, however,

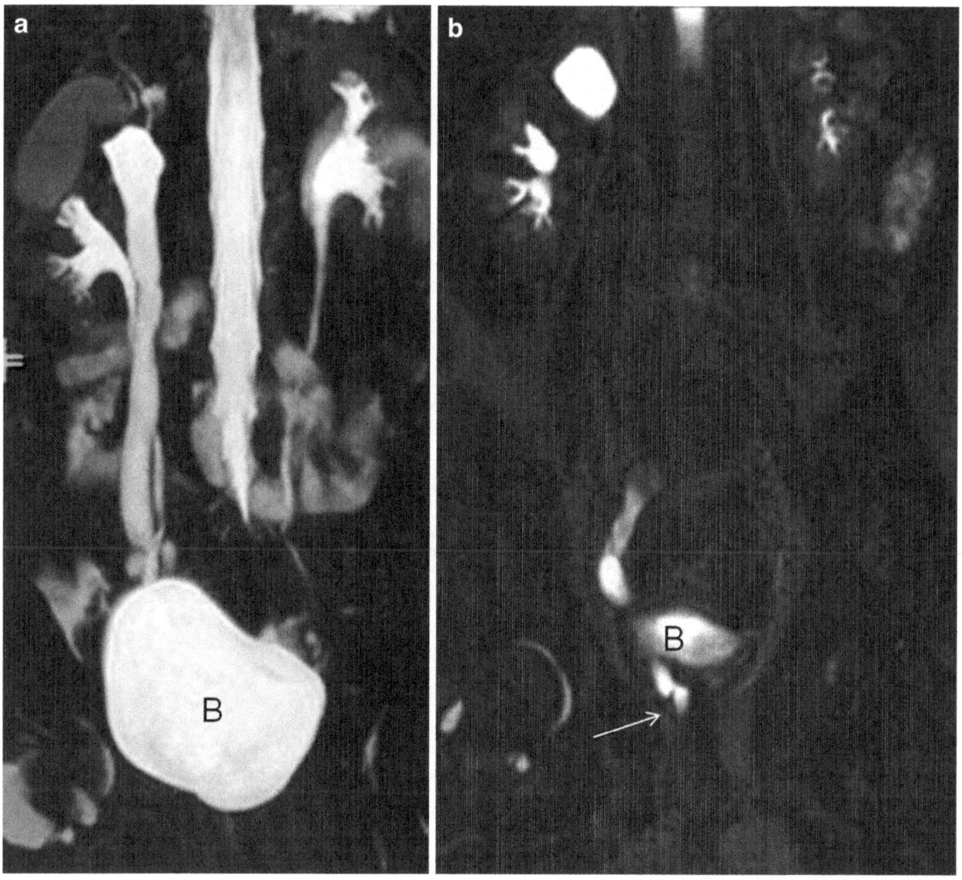

Fig. 10.7 When a dilated upper pole system does not terminate in a ureterocele within the bladder, MRU is an excellent modality for identifying its course and termination. In this example, the duplicated system on the right (**a**) shows a normal lower pole collecting system and dilated upper pole system. With a distended bladder (*B*), the termination is not visualized. In figure (**b**), which is postvoid, the termination (*arrow*) can be seen extending below the level of the bladder

there is any collecting system dilatation, a more detailed evaluation is imperative.

If there is an abnormality, the upper pole is likely dilated secondary to obstruction. The dilated ureter should be followed, and if it cannot be visualized in its entirety, its lower extent can be evaluated relative to the bladder, i.e., whether there is a ureterocele present and where its insertion is located. If there are isolated upper pole hydronephrosis and a normal bladder, the ureter is most likely inserting into an ectopic location. Therefore, the dilated ureter should be followed as distally as possible to attempt to identify its ectopic insertion. Transperineal ultrasound images may localize the ectopic termination of the ureter as being into the urethra or into the vagina.

MRU can be used to assess the anatomy of the ureters in the setting of a duplicated system. It is especially useful in assessing the distal ureteric anatomy and insertion into the bladder or ectopic location (Fig. 10.7) [16].

Ureterocele

A ureterocele is a cystic dilation of the distal ureter. With improving prenatal ultrasound technique and imaging, ureteroceles can be detected prenatally. While most ureteroceles

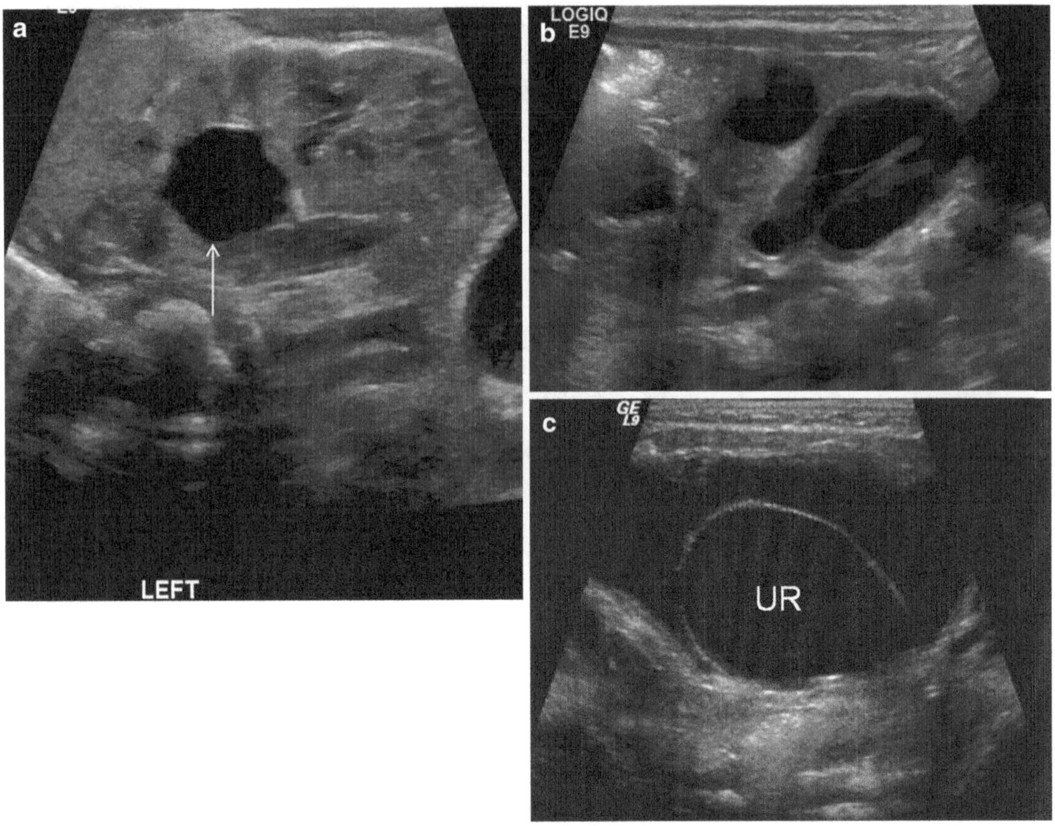

Fig. 10.8 Renal ultrasound (**a**) demonstrates dilation of the upper pole collecting system (*arrow*) and a normal lower pole system. A dilated tortuous ureter is often evident on coronal image obtained from the flank (**b**), and the ureterocele (*UR*) is seen on the transverse image of the bladder (**c**)

are associated with the upper pole of a duplicated system, some are associated with a single system ureter (Fig. 10.8).

Ultrasound is usually the most common imaging modality used to characterize ureteroceles, as the intravesical wall of the ureterocele can usually be seen. Although most ureteroceles are well visualized with proper ultrasound imaging, it can sometimes be difficult to assess a ureterocele in the setting of an overdistended bladder, as the ureterocele may become effaced, or in the setting of an empty bladder, where the wall of the ureterocele can be confused with the wall of the bladder.

Voiding cystourethrography is often performed in the setting of a duplicated system to rule out vesicoureteral reflux. A ureterocele can be detected during the early filling phases of a VCUG as a well-circumscribed, smooth filling defect in the bladder.

Bladder Outlet Obstruction

Bladder outlet obstruction can be a devastating urologic diagnosis in a pediatric patient, as it often affects the prenatal development of the entire urinary tract proximal to the level of obstruction. Additionally, it can also secondarily affect the development of the pulmonary system. It is often due to a congenital abnormality of the urethra. Posterior urethral valves (PUV) are the most common congenital urethral abnormality. However, there are other anomalies including anterior urethral valves, congenital urethral strictures, and urethral polyps (Fig. 10.9). Extrinsic

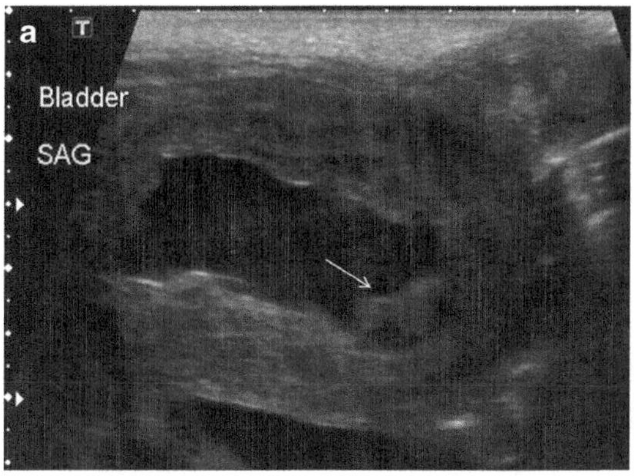

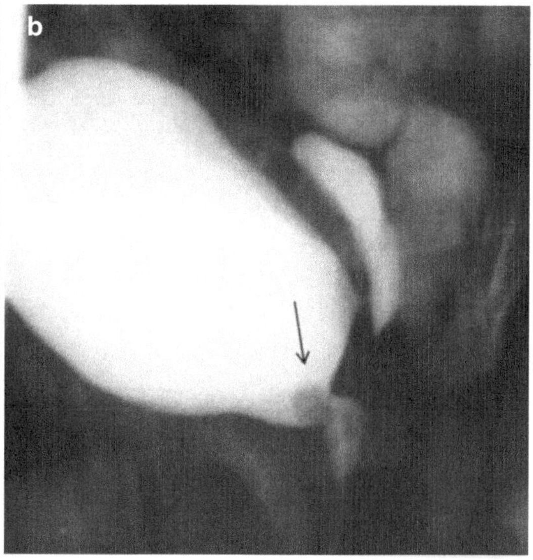

Fig. 10.9 Urethral polyps are an example of bladder outlet obstruction. Ultrasound image demonstrates a thick-walled bladder and a density at the bladder base (**a**, *arrow*=polyp). VCUG shows the polyp in the bladder extending up from the urethra (**b**). Vesicoureteral reflux also seen

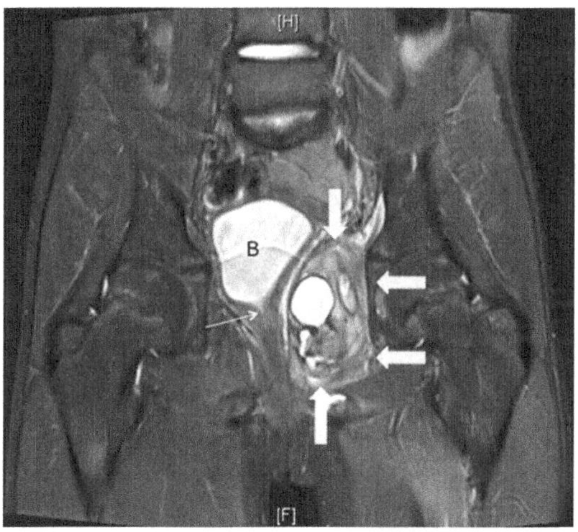

Fig. 10.10 Because of the superb tissue contrast of MRI, relationships of structures are extremely well defined. In this young boy with a pelvic Ewing's sarcoma (*broad arrows*), the compression of the bladder (*B*) and bladder neck (*narrow arrows*) is well defined

compression of the bladder neck and proximal urethral can also lead to bladder outlet obstruction. This can occur with hindgut duplication anomalies, pelvis masses (Fig. 10.10), or a large bladder diverticulum (Fig. 10.11).

Now that prenatal screening ultrasound is more commonly done, bladder outlet obstruction is often diagnosed on prenatal ultrasound imaging. Signs that suggest bladder outlet obstruction are bilateral hydroureteronephrosis, a distended bladder and posterior urethra, oligohydramnios, and increased renal echogenicity. Kaefer et al. demonstrated that 87.5 % of PUV patients demonstrated increased renal echogenicity on prenatal ultrasound at a mean gestational age of 26 weeks. Patients who did not have an obstructive process did not show increased renal echogenicity [17].

In posterior urethral valves, the bladder neck is often noted to be elevated, there is a dilated posterior urethra, and the valve leaflets can be identified (Fig. 10.12). Unilateral or bilateral vesicoureteral reflux can be present in patients with bladder outlet obstruction [18, 19].

Nephrolithiasis and Acute Urinary Obstruction

There is an increasing incidence of kidney stones in children in the United States [20, 21]. The

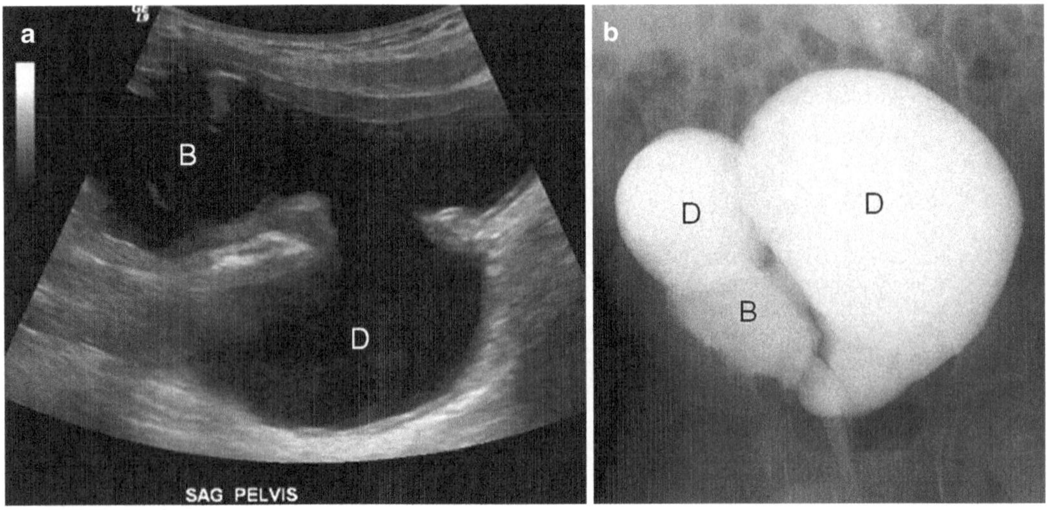

Fig. 10.11 Ultrasound demonstrating a bladder and a large diverticulum (**a**, *D* diverticulum, *B* bladder). VCUG in (**b**) demonstrating two large diverticula with the left obstructing of the bladder neck (*D* diverticulum, *B* bladder)

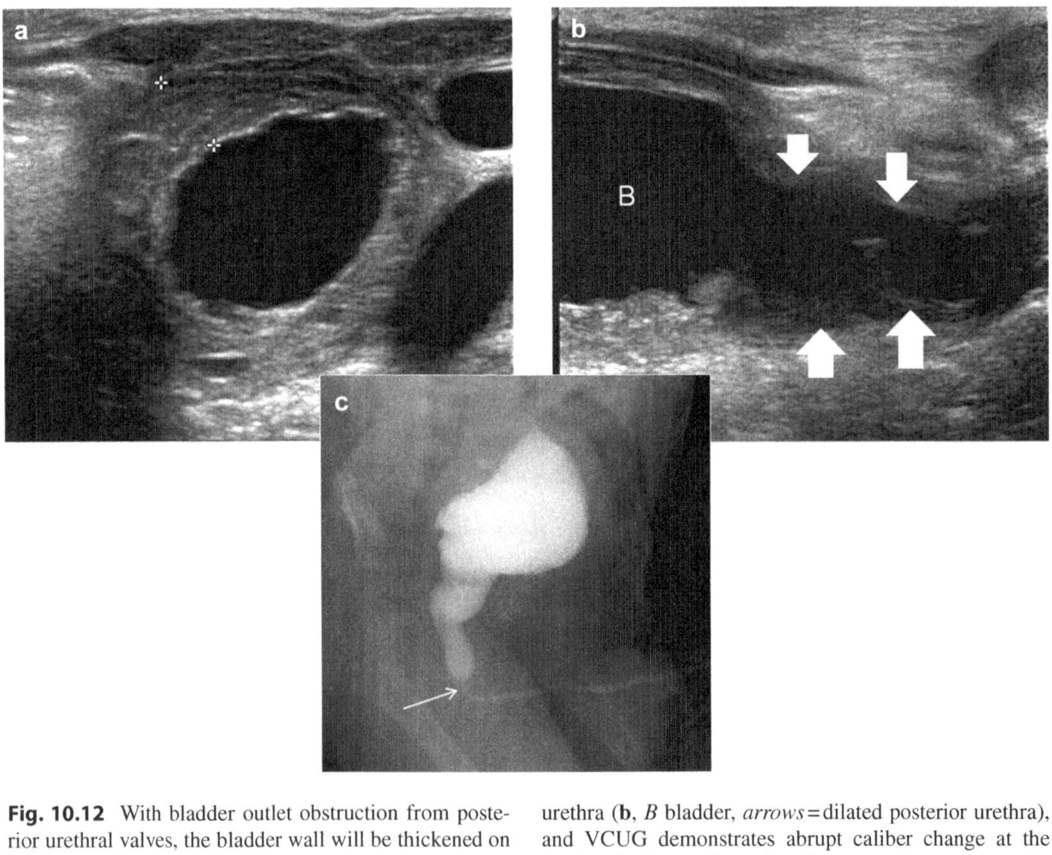

Fig. 10.12 With bladder outlet obstruction from posterior urethral valves, the bladder wall will be thickened on ultrasound (**a**). The bladder develops a keyhole configuration in the sagittal plane secondary to a dilated posterior urethra (**b**, *B* bladder, *arrows* = dilated posterior urethra), and VCUG demonstrates abrupt caliber change at the level of the valves in the posterior urethra (**c**, *arrow* = valves)

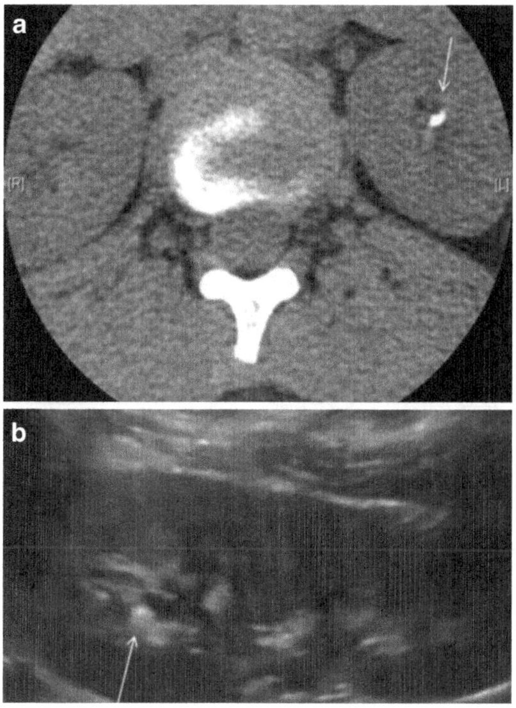

Fig. 10.13 Any opaque calculus, even quite small, is evident on CT (*arrow* in **a**), whereas the same calculus may not as easily be seen on ultrasound when it is too small to produce shadowing and is adjacent to perisinus fat (*arrow* in **b**)

non-contrast computed tomography (NCCT) scan is the gold standard for diagnosis of kidney stones in the adult population. The exposure to radiation, however, is a significant concern in the pediatric population. There is evidence that shows not only an increased risk of radiation-induced cancer for pediatric patients with repeated radiation exposure and increased total lifetime radiation exposure, but there is also evidence demonstrating that the younger the age of initial exposure, the greater the lifetime risk of radiation-induced cancer.

The benefit of CT is that even small calcified calculi are easily identifiable within the kidney as well as along the course of the ureter. Within the pelvis, there can be confusion at times with phleboliths; this, however, is not a significant problem in the pediatric age group. Perirenal or periureteric edema may be seen with acute high-grade obstruction. Small calculi within the kidney that may be easily apparent by CT may be difficult to identify by ultrasound (Fig. 10.13). They may not be dense enough to shadow and, if adjacent to peripelvic fat, may be of similar density. Dense segments of interlobar arteries can be confusing as they may have similar density. One feature that can at times be helpful is to use color Doppler. A stone with this method produces a "twinkle" artifact. Larger more dense calculi will produce posterior shadowing and are more easily identified.

Ureteral calculi which are easily seen on CT are the most difficult to localize on ultrasound. Adequate hydration and a distended urinary bladder may make it possible to visualize especially calculi at or just above the ureterovesical junction (Fig. 10.14). Imaging from a flank approach may identify a ureteral calculus in the mid to upper ureter.

Symptoms of renal colic are due to acute obstruction of the upper urinary tract, and the presence of hydronephrosis is easily identified using ultrasound imaging. However, the ureters are often not well seen, and, therefore, ultrasound may be nondiagnostic in up to 40 % of pediatric stone patients [22]. Most childhood calculi in North America are calcium oxalate and, therefore, are radio-opaque [23]. Consequently X-ray imaging, or KUB, can be used to assess the location and size of the stone. The combination of ultrasound and KUB is often used as opposed to NCCT in order to prevent increased radiation exposure. Johnson et al. evaluated pediatric patients who underwent NCCT imaging in addition to ultrasound and KUB for the diagnosis of nephrolithiasis and found that KUB and ultrasound are sufficient for diagnosis in 90 % of patients who required surgical treatment for stones [24].

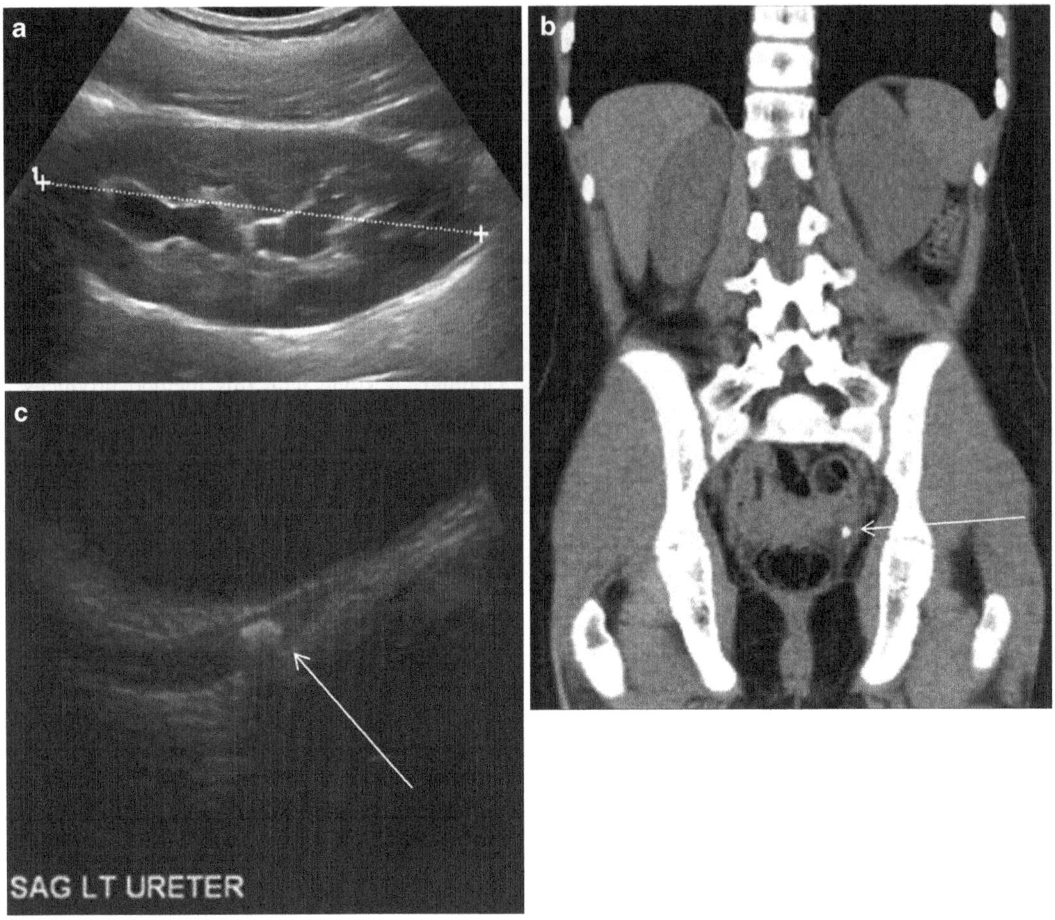

Fig. 10.14 Ultrasound should be the first examination performed in children with a suspected calculus to demonstrate the presence of hydronephrosis (**a**) and shadowing of the left distal ureteral calculus (**b**, *arrow*=calculus) visualized through a full bladder (*B*). Non-contrast CT is the exam of choice in adults when evaluating for urinary calculi but should be utilized in children when ultrasound has failed. An example is shown here (**c**) in a child with a distal left ureteral calculus (*arrow*)

References

1. Mallik M, Watson AR. Antenatally detected urinary tract abnormalities: more detection but less action. Pediatr Nephrol. 2008;23:897.
2. Dietrich RB, Kangarloo H. Kidneys in infants and children: evaluation with MR. Radiology. 1986;159:215–21.
3. Cerwinka WH, Kirsch AJ. Magnetic resonance urography in pediatric urology. Curr Opin Urol. 2010;20:323–9.
4. Nguyen HT, Herndon CD, Cooper C, Gatti J, Kirsch A, Kokorowski P, Lee R, Peres-Brayfield M, Metcalf P, Yerkes E, Cendron M, Campbell JB. The Society for Fetal Urology consensus statement on the evaluation and management of antenatal hydronephrosis. J Pediatr Urol. 2010;6(3):212–31.
5. Anderson N, Clautice-Engle T, Allan R, Abbott G, Wells JE. Detection of obstructive uropathy in the fetus: predictive value of sonographic measurements of renal pelvic diameter at various ages. AJR Am J Roentgenol. 1995;164:719.
6. Babcook CJ, Silvera M, Drake C, Levine D. Effect of maternal hydration on mild fetal pyelectasis. J Ultrasound Med. 1998;17:539.
7. Robinson JN, Tice K, Kolm P, Abuhamad AZ. Effect of maternal hydration on fetal renal pyelectasis. Obstet Gynecol. 1998;92:137.
8. Leung VY, Chu WC, Metreweli C. Hydronephrosis index: a better physiological reference in antenatal ultrasound for assessment of fetal hydronephrosis. J Pediatr. 2009;154:116.
9. Cost GA, Merguerian PA, Cheerasarn SP, Shortliffe LM. Sonographic renal parenchymal and pelvicaliceal areas: new quantitative parameters for renal sonographic follow-up. J Urol. 1996;156: 725–9.

10. Gilbert R, Garra B, Gibbons MD. Renal duplex Doppler ultrasound: an adjunct in the evaluation of hydronephrosis in the child. J Urol. 1993;150: 1192–4.
11. Platt IF, Rubin JM, Ellis HM, DiPietro MA. Duplex Doppler US of the kidney: differentiation of obstructive from nonobstructive dilatation. Radiology. 1989;1:515–17.
12. Whitaker RH. Methods of assessing obstruction in dilated ureters. Br J Urol. 1973;45:15–22.
13. Whitaker RH. Equivocal pelvic-ureteric obstruction. Br J Urol. 1976;47:771–9.
14. Conway JJ, Maizels M. The "well tempered" diuretic renogram: a standard method to examine the asymptomatic neonate with hydronephrosis or hydroureteronephrosis. J Nucl Med. 1992;33:2047–51.
15. Jones RA, Perez-Brayfield MR, Kirsch AJ, Grattan-Smith JD. Renal transit time with MR urography in children. Radiology. 2004;233:41–50.
16. Avni FE, Nicaise N, Hall M. The role of MR imaging for the assessment of complicated duplex kidneys in children: preliminary report. Pediatr Radiol. 2001;31: 215–23.
17. Kaefer M, Peters CA, Retik AB, Benacerraf BR. Increased renal echogenicity: a sonographic sign for differentiating between obstruction and nonobstructive etiologies of in utero bladder distension. J Urol. 1997;158:1026–9.
18. Churchill BM, McLorie GA, Khoury AE, et al. Emergency treatment and long-term follow-up of posterior urethral valves. Urol Clin North Am. 1990;17: 343.
19. Hoover DL, Duckett JW. Posterior urethral valves, unilateral reflux, and renal dysplasia: a syndrome. J Urol. 1982;128:994.
20. Stapleton FB. Childhood stones. Endocrinol Metab Clin North Am. 2002;31:1001.
21. Sas DJ, Hulsey TC, Shatat IF, Orak JK. Increasing incidence of kidney stones in children evaluated in the emergency department. J Pediatr. 2010;157:132.
22. Palmer JS, Donaher ER, O'Riordan M, Dell KM. Diagnosis of pediatric urolithiasis: role of ultrasound and computerized tomography. J Urol. 2005;174: 1413–16.
23. Stapleton FB. Clinical approach to children with urolithiasis. Semin Nephrol. 1996;16:289.
24. Johnson EK, Faerber GJ, Roberts WW, Wolf JS, Park JM, Bloom DA, Wan J. Are stone protocol computed tomography scans mandatory for children with suspected urinary calculi. Pediatr Urol. 2011;78:662.

Renal Imaging: Cystic and Solid Lesions

11

Derek Prabharasuth, Lesli M. LeCompte, and Lori Landau Dyer

Pediatric Tumors of the Kidney

Renal tumors are uncommon in children. Advances in genetic mapping, surgical staging, and chemotherapy have increased cure rates of malignant lesions significantly over the past 20 years. Imaging is vital in these cases for making the initial diagnosis or differential diagnosis as well as for proper staging which will drive the surgical management as well as for follow-up after chemotherapy and/or radiation therapy.

Wilms' Tumor

Etiology and Presentation

Wilms' tumor, also known as nephroblastoma, is the second most common intra-abdominal cancer in childhood [1] and accounts for over 95 % of all pediatric renal tumors [2]. There is an annual incidence of 500 cases in the United States with roughly 75 % of cases occurring in children less than 5 years of age [1]. The peak incidence occurs in years 2 and 3 of life [1]. The most common presentation is that of an incidental palpable abdominal mass [3]. Approximately 5 % of patients present with bilateral synchronous disease [1]. Although Wilms' tumor is rarely invasive, it commonly adheres to the surrounding organs [1]. Local extension into the vena cava and atrium can occur in approximately 5 % [1]. Metastases occur in approximately 12 % of patients at time of diagnosis with lungs being the most common site [1].

Survival for all stages of Wilms' tumor exceeds 90 % owing largely to the multi-cooperative studies of the National Wilms' Tumor Study (NWTS) and the International Society of Paediatric Oncology (SIOP). The main prognostic variables include histopathologic tumor classification (favorable vs. unfavorable) and tumor stage [1].

Two genes have been identified whose presence predisposes to Wilms' tumor development: FWT1 at 17q12–q21 and FWT2 at 19q13 [3]. Patients with familial syndromes and more likely to present with bilateral tumors and present at a younger age. They are also at a higher risk for renal insufficiency [3]. *WT1* is necessary for normal renal and gonadal growth, but heterozygous deletions in *WT1* are linked to WAGR (Wilms' tumor, Aniridia, Genital anomalies, mental Retardation) and Denys-Drash syndrome (male pseudo-hermaphroditism, renal mesangial sclerosis, and nephroblastoma) [3]. Mutations at *WT2* can lead to a number of overgrowth syndromes including hemihypertrophy

D. Prabharasuth, MD
Department of Urology, New York Medical College, Munger Pavilion, Rm 457, Valhalla, NY 10595, USA
e-mail: prabhara@yahoo.com

L.M. LeCompte, MD
Division of Pediatrics, Department of Radiology, Westchester Medical Center, New York Medical College, 100 Woods Rd., Valhalla, NY 10595, USA
e-mail: les99ll@gmail.com

L.L. Dyer, MD (✉)
Department of Urology, Pediatric Urology, New York Medical College, Valhalla, NY, USA
e-mail: doclandau@yahoo.com

L.S. Palmer, J.S. Palmer (eds.), *Pediatric and Adolescent Urologic Imaging*,
DOI 10.1007/978-1-4614-8654-1_11, © Springer Science+Business Media New York 2014

and Beckwith-Wiedemann syndrome (hemihypertrophy, nephromegaly, macroglossia) where the risk of nephroblastoma is 4–10 % with 21 % of children presenting with bilateral disease [3].

Histopathology

Grossly, Wilms' tumor appears as a large, bulky, soft, gray, or tan, solid mass surrounded by a pseudocapsule of compressed renal parenchyma. There may be foci of hemorrhage, necrosis, and cyst formation. Tumors usually arise from the periphery of the kidney sparing the central collecting system [4]. In some cases, an infiltrative growth pattern with a resultant ill-defined and poorly marginated mass is seen [5]. Average tumor size is approximately 11 cm [5]. Local extension into the perinephric fat, renal vein, and hilar lymph nodes is not uncommon [5]. Rarely, fat may comprise a majority of the tumor [5].

Microscopically, classic Wilms' tumor is characterized by the presence of three cell types: blastemal, epithelial, and stromal [6]. Occasionally, the tumor has biphasic or monophasic patterns in which a single cell line is identified. Anaplasia, characterized by marked enlargement of nuclei (at least three times the diameter of adjacent cells), hyperchromatism of the enlarged nuclei, and multipolar mitotic figures, may occur locally or diffusely, denotes unfavorable histology, and portends a worse prognosis.

Imaging (Figs. 11.1 and 11.2)

Preoperative imaging plays a vital role in the management of Wilms' tumor. The NWTS protocol

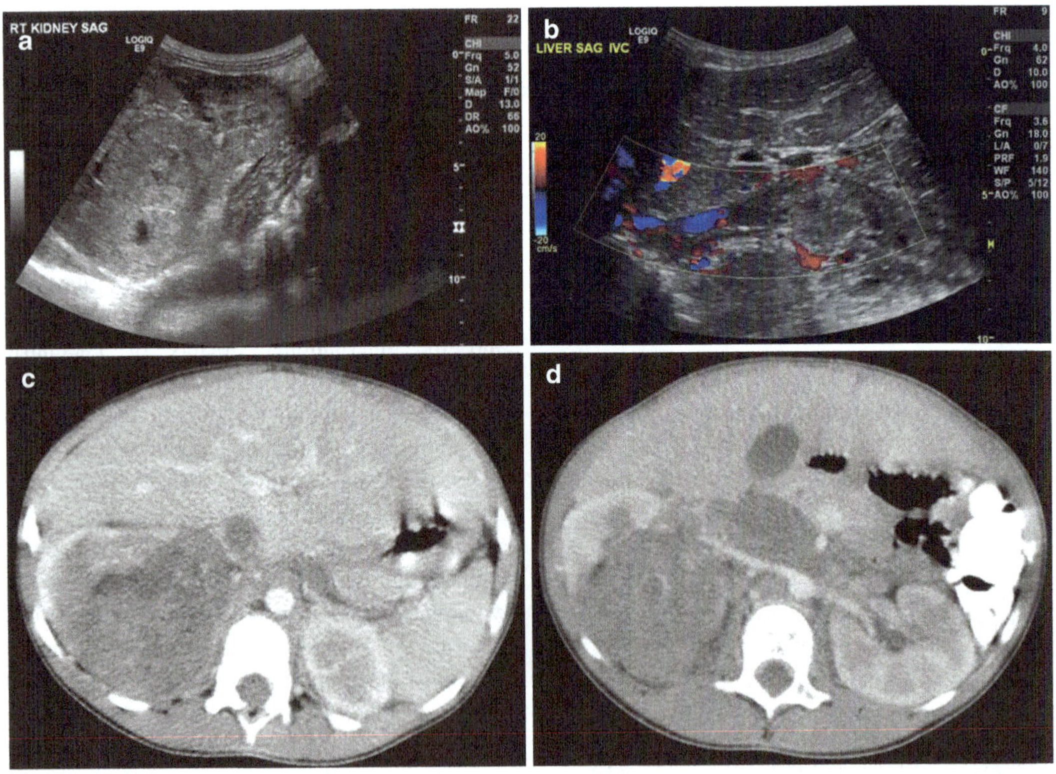

Fig. 11.1 Wilms' tumor. Grayscale ultrasound of the right kidney (**a**). Large heterogeneous echogenic soft tissue mass arising from right upper pole, with small cystic regions representing necrosis. Surrounding hypoechoic edge representing pseudocapsule. Color ultrasound of the IVC (**b**). Focal expansion of infrahepatic IVC by large heterogeneous filling defect representing neoplastic vascular invasion. Flow seen cranial to tumor thrombus. CT Abdomen, axial corticomedullary phase (**c** and **d**) Large heterogeneously enhancing upper-pole mass in the right kidney, with distortion of the right renal artery. Soft tissue expansion of the transhepatic IVC with tumor. Tc99m MDP bone scintigraphy (**e**). Abnormal, asymmetric renal uptake in right kidney

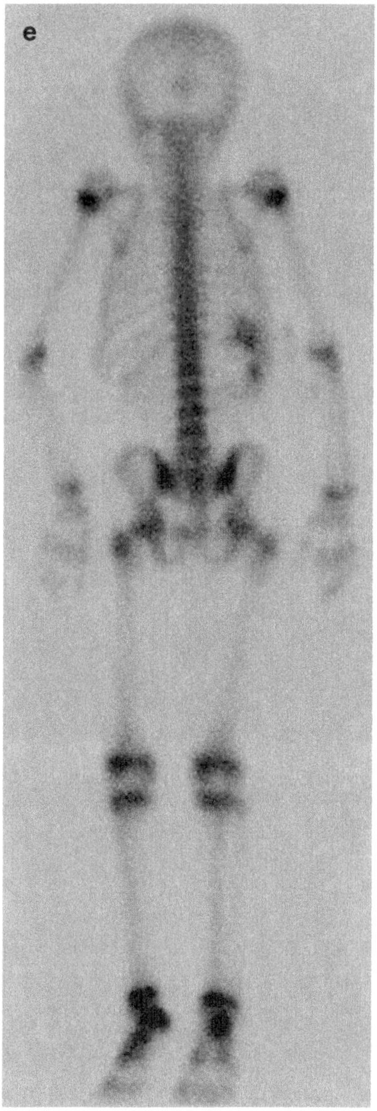

Fig. 11.1 (continued)

advocates imaging prior to radical nephrectomy and adjuvant therapy, while SIOP advocates neoadjuvant chemotherapy based on initial imaging [7]. Recent reports indicate a difficulty in the accurate clinical staging of localized Wilms' tumor when compared to pathologic results [7].

Ultrasound is usually the first imaging modality in the diagnosis of intra-abdominal masses given its safety profile. US may demonstrate an echogenic mass that is partially surrounded by a hypoechoic rim representing the pseudocapsule of Wilms' tumor which is composed of normal compressed renal parenchyma [8]. US may demonstrate a tumor mass of mixed echogenicity with extensive surrounding necrosis. Calcification appears as areas of hyperechogenicity with shadowing [8]. IVC involvement and regional adenopathy may be detected by US although it is less sensitive than CT [8].

CT is the primary imaging modality for staging. On nonenhanced CT imaging, Wilms' tumor appears as a large heterogeneous mass, less dense than the surrounding normal kidney [5]. Low-density areas correspond to areas of necrosis and small areas of intrarenal calcification may be identified. After administration of intravenous contrast, Wilms' tumors show slight enhancement, a pseudocapsule that is usually sharply defined, and areas of necrosis that fail to demonstrate significant uptake of contrast [5]. In infiltrative cases of Wilms' tumor, CT demonstrates an ill-defined mass that completely replaces the kidney with almost no normal parenchyma identified. CT scan may identify regional adenopathy; however, it cannot reliably differentiate reactive from malignant changes. Tumor staging by CT is also likely to overestimate intrarenal disease (stage I) for local extrarenal extension (stage II) [7].

On MRI, Wilms' tumor appears as a large, solid renal tumor. The tumor appears heterogeneous with intermediate signal intensity on T1-weighted images and high signal intensity on T2-weighted images. Variable signal intensity may be due to necrosis, hematoma, or fat. After administration of contrast, the inhomogeneity of the tumor increases. A sharp demarcation of tumor tissue and renal parenchyma can be seen as a pseudocapsule which appears hypointense on T2-weighted sequences. As with CT, local tumor staging has proved difficult with MRI. Lymph node metastases can be difficult to differentiate from reactive changes. Tumor invasion into the renal vein or IVC can be seen on T2 imaging as a high signal surrounded as a filling defect on post-contrast T1 imaging [9].

Nephroblastomatosis

Etiology and Presentation

Nephrogenic rests refer to the persistence of fetal renal embryonic tissue beyond 36 weeks of

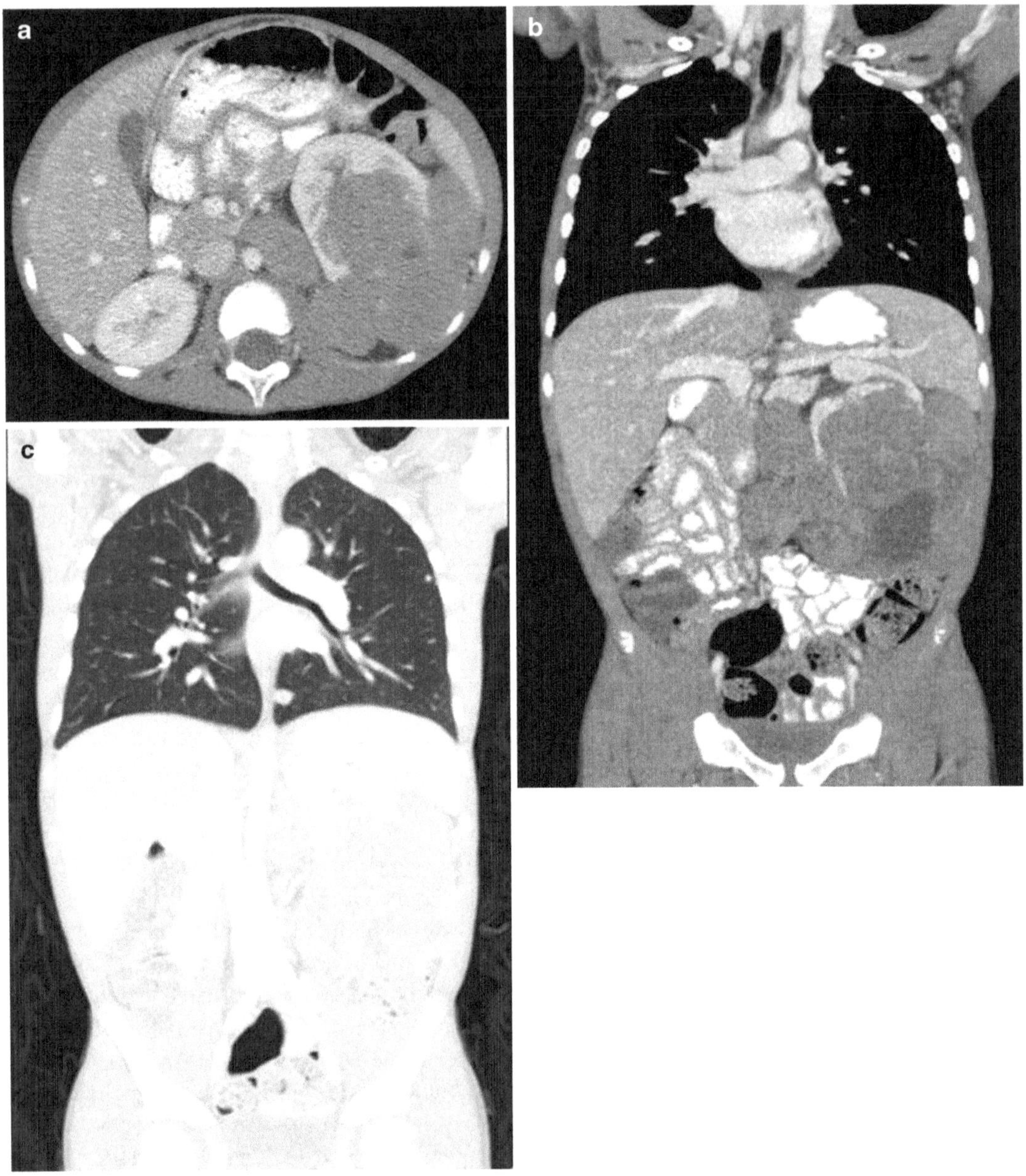

Fig. 11.2 Wilms' tumor, blastemal cell type. CT abdomen and pelvis, axial (**a**) and coronal (**b**) nephrographic phase. Multilobular homogeneously enhancing soft tissue mass arising from the left kidney, with claw sign and distortion of the renal hilum. Retroperitoneal lymph adenopathy in the left periaortic region. Renal vein and IVC patent. CT abdomen and pelvis, coronal in lung window. (**c**) Several small peripheral pulmonary nodules consistent with metastases

gestation. It is present in approximately 1 % of infant kidneys at autopsy [10]. The presence of diffuse or multiple nephrogenic rests is termed nephroblastomatosis [10]. Most nephrogenic rests undergo spontaneous involution; however, malignant transformation to Wilms' tumor represents approximately 30–40 % of Wilms' tumor precursor lesions [10].

Nephrogenic rests may occur in different areas of the kidney, intralobar or perilobar. Intralobar nephrogenic rests occur less commonly than the perilobar type but are more often associated with development of Wilms' tumor [10]. Intralobar nephrogenic rests present with neoplastic changes at a younger age compared to the perilobar type (median 16 vs. 36 months) [10]. Intralobar nephrogenic rests are typically found in conjunction with Wilms' tumor on imaging, while perilobar nephrogenic rests are more often diffuse presenting as unilateral or bilateral flank masses [10].

Perilobar nephrogenic rests are linked to abnormalities in *WT2* and may be associated with Beckwith-Wiedemann syndrome and hemihypertrophy. Intralobar nephrogenic rests are linked to abnormalities in *WT1* and may be associated with WAGR, Denys-Drash syndrome, and sporadic aniridia. Almost 100 % of patients with sporadic aniridia have intralobar nephrogenic rests and 20 % have perilobar rests [10].

Histopathology

Nephrogenic rests are less than 3 cm in diameter and appear as tan nodules within the normal renal parenchyma. In the diffuse form, nephroblastomatosis appears as white plaques replacing much of the renal parenchyma or may form a discrete rind at the kidney periphery. Perilobar nephrogenic rests are found only in the cortex or at the corticomedullary junction. The margins are irregular and indistinct and may interdigitate with normal adjacent renal interstitium. Perilobar rests are composed predominantly of blast cells. Intralobar rests, in contrast, can be located anywhere within the renal parenchyma, and the predominant cell type is either stromal or epithelial [10].

Imaging

Nephroblastomatosis appears on imaging as discrete foci or as diffuse areas of the kidney [11]. On ultrasound, foci appear as homogeneously isoechoic or slightly hypoechoic areas compared to the normal renal cortex. In the diffuse form, nephroblastomatosis appears as a peripheral rim that is homogenous and hypoechogenic compared to the normal renal parenchyma. Because of the similar echogenicities of nephrogenic rests and renal cortex, it may be difficult to demonstrate nephrogenic rests smaller than 1–2 cm in diameter on ultrasound [11].

On unenhanced CT, nephrogenic foci appear as isodense or slightly hyperdense areas compared to renal cortex. Small lesions are nearly impossible to identify. After contrast administration, foci appear as homogenous, hypodense lesions because of poor contrast uptake [11]. Isolated nephrogenic rests have a nodular appearance and enhance less than the adjacent renal parenchyma. If numerous, they may cause the surface of the kidney to appear lobulated [10]. In the diffuse form, the surrounding rim of nephroblastomatosis appears as homogenously hypodense areas compared to the renal cortex (Figs. 11.3 and 11.4) [11].

On MRI, nephrogenic foci appear as isointense or slightly hypointense to the renal cortex on T1- and T2-weighted images. After gadolinium enhancement, the lesions remain homogeneously hypointense compared to the bright enhancing renal cortex [11].

In differentiating Wilms' tumor from nephroblastomatosis, the latter demonstrates near uniform homogeneity, while the former appears heterogenous on CT and MRI imaging especially after contrast or gadolinium administration (Fig. 11.5) [10–12].

Renal Medullary Carcinoma

Etiology and Presentation

Renal medullary carcinoma (RMC) is a rare and fatal pediatric renal tumor that typically affects children of African descent with the sickle cell trait or SC disease. Patients present at 11–39 years with a 3:1 male predilection between 11 and 24 years and then without gender predilection subsequently. RMC most commonly presents as hematuria and less commonly as flank or abdominal pain or a palpable abdominal mass. Approximately 70 % of lesions occur on the right side [13]. The lesion is thought to arise from the collecting system and it grows to invade the surrounding vascular and lymphatic

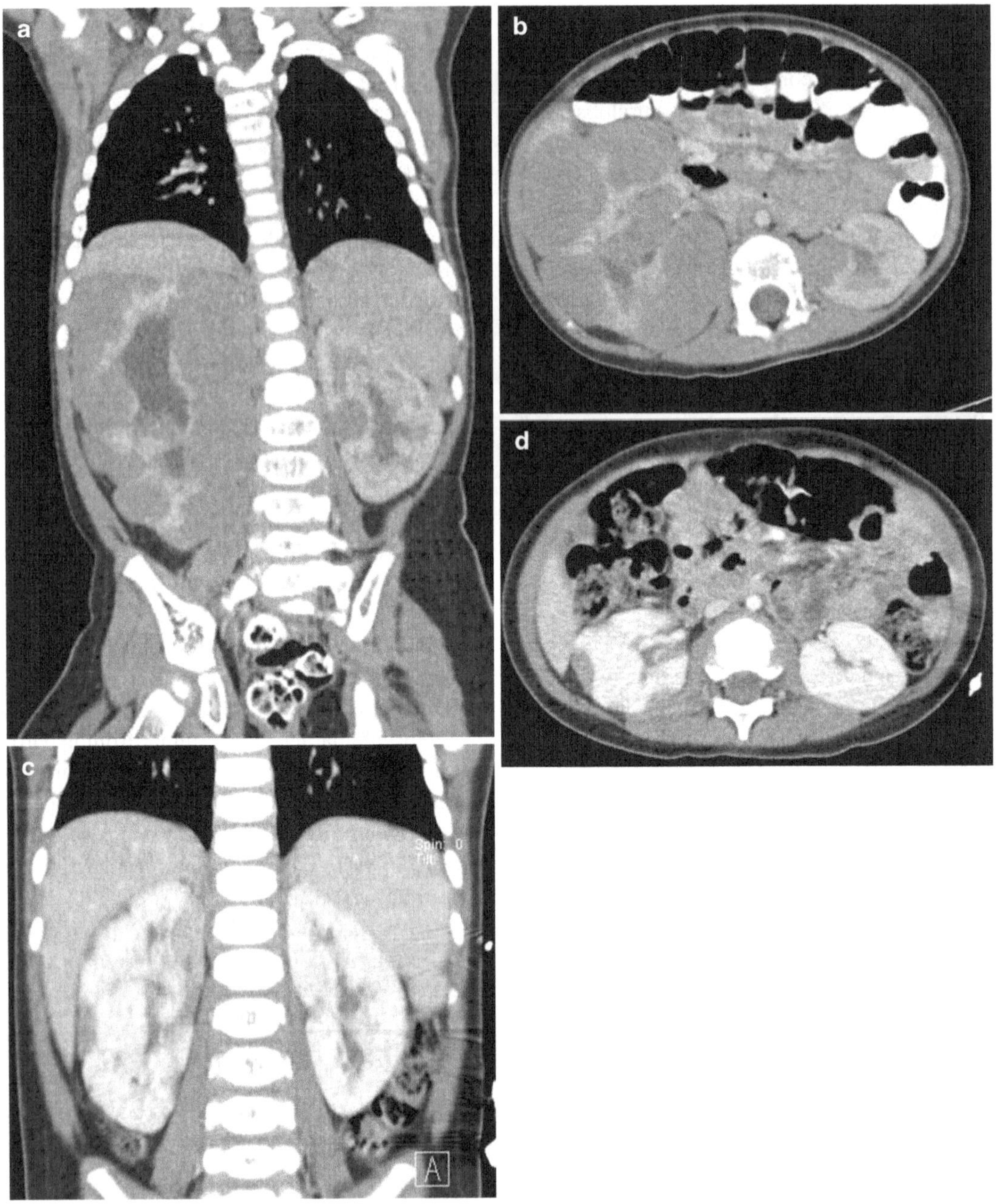

Fig. 11.3 Nephroblastomatosis. CT abdomen, axial and coronal, before (**a** and **b**) and after (**c** and **d**) chemotherapy. Peripheral lobular homogeneous hypodense rim of soft tissue masses in the right kidney, with enlargement of the right kidney and pelvicaliectasis. Solitaire small round soft tissue mass mid left renal pole. Successful response to chemotherapy with interval reduction of tumor bulk in bilateral kidneys

structures [14]. Metastatic disease to the liver, lung, and omentum is often present at diagnosis. Mean time to survival after diagnosis is approximately 15 weeks [15].

Histopathology

Grossly, RMC is a lobulated, tan, firm, or rubbery mass with variable degrees of hemorrhage and necrosis. The lesion has a dominant medullary location and extends into a large portion of the renal parenchyma. Invasion into the surrounding calyces or pelvis, vascular, lymphatic,

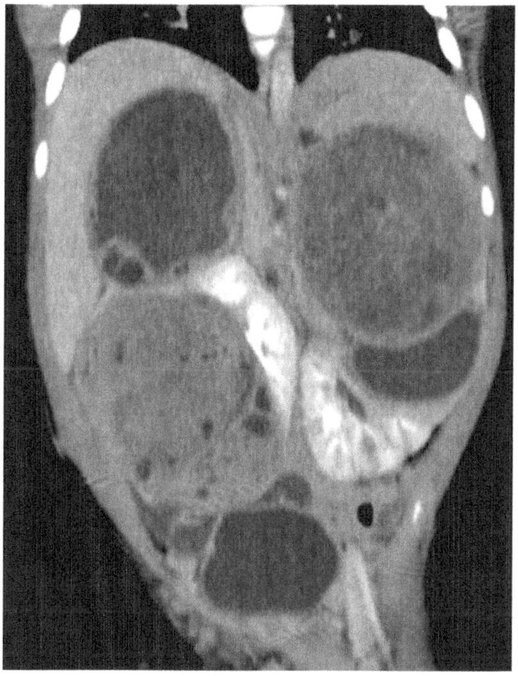

Fig. 11.4 Nephroblastomatosis with bilateral Wilms' tumor. CT abdomen, coronal excretory phase: Several large masses arising off both kidneys, some with increased heterogeneous soft tissue components compatible with Wilms' tumors

and perinephric tissue is often present. Microscopically, RMC demonstrates stromal desmoplasia and inflammation. Satellite lesions are present throughout the renal cortex and pelvic soft tissue. Cells have a dark cytoplasm, clear nuclei, and prominent nucleoli. Hemorrhage and necrosis are often present.

Imaging

There are only a few reported cases of ultrasound findings for RMC given its rarity [13, 16, 17]. Sonogram may detect a heterogenous, hyperechoic renal mass [17] occupying the renal pelvis and most of the renal cortex [16]; however, others have found ultrasound to be unreliable [13].

CT imaging demonstrates an infiltrative, centrally located tumor with caliectasis. Low attenuation areas correspond to areas of necrosis. Hemorrhage, retroperitoneal adenopathy, and metastases are often present. After administration of contrast, renal medullar carcinoma demonstrates heterogeneous contrast enhancement with preservation of the surrounding renal contour.

MRI demonstrates similar findings to CT but is superior in detecting liver metastases, intratumoral hemorrhage [13], and possibly lymphadenopathy [16].

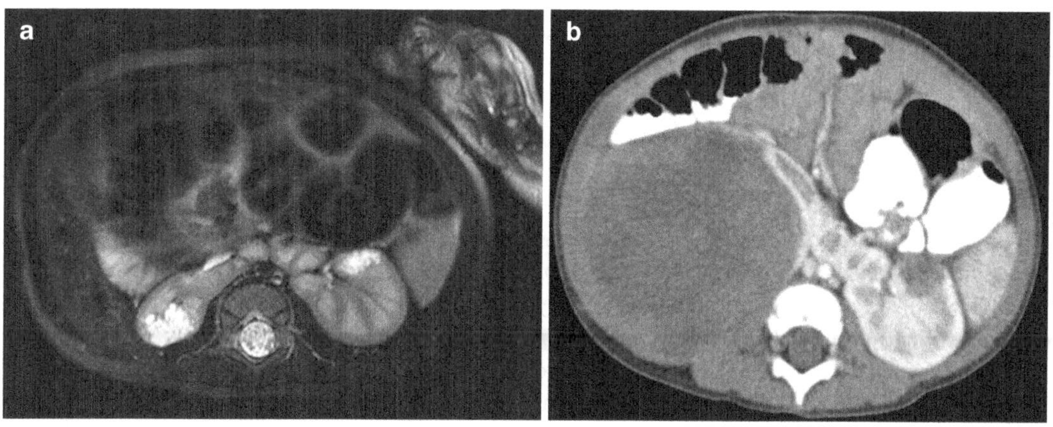

Fig. 11.5 Nephroblastomatosis. MRI abdomen, axial T2 fat saturation with high resolution (**a**) and CT abdomen, corticomedullary phase 7 months later (**b**). Focal perilobar multilocular T2 hyperintense cystic mass in the right moiety of a horseshoe kidney, with interval replacement and development of large soft tissue tumor arising from the same location compatible with malignant transformation of a nephroblastic rest into a Wilms' tumor

Clear Cell Sarcoma of the Kidney

Etiology and Presentation

Clear cell sarcoma of the kidney is classified as an "unfavorable histology" tumor in the National Wilms' Tumor Study Group (NWTSG) [18]. Kidd recognized it as a distinct entity and also noted its proclivity to metastasize to bone [18]. Clear cell sarcoma of the kidney may present as a palpable abdominal mass, as hematuria, or as increasing abdominal girth [19]. Approximately 50 % of cases are diagnosed between years 2 and 3 of life. Mean age at diagnosis is 36 months (range 2 months–14 years) [4]. It shows a 2:1 male to female predominance [4].

Approximately 25 % of patients present with stage I disease, 37 % present as stage II disease, 34 % present as stage III disease, and 4 % present with distant metastases [4]. There are no reported incidences of bilateral disease. Ipsilateral renal hilar lymph node metastases are the most common site of advanced disease at presentation occurring in up to 29 % [4]. Bone metastases are the most common site of disease relapse, but other sites include the lung, abdomen, retroperitoneum, brain, and liver [4]. Long-term follow-up is warranted as approximately 20 % of patients will present with metastases 3 years or more after time of diagnosis. Prognostically, four independent variables affect overall survival: stage at presentation (stage 1 >98 %), treatment with doxorubicin, patient age, and the absence of necrosis [4].

Histopathology

Grossly, clear cell sarcomas are large, tan-gray, soft, mucoid unicentric tumors that distort or nearly completely replace the kidney [4]. They have a well-circumscribed appearance with sharp kidney-tumor borders. Necrosis and hemorrhage are commonly present [4]. Cystic foci are present in nearly all cases. Mean size of tumor is 11.3 cm (range 2.3–24 cm) and mostly the common site of origin is the renal medulla. Microscopically, the classic pattern can be described as cords of plump cells separated by fibrovascular septa, with indistinct cell borders and open chromatin. Cord cells are loosely spaced and separated by extracellular mucopolysaccharide matrix. In addition to the classic appearance, many tumors demonstrate a second morphology that may seamlessly blend with the classic pattern [4].

Imaging

Radiologically, clear cell sarcoma of the kidney appears as a focal mass with a dominant soft tissue component with areas of necrosis [19]. Ultrasonography demonstrates an inhomogeneous pattern of soft tissue echoes and echo-poor areas that correspond to necrosis. Multiple anechoic areas correspond to septated cystic spaces. This may account for the bulk of the tumor and may make differentiation from multilocular cystic nephroma or cystic Wilms' variant difficult [19]. Specular echoes corresponding to calcifications may also be seen.

After contrast administration, CT imaging demonstrates a heterogeneous tumor with attenuation less than that of normal renal parenchyma. Necrotic areas are clearly evident and calcifications or hemorrhage may also be demonstrated [19].

Rhabdoid Tumor of the Kidney

Etiology and Presentation

Rhabdoid tumor of the kidney was originally categorized as an unfavorable histological subtype of Wilms' tumor [6] but was separated out as a distinct entity in 1998 [20]. Malignant rhabdoid tumor of the kidney is one of the most aggressive pediatric renal tumors and accounts for approximately 2 % of all pediatric renal tumors with 80 % occurring under the age of 2 years [21].

These tumors present as a palpable abdominal mass, hematuria, or fever [22] and sometimes with hypercalcemia [20]. Median age at diagnosis is 11 months and occurs more frequently in males (3:2). Extrarenal extension is commonly seen [23] and those presenting with metastases (lung and liver) die of disease progression [4]. Rhabdoid tumors are associated (up to 10 %) with the development of synchronous or metachronous primary tumors of the central nervous system [23]. Most brain lesions are reported as medulloblastoma, but other diagnoses include primitive neuroectodermal tumors, ependymoma, or gliomas [20].

Histopathology

Grossly, rhabdoid tumors resemble a bulky mass, largely replacing the kidney with preservation of a thin rim of peripheral renal tissue. Well-circumscribed boundaries [23] are not commonly seen and they frequently invade [23]. Mean tumor size at time of diagnosis is approximately 9.6 cm (range 3–17 cm). The tumor is soft, friable, gray to pink tan in color with focal areas of necrosis and hemorrhage. The tumor tends to occupy the central portion of the kidney with involvement of the renal hilar structures. The renal vein is often filled with tumor, and involvement of the renal pelvis occurs in some. Most specimens show capsular invasion, intrarenal and intrapelvic involvement, and infiltration of the renal sinus.

Microscopically, rhabdoid tumor of the kidney shows a wide range of morphological diversity. Rhabdoid cells are large with centrally placed nucleoli and abundant cytoplasm with prominent cytoplasmic inclusions [20]. The classical variant shows sheets of solid large, ovoid to polygonal cells, with abundant eosinophilic cytoplasm, intracytoplasmic inclusions, and conspicuous nucleoli [20].

Imaging

CT imaging demonstrates a heterogeneous, lobular, hilar tumor with central hypodense areas corresponding to necrosis and hemorrhage (Fig. 11.6) [22]. Calcification appears linearly and tends to outline the tumor lobule. Crescent-shaped hypodense areas in the periphery of the kidney outline tumor nodules and correspond

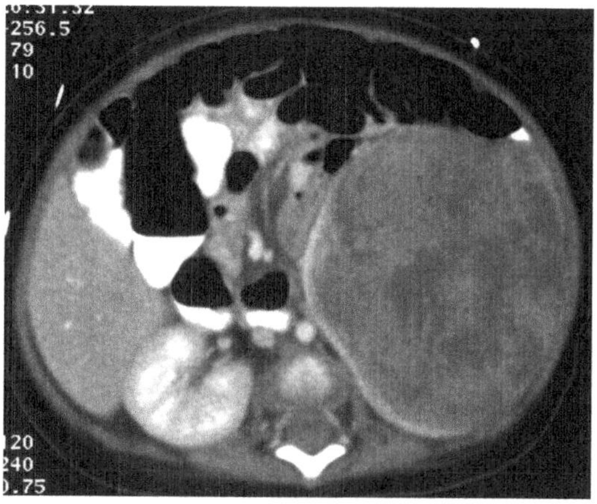

Fig. 11.6 Rhabdoid tumor. CT abdomen, axial late nephrographic phase: large heterogeneously enhancing mass in the left kidney (claw sign) with central necrosis and possible hemorrhage (Courtesy of Dr. Richard D. Bellah, MD at Children's Hospital of Philadelphia)

pathologically to subcapsular hematoma. CT often demonstrates extension into adjacent structures such as the renal vein and inferior vena cava. Distant metastases to the lung may also be present on preoperative imaging. Imaging of the head sometimes demonstrates a synchronous CNS lesion which is not commonly seen in other pediatric renal tumors.

Renal Cell Carcinoma

Etiology and Presentation

Renal cell carcinoma (RCC) accounts for less than 4 % of pediatric renal tumors [24]. The median age at diagnosis is 9–12 years [25] without gender predilection [26]. Most patients present asymptomatically [25, 26]. Symptomatic patients may have hematuria, flank pain, or a palpable abdominal mass. The overall survival rate for children nears 50–60 % but approaches 90 % for those with lower tumor stage. Metastases (lungs, bones, liver, or brain) occur in approximately 20 % [14] and demonstrate survival of approximately 10–15 % at 5 years [25].

Whereas the *von Hippel-Lindau (VHL)* gene is implicated both in familial and sporadic cases of clear cell RCC in adults, recent reports suggest that this mutation is largely absent in children [25]. Translocation carcinomas have recently emerged as the predominant subtype of renal cell carcinoma in children. One such translocation t(X;17)(p11.2;q25) leads to a fusion of the transcription factor gene *TFE3* with the *ASPL* gene on 17q25. Another translocation t(X;1)(p11.2;q21) leads to a fusion *TFE3* transcription factor gene on Xp11.2 with the *PRCC* gene at 1q21.2.

Histopathology

Histologically, RCC are characterized into clear cell, papillary, and chromophobe carcinoma, as in adults. Most tumors are surrounded by a pseudocapsule and angioinvasion is common. Microscopically, translocation carcinomas contain tumor cells resembling conventional clear cell carcinoma but may have areas of papillary features, granular eosinophilic cytoplasm, and calcifications [26]. The architecture may vary but is predominantly solid, tubular, acinar, or alveolar with a hyalinized stroma demonstrating focal inflammatory infiltrates. Cells have voluminous clear cytoplasms with bulging cell borders [24]. Nuclei are vesicular, moderately pleomorphic, and wrinkled [24].

Imaging

RCC commonly appears as large, heterogenous enhancing masses on CT imaging. Many tumors show internal or adjacent hemorrhage, internal calcifications, and neovascularity. On MRI, tumors commonly demonstrate heterogeneous enhancement and intratumoral hemorrhage.

Congenital Mesoblastic Nephroma

Etiology and Presentation

Congenital mesoblastic nephroma (CMN) is the most common pediatric renal tumor diagnosed within the first 3 months of age [26], and roughly 90 % are diagnosed within the first year of life. The tumor shows a male to female predominance of 2:1 [26]. CMN most commonly presents as a palpable abdominal mass, gross hematuria, or as an incidental finding on prenatal sonography. Hypertension and hypercalcemia may occur.

Two morphologic variants exist: classic and cellular. The classical type carries a better prognosis, while the cellular variant has been shown to invade perirenal fat, adjacent organs, and the renal vein and has also been shown to recur locally [27]. Mixed variants, composed of elements of classic and cellular, have also been described. The classic variant is usually diagnosed in the neonatal period, while the cellular variant presents at a later date and is typically larger [28].

Histopathology

Grossly, the classic variant appears as a solid, firm, light yellow mass with no capsule and poorly defined margins, resembling uterine leimyoma [14, 26]. The cellular variant tends to be soft and fleshy, with areas of hemorrhage or necrosis [28]. Other aggressive features of the cellular variant include invasion of surrounding structures such as the colon, small bowel, and pancreas, vascular invasion, tumor thrombus, and extension into the perihilar connective tissue [28].

The classic variant can be described as fibroblastic spindle cells arranged in bundles and fascicles that infiltrate the renal parenchyma [26]. There is low cellularity and atypia is absent [28]. The cellular variant is characterized by increased cellularity, vacuolated cytoplasm [28], plump cells with increased nuclear pleomorphism, a high nuclear/cytoplasmic ratio, and frequent mitotic figures [27]. The tumor cells are larger, fusiform to ovoid, and arranged in sheets with less well-defined bundles [28]. The tumor cells may be surrounded by a highly vascular hyalinizing stroma [28].

Imaging

On prenatal ultrasound, CMN can appear as an enlargement of the kidney [29] or as a large heterogeneous echogenic mass [30] that can sometimes be difficult to discern from the normal renal parenchyma [29] (Fig. 11.7). It is commonly

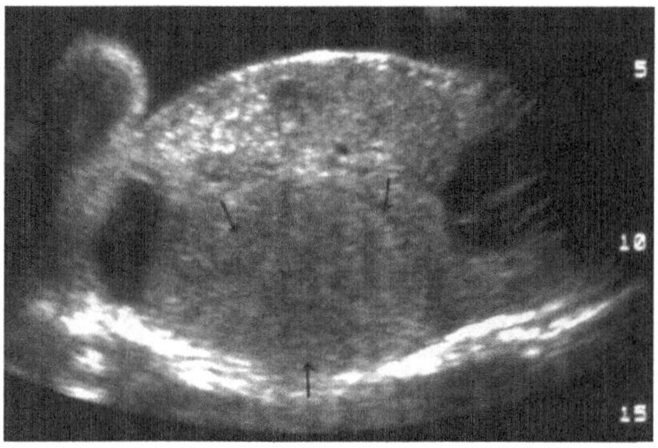

Fig. 11.7 Mesoblastic nephroma. Fetal ultrasound. Large hypo- to isoechoic mass in the renal bed (Courtesy of Dr. Richard D. Bellah, MD at Children's Hospital of Philadelphia)

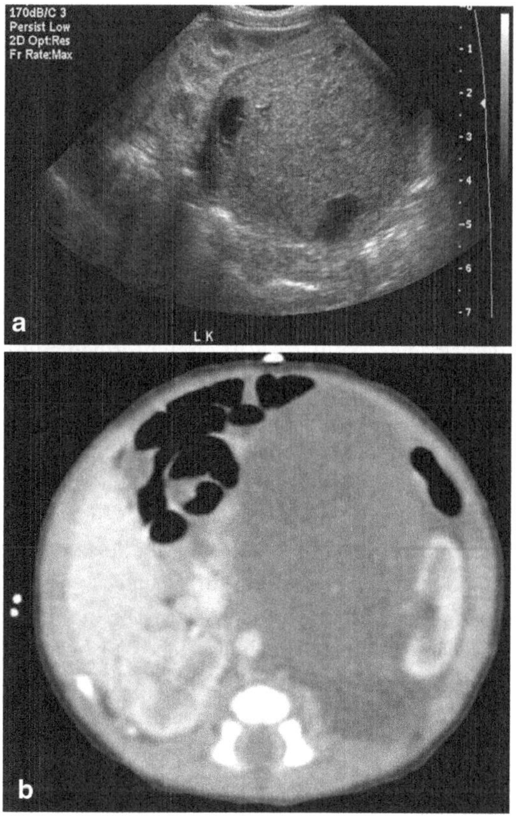

Fig. 11.8 Mesoblastic nephroma. Grayscale ultrasound (**a**) large hypoechoic mass in the left renal bed, with peripheral cystic areas, possibly representing blood vessels and/or necrosis. CT abdomen (**b**), axial corticomedullary phase. CT demonstrates homogeneous enhancement of the left hilar mass distorting and lateral displacing the left kidney

associated with fetal hydrops and polyhydramnios [29]. After birth, CMN appears as a mass with a central poor echoic area surrounded by a thin echogenic rim (ring sign) [28]. This corresponds pathologically to dilated blood vessels at the periphery of the tumor [27] (Fig. 11.8a).

On nonenhanced CT, CMN appears as a large heterogeneous mass with areas of high attenuation which correspond to areas of hemorrhage. After contrast administration, CT demonstrates a heterogeneous mass with enhancement of the solid component and areas of cystic and necrotic changes (Fig. 11.8b). Pathologically, the cellular variant is more likely to be identified if preoperative CT reveals cystic and hemorrhagic areas, while the classic variant is more likely to be a large, uniform, soft tissue mass [27].

MRI before gadolinium administration shows solid components with low signal intensity on T1 and high signal intensity on T2 [27]. High signal intensity on T1 corresponds to areas of hemorrhage. After administration of gadolinium, MRI demonstrates variable heterogeneous enhancement of the solid components.

Multilocular Cystic Renal Tumor

Etiology and Presentation

Multilocular cystic renal tumor refers to two entities that cannot be distinguished on the basis of gross pathology or radiologic findings. Multilocular cystic renal tumor is a benign lesion composed of multiple noncommunicating cysts separated by septa devoid of any blastemal or other embryonal elements. Partially differentiated cystic nephroblastoma refers to a predominant cystic lesion where the septa contain blastemal or other embryonal elements. Multilocular cystic partially differentiated nephroblastoma is typically a benign lesion; however, local recurrence after nephrectomy may occur. The etiology is unclear, but there are several hypotheses. If there are associated nodules of tumorous tissues, the multicystic lesion should be considered malignant. The prognosis for these malignancies is better than their corresponding non-cystic tumors (i.e., Wilms' tumor and RCC).

Multilocular cystic renal tumor presents most commonly as a painless abdominal mass [31]. It shows a bimodal distribution (3 and 25 years) affecting males more commonly than females during childhood, with a ratio of 2:1 and 8:1 in adults.

Histopathology

Grossly, multilocular cystic renal tumor can be described as a solitary, well-circumscribed multiseptated renal lesion containing noncommunicating fluid-filled loculi surrounded by a thick capsule (rind-like) compressing a thin rim of renal parenchyma. Both the capsule and the septations may be thick. The actual cystic spaces may not be very large. Grossly, the lesions may range in size from several millimeters to several centimeters. Mean size is 9.7 cm. The malignant spectrum of this cystic mass tends to be much larger and may be as big as 20 cm. Calcifications may be seen within the septa or mass wall. Hemorrhage, necrosis, and calcification are uncommon.

Microscopically, in multilocular cystic nephroma, the cysts are lined by flattened, cuboidal, or hobnail epithelium. In the well-differentiated, benign subtype, the septa consist of fibrous tissue without blastemal elements. In contrast, the septa in cystic partially differentiated nephroblastoma contain blastemal cells.

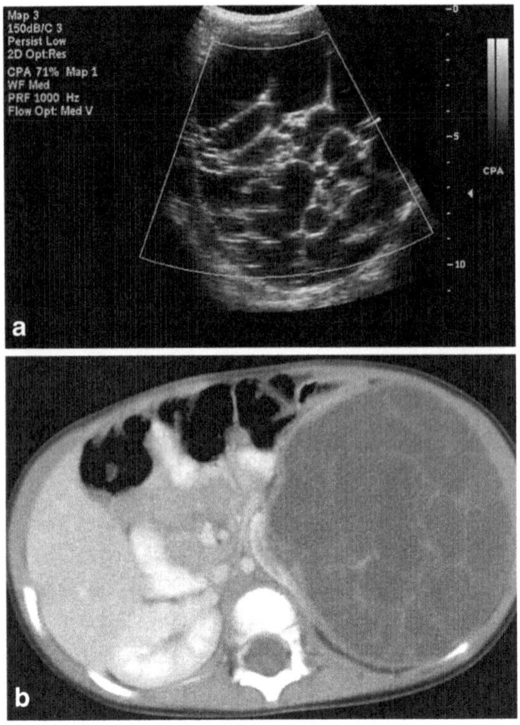

Fig. 11.9 Multilocular cystic renal tumor (1.5-year-old male). Color Doppler ultrasound (**a**) and axial CT (**b**) late nephrographic phase. Large multilocular cystic lesion, without internal vascularity. Lesion resulting in distortion and splaying of the left kidney. No accumulation of contrast on delayed imaging (not shown)

Imaging

Multilocular cystic nephroma and multilocular partially differentiated cystic nephroblastoma cannot be distinguished radiographically. On ultrasound, the kidney appears as a multiloculated mass with thin septa. The renal parenchyma can be compressed by the renal mass forming a thin rim of parenchyma (beak sign).

On nonenhanced CT, multilocular cystic renal tumors appear as sharply circumscribed, multiseptated renal mass. Occasionally, the mass may appear solid when the cysts come in close approximation. The interior of the cysts show attenuation that is consistent with water. With contrast, the septations may enhance; however, the contrast does not accumulate within the individual cysts (Fig. 11.9).

On MRI, the septa and renal capsule appear as low signal intensity on T1-weighted images. The septa enhance after gadolinium administration. On T2-weighted images, the fluid contents of the cyst display high signal intensity (Fig. 11.10).

Metanephric Adenoma

Etiology and Presentation

Metanephric adenoma is typically a benign renal lesion presenting as an incidental, usually unilateral finding on imaging [32, 33]. If symptomatic, metanephric adenoma may present as a palpable mass, abdominal or flank pain, or hematuria [32]. An association with polycythemia is reported in approximately 10 % of cases [34]. Metanephric

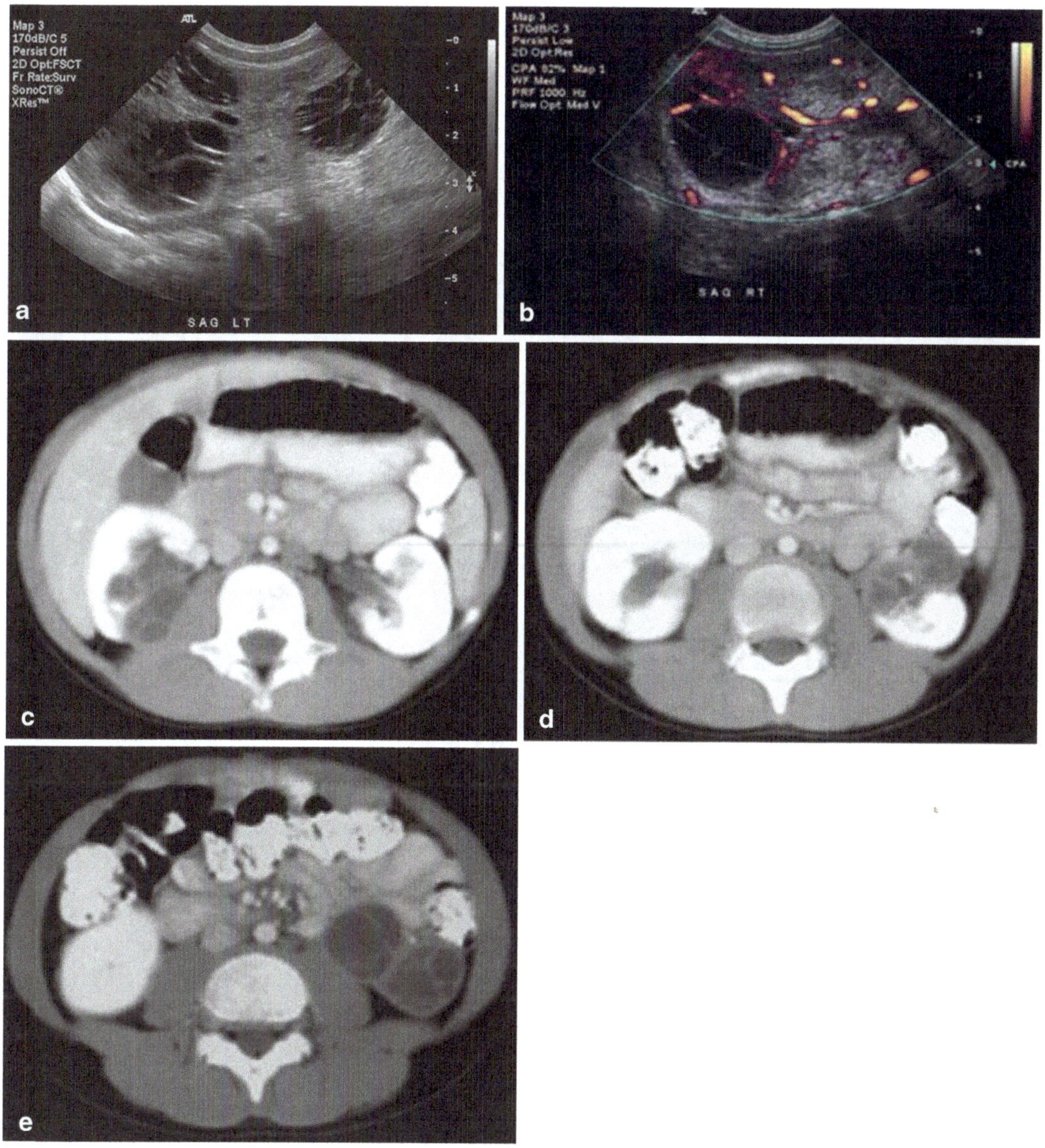

Fig. 11.10 Multilocular cystic renal tumor. Grayscale (**a**) and power Doppler (**b**) ultrasound kidneys. Several multilocular cystic lesions in both kidneys, at least three in the left, with thin avascular septations. CT abdomen, sequential axial images in nephrographic phase. (**c**, **d**, and **e**) Bilateral multilocular cystic masses, with herniation of the right lesion into the renal pelvis

adenoma most commonly occurs in females with a mean age of 41 (range 5–83 years). It demonstrates a female to male ratio of approximately 2:1 [32].

Histopathology

Grossly, metanephric adenoma appears as a well-circumscribed, solid, gray to tan to yellow tumor that is soft to firm [32–34]. Tumors may contain areas of hemorrhage, necrosis, or cystic degeneration [34]. Calcification may occur scattered throughout the tumors, in the cyst walls, or in the center of the tumor [32]. Most tumors are surrounded by a distinct capsule; however, some demonstrate a discontinuous or absent capsule [32].

Microscopically, these tumors are composed predominantly of small uniform epithelial cells

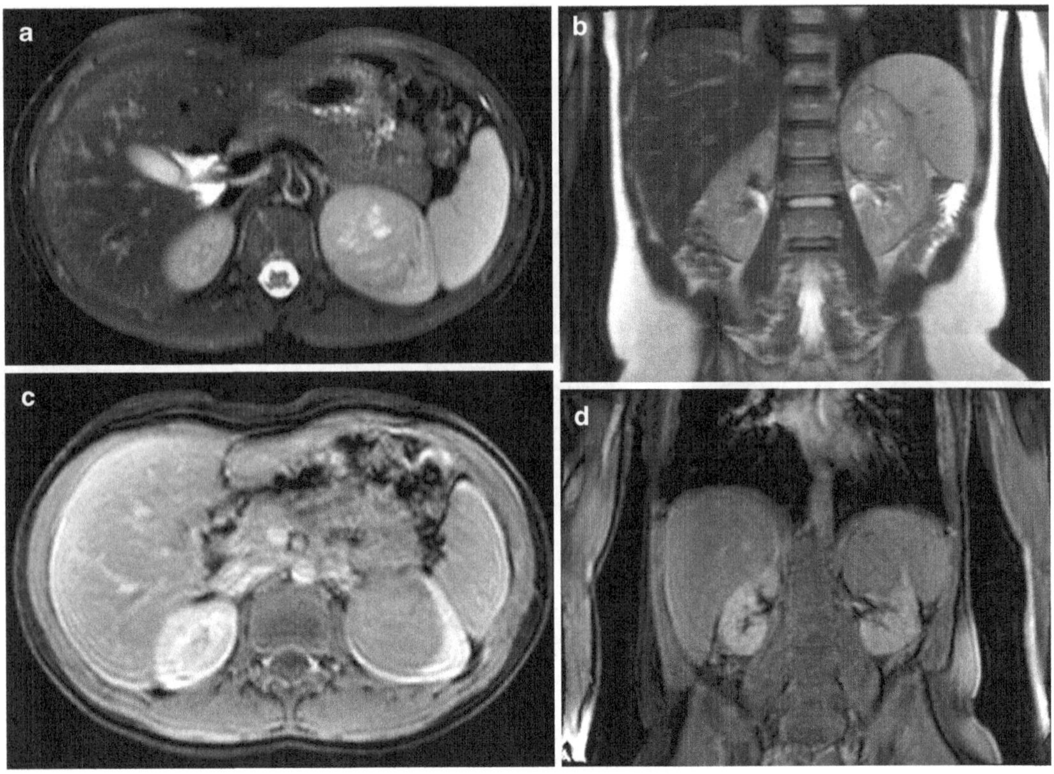

Fig. 11.11 Metanephric adenoma. MRI abdomen, axial T2 fat saturated (**a**), coronal T2 (**b**), axial (**c**), and coronal (**d**) T1 GRE fat saturated post contrast. Large heterogeneous T2 isointense masses in renal cortex arising from the upper pole of the left kidney, with central cystic components. Decreased enhancement relative to remaining kidney post contrast

separated by an acellular stroma [32, 34]. In about 50 % of cases, papillary structures are observed which consist of polypoid fronds or papillary infoldings forming a glomeruloid appearance [34] and are frequently calcified [32]. Cells demonstrate little cytoplasm with irregular rounded or ovoid nuclei with delicate chromatin [32, 34]. Nucleoli are not prominent and pleomorphism and mitotic figures are typically absent [32, 34].

Imaging

On ultrasound, metanephric adenomas appear as hypo-, iso-, or hyperechoic tumors compared to adjacent renal cortex. Color Doppler reveals no vascular flow in the tumor [33].

On unenhanced CT, tumors demonstrate higher attenuation than the adjacent renal parenchyma. With the addition of contrast enhancement, tumors typically demonstrate a lower attenuation than the renal parenchyma reflecting the hypovascular nature of these tumors. Areas of calcifications can frequently be seen.

On MRI, both T1- and T2-weighted images demonstrate lower signal intensity than the renal parenchyma even with the addition of gadolinium (Fig. 11.11).

Angiomyolipoma

Etiology and Presentation

Renal angiomyolipomas (AML) are benign neoplasms composed of adipose tissue, thick-walled blood vessels, and smooth muscle in varying amounts. The arteries in AMLs are deficient in

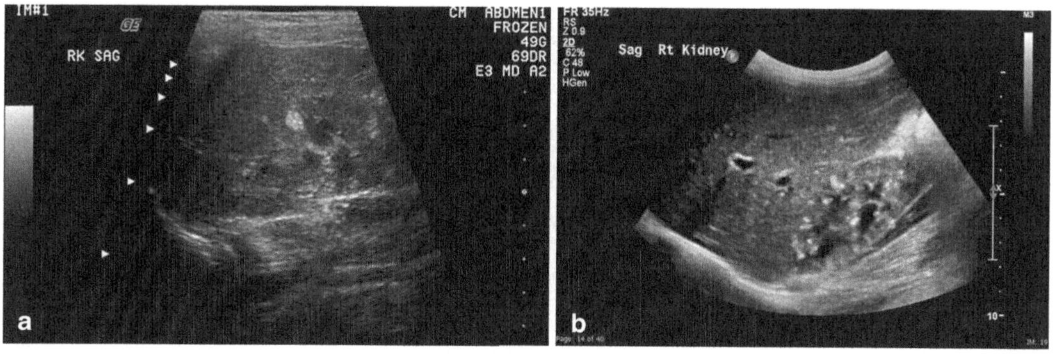

Fig. 11.12 Angiomyolipomas. *Grayscale* ultrasound, right kidney (**a** and **b**). Innumerable small round echogenic foci compatible with fat containing lesions in a patient with underlying tuberous sclerosis

the internal elastic membrane and are consequently torturous and prone to aneurysmal formation and rupture [35]. Approximately 10 % of patients with AML are associated with tuberous sclerosis complex (TS), and up to 80 % of patients with TS develop AML. Deletions of tumor suppressor genes located on chromosomes 9 (TSC1) and 16 (TSC2) are believed to cause AML growth.

Patients with TS are more likely to have numerous bilateral tumors that present at an earlier age and which exhibit increasing size with age [36, 37]. Patients with TS demonstrate three renal phenotypes: AML, renal cysts, and renal carcinoma with AML being the most common phenotype [38]. Many patients with AMLs less than 4 cm in size present incidentally on imaging [35, 39, 40]. Lesions larger than 4 cm commonly present with acute flank or abdominal pain, palpable mass, or hematuria [39]. In some cases, patients may present with Wunderlich syndrome, shock secondary to retroperitoneal bleeding [38]. AMLs are believed to be prone to rupture secondary to the dysplastic elastic tissue leading to aneurysmal formation [14].

Recently, a more aggressive subtype of AML, termed epithelioid, has been described. Tumor size at presentation is much larger than in the classical type [35]. At presentation, epithelioid AMLs may be seen invading local structures such as the renal vein or inferior vena cava or may present with distant metastases.

Histopathology

Grossly, AML is classically described as having a mahogany brown appearance. Microscopically, AMLs contains dysmorphic vascular tissue, smooth muscle, and mature adipose tissues in variable proportions [40]. The epithelioid variant has a large component of polygonal epithelioid cells which can vary in size. Mitotic activity may be seen. Abnormal vessels and fat, in contrast to the classic counterpart, are rarely seen in the epithelioid variant [38].

Imaging

On ultrasonography, AML classically appears as a hyperechoic lesion with posterior acoustic shadowing. The hyperechogenicity is due to the high fat content, multiple tissue interfaces of the tumor, and the extensive vascular tissue present [40]. The difference in acoustic impedance between fat and muscle causes further scatter and adds to the effect (Fig. 11.12) [35].

On CT, AML appears as a fatty heterogeneous mass with varying amounts of tissue density. Hounsfield units of −10 or less correlate to fat content. Surrounding hemorrhage located within or adjacent to a lesion may be seen and appears as a hyperdense, nonenhancing collection on CT [35].

On MRI, AMLs appear hyperintense on both T1- and T2-weighted images due to the fat

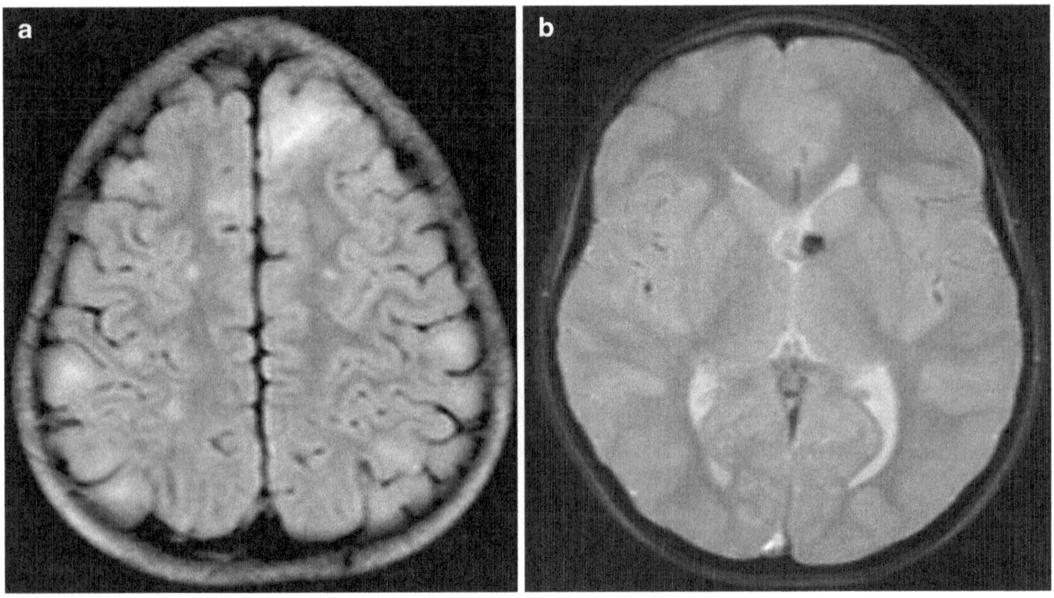

Fig. 11.13 Tuberous sclerosis. MRI brain, axial FLAIR (**a**) and axial GRE (**b**): multiple subcortical FLAIR hyperintense cortical tubers. Small subependymal nodule, with susceptibility artifact, near the foramen of Monroe. Enhancement of nodule raises the possibility of giant cell astrocytoma (not shown)

content with subsequent signal loss on fat suppressed images [40]. In-and-out-of-phase T1-weighted images enhance the ability to detect fat, by utilizing two artifacts: India ink and chemical shift artifacts. The India ink artifact occurs when there is a loss of fat-water interface due to the presence of fat and water protons within the same voxel [35]. The chemical shift artifact occurs because of the difference in precession frequency between fat and water, resulting in high and low signals in the frequency encoding direction on out-of-phase imaging. Imaging of the brain will demonstrate the presence of tubers (Fig. 11.13).

Fat poor AMLs present a diagnostic dilemma as they may resemble other renal lesions such as RCC. On ultrasound, fat poor AMLs are isoreflective to renal parenchyma as they lack fat and a fat-muscle interface. The use of biphasic helical CT (unenhanced, corticomedullary, and early excretory phase) scanning may help differentiate fat poor AML from RCC [35]. On MRI, lipid poor AML demonstrates homogenous enhancement and prolonged enhancement pattern. The use of T2-weighted images may aid in the diagnosis of AML versus RCC, as muscle appears hypointense on T2 imaging, whereas RCC appears hyperintense.

Renal Manifestation of Lymphoma

This is an extremely rare primary tumor in children and is noted exclusively with non-Hodgkin's lymphoma [41]. Reported cases have presented with bilateral or unilateral nephromegaly (Fig. 11.14). Further work-up is usually associated with anemia and/or renal insufficiency or failure. Treatment consists of bilateral biopsy of the masses and subsequent port placement and chemotherapy.

Renal Manifestation of Leukemia

Like lymphoma, primary renal presentation of leukemia is extremely rare in children. There are very few diagnoses that are made on the basis of

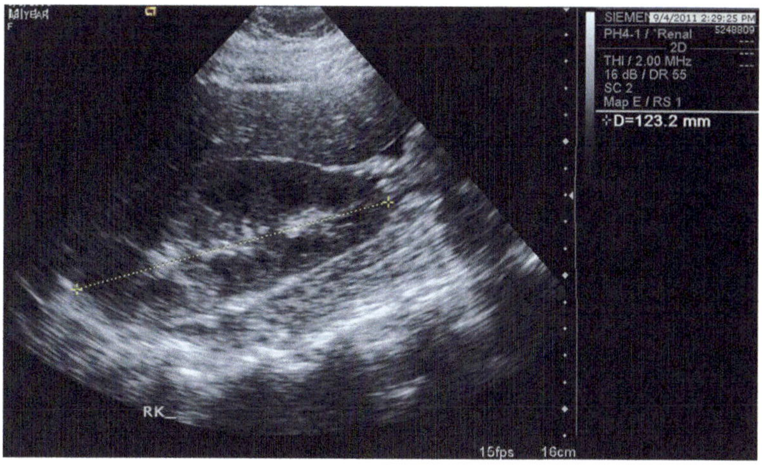

Fig. 11.14 Lymphoma. Grayscale ultrasound right kidney: enlarged right kidney (nl range for age 7.5–11.0) with preservation of corticomedullary differentiation

bilateral renal masses alone [42]. Leukemic infiltration of the kidney is secondary to systemic disease. Reported presenting signs include anemia, tachycardia, neutrophilia, elevated sedimentation rate and increased C-reactive protein, abdominal distention, and urinary tract infection [43]. The kidney is a metastatic site for leukemia in over 50 % of cases [42]. Correlation between renal size and prognostication of the disease at the time of diagnosis has been reported [44]. However, renal failure in ALL is extremely rare. In the rare child who has not already presented with systemic disease when the renal disease manifests, a renal biopsy should be done to confirm the pathologic diagnosis. If ALL has already been diagnosed when a renal mass is detected radiographically, then a biopsy is superfluous.

Histopathology

Leukemic renal infiltration can be nodular or diffuse in presentation. The few reported cases indicate that children usually present with a more diffuse pattern. In all renal ALL, the involvement is cortical and there is periglomerular infiltration [42, 45]. The histopathology on an associated bone marrow biopsy will show a predominance of lymphoblasts and will have precursor B-cell ALL morphology.

Imaging

Radiologic evidence of leukemic infiltration of the kidney is usually detected via ultrasound or CT scan. Bilateral nephromegaly is the most characteristic finding. In addition, when a CT with contrast is done, multiple, bilateral renal nodules (foci) can usually be identified (Figs. 11.15, 11.16, and 11.17).

Pediatric Cystic Diseases of the Kidney

It is currently believed that renal cystic diseases are related to abnormal Wolffian development due to aberrant molecular genetics [46]. Within families, some genetic mutations are heritable in either an autosomal dominant or recessive fashion or have variable penetrance. Children who have inherited these alterations (and associated syndromes) will in time develop a form of the associated disease and its subsequent clinical manifestations. Other genetic alterations are spontaneous mutations that may be a result of environmental or other factors.

As imaging modalities are used with increasing frequency, both heritable and spontaneous mutations are commonly detected on ultrasound or CT scan before they are detected clinically. In

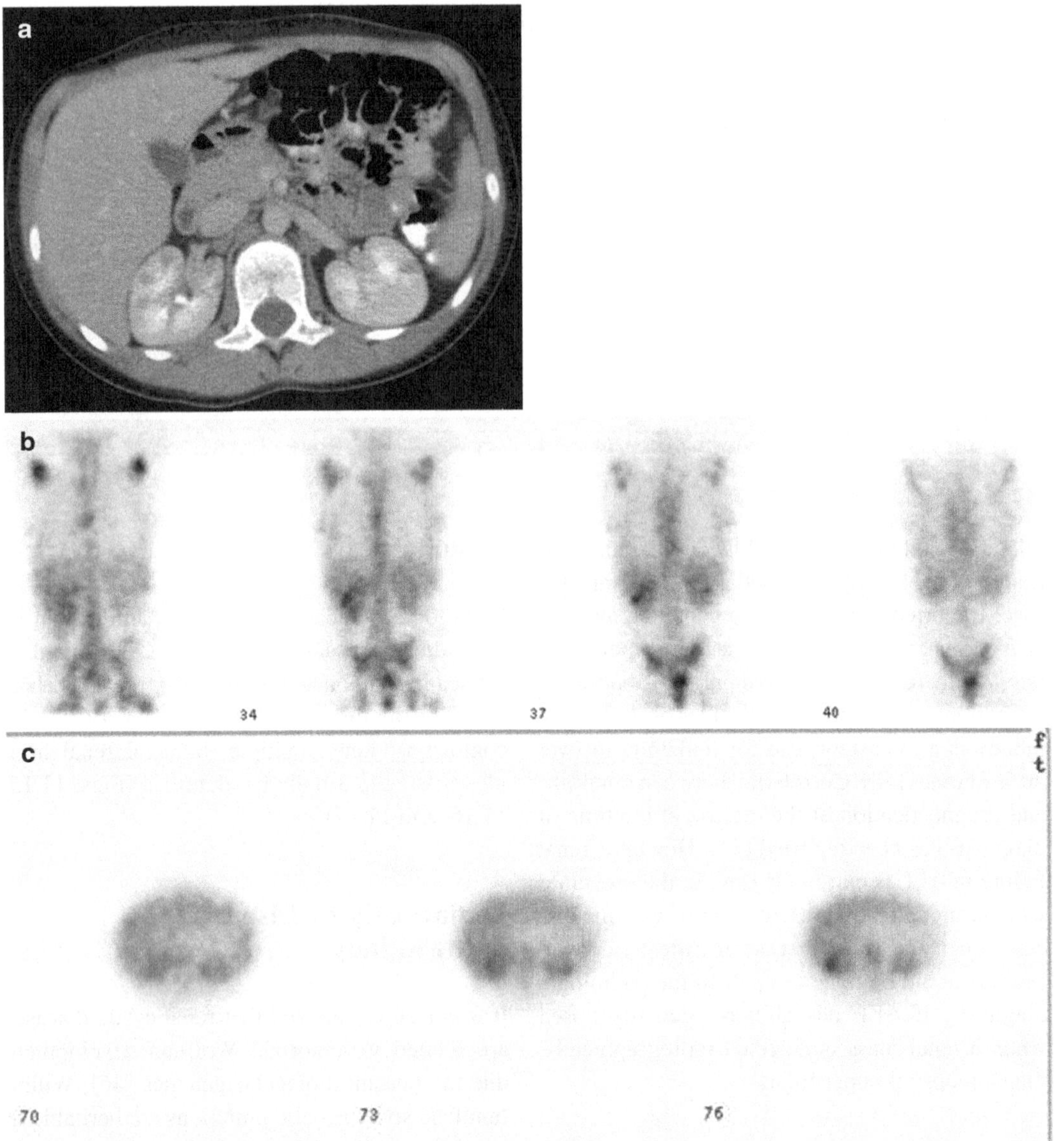

Fig. 11.15 NHL. CT abdomen, axial delayed phase (**a**): scattered small hypointense lesion in both kidneys. Gallium scintigraphy, coronal (**b**) and axial (**c**) static images: small foci of uptake in both kidneys corresponding to leukemic nodules

renal cystic diseases, innovations in radiologic technology have enabled physicians to better advise families regarding their child's prognosis and treatment. Characteristic radiologic findings including number, location, size, wall thickness, associated calcifications, and septations are crucial to determining which disease process or genetic alteration has occurred.

Simple Cysts

A simple cyst is a fluid-filled structure with a surrounding thin wall. Isolated cysts are the most common renal mass found in the adult kidney but are less common in children. Most simple renal cysts in children are asymptomatic and are found incidentally [47]. A single isolated cyst is

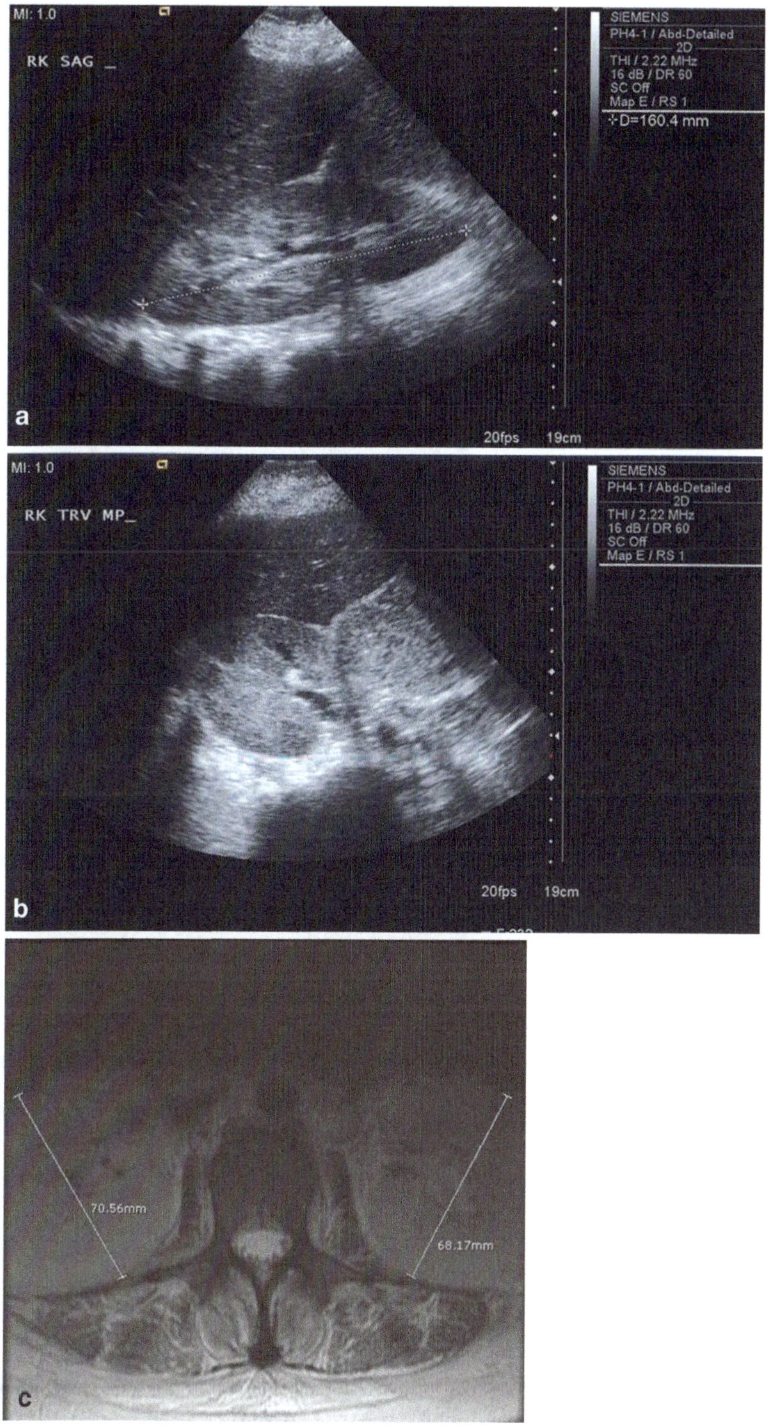

Fig. 11.16 AML. Grayscale ultrasound, sagittal (**a**) and transverse (**b**) right kidney: enlarged echogenic kidneys. MRI lumbosacral spine (**c**), enlarged bilateral kidneys

insignificant in the absence of associated clinical sequelae of pain and hematuria [48]. Clinical symptoms usually only occur if a parapelvic cyst is large enough to obstruct the kidney. A child may have incidental multiple simple cysts or bilateral simple cysts, but if this is noted, a heritable genetic mutation or syndrome should be pursued with a genetic work-up [46, 49, 50].

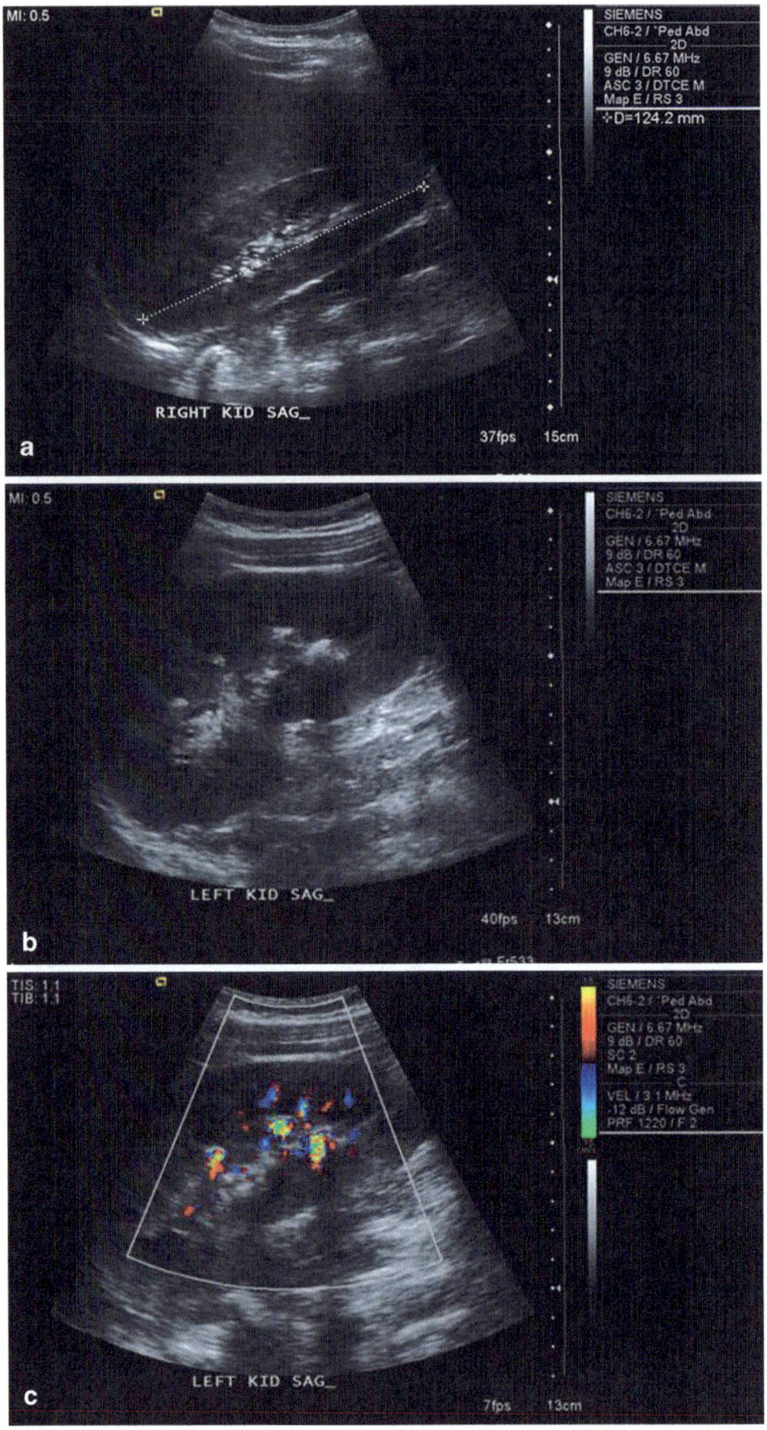

Fig. 11.17 Leukemia. Grayscale and color ultrasound of both kidneys: enlarged kidneys (**a** nl range for age 7.5–11.0), with echogenic foci (**b**) in left renal medulla and pelvis demonstrating posterior acoustic shadowing and twinkle artifact (**c**) compatible with nephrolithiasis

Histopathology

Cysts can be microscopic or macroscopic. Grossly, they appear as thin-walled (1–2 mm) entities encapsulated in straw-colored, clear fluid. They usually stem from the distal convoluted tubule or the collecting duct [51]. They can be saccular or fusiform and arise in any portion of the renal cortex. Simple cysts sometimes occur in association with congenital renal dysplasia. Histologically, the walls of the cysts are lined with cuboidal or flattened epithelium. The capsule is composed of fibrous tissue with collagen and some mononuclear infiltrates. The fluid transudate is similar to plasma.

Imaging

On ultrasound, simple cysts are typical round, unilocular, anechoic lesions with a thin wall and no internal architecture. There is good through transmission with posterior acoustic enhancement, a finding seen with most cystic structures (Fig. 11.18). No associated calcifications, septations, or internal vascularity is seen. Depending on the size of the cyst, it may displace adjacent vessels and collecting system.

On CT, a simple cyst should have a Hounsfield unit measurement in the range of simple fluid, 0–20, a thin or imperceptible wall, and no septations or internal debris/soft tissue. No enhancement or excreted contrast should be seen in the cyst (Fig. 11.19). Lesions less than 1 cm are difficult to accurately measure and are commonly described as lesions that are too small to characterize.

On MRI, homogeneous T1 hypointense and T2 hyperintense signal following that of water

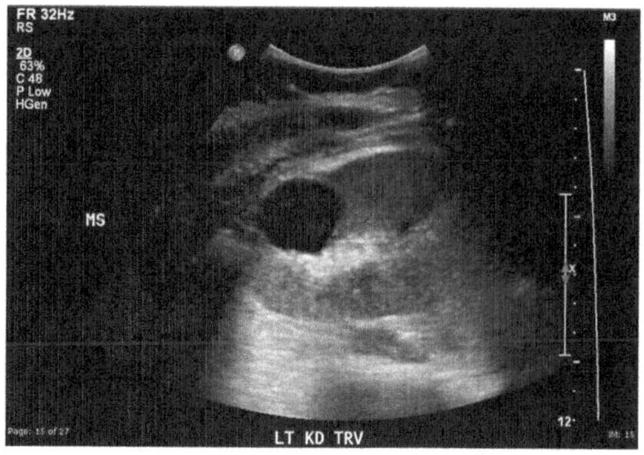

Fig. 11.18 Simple cyst. Ultrasound left kidney: round, anechoic lesion in the upper-pole left kidney, with thin wall, good through transmission and posterior acoustic enhancement

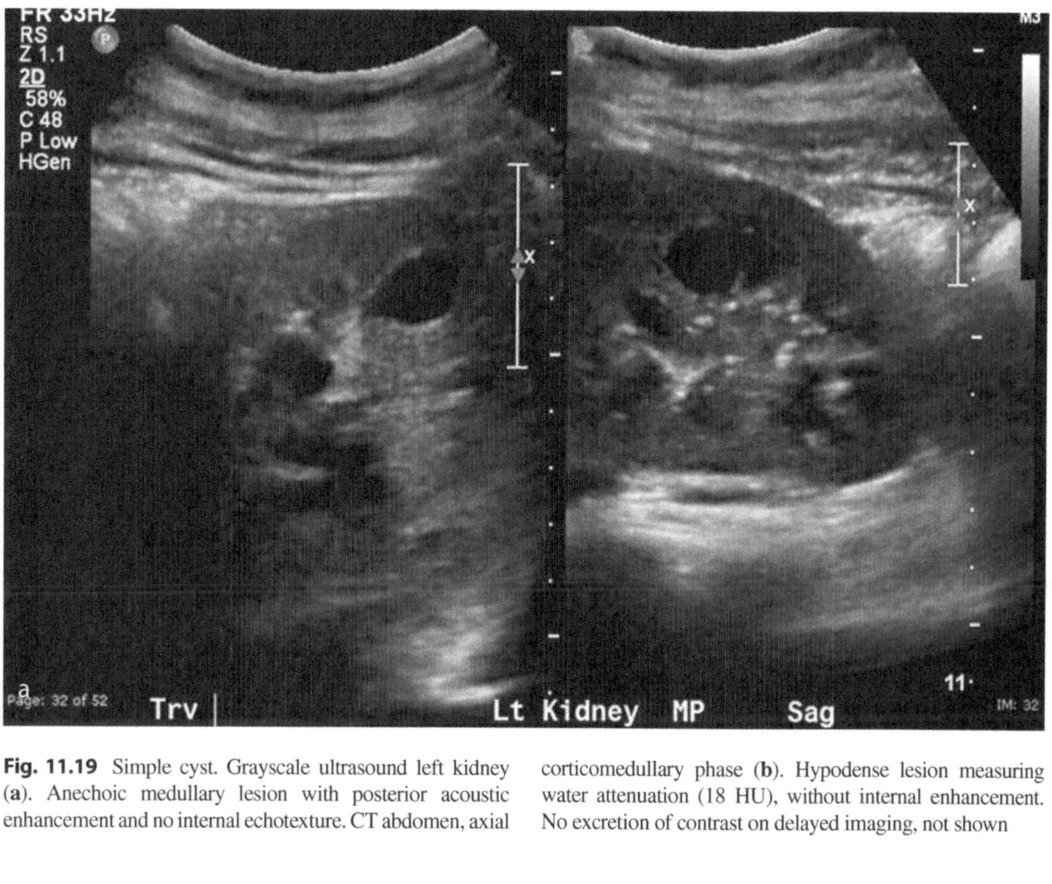

Fig. 11.19 Simple cyst. Grayscale ultrasound left kidney (**a**). Anechoic medullary lesion with posterior acoustic enhancement and no internal echotexture. CT abdomen, axial corticomedullary phase (**b**). Hypodense lesion measuring water attenuation (18 HU), without internal enhancement. No excretion of contrast on delayed imaging, not shown

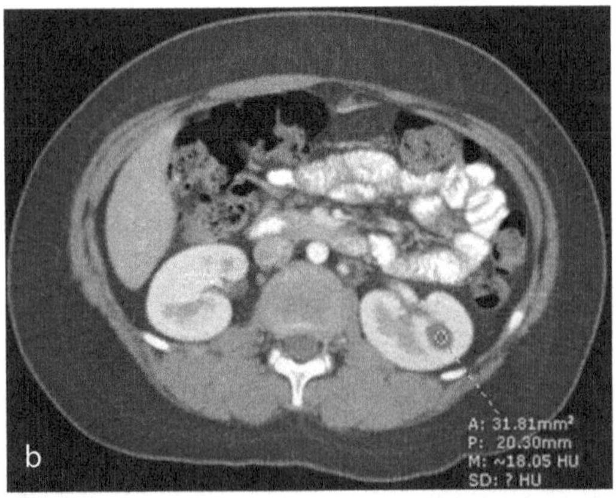

Fig. 11.19 (continued)

(such as CSF). No enhancement or excreted contrast should be seen in the cyst.

A calyceal diverticulum may appear as a simple cyst and in fact may become a cyst once it seals off. Distinction can be made with delayed imaging and layering of contrast (Fig. 11.20).

Hemorrhagic Cysts

Hemorrhagic cysts result when a simple or complex cyst fills with blood following trauma or spontaneous rupture [52]. Six percent of all renal cysts eventually hemorrhage. Hemorrhagic cysts are more likely to become infected then simple cysts.

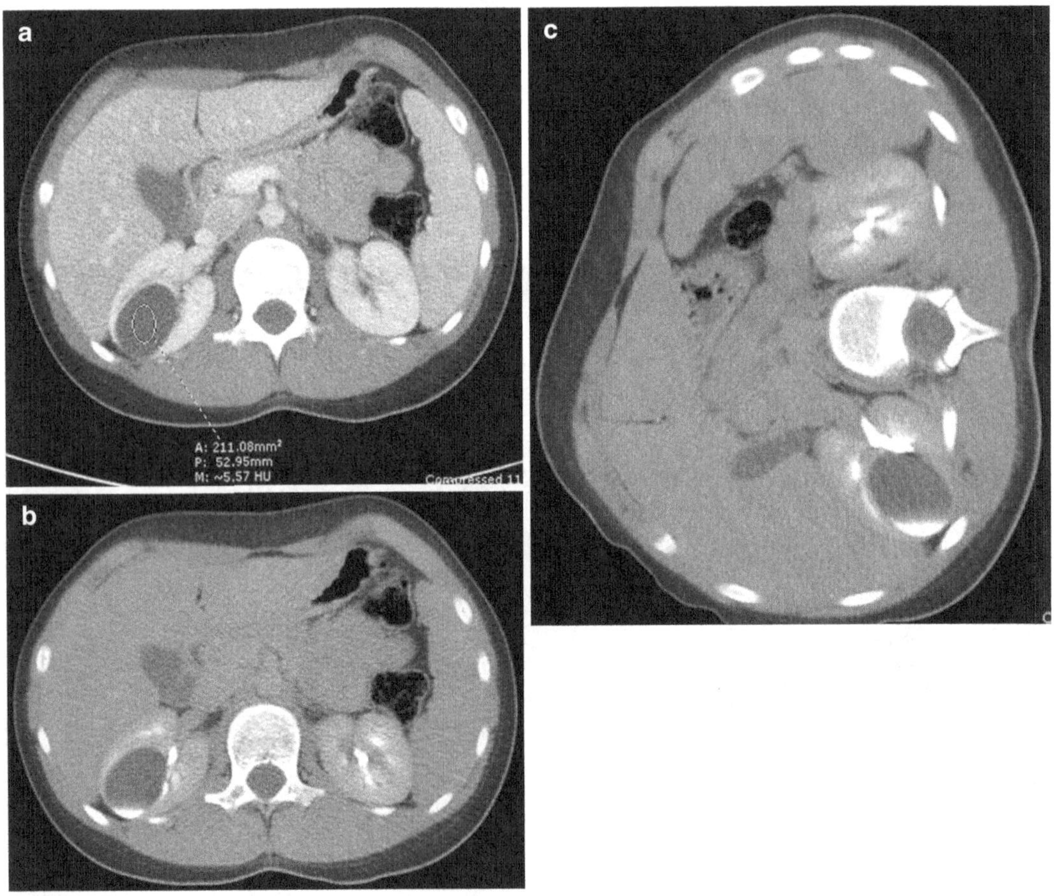

Fig. 11.20 Calyceal diverticulum. CT abdomen, axial nephrographic (**a**) and delayed phase (**b** and **c**). Large hypodense cystic lesion extending from the renal pelvis, measuring simple fluid density on nephrographic phase. Supine delay (**b**), excreted contrast material in the cystic lesion, which layers dependently with repositioning (**c**)

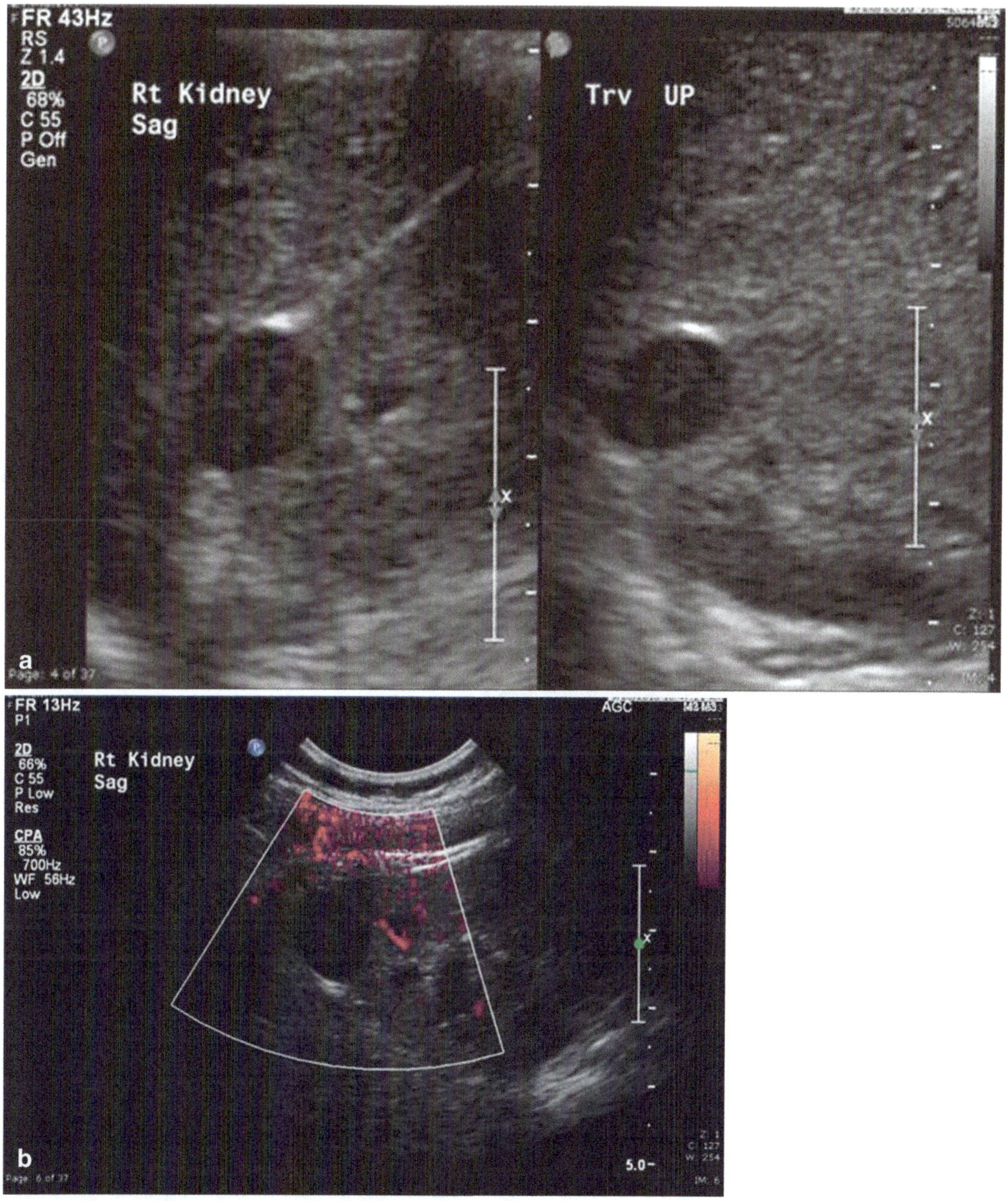

Fig. 11.21 Hemorrhagic cyst. *Grayscale* (**a**) and *power color* Doppler (**b**). Ultrasound right kidney. Hypoechoic lesion, with posterior acoustic enhancement and low-level internal echoes consistent with hemorrhage. No internal vascularity. Resolved on follow-up

Imaging

On ultrasound, a hemorrhagic cyst may contain homogeneous low-level echoes, diffuse, lace-like internal echotexture, or heterogeneous, echogenic debris/clot, depending on timing of imaging. No internal vascularity (Fig. 11.21).

In the acute phase, on non-contrast CT, the hemorrhage attains a Hounsfield unit value of 70–90. As the cyst organizes the Hounsfield units may decrease and the walls or central area of the cyst may become calcified. It is the high attenuation of the cystic structures and the associated calcifications that necessitate routine monitoring of these lesions to ensure that they do not develop true malignant features [51].

On MRI, signal characteristics depend on the stage of the blood products. The most convincing evidence of hemorrhage is a hyperintense T1 signal seen with extracellular methemoglobin. Any signal on T2 other than bright suggests proteinaceous material, including blood products. Calcifications are not typically seen on MRI due to small size (Fig. 11.22).

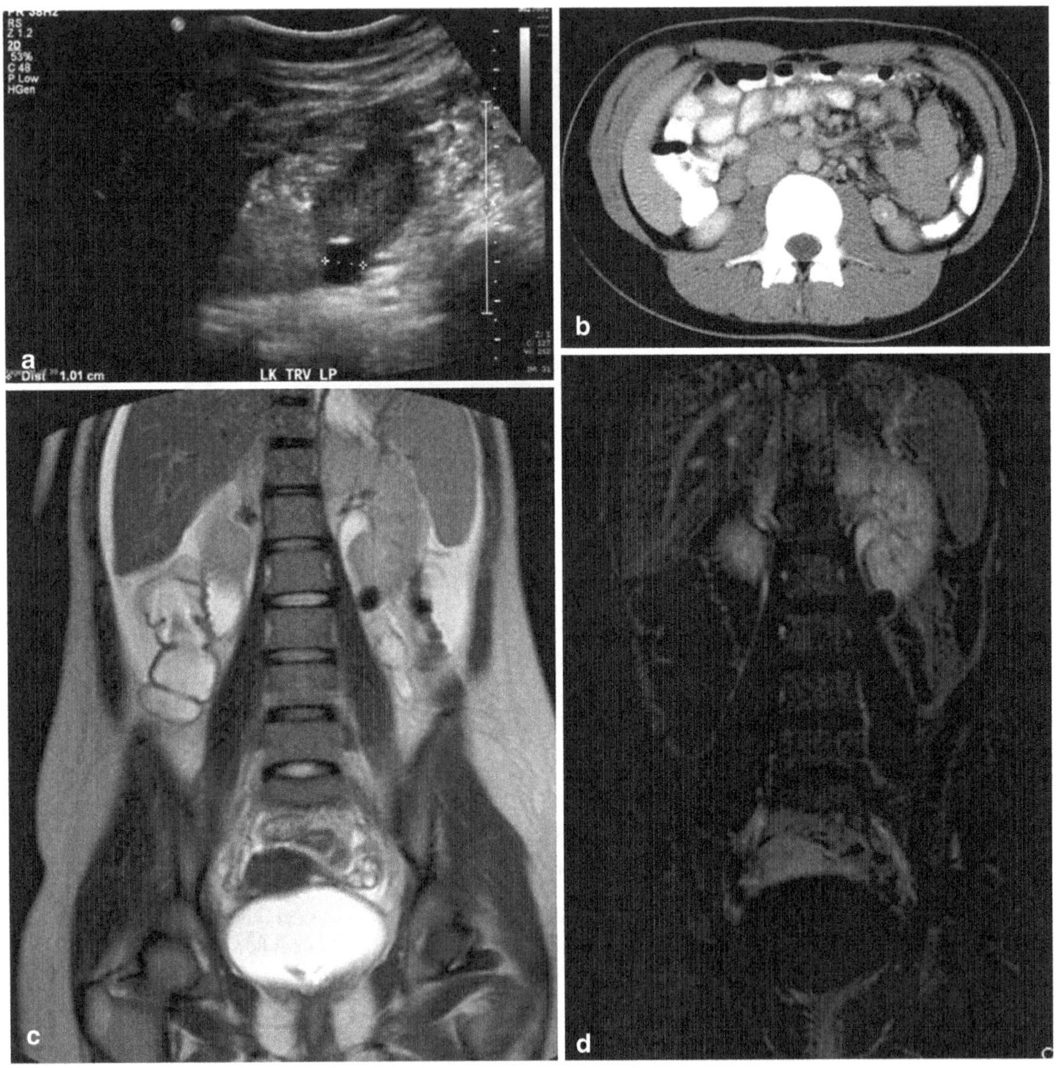

Fig. 11.22 Hemorrhagic cyst. *Grayscale* ultrasound left kidney (**a**) hypoechoic lesion, with posterior acoustic enhancement and low-level internal echoes. Peripheral thin echogenic calcification in the wall. CT abdomen (**b**) hyperdense exophytic lower pole cyst with central dense calcified focus. MRI Abdomen, coronal T2 (**c**) and coronal post-contrast T1 subtraction (**d**), with 1 year follow-up coronal T2 fat saturated. (**e**) Interval change in T2 signal from T2 dark to T2 bright, compatible with evolution of blood product, in a nonenhancing hemorrhagic cyst

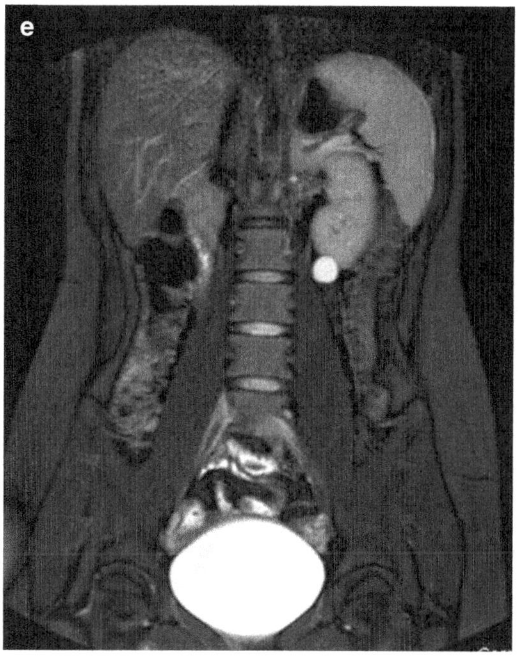

Fig. 11.22 (continued)

Complex Cyst

A complex cyst is a cyst which is associated with septa or hemorrhage (Fig. 11.23). Thickened, irregular septa and walls, coarse calcifications, and vascular soft tissue components are ominous signs within a cystic lesion, and exclusion of neoplasm based on imaging becomes difficult.

On ultrasound, a complex cyst may contain thin septa, thin calcification, and/or debris, including hemorrhage; however, no vascularity is seen within the septa or echogenic components. Cysts have good through transmission and posterior acoustic enhancement. There may be fluid-fluid levels or low-level internal echoes. Cysts containing milk of calcium may demonstrate comet tail artifact. Depending on the size of the calcifications, there may be posterior acoustic shadowing.

Non-contrast CT may demonstrate increased Hounsfield units, greater than 20. CT is the preferred modality for detection of calcifications. Thin septa with minimal enhancement and fluid-fluid levels may be detected.

On MRI, complex cyst can have variable T1/T2 signal depending on the presence of proteinaceous material. There is minimal enhancement of the thin septae and walls. Calcifications are difficult to detect on MRI. Diffusion-weighted imaging is gaining an important role in detecting suspicious soft tissue components within cystic lesions.

Cystic Diseases Associated With Genetic Abnormalities: Juvenile Nephronophthisis (JNPHP) and Medullary Cystic Disease of the Kidney

Etiology and Presentation

These two diseases are typified by small, corticomedullary, and deep medullary cysts (Fig. 11.24). JNPHP is an autosomal recessive mutation mapped to several genes. The infantile form is associated with chromosome 9q, the juvenile form associated with chromosomes 2q and 1p36, and the adolescent chromosome 3q involving a gene product called nephrocystin [48, 53]. The kidneys are usually small at the time of diagnosis, typically in the first decade. Associated presenting signs and symptoms include polyuria (concentrating defect), polydipsia, Fanconi syndrome, and growth retardation [48, 50]. The disease is bilateral and is associated with congenital hepatic fibrosis and end-stage renal disease [54].

Medullary cystic disease of the kidney is inherited in an autosomal dominant fashion. It has an indistinguishable pathologic appearance to JNPHP, but it does not occur in children (age >20 years) and does not have any of the associated systemic abnormalities that are seen in JNPHP [55].

Autosomal Recessive Polycystic Kidney Disease (ARPKD)

Etiology and Presentation

ARPKD is usually diagnosed in the newborn period with either acute renal or liver failure. It can, however, present in the childhood or teenage

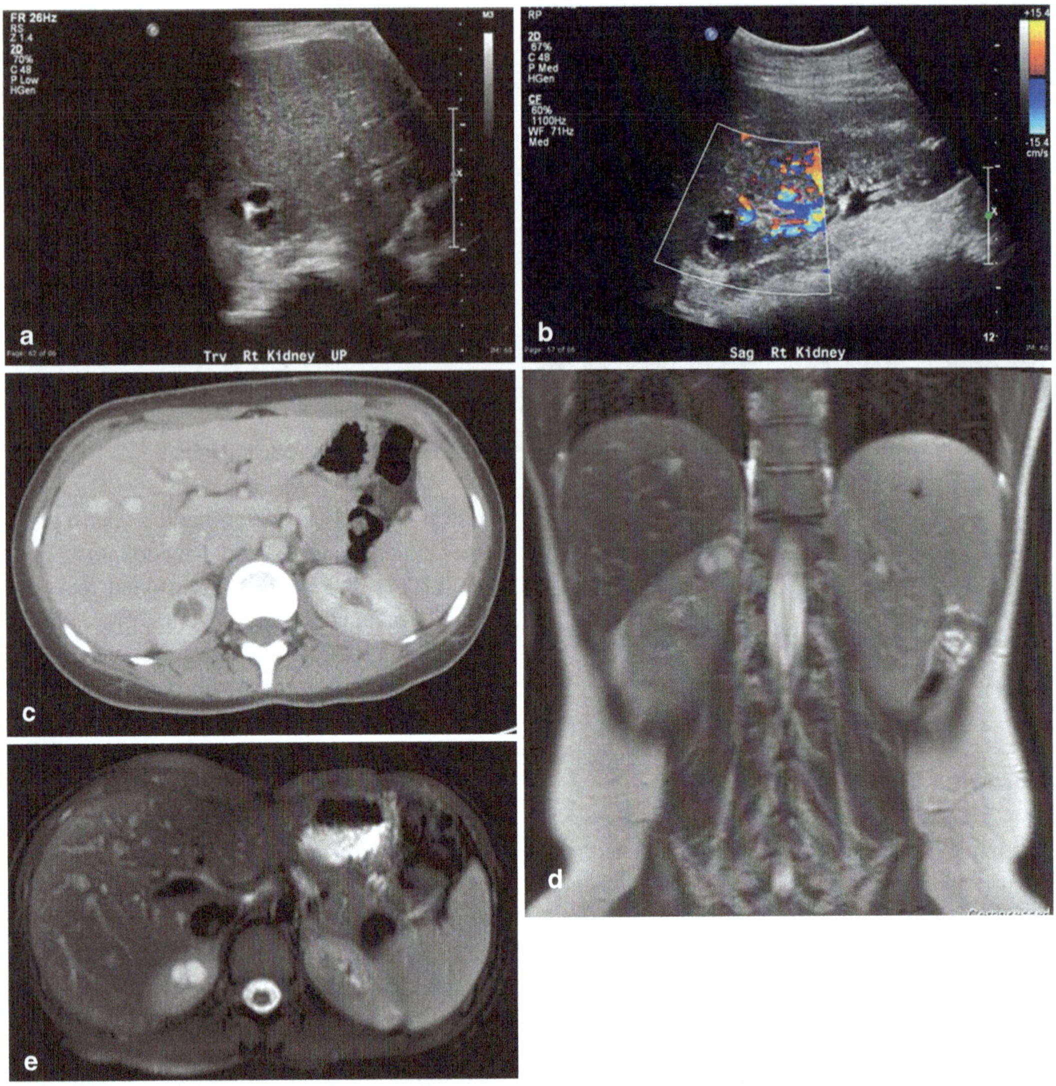

Fig. 11.23 Complex cyst. *Grayscale* (**a**) and *color* Doppler ultrasound (**b**) right kidney: anechoic lesion upper pole, with echogenic septations and no internal vascularity. CT abdomen, axial nephrographic phase. (**c**) Hypodense lesion with thin nonenhancing septation. MRI abdomen, axial T2 fat saturated and coronal T2. (**d** and **e**) Lobular T2 hyperintense lesion with thin septations

years. The severity of the disease is related to age of onset as neonatal presentation correlates with a more severe form of the disease. All affected children have associated liver or pancreatic cysts in addition to some degree of hepatic fibrosis [46]. Usually, one organ (liver or kidney) predominates clinically. The disease stems from a genetic mutation of the PKHD 1 gene located on chromosome 6 (6p21) producing an alteration in the fibrocystin/polyductin protein [56, 57]. Antenatally, there may be a maternal history of oligohydramnios since normal urine output is reduced. The most obvious deformity at birth is the evidence of Potter's facies, which is a result of the decreased amniotic fluid throughout gestation. Pulmonary hypoplasia from a lack of surfactant production is

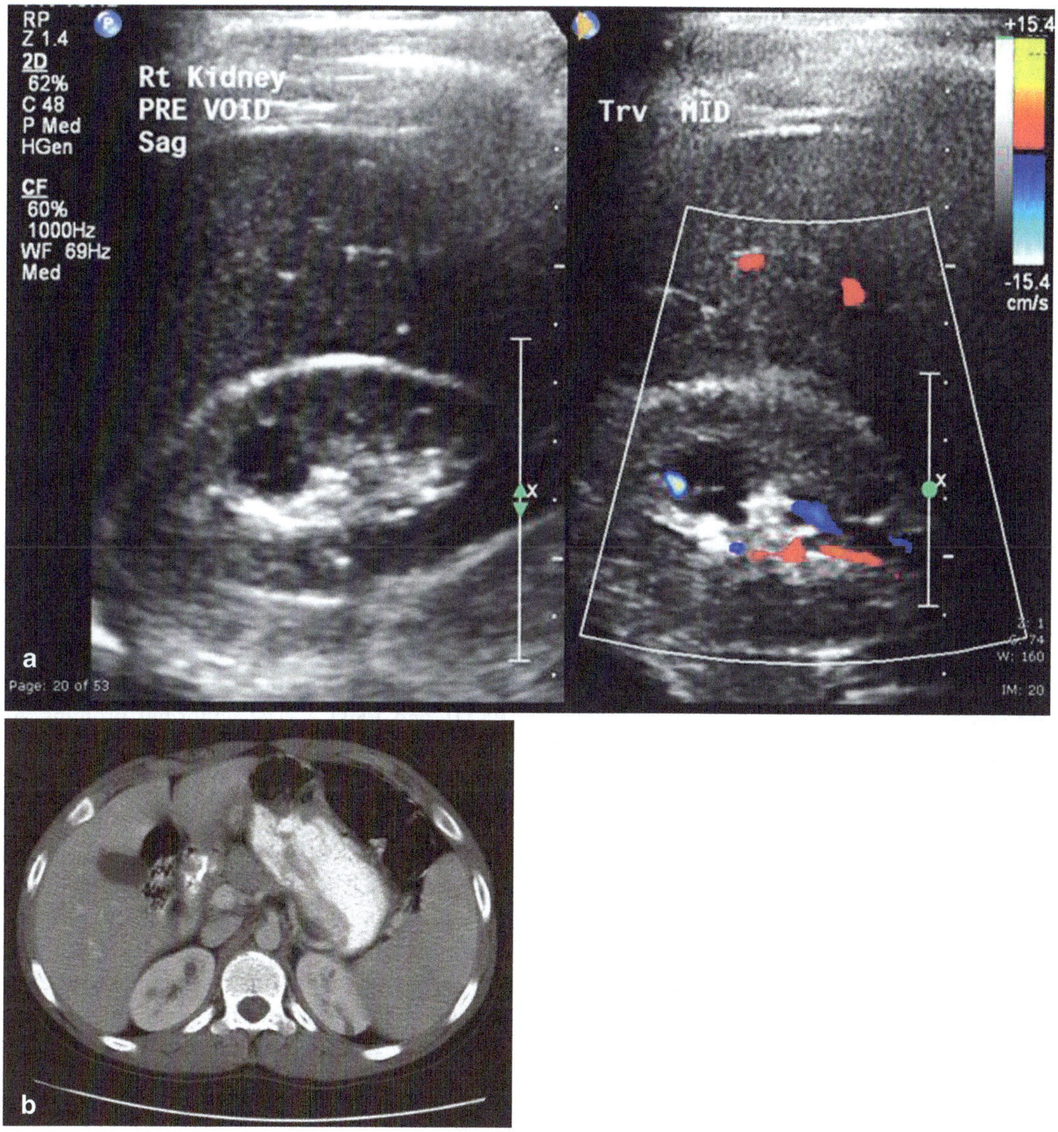

Fig. 11.24 Nephronophthisis (15 years old). (**a**) *Grayscale* and *color* Doppler ultrasound right kidney and (**b**) CT abdomen nephrographic phase. Small right kidney, measuring 7.9 cm (nl range for age 7.5–11.0 cm), with loss of corticomedullary differentiation and medullary cyst. Cyst contains thin septations. Small hypodense cystic lesions in the medulla on the right and at the corticomedullary junction on the left

the most common cause of fetal demise in these children (Fig. 11.25).

There is no cure for ARPKD and supportive therapy including dialysis or renal transplantation must be routinely implemented. In addition to renal failure, children can develop hepatic failure, hypertension, pulmonary disease, and esophageal varices.

Histopathology

Children with ARPKD are born with extremely large kidneys with very small diffuse cortical cysts. The abnormality in the nephron occurs in the collecting ducts, where there is cystic dilation. Grossly, the cysts can be seen upon sectioning the kidney. Microscopic liver findings consist of

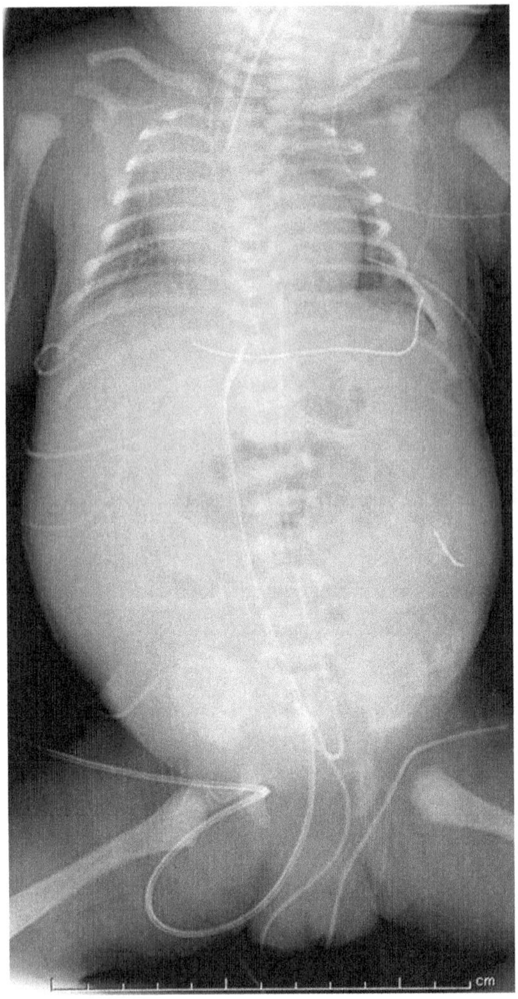

Fig. 11.25 ARPKD. Babygram, DOL 0. Increased abdominal girth, with centralized bowel loops due to enlarged kidneys and ascites fluid. Small thorax secondary to pulmonary hypoplasia, with left-sided chest tube for pneumothorax

periportal cysts in association with fibrosis, but gross lesions are difficult to identify.

Imaging

Ultrasound findings in ARPKD occur prenatally with decreased amniotic fluid and kidneys that may be hyperechoic and large for gestational age. In the neonatal period the sonographic findings of the kidneys include large, hyperechoic kidneys. Additionally, there is loss of the corticomedullary differentiation. In older children with ARPKD, larger cysts may be identified, but they are virtually never identified in younger children. CT scan of the child with ARPKD shows a pooling of contrast peripherally in the collecting ducts. Similarly, MRI shows the cysts as well. The T1-weighted images show fluid as dark where on T2 fluid is bright (Figs. 11.26 and 11.27).

Autosomal Dominant Polycystic Kidney Disease (ADPKD)

Etiology and Presentation

ADPKD is more common than ARPKD. In most affected families, the disease stems from a genetic defect involving chromosomes 4 and 16 and a small subset with an unmapped defect termed PKD3. Genetic testing is available for PKD1 and PKD 2. The abnormal proteins are polycystin-1 and polycystin-2 which are associated with ADPDK1 and 2, respectively [58]. ARKPD occurs in 1 in 500 live births. Clinically significant ADPKD is more common in males than females. The disease is not routinely diagnosed in childhood in patients without a family history since clinical manifestations usually do not occur until adulthood. All people who carry the dominant mutation will eventually develop some clinically relevant finding if they live long enough. In addition to the classic finding of large renal cysts that eventually dominate the kidney, other systemic anomalies including berry aneurysms (40 %); cysts of the spleen, pancreas, and liver; colonic diverticula; aortic aneurysm; and mitral valve prolapse can occur. The most common, clinically significant, presenting sign is hypertension. In addition, most patients have some degree of micro- or macroscopic hematuria that occurs by the fourth decade. Up to 30 % of patients with ADPKD present with nephrolithiasis at some point [59], and almost all patients with cystic disease suffer from flank pain during their lifetime. If the flank pain becomes significant, it can be treated with

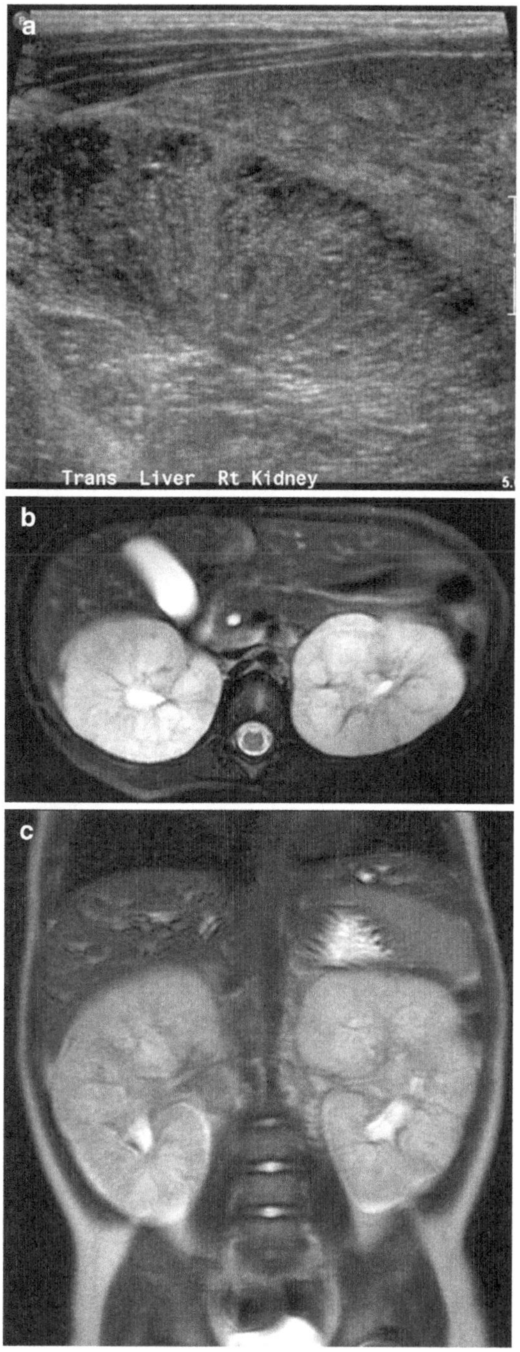

Fig. 11.26 ARPKD. High-frequency ultrasound kidney/liver. (**a**) Enlarged echogenic kidney with radiating dilated collecting ducts extending into the cortex. Also shown, increased liver echogenicity compatible with hepatic fibrosis. MRI kidney, axial T2 fat saturated (**b**) and coronal T2 (**c**). Enlarged T2 hyperintense kidneys, with preservation of reniform architecture

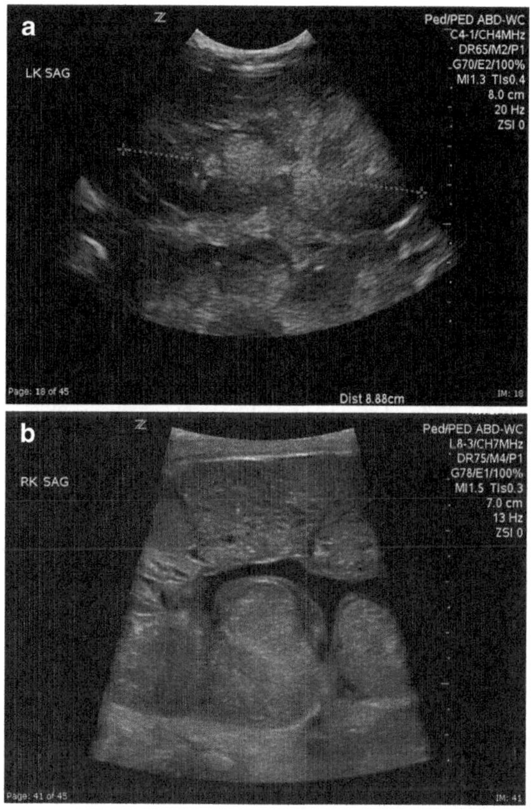

Fig. 11.27 ARPKD. Ultrasound left kidney, low-frequency transducer (**a**) and high-frequency transducer (**b**), DOL 1. Enlarged, echogenic left kidney. Increased echogenicity with small irregular medullary cystic spaces compatible with dilated collecting ducts

aspiration or unroofing [60]. Women with ADPKD have more episodes of pyelonephritis than men. PDK2 has a higher life expectancy and later onset then PKD1.

Histopathology

The abnormality is associated with abnormal epithelial cell polarity and can occur at any point in the nephron, explaining the presence of cysts throughout the medulla and cortex. In addition, the cells secrete excess epithelial growth factor which stimulates epithelial cell proliferation within the cyst walls. Grossly the cysts can range in size from tiny to quite large. Initially, the histological finding is focal tubular proliferation.

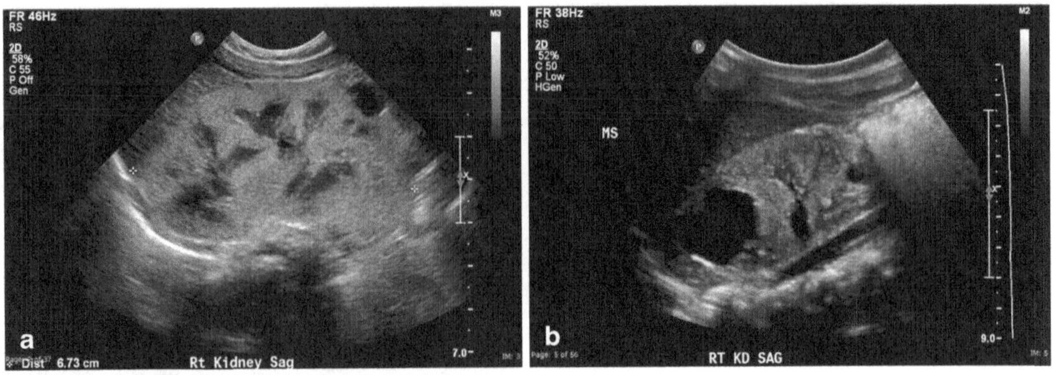

Fig. 11.28 ADPKD. Ultrasound right kidney at 2 months (**a**) and 2 years (**b**). Enlarged echogenic kidney with cortical cysts. Not shown, multiple additional subcentimeter cortical cyst, bilaterally

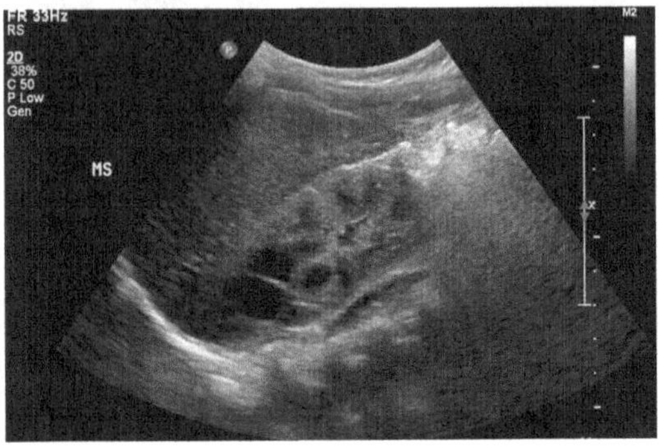

Fig. 11.29 ADPKD. Ultrasound right kidney. Echogenic kidney contains a large upper-pole cyst with thin septation

As the cysts increase and multiply and replace the parenchyma, the typical end-stage renal disease findings are incurred: arteriosclerosis and interstitial fibrosis; hyperplastic polyps are routinely seen. The incidence of renal cell carcinoma is elevated in ADPKD, but no more so than in the general population with ESRD.

Imaging (Figs. 11.28, 11.29, and 11.30)

If renal cysts are seen on the sonogram, then additional abdominal ultrasonography should be done to evaluate the other organs for cysts. Bilateral renal enlargement is typical. In younger children the radiologic appearance may resemble ARPKD, but eventually larger, dominating cysts will develop.

CT and MRI findings are similar to those found on ultrasound. These modalities can also differentiate hemorrhage from rupture during an episode of acute flank pain. For this purpose CT can delineate the fluid medium by distinguishing the Hounsfield units of the liquid. MRI can do the same by determining the signals on T1 and T2. Calcifications within the walls of the kidney are common and depending on their thickness can indicate malignant potential.

Cystic Diseases Not Associated with Genetic Anomalies

Multicystic Dysplastic Kidney (MCDK)

Etiology and Presentation

MCDK is a congenital developmental abnormality that consists of a nonfunctioning kidney formed of smooth cysts. It is usually discovered through antenatal ultrasound in 1/4,300 live births [61]. It has no gender or laterality predilection. It is the most common cause of antenatally detected cystic renal disease [62]. It is the second most common cause of a palpable abdominal mass in a neonate and the most common cause of cystic disease in the infant [63]. Other ipsilateral abnormalities including

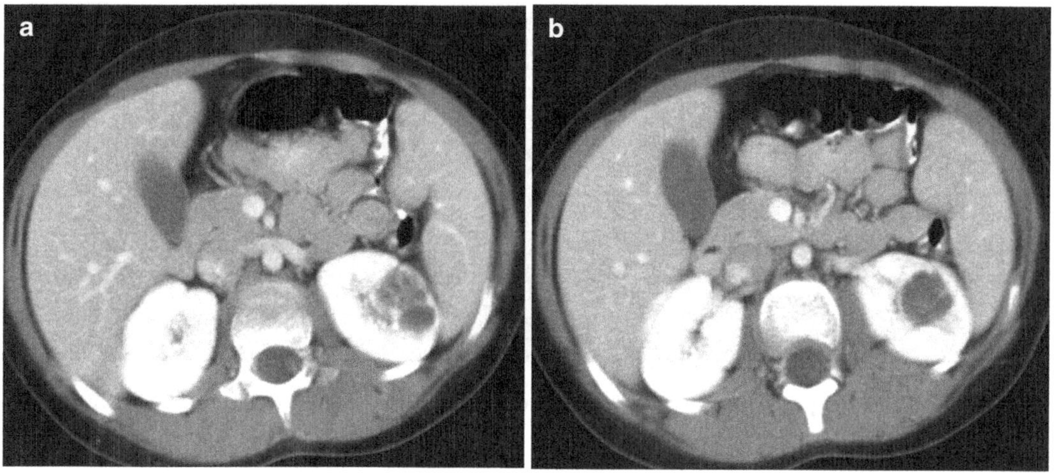

Fig. 11.30 ADPKD. CT Abdomen, sequential axial images nephrographic phase (**a** and **b**). Unilateral multilobular, multilocular hypodense cystic lesion, with thin septations

megaureter, posterior urethral valves, internal cystic structures in the male, and Gartner's cyst in the female can be seen [64]. Compensatory hypertrophy is seen routinely in the functioning kidney. Although children with MCDK are monitored for hypertension and malignancy, it is unclear from the literature if there is a true risk of either [65]. The literature suggests that 40 % of MCDK kidneys involute completely [66, 67]. At this time, nephrectomy is only indicated in patients whom the affected kidney is enlarging instead of decreasing in size and in patients with hypertension [68]. It is debatable whether or not hypertension improves in patients who undergo nephrectomy for MCDK but is still recommended [69]. MCDK can present in older children and adults with hematuria, pain, infection, or hypertension or found incidentally during imaging performed for other purposes.

Histopathology

MCDK is a severe form of dysplasia typically rendering the kidney nonfunctional. The etiology is thought due to dysfunctional cell-cell interactions between the ureteral bud and the metanephric blastema. Kidney size depends upon the configuration and size of the cysts. Potter described two types: type 2b – small cysts with stromal predomination and type 2a – larger cysts with no identifiable parenchyma [66]. Historically, the risk of malignant degeneration is low (1/3,470), but associated reported pathologic diagnosis includes RCC, Wilms' tumor, and mesothelioma. A recent meta-analysis cited no cases of malignancy [70]. Grossly, the kidneys appear as a cluster of grapes [71].

Imaging

The current radiologic work-up in a neonate with MCDK includes a sonogram, voiding cystourethrogram, and a nuclear medicine scan. Historically, MCDK has been followed with interval renal ultrasounds to ensure involution and more importantly lack of solid tissue growth of the affected kidney (Fig. 11.31).

Fetal ultrasound of an MCDK typically shows small round cysts that increase in size and number over the course of the gestation. The kidneys tend to be more echogenic than normal kidneys. The sine qua non of findings are noncommunicating cysts (although they may grossly communicate) that are not centered around a central

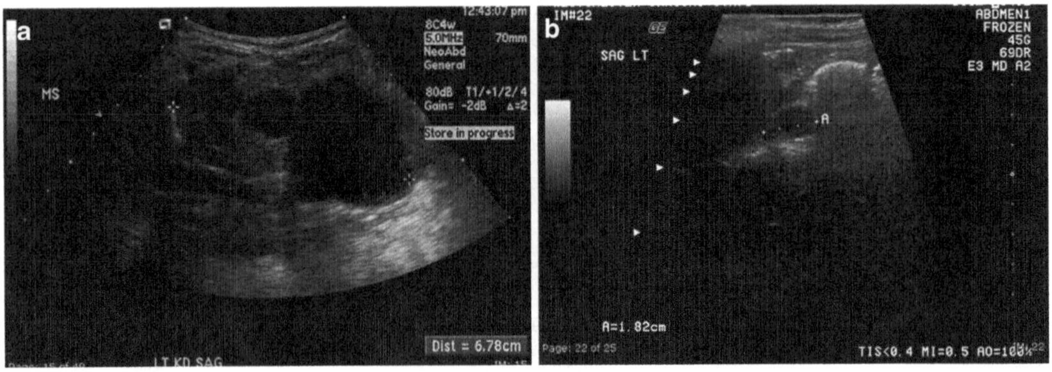

Fig. 11.31 MCDK. Ultrasound left kidney at diagnosis (**a**) and 1 year interval (**b**). Interval decrease in size of kidney and cysts compatible with involution of MCDK (**b**)

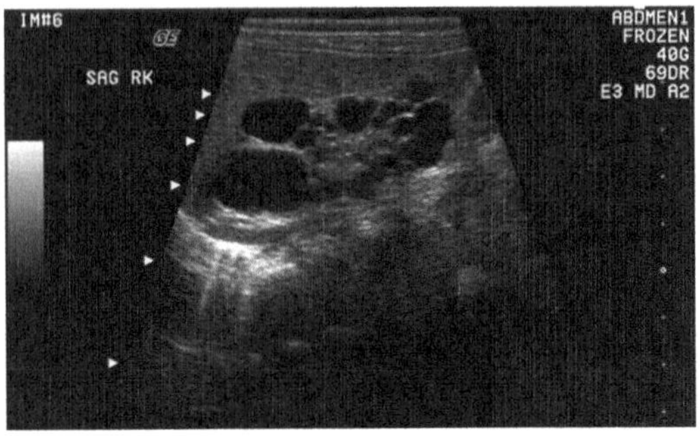

Fig. 11.32 Multicystic dysplastic kidney (*MCDK*). Ultrasound right kidney. Multiple noncommunicating cyst of variable size and no normal reniform parenchyma

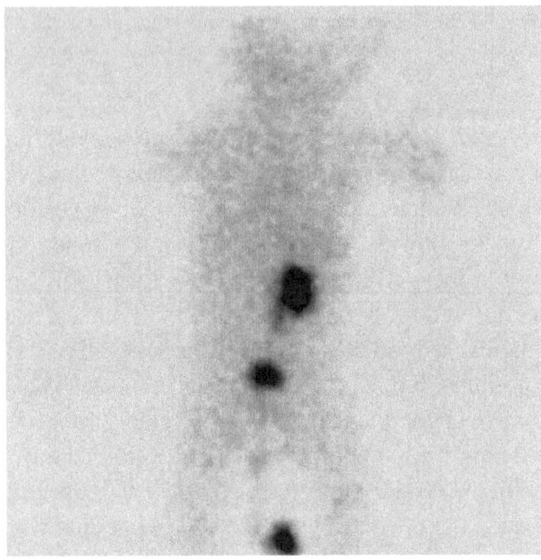

Fig. 11.33 MCDK. Nuclear Medicine Tc99m MAG-3 renogram. Early dynamic image with no activity in the left renal bed

medial cyst (Fig. 11.32). The most distinctive feature of hydronephrosis is the centrally located fluid collection (pelvis) and some identifiable parenchymal tissue. In MCDK, compensatory contralateral renal growth is noted. The use of Doppler may be useful in observing total absence of perfusion [71]. Ultrasound is useful for diagnosing other associated abnormalities, including Gartner's cyst, hemivagina, seminal vesicle cyst, pelvic kidney, megaureter, hydronephrosis, or neurogenic bladder [72].

VCUG is recommended in children with MCDK as there is a reported incidence of 4–25 % of contralateral reflux. Some authors dispute the need of VCUG in children who have had two normal ultrasounds in infancy [73].

A DMSA renal scan can be performed to confirm nonfunction of the kidney and thus distinguish the MCDK definitively from a congenital UPJ obstruction. Nevertheless, there can still be confusion as to the true etiology of the mass, since some MCDKs have minimal (but not absent) uptake on the renal scan (Fig. 11.33).

Distinction between an MCDK and a ureteropelvic junction obstruction may be difficult (Fig. 11.34). When further characterization of the kidneys and collecting systems is needed, one may consider MR urography (MRU). MRU has excellent morphologic delineation of the renal parenchyma and collecting systems, including ureteral course and insertions (Fig. 11.35).

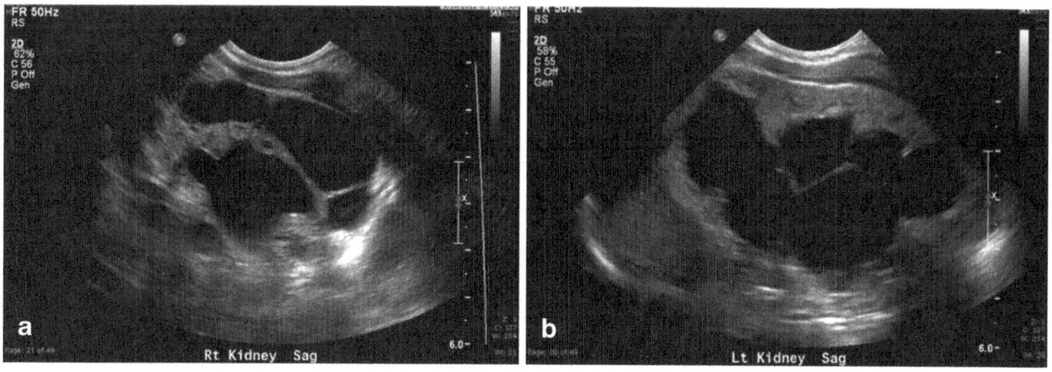

Fig. 11.34 MCDK. Ultrasound bilateral kidneys. Right kidney (**a**): multiple peripheral cyst without communication to renal pelvis compatible with multicystic dysplastic kidney. Left kidney (**b**): grade IV hydronephrosis, with increased renal echotexture and loss of corticomedullary differentiation

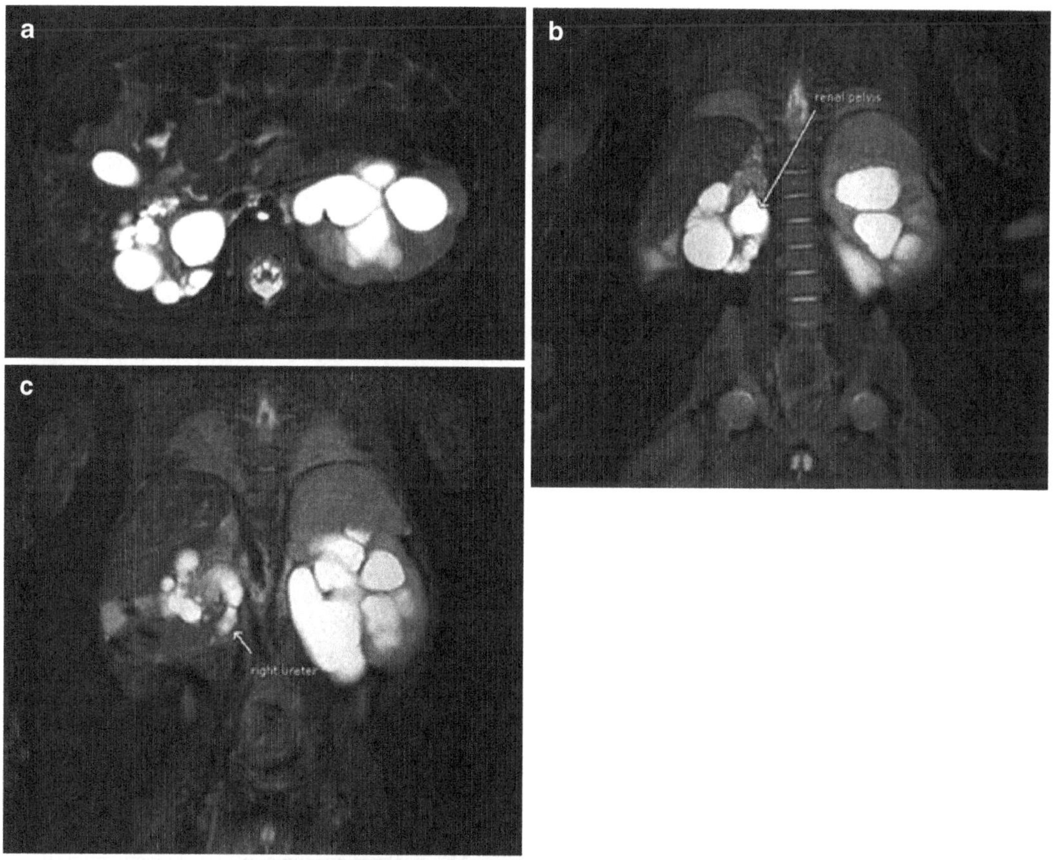

Fig. 11.35 MCDK with contralateral ureteropelvic junction obstruction. MR urogram, axial T2 fat saturation, high resolution (**a**) multiple T2 hyperintense peripheral cystic lesions, of varying size, which do not communicate with central dilated renal pelvis. Grade IV hydronephrosis on the left, with increased T2 renal parenchymal signal and loss of corticomedullary differentiation. Coronal T2 fat saturated (**b** and **c**) proximal ureteral obstruction, on the right, accounting for dysplasia. Abrupt ureteropelvic junction, on the left, with normal caliber ureter (not shown)

References

1. Davidoff AM. Wilms' tumor. Curr Opin Pediatr. 2009;21:357–64.
2. Breslow N, Olshan A, Beckwith JB, Green DM. Epidemiology of Wilms tumor. Med Pediatr Oncol. 1993;21:172–81.
3. Nakamura L, Ritchey M. Current management of Wilms' tumor. Curr Urol Rep. 2010;11:58–65.
4. Geller E, Kochan PS. Renal neoplasms of childhood. Radiol Clin North Am. 2011;49:689–709, vi.
5. Fishman EK, Hartman DS, Goldman SM, Siegelman SS. The CT appearance of Wilms tumor. J Comput Assist Tomogr. 1983;7:659–65.
6. Beckwith JB, Palmer NF. Histopathology and prognosis of Wilms tumors: results from the First National Wilms' Tumor Study. Cancer. 1978;41: 1937–48.
7. Gow KW, Roberts IF, Jamieson DH, Bray H, Magee JF, Murphy JJ. Local staging of Wilms' tumor–computerized tomography correlation with histological findings. J Pediatr Surg. 2000;35:677–9.
8. Reiman TA, Siegel MJ, Shackelford GD. Wilms tumor in children: abdominal CT and US evaluation. Radiology. 1986;160:501–5.
9. Schenk JP, Graf N, Gunther P, et al. Role of MRI in the management of patients with nephroblastoma. Eur Radiol. 2008;18:683–91.
10. Lonergan GJ, Martinez-Leon MI, Agrons GA, Montemarano H, Suarez ES. Nephrogenic rests, nephroblastomatosis, and associated lesions of the kidney. Radiographics. 1998;18:947–68.
11. Rohrschneider WK, Weirich A, Rieden K, Darge K, Troger J, Graf N. US, CT and MR imaging characteristics of nephroblastomatosis. Pediatr Radiol. 1998; 28:435–43.
12. Gylys-Morin V, Hoffer FA, Kozakewich H, Shamberger RC. Wilms tumor and nephroblastomatosis: imaging characteristics at gadolinium-enhanced MR imaging. Radiology. 1993;188:517–21.
13. Blitman NM, Berkenblit RG, Rozenblit AM, Levin TL. Renal medullary carcinoma: CT and MRI features. AJR Am J Roentgenol. 2005;185:268–72.
14. Lowe LH, Isuani BH, Heller RM, et al. Pediatric renal masses: Wilms tumor and beyond. Radiographics. 2000;20:1585–603.
15. Davis Jr CJ, Mostofi FK, Sesterhenn IA. Renal medullary carcinoma. The seventh sickle cell nephropathy. Am J Surg Pathol. 1995;19:1–11.
16. Khan A, Thomas N, Costello B, et al. Renal medullary carcinoma: sonographic, computed tomography, magnetic resonance and angiographic findings. Eur J Radiol. 2000;35:1–7.
17. Pickhardt PJ. Renal medullary carcinoma: an aggressive neoplasm in patients with sickle cell trait. Abdom Imaging. 1998;23:531–2.
18. Argani P, Perlman EJ, Breslow NE, et al. Clear cell sarcoma of the kidney: a review of 351 cases from the National Wilms Tumor Study Group Pathology Center. Am J Surg Pathol. 2000;24:4–18.
19. Glass RB, Davidson AJ, Fernbach SK. Clear cell sarcoma of the kidney: CT, sonographic, and pathologic correlation. Radiology. 1991;180:715–17.
20. Weeks DA, Beckwith JB, Mierau GW, Luckey DW. Rhabdoid tumor of kidney. A report of 111 cases from the National Wilms' Tumor Study Pathology Center. Am J Surg Pathol. 1989;13:439–58.
21. Agrons GA, Kingsman KD, Wagner BJ, Sotelo-Avila C. Rhabdoid tumor of the kidney in children: a comparative study of 21 cases. AJR Am J Roentgenol. 1997;168:447–51.
22. Chung CJ, Lorenzo R, Rayder S, et al. Rhabdoid tumors of the kidney in children: CT findings. AJR Am J Roentgenol. 1995;164:697–700.
23. Panuel M, Bourliere-Najean B, Scheiner C, et al. Radiologic features of rhabdoid tumor of the kidney. Eur J Radiol. 1992;14:204–6.
24. Bruder E, Passera O, Harms D, et al. Morphologic and molecular characterization of renal cell carcinoma in children and young adults. Am J Surg Pathol. 2004;28: 1117–32.
25. Spreafico F, Collini P, Terenziani M, Marchiano A, Piva L. Renal cell carcinoma in children and adolescents. Expert Rev Anticancer Ther. 2010;10:1 967–78.
26. Ahmed HU, Arya M, Levitt G, Duffy PG, Mushtaq I, Sebire NJ. Part I: primary malignant non-Wilms' renal tumours in children. Lancet Oncol. 2007;8:730–7.
27. Chaudry G, Perez-Atayde AR, Ngan BY, Gundogan M, Daneman A. Imaging of congenital mesoblastic nephroma with pathological correlation. Pediatr Radiol. 2009;39:1080–6.
28. Chan HS, Cheng MY, Mancer K, et al. Congenital mesoblastic nephroma: a clinicoradiologic study of 17 cases representing the pathologic spectrum of the disease. J Pediatr. 1987;111:64–70.
29. Irsutti M, Puget C, Baunin C, Duga I, Sarramon MF, Guitard J. Mesoblastic nephroma: prenatal ultrasonographic and MRI features. Pediatr Radiol. 2000;30: 147–50.
30. Chen YF, Li YW, Sheih CP, Hsu CY. Renal cell carcinoma: unusual pediatric renal tumors. J Formos Med Assoc. 1999;98:118–21.
31. Madewell JE, Goldman SM, Davis Jr CJ, Hartman DS, Feigin DS, Lichtenstein JE. Multilocular cystic nephroma: a radiographic-pathologic correlation of 58 patients. Radiology. 1983;146:309–21.
32. Davis Jr CJ, Barton JH, Sesterhenn IA, Mostofi FK. Metanephric adenoma. Clinicopathological study of fifty patients. Am J Surg Pathol. 1995;19:1101–14.
33. Bastide C, Rambeaud JJ, Bach AM, Russo P. Metanephric adenoma of the kidney: clinical and radiological study of nine cases. BJU Int. 2009;103: 1544–8.
34. Hartman DJ, Maclennan GT. Renal metanephric adenoma. J Urol. 2007;178:1058.
35. Halpenny D, Snow A, McNeill G, Torreggiani WC. The radiological diagnosis and treatment of renal angiomyolipoma-current status. Clin Radiol. 2010;65: 99–108.

36. Ewalt DH, Sheffield E, Sparagana SP, Delgado MR, Roach ES. Renal lesion growth in children with tuberous sclerosis complex. J Urol. 1998;160:141–5.
37. Casper KA, Donnelly LF, Chen B, Bissler JJ. Tuberous sclerosis complex: renal imaging findings. Radiology. 2002;225:451–6.
38. Bissler JJ, Kingswood JC. Renal angiomyolipomata. Kidney Int. 2004;66:924–34.
39. Oesterling JE, Fishman EK, Goldman SM, Marshall FF. The management of renal angiomyolipoma. J Urol. 1986;135:1121–4.
40. Lienert AR, Nicol D. Renal angiomyolipoma. BJU Int. 2012;110 Suppl 4:25–7.
41. Arranz Arija JA, Carrion JR, Garcia FR, et al. Primary renal lymphoma: report of 3 cases and review of the literature. Am J Nephrol. 1994;14:148–53.
42. Pradeep R, Madhumathi DS, Lakshmidevi V, et al. Bilateral nephromegaly simulating Wilms tumor: a rare initial manifestation of acute lymphoblastic leukemia. J Pediatr Hematol Oncol. 2008;30:471–3.
43. Erdem E, Kayiran P, Ozcelik G, Ozel A, Yildiz YZ. Rare presentation of pediatric acute lymphoblastic leukemia: nephromegaly at time of diagnosis. Indian J Hematol Blood Transfus. 2011;27:43–5.
44. Rajantie J, Jaaskelainen J, Perkkio M, Siimes MA. Kidneys very large at diagnosis are associated with poor prognosis in children with acute lymphoblastic leukemia. Am J Pediatr Hematol Oncol. 1986;8:87–90.
45. Richmond J, Sherman RS, Diamond HD, Craver LF. Renal lesions associated with malignant lymphomas. Am J Med. 1962;32:184–207.
46. Campbell MF, Wein AJ, Kavoussi LR. Campbell-Walsh urology, editor-in-chief, Alan J. Wein; editors, Louis R. Kavoussi … [et al.]. 9th ed. Philadelphia: W.B. Saunders; 2007.
47. Dugougeat F, Navarro O, Soares Souza AS, Geary D, Daneman A. Multiple unilateral renal cysts in two children. Pediatr Radiol. 2000;30:346–8.
48. McHugh K, Stringer DA, Hebert D, Babiak CA. Simple renal cysts in children: diagnosis and follow-up with US. Radiology. 1991;178:383–5.
49. Terada N, Ichioka K, Matsuta Y, Okubo K, Yoshimura K, Arai Y. The natural history of simple renal cysts. J Urol. 2002;167:21–3.
50. Blazer S, Zimmer EZ, Blumenfeld Z, Zelikovic I, Bronshtein M. Natural history of fetal simple renal cysts detected in early pregnancy. J Urol. 1999;162:812–14.
51. Bisceglia M, Galliani CA, Senger C, Stallone C, Sessa A. Renal cystic diseases: a review. Adv Anatomic Pathol. 2006;13:26–56.
52. Eknoyan G. A clinical view of simple and complex renal cysts. J Am Soc Nephrol. 2009;20:1874–6.
53. Gascue C, Katsanis N, Badano JL. Cystic diseases of the kidney: ciliary dysfunction and cystogenic mechanisms. Pediatr Nephrol. 2011;26:1181–95.
54. Witzleben CL, Sharp AR. "Nephronophthisis-congenital hepatic fibrosis": an additional hepatorenal disorder. Human Pathol. 1982;13:728–33.
55. Scolari F, Puzzer D, Amoroso A, et al. Identification of a new locus for medullary cystic disease, on chromosome 16p12. Am J Hum Genet. 1999;64:1655–60.
56. Harris PC, Rossetti S. Molecular genetics of autosomal recessive polycystic kidney disease. Mol Genet Metabol. 2004;81:75–85.
57. Zerres K, Mucher G, Bachner L, et al. Mapping of the gene for autosomal recessive polycystic kidney disease (ARPKD) to chromosome 6p21-cen. Nat Genet. 1994;7:429–32.
58. Gabow PA. Autosomal dominant polycystic kidney disease. N Engl J Med. 1993;329:332–42.
59. Torres VE, Erickson SB, Smith LH, Wilson DM, Hattery RR, Segura JW. The association of nephrolithiasis and autosomal dominant polycystic kidney disease. Am J Kidney Dis. 1988;11:318–25.
60. Brown JA, Torres VE, King BF, Segura JW. Laparoscopic marsupialization of symptomatic polycystic kidney disease. J Urol. 1996;156:22–7.
61. Gordon AC, Thomas DF, Arthur RJ, Irving HC. Multicystic dysplastic kidney: is nephrectomy still appropriate? J Urol. 1988;140:1231–4.
62. Pollack HM. Clinical urography: an atlas and textbook of urological imaging. Philadelphia: Saunders; 1990.
63. Hartman GE, Shochat SJ. Abdominal mass lesions in the newborn: diagnosis and treatment. Clin Perinatol. 1989;16:123–35.
64. Merrot T, Lumenta DB, Tercier S, Morisson-Lacombes G, Guys JM, Alessandrini P. Multicystic dysplastic kidney with ipsilateral abnormalities of genitourinary tract: experience in children. Urology. 2006;67:603–7.
65. Onal B, Kogan BA. Natural history of patients with multicystic dysplastic kidney-what follow up is needed? J Urol. 2006;176:1607–11.
66. Osathanondh V, Potter EL. Pathogenesis of polycystic kidneys. Type 2 Due to inhibition of ampullary activity. Arch Pathol. 1964;77:474–84.
67. Kessler OJ, Ziv N, Livne PM, Merlob P. Involution rate of multicystic renal dysplasia. Pediatrics. 1998;102:E73.
68. Snodgrass WT. Hypertension associated with multicystic dysplastic kidney in children. J Urol. 2000;164:472–3;discussion 3–4.
69. Goldfarb DA. The renin-angiotensin system. New concepts in regulation of blood pressure and renal function. Urol Clin North Am. 1994;21:187–94.
70. Narchi H. Risk of Wilms' tumour with multicystic kidney disease: a systematic review. Arch Dis Child. 2005;90:147–9.
71. Riccabona M, Ring E, Fueger G, Petritsch P, Villits P. Doppler sonography in congenital ureteropelvic junction obstruction and multicystic dysplastic kidneys. Pediatr Radiol. 1993;23:502–5.
72. Walker D, Fennell R, Garin E, Richard G. Spectrum of multicystic renal dysplasia: diagnosis and management. Urology. 1978;11:433–6.
73. Ismaili K, Avni FE, Alexander M, Schulman C, Collier F, Hall M. Routine voiding cystourethrography is of no value in neonates with unilateral multicystic dysplastic kidney. J Pediatr. 2005;146:759–63.

12 Renal Imaging: Infection

Dana C. Rice, Massoud Majd, and H. Gil Rushton

Introduction

Principles of pediatric uroradiology are trending towards decreased or no radiation exposure with combined morphologic and functional imaging [1]. One of the major advances in non-radiation-based imaging technology has been in ultrasound [2] including motion mode, harmonic imaging, color Doppler sonography, duplex Doppler sonography, and three-dimensional (3D) techniques [3–5]. Reconstructed 3D ultrasound images are comparable to intravenous urography (IVU) or magnetic resonance urography (MRU), as well as allowing visualization of the bladder surface which is considered virtual cystoscopy [6, 7]. Additional advancements in ultrasonography enable functional studies such as contrast-enhanced voiding urosonography (VUS), which reportedly has the potential to become an alternative for voiding cystourethrography (VCUG) [8]. However, there are still limitations including limited evaluation of the urethra and bladder as well as longer study time [9].

MRU enables detailed functional and anatomic evaluation of the urinary system in a single test without radiation exposure. However, functional MRU studies are not yet standardized [1]. In addition, many younger children will require sedation or general anesthesia to successfully complete the study. Severe adverse reactions to gadolinium-based contrast agents are rare, but mild reactions such as headaches, nausea, and taste perversion occur in up to 8 % of patients [10]. Nephrogenic systemic fibrosis has been reported rarely in pediatric patients with acute or chronic renal failure. MRI compatible foreign bodies, such as ureteral stents, surgical clips, and prosthesis, may cause significant artifacts on the images which can decrease effectiveness of the study [10]. Even with its limitations, MRU has the potential to emerge as the imaging technique of choice for the evaluation of pediatric GU disorders.

Renal scintigraphy is often an underused imaging modality in the pediatric population. Understanding of pharmacologic properties of different renal radiopharmaceuticals and their relationship to renal physiologic principles are essential in appropriate use of this imaging modality. The administered dose of the radiopharmaceutical

D.C. Rice, MD
Department of Urology, George Washington University School of Medicine, Washington, DC, USA

M. Majd, MD, FACR
Section of Nuclear Medicine, Department of Radiology, Children's National Medical Center, 111 Michigan Avenue, NW, Washington, DC 20010, USA

Radiology and Pediatrics, George Washington University School of Medicine, Washington, DC, USA

H.G. Rushton, MD, FAAP (✉)
Division of Pediatric Urology, Children's National Medical Center, 111 Michigan Avenue, NW, Washington, DC 20010, USA

Urology and Pediatrics, George Washington University School of Medicine, Washington, DC, USA
e-mail: hrushton@childrensnational.org

L.S. Palmer, J.S. Palmer (eds.), *Pediatric and Adolescent Urologic Imaging*,
DOI 10.1007/978-1-4614-8654-1_12, © Springer Science+Business Media New York 2014

should be kept as low as possible. When used appropriately, radionuclide imaging provides insight into both anatomical and functional aspects of the genitourinary system with a low radiation dose and negligible side effects [11].

CT scanning is a widely available, quick and easy imaging technique for evaluation of many medical and surgical disorders. Both non-contrast stone protocols and contrast-enhanced CT urography are commonly used in the adult population. However, due to its high radiation dose, its use in children should be limited to complex cases or situations when MRI is not available [1, 12]. In fact, many institutions are currently conducting risk/benefit analysis for CT scan radiation dose. At this time in the United States, it is estimated that only 40 % of CT scanners are accredited [13]. Also being debated is the total dosage of radiation that puts someone at higher risk for oncologic side effects. In children in particular there are concerns that some settings for dosage safety are not being adjusted appropriately to weight-based criteria. Regulation is beginning to be legally enforced in some states. For instance, since July of 2012, California state law will require radiologists to record the dose of radiation each patient receives [13].

Acute Pyelonephritis

Acute pyelonephritis (APN) represents the most serious type of urinary tract infection (UTI) in children. It is not only responsible for acute morbidity, but it may lead to irreversible renal parenchymal damage. Approximately 8 % of girls and 2 % of boys will have a UTI during their first 8 years of life with febrile UTIs having the highest incidence within the first year of life [14, 15]. The diagnosis of APN in older children traditionally has been made on the basis of the classic signs and symptoms of fever and flank pain or tenderness associated with pyuria and positive urine culture. However, accurate diagnosis based solely on these parameters is often difficult, particularly in neonates and infants who may present with nonspecific symptoms such as irritability, poor feeding, failure to thrive, vomiting, and diarrhea [16, 17]. Despite the fact that the majority of patients (50–80 %) with fever and systemic clinical findings consistent with APN have abnormal DMSA scan findings, there is still a high false-positive and/or false-negative rate based on routine clinical and laboratory parameters [18].

Pathophysiology of Acute Pyelonephritis

Experimental studies by Roberts and others found that bacterial adherence to uroepithelium elicits an inflammatory cascade proportional to the virulence of the infecting organism. The acute inflammatory response responsible for the eradication of bacteria may lead to damage of interstitial renal tissue and result in subsequent renal scarring [19]. Studies have reported that focal ischemia from vascular occlusion [20], vasoconstriction [21], or vascular compression [22] may result from APN. In the refluxing piglet model, Majd and Rushton found reduced renal blood flow in sites of APN identified by diminished uptake of DMSA and subsequently confirmed by histopathology. Uninvolved areas of the affected kidneys demonstrated normal blood flow comparable to the contralateral normal kidney [23].

Imaging of Acute Pyelonephritis

Sonography

Standard ultrasound imaging in the pediatric population utilizes a variety of machines with transducers ranging between 3.5 megahertz (MHz) and 10 MHz, with the majority of children requiring 3.5–5 MHz transducers [24]. Criteria for diagnosis of APN on ultrasound include one or more areas of increased or decreased cortical echogenicity and/or loss of corticomedullary differentiation with or without focal or diffuse renal enlargement [25] (Fig. 12.1).

Several clinical studies have clearly demonstrated that renal sonography is not as reliable as DMSA scintigraphy for the detection of APN [26–32]. In one prospective study of 91 children with culture-documented febrile UTIs, DMSA

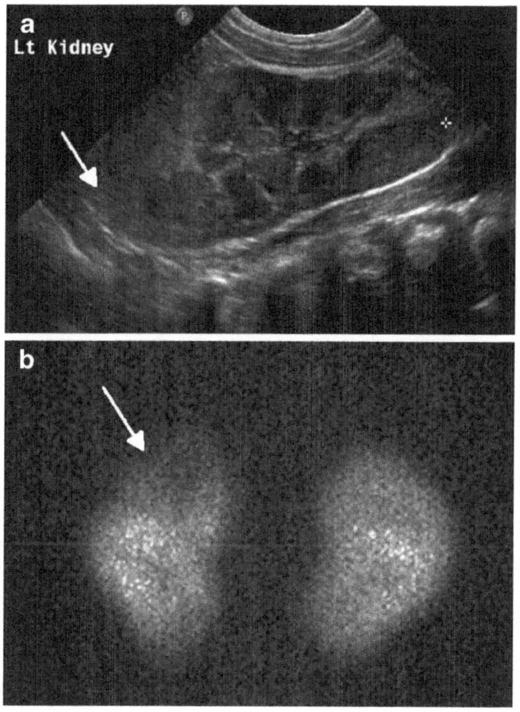

Fig. 12.1 Acute pyelonephritis in the upper pole of the left kidney of a 5-week-old male with urosepsis. (**a**) Longitudinal sonogram shows hyperechoic left upper pole with loss of corticomedullary differentiation (*arrow*). (**b**) DMSA scan obtained the same day demonstrates decreased uptake in the left upper pole without loss of volume (*arrow*)

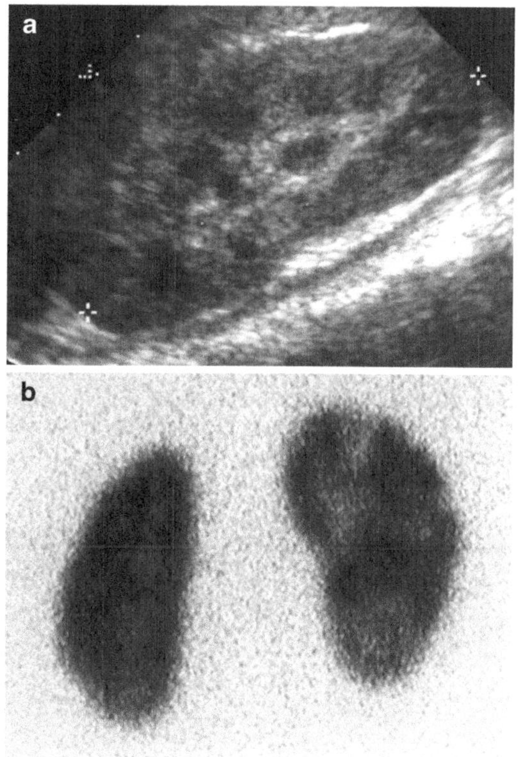

Fig. 12.2 False-negative sonogram of the right kidney of a child with multifocal acute pyelonephritis. (**a**) Longitudinal sonogram of the right kidney shows normal echogenicity and corticomedullary differentiation. (**b**) DMSA scan demonstrate swollen right kidney with multiple foci of decreased uptake

renal scans showed changes consistent with APN in 63 % of patients, while sonography revealed changes consistent with APN in only 39 % of the same patients [26]. In another prospective study of 112 children with their first documented symptomatic UTI, ultrasound was effective in detecting dilatation of the collecting system and renal swelling but failed to detect over half of those patients with DMSA evidence of APN [27] (Fig. 12.2).

Power Doppler Sonography

As focal ischemia is an early event in APN, it seems logical to expect high sensitivity for Doppler sonography in its detection. The classic color Doppler ultrasound of the kidney outlines the speed and direction of moving blood through the larger intrarenal blood vessels but does not visualize smaller cortical vessels resulting in poor sensitivity in detection of APN. In contradistinction, power Doppler sonography displays the strength of the Doppler signal from all moving blood cells regardless of speed or direction and is therefore more sensitive than color Doppler for detection of blood flow in the small vessels (Fig. 12.3). Stogianni et al. described effective use of power Doppler in the diagnosis of APN utilizing linear 5–10 MHz transducers in children less than 3 months old and convex 5 MHz transducers in children older than 3 months [33]. Axial and longitudinal images were obtained to develop intricate vascular maps of the kidneys. APN was defined by the decreased or absent blood flow in specific zones of the renal parenchyma as well as renal swelling and loss of corticomedullary differentiation [33] (Fig. 12.4).

Recently Brader et al. retrospectively studied a combination of grayscale and power Doppler

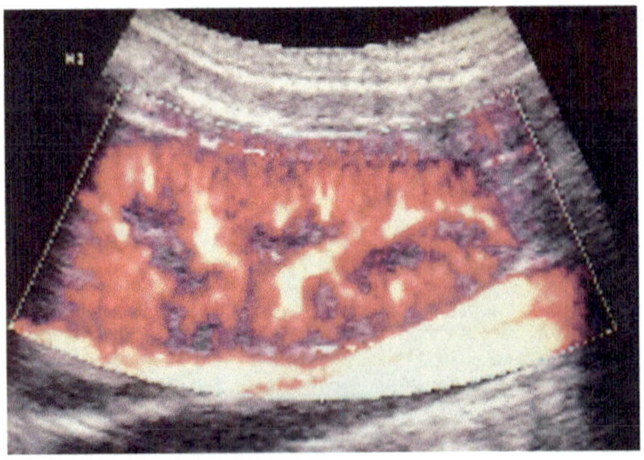

Fig. 12.3 Normal power Doppler renal sonogram. Coronal image of the right kidney of a piglet shows normal perfusion of the renal parenchyma

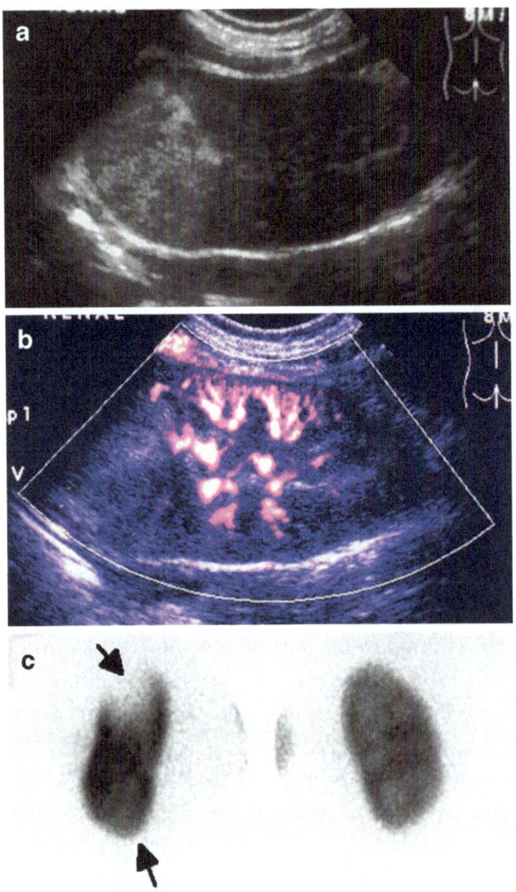

Fig. 12.4 Abnormal power Doppler renal sonogram and DMSA scan of a child with left acute pyelonephritis. (**a**) Grayscale longitudinal sonogram of the left kidney shows hyperechoic upper pole, but no definite abnormality in the lower pole. (**b**) Power Doppler sonogram demonstrates decreased/absent perfusion of the upper and lower poles. (**c**) DMSA scan shows a large photopenic area in the upper pole of the left kidney and mild decreased uptake in the lower pole (*arrows*)

renal sonography in children with clinical APN and compared the findings with DMSA scans [34]. Expanding criteria for APN to include changes in flow characteristics on power Doppler in addition to changes on grayscale sonography, they found combined sensitivity of 92.1 %, specificity of 97.8 %, and positive predictive value of 88–92 %. When compared with DMSA scan, they found sensitivity and specificity of 94 and 100 %, respectively. However, in an experimentally induced APN in piglets, sensitivity of power Doppler for the detection of histopathologically confirmed lesions was significantly lower than DMSA SPECT, CT, and MRI [35].

Renal Cortical Scintigraphy

Renal cortical scintigraphy with 99m Tc dimercaptosuccinic acid (DMSA) is considered the imaging modality of choice for detecting renal parenchymal involvement in children with UTI and as a marker to assess the extent and progression of renal damage [36]. Approximately 60 % of administered radiolabeled DMSA is picked up by the proximal tubular cells, and the remaining is filtered and excreted at a low concentration. Therefore, the delayed images show excellent visualization of the renal cortex without any significant tracer activity in the pelvicalyceal systems.

Approximately 2 h after intravenous administration DMSA ($\leq$0.05 mCi/kg body weight; minimum 0.03 mCi, maximum 3 mCi), images of the kidneys are obtained. Basically two imaging techniques can be used: planar imaging with magnification or single-photon emission computerized tomography (SPECT).

For planar imaging with pinhole magnification, a high-resolution, parallel-hole collimator is used to obtain posterior image of both kidneys together for calculation of differential renal function. In addition posterior and posterior-oblique images of each kidney are acquired using a pinhole collimator with 3–4 mm aperture insert (Fig. 12.5).

For SPECT imaging, usually a dual detector rotating gamma camera equipped with high-resolution, low-energy collimators is used to acquire 120 images of the kidneys (3° apart). Data acquisition takes approximately 20 min. The images are then reconstructed in coronal, transverse, and axial planes (Fig. 12.6).

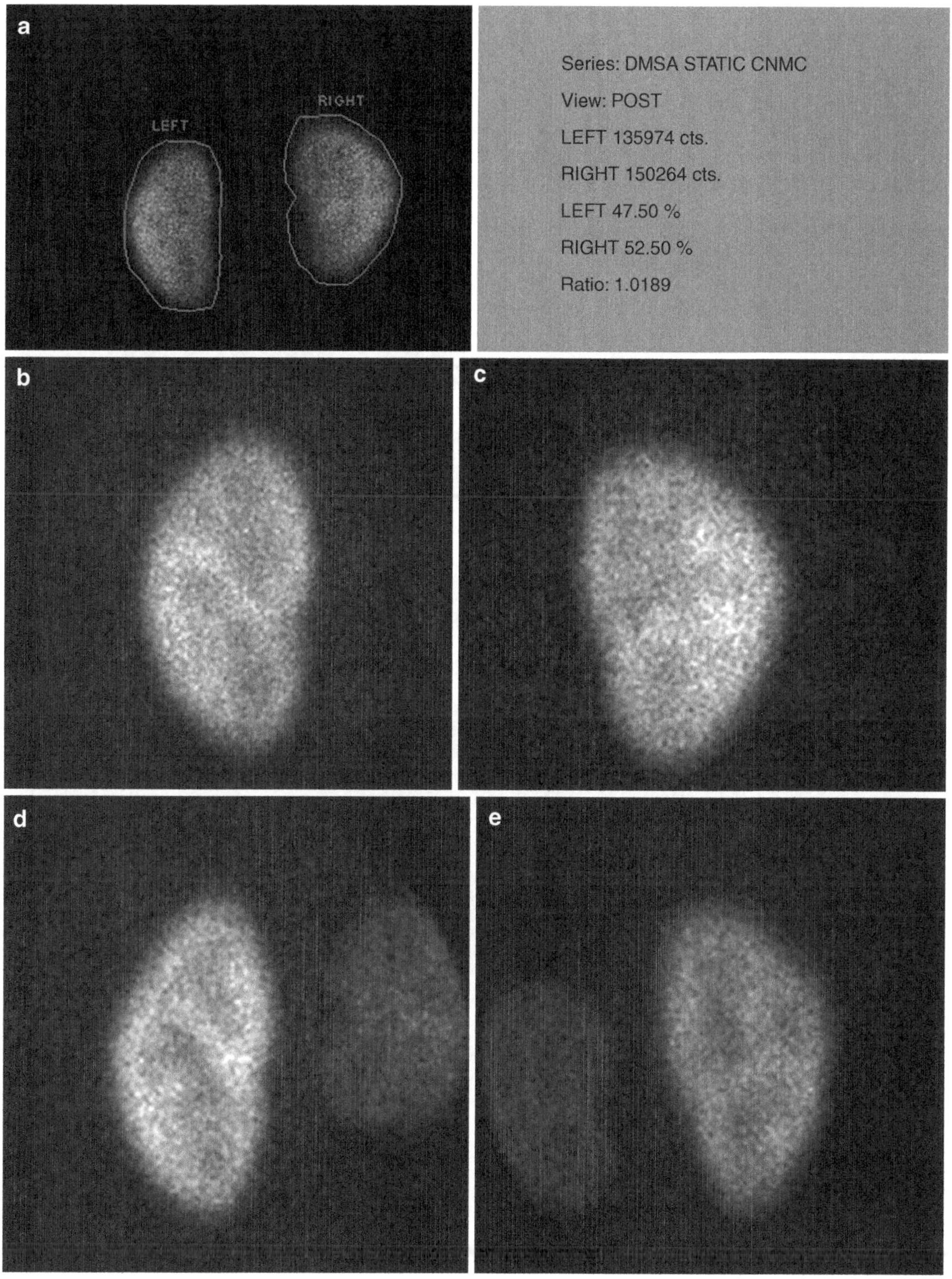

Fig. 12.5 Normal planar DMSA scan with pinhole magnification in a 5-year-old child. (**a**) Posterior image using parallel-hole collimator shows normal cortical uptake bilaterally with the calculated differential function of 47.5 % on the left and 52.5 % on the right. (**b**, **c**, **d**, and **e**) Magnified pinhole posterior and posterior-oblique images of the kidneys show normal cortical uptake of DMSA with relative central photopenia corresponding to the medulla and collecting systems

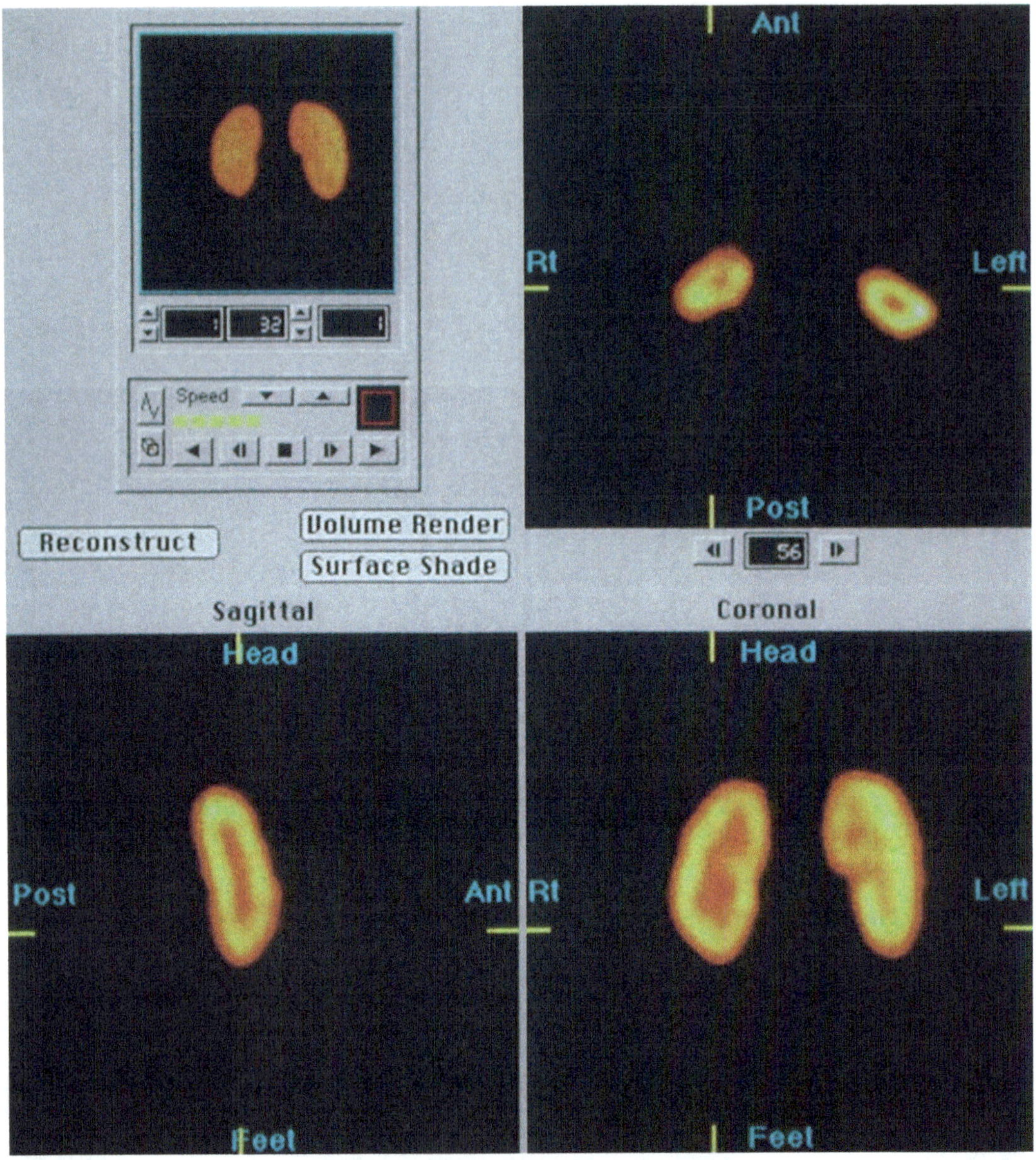

Fig. 12.6 Normal SPECT: selected reconstructed transverse, sagittal, and coronal images show normal cortical DMSA uptake

Normal DMSA Scan

Uptake of DMSA in normal kidneys reflects the morphology of renal cortex. High-resolution images show the details of the cortex and cortical columns with good differentiation from the collecting systems and medulla. Irregularities in the contour of the kidneys due to fetal lobulation may be present between the medullary pyramids (over cortical columns) and can be differentiated from the cortical scars which occur over the pyramids (between cortical columns) (Fig. 12.7).

Acute Pyelonephritis and Renal Scar

The typical manifestation of APN on DMSA scan is decreased cortical uptake, usually focal or

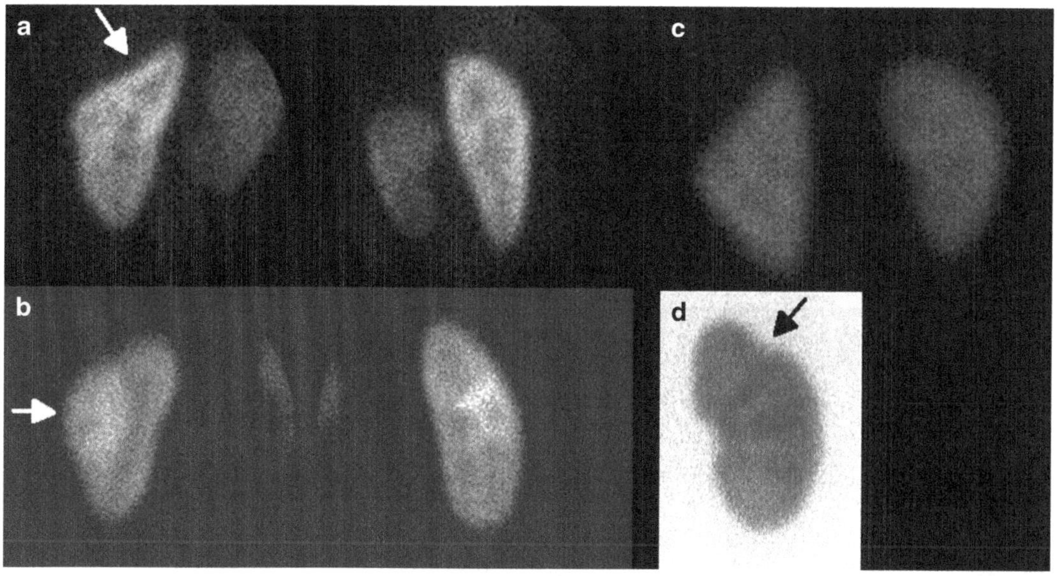

Fig. 12.7 Normal variants on DMSA scan: splenic impression (*arrow*) (**a**), column of Bertin (*arrow*) (**b**), triangular left kidney (**c**), and fetal lobulation (*arrow*) (**d**). Note cortical column under the fetal lobulation

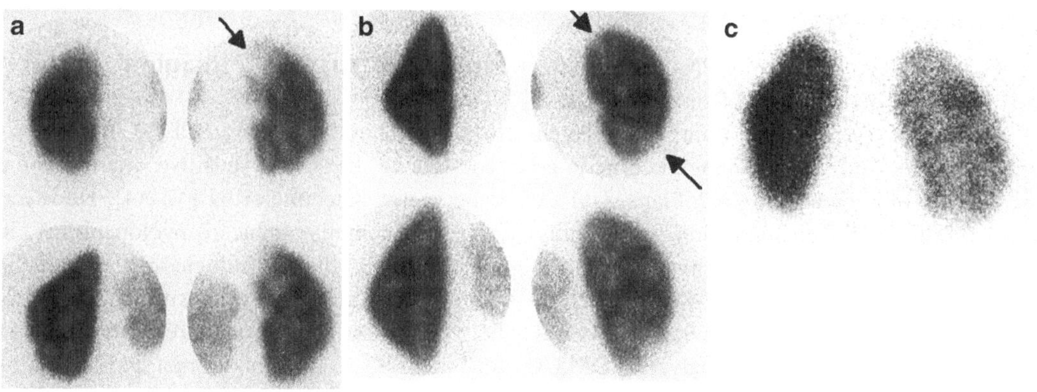

Fig. 12.8 Scintigraphic patterns of acute pyelonephritis: acute pyelonephritis usually presents either as a single focus (**a**) or multiple foci (**b**) of decreased uptake without volume loss (*arrows*). A less common pattern is panpyelonephritis manifesting as diffusely decreased uptake in an enlarged kidney (**c**)

multifocal, without volume loss or contraction of the renal cortex. In severe cases diffusely decreased uptake of DMSA may be observed (Fig. 12.8).

A mature cortical scar is usually associated with contraction and loss of volume of the involved cortex manifested as wedge-shaped defect, cortical thinning, or flattening of the renal contour (Fig. 12.9).

Sensitivity and Specificity of DMSA for Detection of Acute Pyelonephritis

Early clinical reports showed that renal cortical scintigraphy using 99m Tc DMSA was significantly more sensitive than intravenous urogram (IVU) and renal sonography in the detection of APN [37–39]. To evaluate the true sensitivity and specificity of renal cortical scintigraphy for the

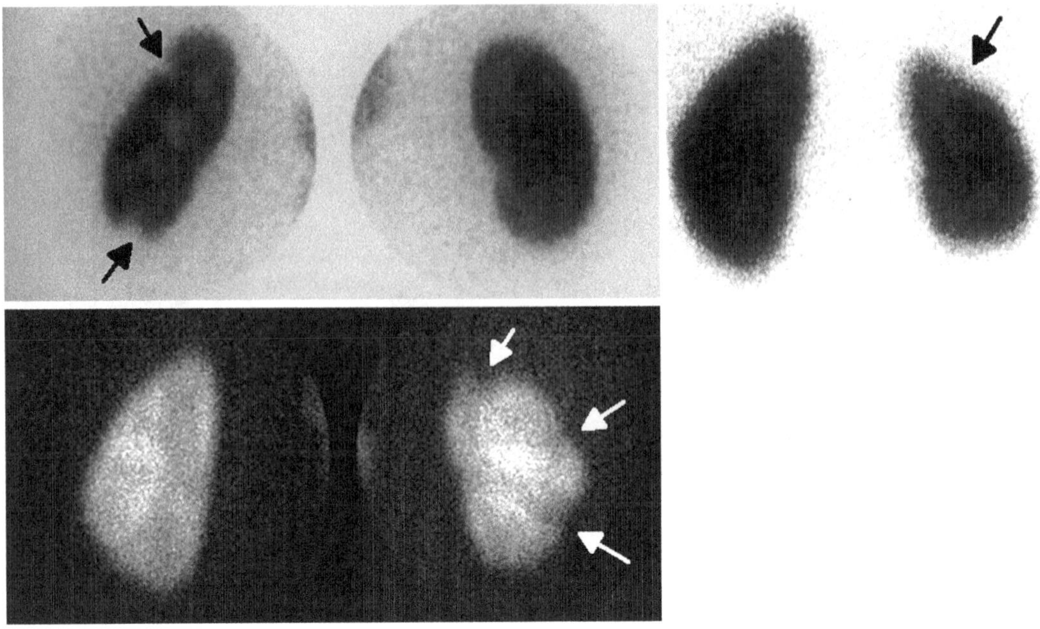

Fig. 12.9 Scintigraphic patterns of cortical scars in three different patients: cortical scars appear either as focal areas of decreased uptake with volume loss, cortical thinning, or as a more extensive polar or global volume loss (*arrows*)

detection and localization of APN, studies were conducted in a piglet model of surgically inducing unilateral vesicoureteral reflux of infected urine and using strict histopathologic criteria as the standard of reference [40, 41]. Planar DMSA scans using pinhole magnification were highly reliable for detecting and localizing experimental APN with a sensitivity of 87–89 % and specificity of 100 % in both studies. When individual pyelonephritic lesions were analyzed, DMSA scan findings correlated with histopathological changes with an agreement rate of 89–94 %. Those lesions not detected were microscopic foci of inflammation not evident on gross examination and not associated with significant parenchymal damage.

Not only is DMSA scintigraphy highly sensitive and specific for the diagnosis of APN, but it also provides important information regarding renal function and the extent of renal parenchymal inflammation. Documentation of renal parenchymal damage associated with APN is fundamental to understanding the relative roles of infection and vesicoureteral reflux in the etiology of pyelonephritis and renal scarring.

Pinhole Versus SPECT Imaging

In some clinical studies, SPECT imaging is reported to be more sensitive than pinhole imaging for detecting APN [42–44]. However, in experimentally induced pyelonephritis in piglets, using histopathologic criteria as the standard of reference, the sensitivity and specificity for detecting affected renal zones were 86 % and 95 % for pinhole imaging and 91 % and 82 % for SPECT. The overall accuracy was 88 % for both techniques in assessing kidney involvement [45] (Fig. 12.10). Thus, SPECT imaging appears to be slightly more sensitive than standard pinhole imaging but may result in more false-positive findings. Furthermore, it may be easier to differentiate acute inflammatory changes from chronic renal scarring with pinhole imaging.

MAG 3 Renal Scan

Technetium-99 m labeled mercaptoacetyl triglycine is a renal imaging radiopharmaceutical which is rapidly picked up and secreted by the tubular cells yielding excellent visualization of

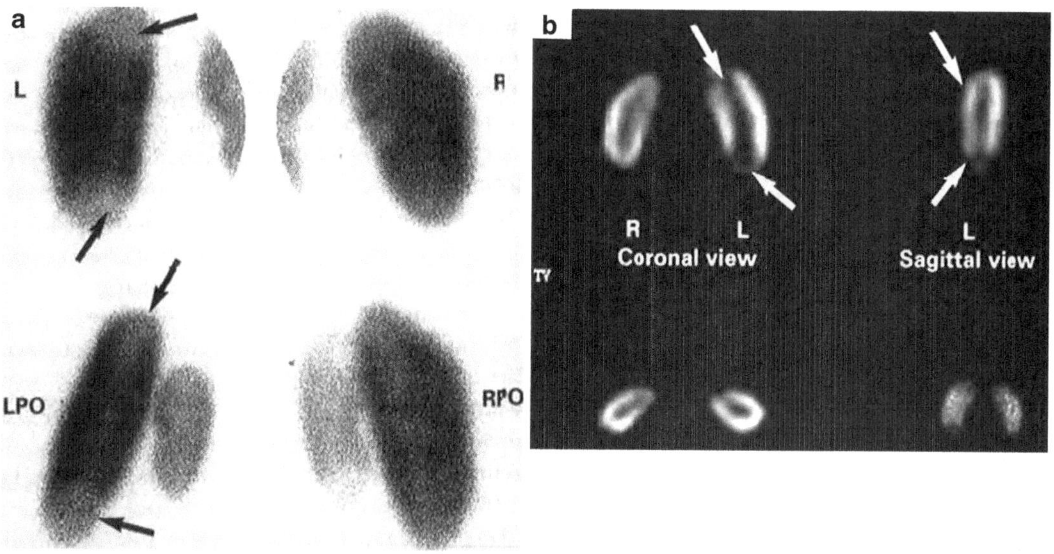

Fig. 12.10 (**a**) Posterior-oblique pinhole and (**b**) coronal and sagittal SPECT images of ^{99m}Tc-DMSA renal scan in a young pig with bilateral vesicoureteral reflux and acute pyelonephritis 48 h after introduction of *E. coli* broth into the bladder. Photopenic lesions in the left upper and lower poles are demonstrated by both techniques (*arrows*) (From Pohl et al. [142]. Reprinted with permission from Informa Healthcare)

pelvicalyceal systems and ureter making it the radiopharmaceutical of choice for dynamic renal imaging such as diuresis renography and captopril renography. However, its high cortical concentration during the first few minutes after injection and subsequent rapid clearance may allow detection of focal cortical functional abnormalities. The expected finding in APN would be focal decreased uptake on the early images with subsequent poor clearance (cortical retention) in the same area.

In a clinical comparative study, Piepz et al. concluded that the accuracy of the MAG3 renal scan was population dependent. When the DMSA scan was normal or very abnormal, the MAG3 image correctly reflected the findings of the DMSA renal scan. However, when the DMSA abnormalities were less pronounced, the early MAG3 scan failed to detect about half of the cases [46].

Computed Tomography (CT) Scans

Abdominal CT scanning is an effective rapid imaging technique for documenting the nature and extent of renal parenchymal involvement and for evaluation of perinephric space as well as other abdominal viscera. However, because of high radiation dose and the need for rapid IV administration of iodinated contrast media, its routine use in evaluating children with UTI is impractical and should be reserved for complicated cases.

APN lesions typically appear as wedge-shaped, ill-defined, or striated areas of decreased attenuation (Fig. 12.11). In an experimental refluxing piglet study performed by Majd et al., the CT scan proved to be highly accurate for the detection of pyelonephritic lesions with sensitivity and specificity similar to DMSA SPECT and MRI [35].

Magnetic Resonance Imaging (MRI)

Magnetic resonance imaging (MRI) with IV administration of gadolinium has been shown to be highly accurate for the detection of pyelonephritic lesions both in clinical and experimental studies. The fast inversion recovery sequence markedly decreases the signal intensity of normal parenchyma and allows pyelonephritic lesions to be seen as foci of medium or high signal intensity

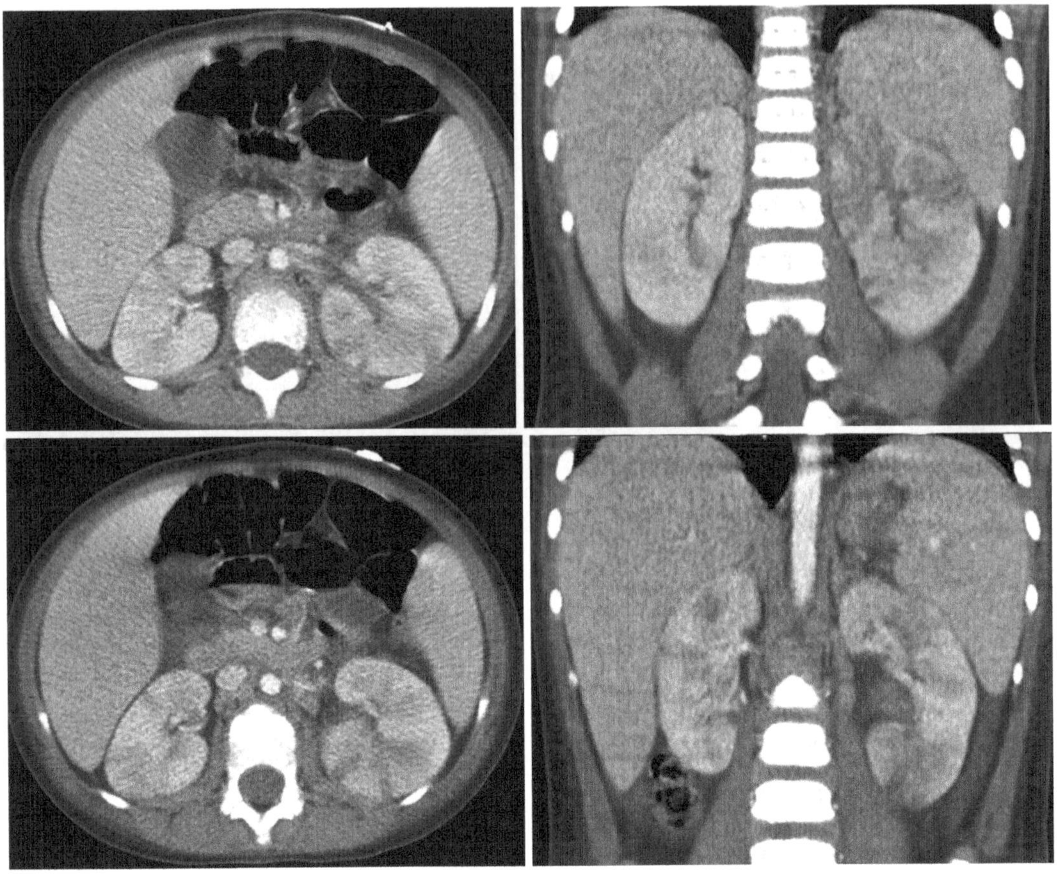

Fig. 12.11 Bilateral multifocal acute pyelonephritis in a 4-year-old female with fever, abdominal pain, and shock. Transverse and coronal CT images demonstrate multiple striated areas of hypoattenuation in the swollen left kidney and less severe involvement of the right kidney

(Fig. 12.12). In a clinical study, the sensitivity of MRI was similar to that of DMSA scan [47]. In an experimental refluxing piglet study, MRI showed high sensitivity and specificity for detection of pyelonephritic lesion similar to DMSA SPECT and CT [35] (Table 12.1).

Renal scars appear as a focal area of parenchymal volume loss with deformity of the renal contour and can be easily differentiated from APN [48]. Renal function can be estimated on MRI without ionizing radiation and iodinated contrast media. In one study of children with febrile UTIs, the cortical phase of contrast-enhanced MRI demonstrated greater interobserver agreement and cost-effectiveness when compared with DMSA for the diagnosis of pyelonephritis [10].

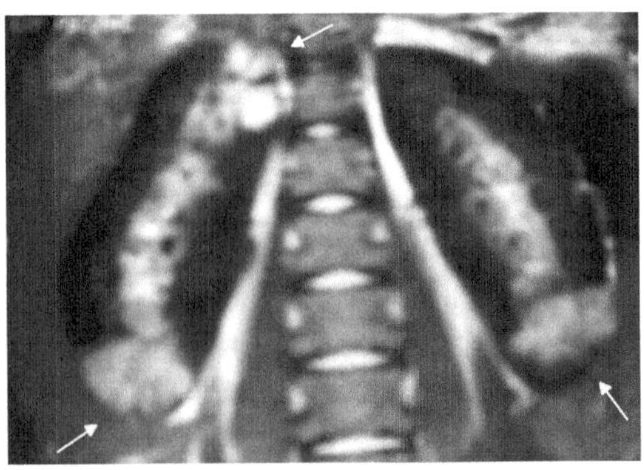

Fig. 12.12 MRI manifestation of acute pyelonephritis: coronal post-gadolinium fast multiplanar inversion recovery images demonstrate foci of high signal intensity in the upper and lower poles of the right kidney and the lower pole of the left kidney against a background of low signal in the normal cortex (*arrows*)

Table 12.1 Diagnosis of experimental acute pyelonephritis in piglets: comparison of DMSA, MRI, CT, and power Doppler

	SPECT DMSA (%)	Gadolinium MRI (%)	Spiral CT (%)	Doppler Sono (%)
Sensitivity	94	91	87	56
Specificity	98	92	92	81
Overall accuracy	96	91	90	69

Source: Majd et al. [35]

Fungal Infections

Renal fungal infections are most often recognized in high-risk groups of neonates and infants. Reported mortality rates in children with candidemia range from 19 to 31 % and with invasive aspergillosis from 68 to 77 % [49]. Premature, low-birth-weight infants are at highest risk for disseminated candidiasis secondary to immature immune systems, increased invasive procedures, use of H2 blockers, and multiple courses of antibiotics [50].

Renal candidiasis is a combination of candiduria and ultrasound evidence of renal parenchymal infiltration or fungal bezoars in the collecting system. Fungal bezoars are a rare complication that may cause urinary obstruction [51]. In neonates with candiduria, the reported incidence of renal candidiasis varies between 35 and 58 %, whereas patients with candidemia have a 61–70 % prevalence of candiduria and 5–33 % incidence of renal candidiasis [51]. Term infants and older children with congenital abnormalities of the urinary tract are also at higher risk for candiduria [52].

The presentation of candiduria may be asymptomatic or as an acute urinary infection with symptoms of dysuria, cloudy urine, fever, or failure to thrive. Currently there is no standard definition used for diagnosis of candida UTI; however, most of the reported literature uses 10^4 colony-forming units/mL via catheterized specimen. Obstructive renal candidiasis may present with sepsis, acute renal failure, or palpable flank mass. The clinical presentation of systemic candidemia is similar to bacterial sepsis with lethargy, feeding intolerance, apnea, and/or respiratory distress [51]. Neonatal candidemia often involves multiple organ systems. Due to the invasive nature of this disease work-up should be performed to rule out systemic fungal infection if candida UTI is found. This includes blood, urine, and cerebral spinal fluid cultures, eye examination, echocardiogram, and imaging of the liver, spleen, and kidneys [53].

Imaging of Renal Fungal Infections

Sonography and IVP

Renal ultrasonography is performed routinely in cases of candiduria and systemic candidemia. In obstructive renal candidiasis dilation of the upper urinary tract is visualized as well as fungal masses (bezoars). It is possible to see focal or diffuse parenchymal changes in nonobstructing renal candidiasis [51]. Fungal masses on ultrasound are hyperechoic structures within the collecting system that do not have acoustic shadowing [54] (Fig. 12.13). The differential for these findings includes urolithiasis, nephrocalcinosis, clot, debris, and tumor. Fungal infiltration of the kidney may be seen on ultrasound in the presence of positive urine and/or blood cultures. The ultrasound findings are characterized by enlarged kidneys with diffusely increased echogenicity [55].

DMSA

Use of DMSA for renal candidiasis was reported in one case study, and it did not aid in diagnosis but did demonstrate decrease uptake and corresponding renal parenchymal damage [56]. In cases where fungal bezoars persist following treatment and lead to reinfection, DMSA may be helpful in determining differential renal function. If the affected kidney is poorly functioning, then surgical planning for nephrectomy, endoscopic manipulation, or percutaneous resection may be considered.

CT Scans

Although ultrasonography is used more commonly in critically ill neonates, occasionally CT

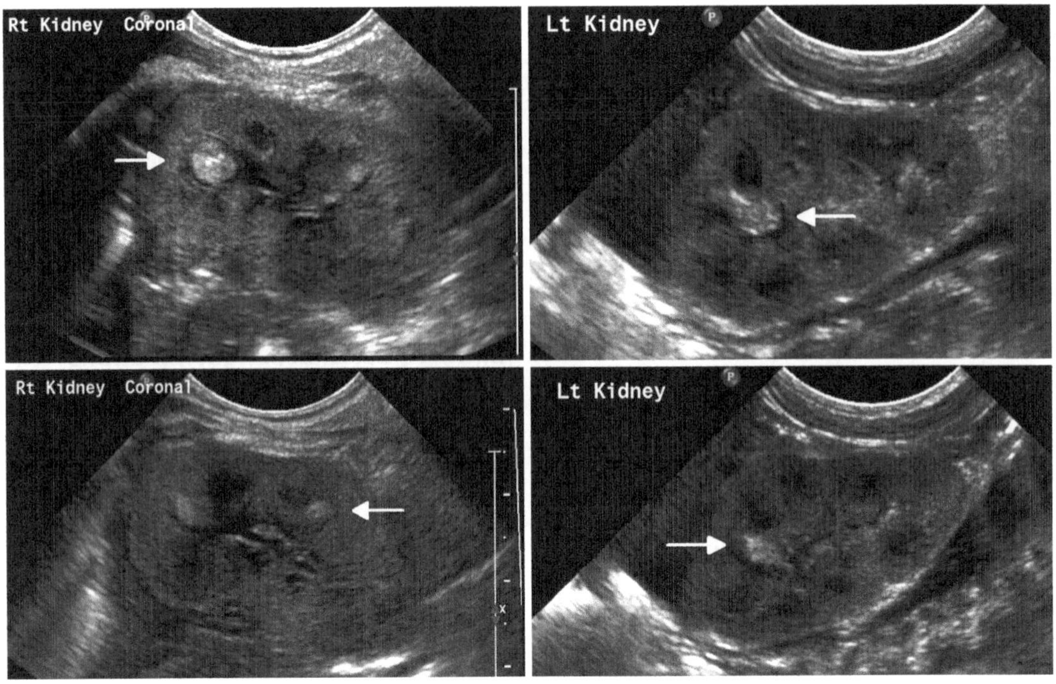

Fig. 12.13 Bilateral renal fungal infection in an infant with candidemia: sonogram shows multiple discrete nonshadowing echogenic foci within the calyces of both kidneys (fungus balls)

scans have been used to diagnose renal candidiasis. The appearance of fungal bezoars is that of a soft tissue masses in the collecting system [55]. CT scan with delayed urogram was reported to assist in the rare diagnosis of a neonate with candida infection and urinary ascites secondary to fungal obstruction and forniceal rupture [57].

MRI

MRI imaging was reported to be superior to CT scan for imaging of fungal balls in the collecting system. On the T2-weighted phase and STIR (short TI inversion recovery) images, the bezoars were hyperintense compared to renal parenchyma [58]. While this modality is excellent for demonstrating fungal bezoars, it often requires anesthesia and is a lengthy test that is risky in critically ill patients such as septic neonates. Other studies have shown, however, that MRI imaging was less effective than ultrasound at detecting fungal bezoars [56].

Tuberculosis (TB)

Genitourinary tuberculosis (GUTB) is the second most common site of extrapulmonary tuberculosis. While 90 % of GUTB cases occur in non-westernized populations where TB is still endemic [59], a resurgence is anticipated in western countries due to the spread of HIV and acquired immunodeficiency syndrome (AIDS) [60]. The classic presentation of renal TB is kidney damage from obstruction or massive caseous destruction [62]. TB infection occurs through inhalation of aerosolized Mycobacterium tuberculosis bacilli. The kidneys are infected through hematogenous spread of the bacilli. The bacilli pass down the renal tubules involving the renal calyces and can eventually enter the renal pelvis and attach to the urothelium. Stricture formation commonly results in hydroureter or hydronephrosis, and up to 10 % of patients with renal TB have bladder contractures [59]. In addition, GUTB may spread to the prostate and epididymis.

Imaging of Renal Tuberculosis

Sonography and IVP

Ultrasonography is the least specific imaging technique when compared with IVU and CT scan, particularly when evaluating the renal parenchyma. It is still particularly useful in diagnosis of epididymal involvement and TB orchitis [67]. IVP is similar to CT scan in the ability to demonstrate focal scars and hydronephrosis and is reported to be superior to CT scan for showing abnormalities of the bladder [59]. In late-stage disease, IVP demonstrates distortion of the calyces, strictures of the ureters, and bladder fibrosis [63]. Irregularities of the calyceal or parenchymal contour, calcification, or autonephrectomy can also be demonstrated [59] (Fig. 12.14).

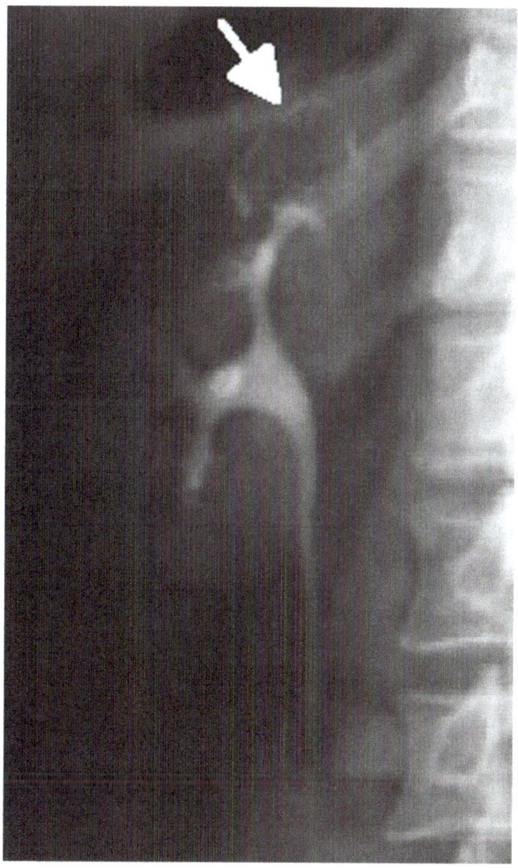

Fig. 12.14 IVP demonstration of renal tuberculosis: a calcification rimmed cavity does not fill with IV contrast (*arrow*) (From Patterson et al. [143]. Reprinted with permission from Blackwell Publishing)

CT Scans

CT scan has the benefit of demonstrating abnormalities and lesions within and outside the urinary tract that are suggestive of GUTB. CT scan is the most sensitive method for detecting renal calcification. It is also best for detection of thickening, fibrosis, and ulceration along the renal tract. Findings of thickening and fibrosis of the bladder wall may be suggestive of tuberculosis cystitis [59]. Due to the rarity of pediatric renal TB, there is a paucity of literature regarding routine diagnostic use of CT scan in children for TB (Fig. 12.15).

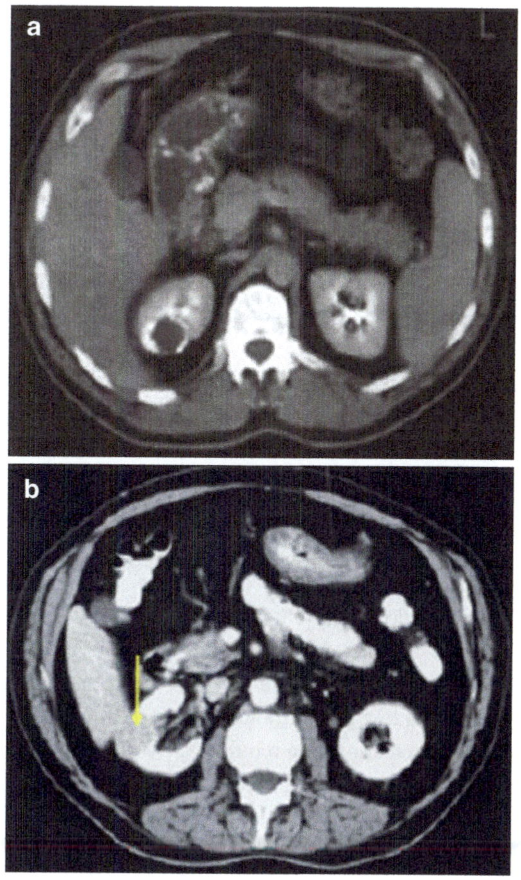

Fig. 12.15 CT scan in same patient as Fig. 12.14: (**a**) CT scan with IV contrast shows a calcified caseation of an upper pole lesion which does not fill with contrast. (**b**) CT nephrogram phase showing a calcified granulomatous lesion (*arrow*) (From Patterson et al. [143]. Reprinted with permission from Blackwell Publishing)

DMSA

A DMSA scan may be helpful in guiding surgical management of patients who are being evaluated for nephrectomy. If a nonfunctioning kidney is present often nephrectomy will be performed to eradicate disease.

MRI

Due to the cost limitations and availability of MRI in areas where GUTB is prevalent, MRI has been a rarely used imaging modality.

Renal Abscess

Renal abscess is a rare form of pediatric infection. The three basic pathophysiologic mechanisms of renal abscess formation are hematogenous spread, ascending infection, and contamination by proximity to an infected area [68]. In the past, the majority of renal abscesses were not thought to be caused by ascending infection. Historically, Staphylococcus aureus was the most common reported offending agent presumably as a result of hematogenous seeding from a peripheral cutaneous site of origin [69, 70]. More cases of gram-negative infections in the presence of vesicoureteral reflux or other anatomic abnormalities of the urinary tract are now being seen [71].

Abscesses can originate in the corticomedullary portion of the kidney, the renal cortex, or within layers of Gerota's fascia [68]. Symptoms of renal abscess are often nonspecific which may lead to a delay in treatment. It can mimic symptoms of appendicitis or, when a palpable mass is present, may be mistaken for neoplasm, i.e., Wilms' tumor or neuroblastoma. The most common presentation of a renal abscess includes high fever, lethargy, and flank pain associated with laboratory findings of leukocytosis and elevated ESR. Dysuria and/or foul-smelling urine is not regularly seen with initial presentation, and the patient may have sterile urine cultures, particularly in cases of hematogenous seeding. A variety of imaging techniques have been used to diagnose renal abscesses, including IVP, angiography, gallium-67 scintigraphy, sonography, and CT [72–76].

Imaging or Renal Abscesses

Sonography and IVP

Traditionally IVP and occasionally angiography were used to diagnose a renal abscess [69]. Findings suggestive of renal abscess were intrinsic masses with calyceal deformity and diminished renal function. However, with advances in imaging, ultrasound and CT have become the most common diagnostic imaging for renal abscesses [76]. In children, ultrasound is the primary imaging modality of choice to help limit radiation exposure. Typical findings on renal ultrasound consistent with renal abscess are presence of anechoic or septated renal masses [76] (Fig. 12.16). Ultrasound may also be used to assist therapeutically; ultrasound-guided sampling for culture of a renal abscess can help dictate specific antibiotic therapy. It can also be used to facilitate treatment with complete abscess percutaneous aspiration and/or drain placement. Ultrasound is also useful for follow-up and determining resolution of abscess during the course of treatment as it is noninvasive and does not expose the patient to radiation.

VCUG

VCUGs are often obtained in children with renal abscesses as part of an evaluation to determine if any genitourinary abnormality is present. This information is necessary for prevention and management of future infections. A VCUG is not useful in acute diagnosis of renal abscess and is contraindicated at time of infection. When VUR is associated with renal abscess, the causative organism is often found to be gram-negative bacteria [69].

CT Scan

Although CT scans are less often used in children, renal abscess cavities can have varying levels of necrosis and septation, at times, making it difficult to distinguish from renal neoplasm on sonography. CT scans maybe utilized for clarification when MRI is not available or sedation of the patient is not desired [77]. Findings on CT scan consistent with renal abscess are well-defined areas of low attenuation which develop a

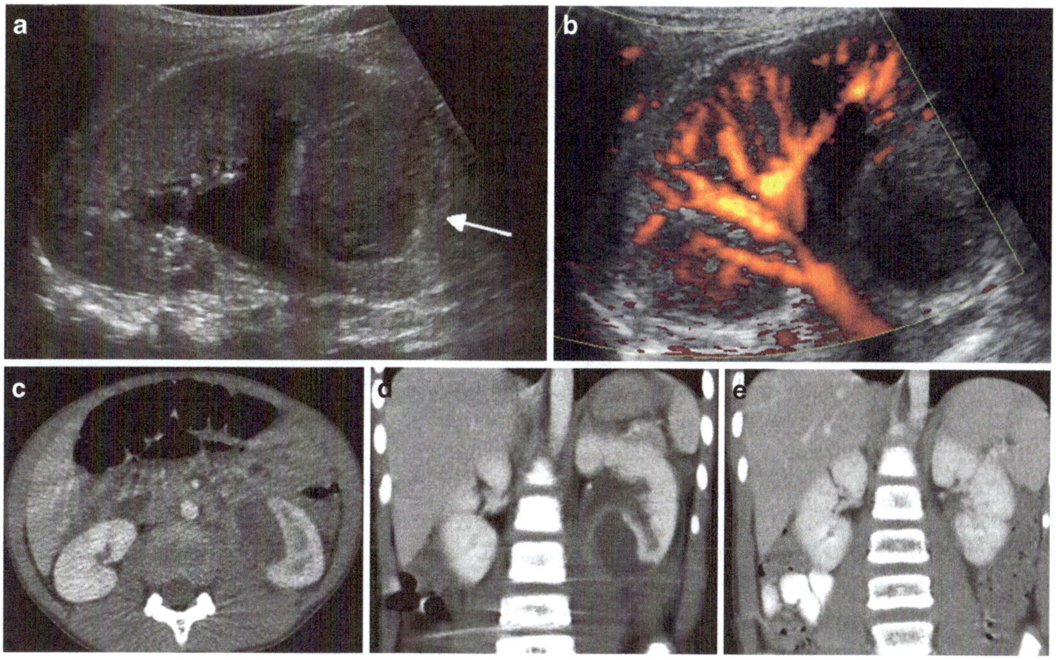

Fig. 12.16 Subcapsular abscess in a 6-year-old male with flank pain and low-grade fever: the renal sonogram shows a circumscribed area of mixed echogenicity (*arrow*) (**a**) with absent perfusion on Doppler image (**b**). Transverse (**c**) and coronal (**d**) CT images demonstrate a large collection of fluid compressing the medial aspect of the lower pole of the left kidney. Follow-up CT scan (**e**) 2 weeks after percutaneous drainage and intravenous antibiotics shows complete resolution of the abscess and re-expansion of the renal parenchyma

rim of peripheral enhancement after infusion of intravenous contrast; however, the lesion itself does not enhance [76] (Fig. 12.16).

MRI

At this point in time, there are no studies in children demonstrating a definitive benefit of MRI for managing renal abscesses and is therefore not being used routinely in their evaluation. The use of MRI has been reported in the adults where lesions are concerning for malignancy and need to be distinguished from abscess.

Treatment of Renal Abscess

The classic treatment of renal abscess has been surgical drainage in addition to appropriate antibiotic therapy. However, improved antibiotics and diagnostic techniques, together with the ability to obtain culture by percutaneous aspiration or drainage under ultrasonic control, have often obviated the necessity for surgical intervention. Currently, most cases of renal abscess initially can be managed initially with parenteral antibiotics, with percutaneous drainage being reserved for persistent infection. If percutaneous drainage of the renal abscess and antibiotic treatment fail to successfully eradicate the abscess, open exploration or even nephrectomy may be necessary.

Xanthogranulomatous Pyelonephritis

Xanthogranulomatous pyelonephritis (XGP) was first reported in 1916 by Schlagenhaufer [78]. The etiology of XGP remains unknown but is often associated with urinary tract obstruction, infection, and/or renal stones. XGP is an atypical form of severe chronic renal parenchymal infection characterized by unilateral destruction of parenchyma and accumulation of lipid-laden macrophages either surrounding abscess cavities or as discrete yellow nodules. While it predominately affects middle-aged women, it may occur in all ages. It is rare in children with only 265 reported cases since 1960 [79]. The age of presentation has ranged from infancy to 16 years with the most common age of presentation less than 8 years old and rare presentations in infancy [78]. XGP is focal in only about 10 % of cases and is most commonly caused by Proteus mirabilis or Escherichia coli infection with 50–75 % of patients having positive urine cultures [78, 80].

Most patients present with nonspecific symptoms of chronic infection, including weight loss, recurrent fever, failure to thrive, pallor, and lethargy, although those with the focal form often appear healthy [81, 82]. Urinary symptoms are uncommon, and less than half of the patients present with hypertension [83]. A palpable abdominal mass is present in approximately one-third of cases.

Both diffuse and focal forms of the disease have been reported, with the focal form being more common in children [81, 84]. Calcification or stones may be present in 70–79 % of patients with staghorn calculi being common, although this is less often seen in the focal XGP [78]. In children less than 8 years of age, the disease is usually focal, unilateral with left predominance, and without calculus [78]. The pathologic and radiologic differences between focal and diffuse XGP have been described [86]. No radiologic feature is diagnostic of XGP.

Imaging of Xanthogranulomatous Pyelonephritis

Sonography and Intravenous Pyelography (IVP)

In the diffuse form of XGP, the typical ultrasound findings are increased renal size, replacement of normal parenchyma with multiple fluid-filled masses, and posterior acoustic shadowing due to calcifications [87]. In the focal form, hypoechoic areas due to distended calyces and an inflammatory mass with a central hyperechoic area consisting of granulomatous tissue are noted [78].

Power Doppler

It has been suggested that use of a power color Doppler may be useful in the differentiation of XGP from neoplasm. In a retrospective examination of patients found to have XGP following nephrectomy, it was noted that both patients had lack of perfusion for the expanding intrarenal process [88]. This is directly contrasted to a renal neoplasm in which increased perfusion is found on color Doppler.

DMSA or MAG-3 Scintigraphy

While Tc-99 DMSA renal scintigraphy is the imaging of choice to assist in estimating relative renal function [78]. Tc-99m MAG3 can be used [88]. These studies can be especially helpful when attempting to determine surgical benefits of partial versus total nephrectomy.

CT Scan

Characteristic sonographic or CT appearances of XGP also have been reported [89]. Typically, this is characterized by dilated calyceal spaces producing the "bear paw sign" [78]. CT scan enables excellent cross-sectional imaging which helps determine extrarenal extension. Some studies have demonstrated that four-phase CT scan is as accurate as MRI for the preoperative diagnosis of XGP [90] (Fig. 12.17).

MRI

MRI generally demonstrates an enlarged, multiloculated kidney. It has the benefit of distinguishing fatty tissue and detection of abscess and fistula formation as well as providing MR angiography that aids in surgical planning [78]. Chemical shift MR imaging (in and out of phase) is useful to detect small amounts of intracellular fat and with known lipid-laden macrophages being a hallmark of XGP. MRI may benefit in the differentiation of XGP from a neoplasm [91].

The abovementioned radiologic features are nonspecific and often mimic neoplasia or other forms of chronic inflammatory renal parenchymal disease. Consequently, the correct diagnosis is seldom made preoperatively, although with the increased sensitivity of radiologic investigations, preoperative diagnosis is becoming more

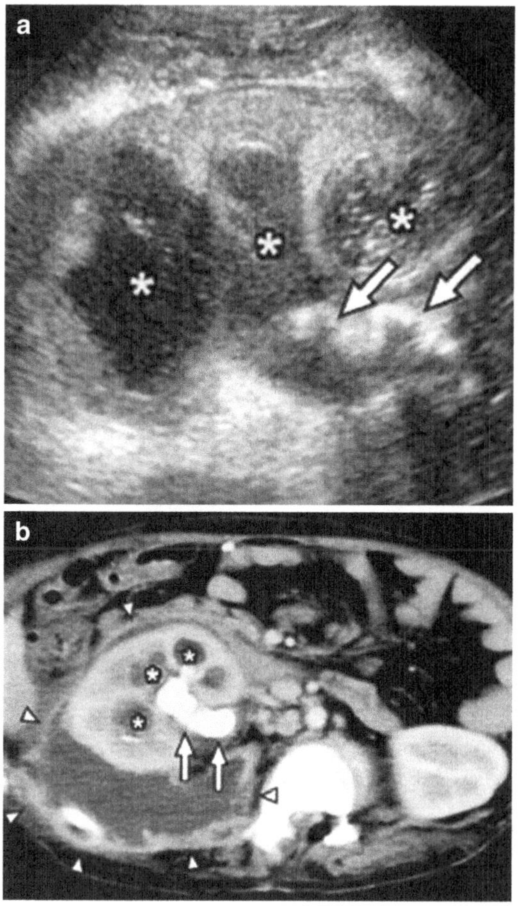

Fig. 12.17 A 3-year-old girl with XGP. (**a**) Sonographic image demonstrating an enlarged left kidney as well as multiple dilated calyces filled with debris (*asterisks*). An echogenic, shadowing calculus (*arrow*) is seen within the renal pelvis. (**b**) Axial contrast-enhanced CT image showing multiple hypoattenuating areas within an enlarged left kidney. Larger, more central low-attenuation areas likely represent debris-filled calyces (*asterisks*), while more peripheral, smaller low-attenuation areas (*arrowheads*) likely relate to parenchymal necrosis. A hyperattenuating calculus is seen within the left renal pelvis (*arrow*). There is left perinephric fat inflammatory stranding and multiple enlarged retroperitoneal lymph nodes (From Styne et al. [144]. Reprinted with permission from Springer-Verlag)

common [78, 85, 90]. Differential diagnosis in children includes Wilms' tumor, renal cell carcinoma, mesoblastic nephroma, renal abscess, tuberculosis, hydronephrosis, and cystic renal disease. Fine-needle aspiration biopsy has been used to assist in preoperative diagnosis, with success limited to the diffuse form [92].

Renal Scarring

It has become increasingly clear that the term renal scarring has been applied to the end result of more than one type of pathophysiological process, including abnormalities that are both congenital and those that are acquired postnatally, i.e., following infection. Partly because most renal scars detected in children with prior urinary tract infection(s) are established by the time of initial evaluation, their pathogenesis remains controversial [93–95]. Although the vast majority of cases of renal scarring associated with VUR are detected during the evaluation of children with UTI, DMSA studies of prenatally detected hydronephrosis secondary to high-grade VUR also have confirmed cases of congenital functional abnormalities even in the absence of infection [96–101] (see Fig. 12.18). Furthermore, a higher prevalence of renal scarring has been reported in children with secondary VUR associated with functional or anatomical bladder outlet obstruction, including posterior urethral valves and neuropathic bladders, than in children with primary VUR [102]. Lumping renal sequelae from all of these pathophysiologic entities under the terms "renal scarring" or "reflux nephropathy" has hampered attempts at understanding the pathogenic mechanisms involved.

The critical role that infection plays in the pathogenesis of renal scarring associated with reflux was clarified in Ransley and Risdon's classic experimental studies of VUR in piglets [103]. They demonstrated that in the face of VUR and normal voiding pressures, renal scarring occurs only when urinary infection is present. Reflux in the absence of infection caused renal changes only when bladder outlet resistance was increased, i.e., obstruction, not reflux, was the pathophysiologic explanation for renal damage. It was suggested that the portions of the kidney at risk for scarring are those susceptible to pyelotu bular backflow (intrarenal reflux), based on papillary morphology and configuration.

Clinically, new or progressive scarring is almost always associated with a history of UTI. Experimental studies and clinical experience have shown that even a single episode of

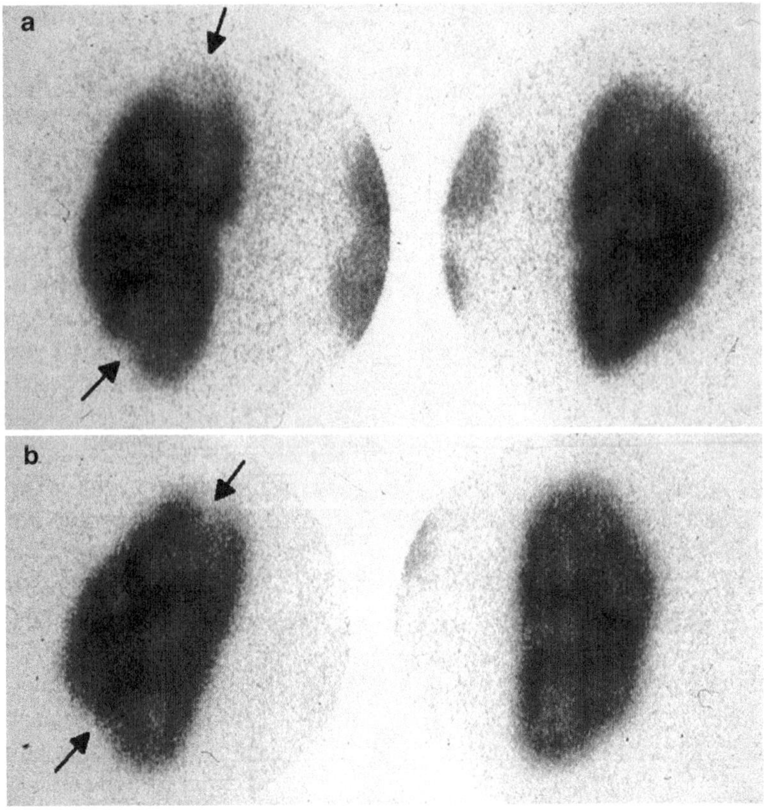

Fig. 12.18 Progression of acute pyelonephritis to renal scar: initial scan shows acute pyelonephritis (AP) in the left upper pole (**a**) and smaller photopenic focus in the lateral aspect of the lower pole (*arrows*). Follow-up DMSA scan several months later demonstrates discrete renal scars with loss of cortex in the same areas of the kidney (*arrows*) (**b**)

pyelonephritis can lead to significant renal damage [104, 105]. There is a clear association between the number of pyelonephritic attacks and incidence of renal scarring [106–109] and a correlation between the severity of VUR and renal scarring [106, 109–112]. Both experimental and clinical studies have shown that some renal scarring can be prevented or diminished by early antibiotic treatment [104, 113–115]. When VUR is present, progressive renal scarring can be successfully prevented by keeping the patient free of infection [111, 112, 116].

Imaging of Renal Scarring

In the past, the primary imaging modality for detecting renal scarring was the intravenous pyelogram. Although relatively sensitive for the detection of renal scarring, the IVP is not sensitive in the detection of APN [117]. Furthermore, pyelographic evidence of new renal scarring may take two or more years to develop after a documented urinary tract infection [107, 118]. IVP has been replaced by nuclear scintigraphy and MRI as improved modalities for demonstrating the presence of renal scarring.

DMSA

DMSA renal cortical scintigraphy is capable of detecting both the inflammatory changes of acute pyelonephritis and renal scarring. Several studies comparing the DMSA renal scan to the IVP in the detection of renal scarring have demonstrated a greater sensitivity with DMSA imaging, especially in younger children [30, 119–124]. Merrick et al. compared the findings of IVP to DMSA scans in 79 children who had proven urinary tract infection and had been followed for a period of 1–4 years [119]. Sensitivity of IVP for the detection of renal scars was 80 % and specificity was 92 %, whereas cortical scintigraphy had a sensitivity of 92 % and specificity of 98 %. When both IVP and DMSA scintigraphy demonstrate scars, an excellent correlation on a site-by-site basis has been reported [119–121, 123, 125]. When compared with histology in an animal model, the sensitivity of the DMSA scan for the detection of renal scarring in 60 piglets with reflux and infected urine was 85 % and the specificity was 97 % [126]. Thus, DMSA renal cortical scintigraphy offers a superior opportunity to study the progression of renal damage or functional loss from the time of the initial insult until either complete healing or irreversible scarring develops.

Studies comparing ultrasonography with DMSA scintigraphy for the detection of renal scarring, consistently report greater sensitivity with DMSA renal scans [27, 30, 31]. In one study, Yen and associates compared ultrasound, IVP, and both planar and SPECT DMSA renal scintigraphy in the evaluation of 130 children with UTI (42 patients), VUR (37 patients), and unilateral or bilateral small kidneys (51 patients) [32]. SPECT imaging of DMSA scans detected the highest number of defects, followed by planar imaging.

Renal scars detected by DMSA scintigraphy appear as focal or generalized areas of diminished uptake of DMSA associated with loss or contraction of functioning renal cortex. This may appear as thinning or flattening of the cortex in some kidneys, while in others renal scars appear as classic discrete wedge-shaped parenchymal defects (Fig. 12.9). In more severe cases, generalized damage may be associated with multifocal or diffusely scarred kidneys and reduced differential renal function. In contrast, defects associated with APN are more typically characterized by focal areas of diminished uptake but with preservation of the normal renal contour (Fig. 12.8). Although it is often possible for an experienced observer to distinguish acute versus chronic lesions, it should be recognized that this differentiation may be less apparent in those kidneys with APN superimposed on preexistent renal scarring.

MRI

Renal scarring can be seen easily on MRU. It appears as focal areas of parenchymal volume loss with deformity of the renal contour, with or without associated deformity of the underlying calyx [48]. The cost, availability, length of exam time, and need for anesthesia in many children are limiting factors for utilizing this modality routinely for renal scarring evaluation. However, it does have the benefit of both functional and anatomic studies in one examination so it may be useful in some pediatric evaluations [127].

Congenital Renal Scarring Associated with Reflux

With increasing access and usage of antenatal ultrasonography, it has become apparent that many of the scars attributed to VUR actually occur in utero and represent a developmental abnormality and not acquired pyelonephritic changes [128, 129]. Acquired damage is the dominant etiology in girls with febrile UTI, while congenital damage is mostly seen in boys. Severe reflux may be associated with significant renal dysplasia thought to result from abnormal induction of the nephrogenic cord during embryogenesis [130, 139]. Several reports have described DMSA scan renal functional abnormalities in patients with primary vesicoureteral reflux detected prenatally [96–100, 132]. The reported incidence of renographic abnormalities in these studies has varied widely, ranging from 17 to 60 % [96, 97, 99]. Many of these infants were evaluated by renal scintigraphy prior to any known episodes of infection, confirming that the functional abnormalities present at birth represent a congenital fetal nephropathy rather than a secondary acquired abnormality.

New or Acquired Scarring

Historically, a common assumption was that VUR was an absolute prerequisite for new or acquired renal scarring. This mindset was perpetuated by earlier investigations of new or acquired renal scarring, most of which focused retrospectively on patients with known VUR. Several investigators have now evaluated the evolution of the acute inflammatory changes associated with

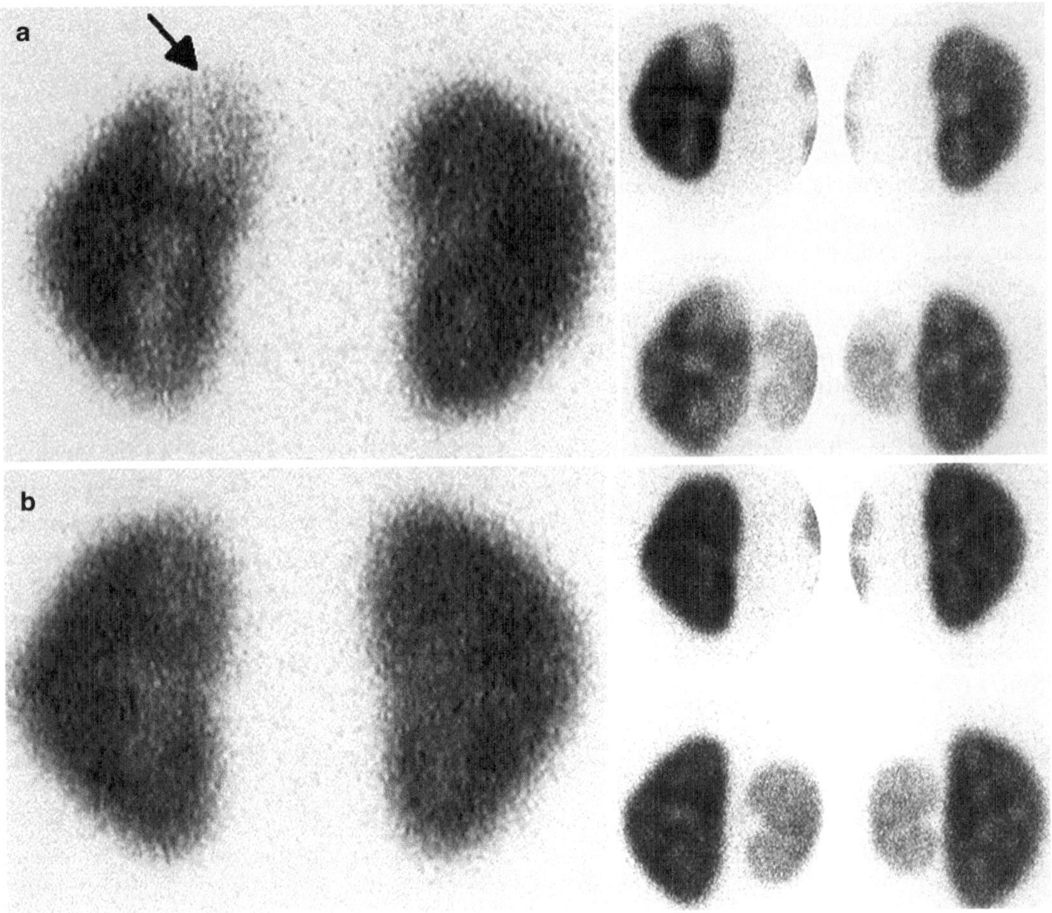

Fig. 12.19 Resolution of acute pyelonephritis: initial scan demonstrates a large photopenic area in the left upper pole (*arrow*) (**a**). Repeat DMSA scan 8 months later shows complete resolution of acute inflammatory changes without renal scarring (**b**)

pyelonephritis using serial DMSA renal scans [133–137]. The interval from the initial DMSA scan obtained at the time of acute infection until the repeat scan has ranged from 3 months to 2 years. The majority of acute pyelonephritic defects resolved after prompt treatment with antibiotics (Fig. 12.18). Acute DMSA renal scan defects persisted as renal scarring in 36–52 % of kidneys. The sites of new renal scarring corresponded exactly to those sites of APN seen on the initial DMSA renal scans, confirming the primary role of the acute inflammatory response to infection in the etiology of acquired renal scarring (Fig. 12.19). Contralateral normal kidneys and initially uninvolved areas of abnormal kidneys have almost always remained normal on follow-up DMSA renal scans. Surprisingly, reflux has been present in only 25–50 % of kidneys that developed new renal scarring. This is attributable in part to the fact that the majority of patients (63–75 %) with acute inflammatory changes on the initial DMSA renal scans did not have VUR. These observations provide convincing clinical evidence that renal parenchymal infection, rather than vesicoureteral reflux, is the prerequisite for acquired (postnatal) renal scarring. Once bacteria have invaded the renal parenchyma, causing inflammation demonstrated by DMSA scans, the propensity for renal scarring can be equally as great whether or not reflux is present, depending on the extent of the initial inflammatory response.

Despite these findings, the importance of VUR (particularly grades III or higher) as a risk factor for renal scarring should not be discounted.

Clearly, patients with moderate and severe reflux are much more likely to develop acute pyelonephritic damage than children with mild or no reflux [16, 138]. Furthermore, although 62 % of the kidneys with post-pyelonephritic renal scarring in one study were drained by nonrefluxing ureters, renal scarring was still significantly more common in those kidneys with grade III or higher VUR compared with kidneys with mild or no reflux [139]. Thus, the increased propensity for scarring in patients with higher grades of VUR is attributable in part to the increased risk of these kidneys for acute inflammatory damage at the time of the initial infection [28, 138, 140]. When present, moderate or severe reflux (grade > III) remains the most significant host risk factor for APN and renal scarring.

Other risk factors for the development of renal scarring include associated bladder pathology, regardless of whether reflux is present. In one study, the frequency of new renal scarring was significantly higher in kidneys associated with overt bladder pathology compared with those with normal bladders (86 % versus 32 %; $p=0.028$) [136]. Urodynamic evaluation of children with neuropathic bladders associated with spina bifida has demonstrated that increased intravesical pressure may lead to upper tract deterioration, with or without vesicoureteral reflux [141]. Animal studies have also shown an increased propensity for renal scarring when infection and reflux occur in the presence of bladder outlet obstruction [103].

Summary

There are many choices for imaging for pediatric patients with renal infections. There have been numerous studies examining which studies are best for which diseases and patients. Overall it is preferred in the pediatric population to begin with noninvasive, no radiation studies such as the ultrasound; however, the decreased accuracy of sonography for the detection of APN and renal scarring limits its applicability. DMSA scans, CT scan, and MRI are generally equivalent in ability to detect renal parenchymal abnormalities beyond ultrasonic evaluation, but the argument ensues whether long-term risk of radiation exposure in CT scans and DMSA scans is more of a concern than the costs and need for heavy sedation or anesthesia for MRI. Availability and cost are also increasingly popular topics of discussion in the medical community.

Ultimately the advances in imaging modalities over the past few decades have undeniably influenced physician's ability to successfully care for and treat their patients. The accuracy of imaging enables clinicians to diagnose and treat patients early in their course of disease. However, even with all of the changes, there are still many philosophies regarding which tests should be performed and at what point in the course of treatment. The ideal imaging modality would be noninvasive, cost-efficient, without risk, and readily available in all areas of the country. In addition, it would be able to perform both anatomical and functional studies in one test and have randomized trials to prove its benefits over traditional imaging methods. Until the point in time where such an exam and clinical trials exist, we will have to rely on current and historical data evaluating sonography, DMSA, CT scans, and MRI for our current standard of care models.

References

1. Darge K, Grattan-Smith JD, Riccabona M. Pediatric uroradiology: state of the art. Pediatr Radiol. 2011;41(1):82–91.
2. Riccabona M, Avni FE, Blickman JG, Dacher J, Darge K, Lobo ML, et al. Imaging recommendations in paediatric uroradiology: minutes of the ESPR uroradiology task force session on childhood obstructive uropathy, high-grade fetal hydronephrosis, childhood haematuria, and urolithiasis in childhood. ESPR Annual Congress, Edinburgh, UK, June 2008. Pediatr Radiol. 2009;39(8):891–8.
3. Riccabona M. Pediatric three-dimensional ultrasound: basics and potential clinical value. Clin Imaging. 2005;29(1):1–5.
4. Riccabona M, Sorantin E, Ring E. Application of M-mode sonography to functional evaluation in pediatric patients. Eur Radiol. 1998;8(8):1457–61.
5. Bartram U, Darge K. Harmonic versus conventional ultrasound imaging of the urinary tract in children. Pediatr Radiol. 2005;35(7):655–60.
6. Moon MH, Kim SH, Lee YH, Cho JY, Jung SI, Park SH, et al. Diagnostic potential of three-dimensional ultrasound-based virtual cystoscopy: an experimental study using pig bladders. Invest Radiol. 2006;41(12):883–9.

7. Riccabona M, Fritz G, Ring E. Potential applications of three-dimensional ultrasound in the pediatric urinary tract: pictorial demonstration based on preliminary results. Eur Radiol. 2003;13(12):2680–7.
8. Darge K. Voiding urosonography with ultrasound contrast agents for the diagnosis of vesicoureteric reflux in children: I. Procedure. Pediatr Radiol. 2008;38(1):40–53.
9. Darge K. Voiding urosonography with US contrast agents for the diagnosis of vesicoureteric reflux in children: II. Comparison with radiological examinations. Pediatr Radiol. 2008;38(1):54–63.
10. Cerwinka WH, Kirsch AJ. Magnetic resonance urography in pediatric urology. Curr Opin Urol. 2010;20(4):323–9.
11. Sty JR, Pan CG. Genitourinary imaging techniques. Pediatr Clin North Am. 2006;53(3):339–61.
12. Maudgil DD, McHugh K. The role of computed tomography in modern paediatric uroradiology. Eur J Radiol. 2002;43(2):129–38.
13. Goske MJ. Getting it right: are regulation and registries for CT radiation dose in children the answer? Pediatr Radiol. 2011;41 Suppl 2:567–70.
14. Hellström A, Hanson E, Hansson S, Hjälmås K, Jodal U. Association between urinary symptoms at 7 years old and previous urinary tract infection. Arch Dis Child. 1991;66(2):232–4.
15. Mårild S, Jodal U. Incidence rate of first-time symptomatic urinary tract infection in children under 6 years of age. Acta Paediatr. 1998;87(5):549–52.
16. Majd M, Rushton HG, Wiedermann BL. Relationship among vesicoureteral reflux, P-fimbriated Escherichia coli, and acute pyelonephritis in children with febrile urinary tract infection. J Pediatr. 1991;119(4):578–85.
17. Busch R, Huland H. Correlation of symptoms and results of direct bacterial localization in patients with urinary tract infections. J Urol. 1984;132(2):282–5.
18. Rushton HG. The evaluation of acute pyelonephritis and renal scarring with technetium 99m-dimercaptosuccinic acid renal scintigraphy: evolving concepts and future directions. Pediatr Nephrol. 1997;11(1):108–20.
19. Roberts JA. Etiology and pathophysiology of pyelonephritis. Am J Kidney Dis. 1991;17(1):1–9.
20. Kaack MB, Dowling KJ, Patterson GM, Roberts JA. Immunology of pyelonephritis. VIII. E. coli causes granulocytic aggregation and renal ischemia. J Urol. 1986;136(5):1117–22.
21. Hill GS, Clark RL. A comparative angiographic, microangiographic, and histologic study of experimental pyelonephritis. Invest Radiol. 1972;7(1):33–47.
22. Androulakakis PA, Ransley PG, Risdon RA, Sorger K, Hohenfellner R. Microvascular changes in the early stage of reflux pyelonephritis. An experimental study in the pig kidney. Eur Urol. 1987;13(4):219–23.
23. Majd M, Rushton HG. Renal cortical scintigraphy in the diagnosis of acute pyelonephritis. Semin Nucl Med. 1992;22(2):98–111.
24. Piccoli G, Consiglio V, Deagostini M, Serra M, Biolcati M, Ragni F, et al. The clinical and imaging presentation of acute "non complicated" pyelonephritis: a new profile for an ancient disease. BMC Nephrol. 2011;12(1):68.
25. Jaksic E, Bogdanovic R, Artiko V, Saranovic DS, Petrasinovic Z, Petrovic M, et al. Diagnostic role of initial renal cortical scintigraphy in children with the first episode of acute pyelonephritis. Ann Nucl Med. 2011;25(1):37–43.
26. Björgvinsson E, Majd M, Eggli KD. Diagnosis of acute pyelonephritis in children: comparison of sonography and 99mTc-DMSA scintigraphy. Am J Roentgenol. 1991;157(3):539–43.
27. MacKenzie JR, Fowler K, Hollman AS, Tappin D, Murphy AV, Beattie TJ, et al. The value of ultrasound in acute urinary tract infection. Br J Urol. 1994;74(2):240–4.
28. Stokland E, Hellstrom M, Jacobsson B, Jodal U, Lundgren P, Sixt R. Early 99m Tc-dimercaptosuccinic acid scintigraphy insympptomatic first time urinary tract infection. Acta Pediatr. 1996;85(4):430–6.
29. Benador D, Benador N, Slosman DO, Nusslé D, Mermillod B, Girardin E. Cortical scintigraphy in the evaluation of renal parenchymal changes in children with pyelonephritis. J Pediatr. 1994;124(1):17–20.
30. Shanon A, Feldman W, McDonald P, Martin DJ, Matzinger MA, Shillinger JF, et al. Evaluation of renal scars by technetium-labeled dimercaptosuccinic acid scan, intravenous urography, and ultrasonography: a comparative study. J Pediatr. 1992;120(3):399–403.
31. Tasker AD, Lindsell DR, Moncrieff M. Can ultrasound reliably detect renal scarring in children with urinary tract infection? Clin Radiol. 1993;47(3):177–9.
32. Yen TC, Chen WP, Chang SL, Huang YC, Hsieh CP, Yeh SH, et al. A comparative study of evaluating renal scars by 99mTc-DMSA planar and SPECT renal scans, intravenous urography, and ultrasonography. Ann Nucl Med. 1994;8(2):147–52.
33. Stogianni A, Nikolopoulos P, Oikonomou I, Gatzola M, Balaris V, Farmakiotis D, et al. Childhood acute pyelonephritis: comparison of power Doppler sonography and Tc-DMSA scintigraphy. Pediatr Radiol. 2007;37(7):685–90.
34. Brader P, Riccabona M, Schwarz T, Seebacher U, Ring E. Value of comprehensive renal ultrasound in children with acute urinary tract infection for assessment of renal involvement: comparison with DMSA scintigraphy and final diagnosis. Eur Radiol. 2008;18(12):2981–9.
35. Majd M, Nussbaum Blask AR, Markle BM, Shalaby-Rana E, Pohl HG, Park J, et al. Acute pyelonephritis: comparison of diagnosis with 99mTc-DMSA SPECT, spiral CT, MR imaging, and power Doppler US in an experimental pig model. Radiology. 2001;218(1):101–8.
36. Lavocat MP, Granjon D, Allard D, Gay C, Freycon MT, Dubois F. Imaging of pyelonephritis. Pediatr Radiol. 1997;27(2):159–65.
37. Handmaker H. Nuclear renal imaging in acute pyelonephritis. Semin Nucl Med. 1982;12(3):246–53.

38. Traisman ES, Conway JJ, Traisman HS, Yogev R, Firlit C, Shkolnik A, et al. The localization of urinary tract infection with 99mTc glucoheptonate scintigraphy. Pediatr Radiol. 1986;16(5):403–6.
39. Sty JR, Wells RG, Starshak RJ, Schroeder BA. Imaging in acute renal infection in children. AJR Am J Roentgenol. 1987;148(3):471–7.
40. Rushton HG, Majd M, Chandra R, Yim D. Evaluation of 99mtechnetium-dimercapto-succinic acid renal scans in experimental acute pyelonephritis in piglets. J Urol. 1988;140(5 Pt 2):1169–74.
41. Parkhouse HF, Godley ML, Cooper J, Risdon RA, Ransley PG. Renal imaging with 99Tcm-labelled DMSA in the detection of acute pyelonephritis: an experimental study in the pig. Nucl Med Commun. 1989;10(1):63–70.
42. Tarkington MA, Fildes RD, Levin K, Ziessman H, Harkness B, Gibbons MD. High resolution single photon emission computerized tomography (SPECT) 99mtechnetium-dimercapto-succinic acid renal imaging: a state of the art technique. J Urol. 1990;144(2 Pt 2):598–600.
43. Itoh K, Asano Y, Tsukamoto E, Kato C, Nakada K, Nagao K, et al. Single photon emission computed tomography with Tc-99m-dimercaptosuccinic acid in patients with upper urinary tract infection and/or vesicoureteral reflux. Ann Nucl Med. 1991;5(1):29–34.
44. Itoh K, Yamashita T, Tsukamoto E, Nonomura K, Furudate M, Koyanagi T. Qualitative and quantitative evaluation of renal parenchymal damage by 99mTc-DMSA planar and SPECT scintigraphy. Ann Nucl Med. 1995;9(1):23–8.
45. Majd M, Rushton HG, Chandra R, Andrich MP, Tardif CP, Rashti F. 99mTc-DMSA renal cortical scintigraphy for the detection of experimental acute pyelonephritis in piglets: comparison of planar (pinhole) and SPECT imaging. J Nucl Med. 1996;37(10):1731–4.
46. Piepsz A, Pintelon H, Verboven M, Keuppens F, Jacobs A. Replacing 99mTcm-DMSA for renal imaging? Nucl Med Commun. 1992;13(7):494–6.
47. Lonergan GJ, Pennington DJ, Morrison JC, Haws RM, Grimley MS, Kao TC. Childhood pyelonephritis: comparison of gadolinium-enhanced MR imaging and renal vortical scintigraphy for diagnosis. Radiology. 1998;207(2):377–85.
48. Renjen P, Bellah R, Hellinger JC, Darge K. Advances in uroradiologic imaging in children. Radiol Clin North Am. 2012;50(2):207–18.
49. Blyth CC, Palasanthiran P, O'Brien TA. Antifungal therapy in children with invasive fungal infections: a systematic review. Pediatrics. 2007;119(4):772–84.
50. Saiman L, Ludington E, Pfaller M, Rangel-Frausto S, Wiblin RT, Dawson J, et al. Risk factors for candidemia in neonatal intensive care unit patients. Pediatr Infect Dis J. 2000;19(4):319–24.
51. Bisht V, Voort JV. Clinical practice: obstructive renal candidiasis in infancy. Eur J Pediatr. 2011;170(10):1227–35.
52. Johnson KC, Barone JG. Management of obstructing fungal pyelonephritis in infants. Urology. 2006;67(2):424.e7–9.
53. Pappas PG, Kauffman CA, Andes D, Benjamin Jr DK, Calandra TF, Edwards Jr JE, et al. Clinical practice guidelines for the management of candidiasis: 2009 update by the Infectious Diseases Society of America. Clin Infect Dis. 2009;48(5):503–35.
54. Kintanar C, Cramer BC, Reid WD, Andrews WL. Neonatal renal candidiasis: sonographic diagnosis. Am J Roentgenol. 1986;147(4):801–5.
55. Karlowicz MG. Candidal renal and urinary tract infection in neonates. Semin Perinatol. 2003;27(5):393–400.
56. Rebhandl W, Saadi S, Herneth AM, Presterl E, Kurosh P, Wandl-Vergesslich K, et al. Successful conservative treatment of severe renal candidosis with fungus balls. Pediatr Nephrol. 1999;13(8):688–92.
57. Sie AHI, Patel N, Spenceley N. Neonatal urinary ascites in renal candidal infection. J Paediatr Child Health. 2006;42(6):387–8.
58. Erden A, Fitoz S, Karagulle T, Tukel S, Akyar S. Radiological findings in the diagnosis of genitourinary candidiasis. Pediatr Radiol. 2000;30(12):875–7.
59. Abbara A, Davidson RN. Etiology and management of genitourinary tuberculosis. Nat Rev Urol. 2011;8(12):678–88.
60. Chattopadhyay A, Bhatnagar V, Agarwala S, Mitra DK. Genitourinary tuberculosis in pediatric surgical practice. J Pediatr Surg. 1997;32(9):1283–6.
61. Nzerue C, Drayton J, Oster R, Hewan-Lowe K. Genitourinary tuberculosis in patients with HIV infection: clinical features in an inner-city hospital population. Am J Med Sci. 2000;320(5):299–303.
62. Nourse PJ, Cotton MF, Bates WD. Renal manifestations in children co-infected with HIV and disseminated tuberculosis. Pediatr Nephrol. 2010;25(9):1759–63.
63. Eastwood JB, Corbishley CM, Grange JM. Tuberculosis and the kidney. J Am Soc Nephrol. 2001;12(6):1307–14.
64. Nerli RB, Kamat GV, Alur SB, Koura A, Vikram P, Amarkhed SS. Genitourinary tuberculosis in pediatric urological practice. J Pediatr Urol. 2008;4(4):299–303.
65. García-Rodríguez JA, García Sánchez JE, Muñoz Bellido JL, Montes Martínez I, Rodríguez Hernández J, Fernández Gorostarzu J, et al. Genitourinary tuberculosis in Spain: review of 81 cases. Clin Infect Dis. 1994;18(4):557–61.
66. Boehme CC, Nabeta P, Hillemann D, Nicol MP, Shenai S, Krapp F, et al. Rapid molecular detection of tuberculosis and rifampin resistance. N Engl J Med. 2010;363(11):1005–15.
67. Chung JJ, Kim MJ, Lee T, Yoo HS, Lee JT. Sonographic findings in tuberculous epididymitis and epididymo-orchitis. J Clin Ultrasound. 1997;25(7):390–4.
68. Angel C, Shu T, Green J, Orihuela E, Rodriquez G, Hendrick E. Renal and peri-renal abscesses in

children: proposed physio-pathologic mechanisms and treatment algorithm. Pediatr Surg Int. 2003; 19(1–2):35–9.

69. Rote AR, Bauer SB, Retik AB. Renal abscess in children. J Urol. 1978;119(2):254–8.
70. Vachvanichsanong P, Dissaneewate P, Patrapinyokul S, Pripatananont C, Sujijantararat P. Renal abscess in healthy children: report of three cases. Pediatr Nephrol. 1992;6(3):273–5.
71. Timmons JW, Perlmutter AD. Renal abscess: a changing concept. J Urol. 1976;115(3):299–301.
72. Koehler PR. The roentgen diagnosis of renal inflammatory masses-special emphasis on angiographic changes. Radiology. 1974;112(2):257–66.
73. Hopkins GB, Hall RL, Mende CW. Gallium-67 scintigraphy for the diagnosis and localization of perinephric abscesses. J Urol. 1976;115(2):126–8.
74. Kumar B, Coleman RE, Alderson PO. Gallium citrate Ga 67 imaging in patients with suspected inflammatory processes. Arch Surg. 1975;110(10): 1237–42.
75. Gerzof SG, Gale ME. Computed tomography and ultrasonography for diagnosis and treatment of renal and retroperitoneal abscesses. Urol Clin North Am. 1982;9(1):185–93.
76. Wippermann C, Schofer O, Beetz R, Schumacher R, Schweden F, Riedmiller H, et al. Renal abscess in childhood: diagnostic and therapeutic progress. Pediatr Infect Dis J. 1991;10(6):446–50.
77. Lee EY. CT imaging of mass-like renal lesions in children. Pediatr Radiol. 2007;37(9):896–907.
78. Chang JW, Chen SJ, Chin TW, Tsai H, Pan CC, Chu YK, et al. Xanthogranulomatous pyelonephritis treated by partial nephrectomy. Pediatr Nephrol. 2004;19(10):1164–7.
79. Hendrickson RJ, Lutfiyya WL, Karrer FM, Furness III PD, Mengshol S, Bensard DD. Xanthogranulomatous pyelonephritis. J Pediatr Surg. 2006;41(2):E15–7.
80. Rao AG, Eberts PT. Xanthogranulomatous pyelonephritis: An uncommon pediatric renal mass. Pediatr Radiol. 2011;41(5):671–2.
81. Watson AR, Marsden HB, Lendon M, Jones PH. Renal pseudotumors caused by xanthogranulomatous pyelonephritis. Arch Dis Child. 1982;57(8): 635–7.
82. Yazaki T, Ishikawa S, Ogawa Y, Takahashi S, Nemoto S, Rinsho K, et al. Xanthogranulomatous pyelonephritis in childhood: case report and review of English and Japanese literature. J Urol. 1982;127(1):80–3.
83. Levy M, Baumal R, Eddy AA. Xanthogranulomatous pyelonephritis in children: etiology, pathogenesis, clinical and radiologic features, and management. Clin Pediatr. 1994;33(6):360–6.
84. Schulman CC, Denis R. Re: xanthogranulomatous pyelonephritis in childhood. J Urol. 1977;117(3):398.
85. Malek RS, Elder JS. Xanthogranulomatous pyelonephritis: a critical analysis of 26 cases and of the literature. J Urol. 1978;119(5):589–93.
86. Bagley FH, Stewart AM, Jones PF. Diffuse xanthogranulomatous pyelonephritis in children: an unrecognized variant. J Urol. 1977;118(3):434–5.
87. Cousins C, Somers J, Broderick N, Rance C, Shaw D. Xanthogranulomatous pyelonephritis in childhood: ultrasound and CT diagnosis. Pediatr Radiol. 1994;24(3):210–2.
88. Eckoldt F, Riebel T, Wolke S. Xanthogranulomatous pyelonephritis in children: diagnostic and therapeutic aspects. J Med Ultrason. 2009;36(1):33–7.
89. Subramanyam BR, Megibow AJ, Raghavendra BN, Bosniak MA. Diffuse xanthogranulomatous pyelonephritis: analysis by computed tomography and sonography. Urol Radiol Urol Radiol. 1982; 4(1):5–9.
90. Zugor V, Schott GE, Labanaris AP. Xanthogranulomatous pyelonephritis in childhood: a critical analysis of 10 cases and of the literature. Urology. 2007;70(1):157–60.
91. Goyal A, Gadodia A, Sharma R. Xanthogranulomatous pyelonephritis: an uncommon pediatric renal mass. Pediatr Radiol. 2010;40(12):1962–3.
92. Sease WC, Elyaderani MK, Belis JA. Ultrasonography and needle aspiration in diagnosis of xanthogranulomatous pyelonephritis. Urology. 1987;29(2):231–5.
93. Asymptomatic bacteriuria in schoolchildren in Newcastle upon Tyne. Arch Dis Child. 1974;50(2): 90–102.
94. McLachlan MS, Meller ST, Jones ER, Asscher AW, Fletcher EW, Mayon-White RT, et al. Urinary tract in schoolgirls with covert bacteriuria. Arch Dis Child. 1975;50(4):253–8.
95. Smellie JM, Normand IC, Katz G. Children with urinary infection: a comparison of those with and those without vesicoureteric reflux. Kidney Int. 1981;20(6):717–22.
96. Crabbe DC, Thomas DF, Gordon AC, Irving HC, Arthur RJ, Smith SE. Use of 99mtechnetium-dimercaptosuccinic acid to study patterns of renal damage associated with prenatally detected vesicoureteral reflux. J Urol. 1992;148(4):1229–31.
97. Sheridan M, Jewkes F, Gough DCS. Reflux nephropathy in the 1st year of life – the role of infection. Pediatr Surg Int. 1991;6(3):214–6.
98. Burge DM, Griffiths MD, Malone PS, Atwell JD. Fetal vesicoureteral reflux: outcome following conservative postnatal management. J Urol. 1992;148(5 Pt 2):1743–5.
99. Anderson PA, Rickwood AM. Features of primary vesicoureteric reflux detected by prenatal sonography. Br J Urol. 1991;67(3):267–71.
100. Najmaldin A, Burge DM, Atwell JD. Reflux nephropathy secondary to intrauterine vesicoureteric reflux. J Pediatr Surg. 1990;25(4):387–90.
101. Gordon I. Urinary tract infection in paediatrics: the role of diagnostic imaging. Br J Radiol. 1990;63(751):507–11.
102. Rushton HG, Majd M, Jantausch BA, Wiedermann BL, Belman AB. Renal scarring following reflux and

nonreflux pyelonephritis in children: evaluation with 99mtechnetium-dimercaptosuccinic acid scintigraphy. J Urol. 1992;147(5):1327–32.
103. Ransely PG, Risdon RA. Reflux and renal scarring. Br J Radiol (Suppl). 1978;51(14):1–35.
104. Ransley PG, Risdon RA. Reflux nephropathy: effects of antimicrobial therapy on the evolution of the acute pyelonephritic scar. Kidney Int. 1981;20(6):733–42.
105. Smellie JM, Preece MA, Paton AM. Somatic growth in girls receiving low dose prophylactic co-trimoxazole. Br Med J (Clin Res Ed). 1983;287(6396):875.
106. Jodal U. The natural history of bacteriuria in childhood. Infect Dis Clin North Am. 1987;1(4):713–29.
107. Smellie JM, Ransely PG, Normand IC, Prescod N, Edwards D. Development of new renal scars: a collaborative study. Br Med J (Clin Res Ed). 1985;290(6486):1957–60.
108. Martinell J, Lidin-Janson G, Jagenburg R, Sivertsson R, Claesson I, Jodal U. Girls prone to urinary infections followed into adulthood. Indices of renal disease. Pediatr Nephol. 1996;10(2):139–42.
109. Swerkersson S, Jodal U, Sixt R, Stokland E, Hansson S. Relationship among vesicoureteral reflux, urinary tract infection and renal damage in children. J Urol. 2007;178(2):64751.
110. Bisset 3rd GS, Strife JL, Dunbar JS. Urography and voiding cystourethrography: findings in girls with urinary tract infection. AJR Am J Roentgenol. 1987;148(3):479–82.
111. Skoog SJ, Belman AB, Majd M. A nonsurgical approach to the management of primary vesicoureteral reflux. J Urol. 1987;138(4 Pt 2):941–6.
112. Bellinger MF, Duckett JW. Vesicoureteral reflux: a comparison of non-surgical and surgical management. Contrib Nephrol. 1984;39:81–93.
113. Glauser MP, Lyons JM, Braude AI. Prevention of chronic experimental pyelonephritis by suppression of acute suppuration. J Clin Invest. 1978;61(2):403–7.
114. Winberg J, Bollgren I, Källenius G, Möllby R, Svenson SB. Clinical pyelonephritis and focal renal scarring. A selected review of pathogenesis, prevention, and prognosis. Pediatr Clin North Am. 1982;29(4):801–14.
115. Winter AL, Hardy BE, Alton DJ, Arbus GS, Chruchill BM. Acquired renal scars in children. J Urol. 1983;129(6):1190–4.
116. Edwards D, Normand IC, Prescod N, Smellie JM. Disappearance of vesicoureteric reflux during long-term prophylaxis of urinary tract infection in children. Br Med J. 1977;2(6082):285–8.
117. Silver TM, Kass EJ, Thornbury JR, Konnak JW, Wolfman MG. The radiological spectrum of acute pyelonephritis in adults and adolescents. Radiology. 1976;118(1):65–71.
118. Filly R, Friedland GW, Govan DE, Fair WR. Development and progression of clubbing and scarring in children with recurrent urinary tract infections. Radiology. 1974;113(1):145–53.
119. Merrick MV, Uttley WS, Wild SR. The detection of pyelonephritic scarring in children by radioisotope imaging. Br J Radiol. 1980;53(630):544–56.
120. Goldraich NP, Ramos OL, Goldraich IH. Urography versus DMSA scan in children with vesicoureteral reflux. Pediatr Nephrol. 1989;3(1):1–5.
121. Monsour M, Azmy AF, MacKenzie JR. Renal scarring secondary to vesicoureteric reflux. Critical assessment and new grading. Br J Urol. 1987;60(4):320–4.
122. Elison BS, Taylor D, Van der Wall H, Pereira JK, Cahill S, Rosenberg AR, et al. Comparison of DMSA scintigraphy with intravenous urography for the detection of renal scarring and its correlation with vesicoureteric reflux. Br J Urol. 1992;69(3):294–302.
123. Farnsworth RH, Rossleigh MA, Leighton DM, Bass SJ, Rosenberg AR. The detection of reflux nephropathy in infants by 99mtechnetium dimercaptosuccinic acid studies. J Urol. 1991;145(3):542–6.
124. Stoller ML, Kogan BA. Sensitivity of 99mtechnetium-dimercaptosuccinic acid for the diagnosis of chronic pyelonephritis: clinical and theoretical considerations. J Urol. 1986;135(5):977–80.
125. Stokland E, Hellström M, Jacobsson B, Jodal U, Sixt R. Evaluation of DMSA scintigraphy and urography in assessing both acute and permanent renal damage in children. Acta Radiol. 1998;39(4):447–52.
126. Arnold AJ, Brownless SM, Carty HM, Rickwood AM. Detection of renal scarring by DMSA scanning–an experimental study. J Pediatr Surg. 1990;25(4):391–3.
127. Renjen P, Bellah R, Hellinger JC, Darge K. Pediatric urologic advanced imaging: techniques and applications. Urol Clin North Am. 2010;37(2):307–18.
128. Brandström P, Nevéus T, Sixt R, Stokland E, Jodal U, Hansson S. The Swedish reflux trial in children: IV. Renal damage. J Urol. 2010;184(1):292–7.
129. Koyle MA, Elder JS, Skoog SJ, Mattoo TK, Pohl HG, Reddy PP, et al. Febrile urinary tract infection, vesicoureteral reflux, and renal scarring: current controversies in approach to evaluation. Pediatr Surg Int. 2011;27(4):337–46.
130. Mackie GG, Stephens FD. Duplex kidneys: a correlation of renal dysplasia with position of the ureteral orifice. J Urol. 1974;114(2):274–80.
131. Sommer JT, Stephens FD. Morphogenesis of nephropathy with partial ureteral obstruction and vesicoureteral reflux. J Urol. 1981;125(1):67–72.
132. Gordon AC, Thomas DF, Arthur RJ, Irving HC, Smith SE. Prenatally diagnosed reflux: a follow-up study. Br J Urol. 1990;65(4):407–12.
133. Jakobsson B, Svensson L. Transient pyelonephritic changes on 99mTechnetium-dimercaptosuccinic acid scan for at least five months after infection. Acta Paediatr. 1997;86(8):803–7.
134. Rosenberg AR, Rossleigh MA, Brydon MP, Bass SJ, Leighton DM, Farnsworth RH. Evaluation of acute urinary tract infection in children by dimercaptosuccinic acid scintigraphy: a prospective study. J Urol. 1992;148(5 Pt 2):1746–9.

135. Wallin L, Bajc M. Typical technetium dimercaptosuccinic acid distribution patterns in acute pyelonephritis. Acta Paediatr. 1993;82(12):1061–5.
136. Rushton HG, Majd M. Dimercaptosuccinic acid renal scintigraphy for the evaluation of pyelonephritis and scarring: a review of experimental and clinical studies. J Urol. 1992;148(Pt 2):1726–32.
137. Stokland E, Hellström M, Hansson S, Jodal U, Odén A, Jacobsson B. Reliability of ultrasonography in identification of reflux nephropathy in children. Br Med J. 1994;309(6949):235–9.
138. Jakobsson B, Nolstedt L, Svensson L, Söderlundh S, Berg U. 99mTechnetium-dimercaptosuccinic acid scan in the diagnosis of acute pyelonephritis in children: relation to clinical and radiological findings. Pediatr Nephrol. 1992;6(4):328–34.
139. Jakobsson B, Berg U, Svensson L. Renal scarring after acute pyelonephritis. Arch Dis Child. 1994; 70(2):111–5.
140. Majd M, Rushton HG, Jantausch B, Wiedermann BL. Relationship among vesicoureteral reflux, P-fimbriated Escherichia coli, and acute pyelonephritis in children with febrile urinary tract infection. J Pediatr. 1991;119(4):578–85.
141. McGuire EJ, Woodside JR. Diagnostic advantages of fluoroscopic monitoring during urodynamic evaluation. J Urol. 1981;125(6):830–4.
142. Pohl HG, Rushton HG. Urinary tract infections in children. In: Docimo S, Canning D, Khoury A, editors. The Kelalis-King-Belman textbook of clinical pediatric urology. 5th ed. London: CRC Press; 2007. p. 103–66.
143. Patterson IYL, Robertus LM, Gwynne RA, Gardiner RA. Genitourinary tuberculosis in Australia and New Zealand. BJU Int. 2012;109 Suppl 3:27–30.
144. Styne N et al. Xanthogranulomatous pyelonephritis: an uncommon pediatric renal mass. Pediatr Radiol. 2011;41(5):671–2.

13 Urolithiasis

Christina B. Ching, Gabriella L. Crane, and John C. Pope IV

Abbreviations

US	Ultrasound
CT	Computed tomography
IVP	Intravenous pyelography
UPJ	Ureteropelvic junction
SWL	Shock wave lithotripsy
MRI	Magnetic resonance imaging
MCDK	Multicystic dysplastic kidney

Overview of Urolithiasis in the Pediatric Patient

There has been a surge in pediatric stone disease over the past decade, partially attributed to changing diets high in sodium and protein, increasing obesity, and decreasing fluid intake [1–3]. A study of the Pediatric Health Information Database found a threefold increase in the diagnosis of pediatric urolithiasis between 1999 and 2008 in the United States, with a mean annual increase in diagnosis of 10.6 % [1]. This statistic, coupled with the fact that pediatric stone disease is often a sign of an underlying metabolic disorder [2, 4], necessitates a good method of patient evaluation in suspected stone disease. Imaging plays an important role in accurately and expeditiously identifying and localizing stones in order to enable prompt work-up and management. In addition, imaging may help to rule out other pathology responsible for a patient's symptoms and to evaluate specific anatomical anomalies perhaps predisposing a child to stone formation, such as ureteropelvic junction (UPJ) obstruction or nephrocalcinosis.

Pediatric stone disease is related to metabolic abnormalities more than half the time [2, 4–6], resulting in a high probability of recurrent disease. These young patients are thus likely to require multiple follow-up imaging examinations during their lifetimes. As a result, a keen understanding of the different modalities available is imperative in order to most effectively and safely follow this population.

Drawbacks of Ionizing Radiation

While imaging is integral in the diagnosis and management of stone disease, there is growing concern over its frequent use and the harmful effects of excessive ionizing radiation. Adult stone formers are known to be exposed to high

C.B. Ching, MD • J.C. Pope IV, MD (✉)
Urologic Surgery and Pediatrics,
Division of Pediatric Urology,
Monroe Carell Jr. Children's Hospital at Vanderbilt,
2200 Children's Way, 4102-DOT, Nashville, TN
37232-9820, USA
e-mail: christina.b.ching@vanderbilt.edu;
john.pope@vanderbilt.edu

G.L. Crane, MD
Diagnostic Imaging,
Monroe Carell Jr. Children's Hospital at Vanderbilt,
2200 Children's Way, Nashville, TN 37232-9820, USA
e-mail: gabriella.l.crane@vanderbilt.edu

L.S. Palmer, J.S. Palmer (eds.), *Pediatric and Adolescent Urologic Imaging*,
DOI 10.1007/978-1-4614-8654-1_13, © Springer Science+Business Media New York 2014

levels of radiation over the course of their disease due to excessive use of ionizing radiation [7, 8]. For this reason, the American Urological Association published guidelines in 2012 to help establish an appropriate protocol to address these concerns and to limit radiation exposure and cost of high-resolution imaging in adult patients [9].

Children are especially susceptible to the harmful effects of radiation. Their developing tissues are more radiosensitive [10], and care must be taken to prevent damage to gonadal tissue causing problems with future fertility as well as risking the passage of radiation-induced genetic changes to future generations. Simply by virtue of their age, they have a longer expected life span during which they may develop radiation-induced cancers [11]. A study comparing lifetime cancer risk from a single computed tomography (CT) examination for pediatric stone disease to lifetime risk of developing cancer otherwise found a risk ratio of 0.2–0.3 % [12]. A recent study from the United Kingdom found that children receiving a cumulative dose of at least 30 mGy and 50–74 mGy were 3 times as likely to develop leukemia and brain cancer as compared to patients receiving <5 mGy [10]. Since patients diagnosed with stone disease at a young age have an increased risk of recurrent disease and may require more frequent imaging, the purpose and contribution of each imaging study should be considered carefully as the cumulative radiation dose to these patients can add up quickly.

Given concern over the impact of radiation on the pediatric population, the Alliance for Radiation Safety in Pediatric Imaging instituted the *Image Gently* campaign to remind practitioners of the harmful effects of excessive ionizing radiation and to encourage the use of pediatric protocols for CT imaging [13]. The use of low-dose CT techniques will be discussed more in depth later; however, other methods for decreasing radiation exposure include simply decreasing the number of radiographic studies performed by selectively imaging based on good clinical judgment and by choosing nonionizing modalities when possible.

Stone Imaging Modalities

The primary purpose of imaging urolithiasis is to make an initial diagnosis. Other important information, however, can be gathered with imaging, such as stone location and composition, presence of obstruction, changes in location or number of stones following surgical intervention or medical therapy, and the presence of anomalous anatomy that may coexist with stone formation. The best imaging modality which provides this information is one that is accurate, efficient, and safe.

The initial indication for imaging a patient suspected of having stones is the presence of symptoms. Stone disease most commonly presents in children as flank/abdominal pain (60–75 % of children/adolescents) but can also present as gross hematuria (30 %) and dysuria (13 %) [6, 14]. It is usually in evaluating such symptoms that stone disease is identified; 13 % of children, however, may have a stone discovered incidentally [15]. Symptoms can also be nonspecific, creating concern for other pathology such as appendicitis which can be evaluated at the time of imaging [16]. While imaging may be useful for the initial diagnosis, it is also an important tool for the follow-up of a patient with a known stone that is being observed – monitoring the stone for growth, obstruction, or passage and helping to guide the timing of intervention if necessary. Imaging may also be used to follow a patient after intervention for efficacy of the procedure and for recurrence.

The ability to image a stone partly depends on its composition. Luckily, the majority of stones in children are calcium based (specifically calcium oxalate and/or calcium phosphate) and thus opaque when using x-ray [3, 16]. These stones are very dense and therefore readily visible on both abdominal radiography and noncontrast CT. On the other hand, uric acid stones are radiolucent and therefore not visible on abdominal radiography; they may be seen as low-density structures on noncontrast CT. In these cases, contrast material administered intravenously and then excreted by the kidneys into the collecting system may be required in order to create a "filling defect" whereby the radiopaque contrast is displaced by the low-density stone. Struvite and cystine stones are of intermediate density, resulting in some difficulty seeing small stones on abdominal radiography. Drug stones (indinavir, ceftriaxone, sulfadiazine) and matrix/protein stones have variable densities and may be indistinguishable from surrounding tissue and not visible even on noncontrast CT [16].

The location of the stone will also affect how it is seen on various imaging modalities. For example, ultrasound (US) often fails to identify ureteral stones, particularly if the ureter is not dilated or if there is overlying bowel gas which prevents penetration of the ultrasound beam. Identifying stones on CT, on the other hand, is unaffected by stone location or bowel gas. The most common location for pediatric stone disease is in the upper tract (94 % of 54 children evaluated at Hopkins), with approximately 50 % being in the kidney alone [6]. In reality, stones can be located anywhere: from the kidney and ureter, down to the bladder and urethra. The location of the stone, therefore, may dictate the type of examination used to follow it.

Intravenous Pyelography

In the past, intravenous pyelography (IVP) was the technique of choice for evaluating the urinary tract. An IVP consists of a scout radiograph of the abdomen, an image obtained immediately after bolus of intravenous contrast (nephrographic phase), and subsequent delayed images at 5-min intervals (excretory phase). These various phases allow evaluation of bony, soft tissue, calcific, or gaseous abnormalities as well as renal function and urinary tract anomalies. It has been largely replaced with more precise and efficient techniques such as CT and is not commonly performed at tertiary care centers where other modalities are available.

It is, however, still useful in select cases to identify ureteral insertion or kidney location or in the evaluation of urinary tract reconstruction. In regard to stone disease, the simple plain film can identify radiopaque (calcium containing) calculi prior to contrast administration, while radiolucent stones can be identified as filling defects in the excretory phase. The nephrographic phase can demonstrate asymmetry in renal function which may occur secondary to obstruction. This is inferred by delayed uptake of contrast by the renal parenchyma and delayed excretion. The excretory phase can show the integrity of the renal collecting system and the degree and level of ureteral obstruction and can provide a map of the ureters, which is particularly important in cases of congenital urinary tract anomalies when ureteral ectopia is suspected. IVP is also easily used intraoperatively in the case of shock wave lithotripsy (SWL) or in guiding percutaneous access of the collecting system [17].

Some disadvantages to IVP are that it utilizes ionizing radiation and requires intravenous contrast administration, placing the patient at risk for nephrotoxicity and allergic reactions. Performing IVPs can also be relatively time intensive and reliant on a good bowel preparation [18]. In general, this procedure has fallen out of favor in the evaluation of renal stones.

Radiography

Radiography or plain film is quick, easy, and readily accessible. The radiation dose for a single radiograph is also minimal. Alone, however, abdominal radiographs only have a sensitivity of 62 % and specificity of 67 % in stone diagnosis [19]. This is partly because only radiopaque stones can be seen on radiographs (Fig. 13.1). Radiolucent stones (such as pure uric acid, xanthine, struvite, matrix stones) are not visible. Also, small radiopaque stones (<3 mm) may be obscured by overlying soft tissue densities, such as colonic stool, or superimposed by bony structures [18]. Other calcifications such as pelvic phleboliths and appendicoliths can be confused for distal ureteral stones, although classically

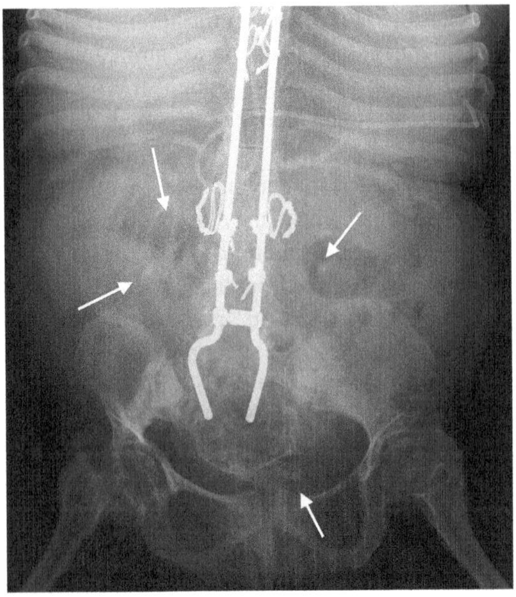

Fig. 13.1 Abdominal radiograph demonstrates bilateral renal stones and bladder stones which are radiopaque (*arrows*)

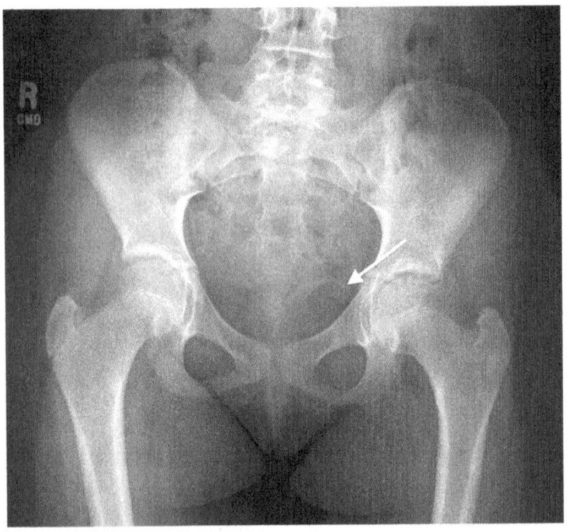

Fig. 13.2 Abdominal radiograph demonstrates a round calcification in the left pelvis (*arrow*). This calcification is more radiolucent in the center as compared to the periphery, consistent with a phlebolith. A ureteral stone would be most dense/radiopaque at its center

phleboliths appear as rounded calcifications with a relatively radiolucent center on abdominal radiography (Fig. 13.2). Unfortunately, radiography offers no information about obstruction [18]. As a result, abdominal radiographs are of little utility in the acute evaluation of a kidney stone [19].

In the case of a known stone former with radiopaque stones, radiography can be used effectively to follow stone size progression or change in stone location. Abdominal radiographs can also be used preoperatively in preparation for SWL to ensure good visualization of the stone on fluoroscopy during the procedure and postoperatively to determine resolution or stone passage (Fig. 13.3). The sensitivity and specificity of radiography are improved when used in conjunction with ultrasound.

Ultrasound

Given its lack of ionizing radiation, ultrasound (US) is often the initial modality of choice in evaluating a pediatric patient with suspected urolithiasis and nonemergent abdominal or flank pain [20, 21]. It is also lower in cost than CT, is noninvasive, does not require sedation, and can be performed portably, allowing bedside evaluation of sick patients.

The greatest strength of US in the setting of stone disease is in evaluating for obstruction, or hydronephrosis, easily depicted as fluid distension of the renal pelvis and calices [15] (Fig. 13.4). It can also provide extensive anatomical detail in patients with congenital duplications and other anomalies contributing to stone formation. US can also directly demonstrate stones. Typically, a renal stone appears as a very bright, or echogenic, rounded structure. Due to its high density, the stone will block penetration of the US beam, resulting in a black shadow behind it. This is referred to as posterior acoustic shadowing [2, 16] (Figs. 13.5 and 13.6). The exceptions are drug stones or matrix/protein stones which are of variable density and may not be distinguishable from surrounding soft tissue on ultrasound [16].

Stones are most easily identified in the kidney and in the distended urinary bladder (Fig. 13.7).

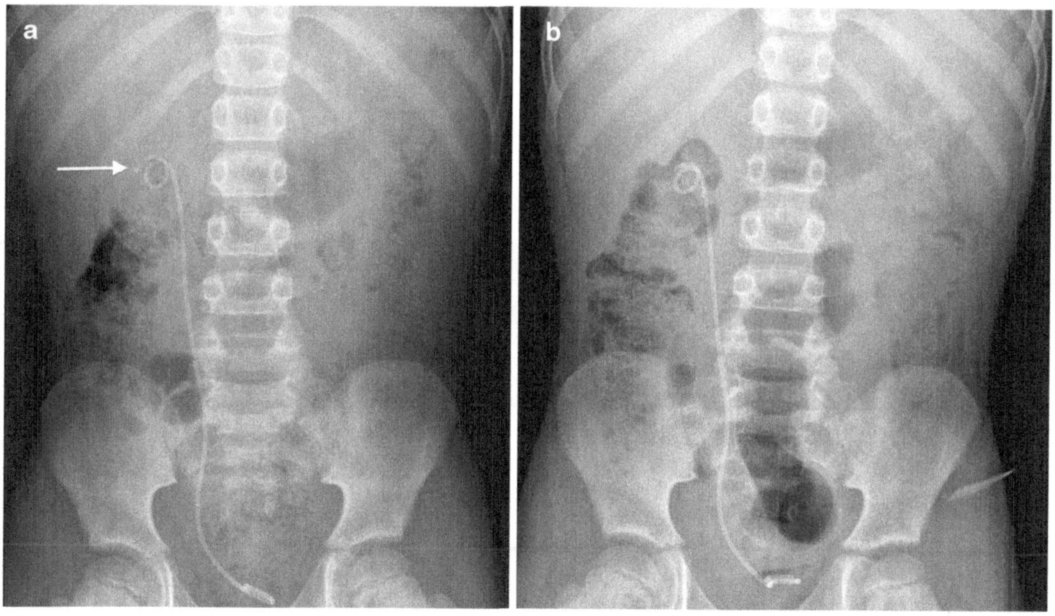

Fig. 13.3 A 7-year-old boy presenting with right flank pain was found to have an obstructing right ureteropelvic junction stone. (**a**) Abdominal radiograph after preoperative stent placement demonstrates a radiopaque stone in the right kidney (*arrow*). (**b**) Abdominal radiograph 2 weeks after SWL demonstrates eradication of the stone

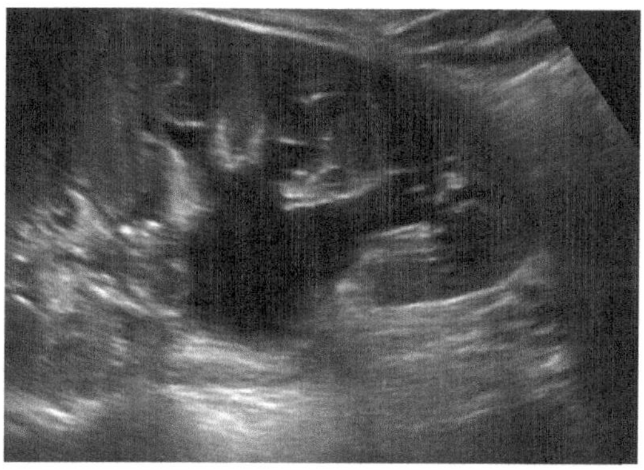

Fig. 13.4 A 15-year-old female with hydronephrosis due to an obstructing distal stone. This US shows a dilated renal pelvis communicating with dilated calyces. This patient required a ureteral stent for her obstruction

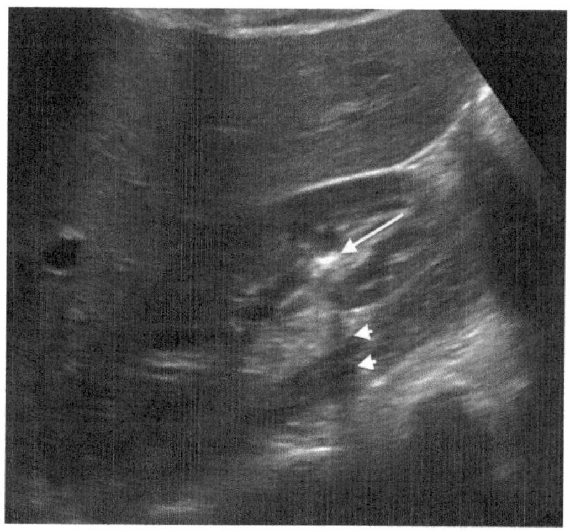

Fig. 13.5 A 15-year-old female with a nonobstructing lower pole renal stone. The stone is echogenic (*long arrow*) and causes posterior acoustic shadowing (*arrow heads*)

In general, US is poor at localizing ureteral stones, especially in the absence of ureteral dilatation. Palmer et al. found that the detection rate for ureteral calculi was only 38 % as compared to 90 % for renal stones [22]. Hydronephrosis may suggest a ureteral stone, but even in the presence of hydroureter, it is often difficult to see the ureteral stone if there is overlying bowel gas or surrounding soft tissue which obscures the ureter [2–15] (Figs. 13.8 and 13.9). If the dilated ureter at the level of obstruction can be seen, then the stone may be visible (Fig. 13.10).

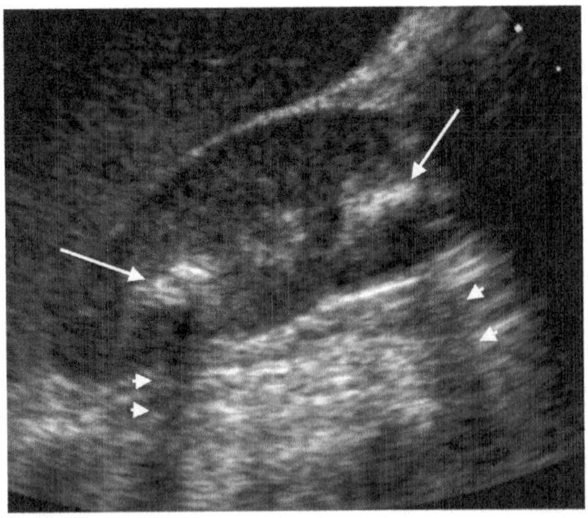

Fig. 13.6 An 8-year-old female with renal stones in the upper and lower poles. Both stones are echogenic (*long arrows*) with posterior acoustic shadowing (*arrow heads*)

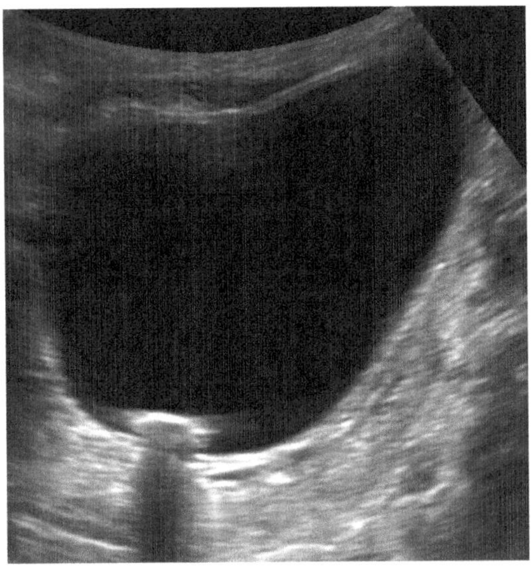

Fig. 13.7 Bladder stone on US. Similar to the renal stones, the bladder stone is echogenic and demonstrates clear posterior acoustic shadowing

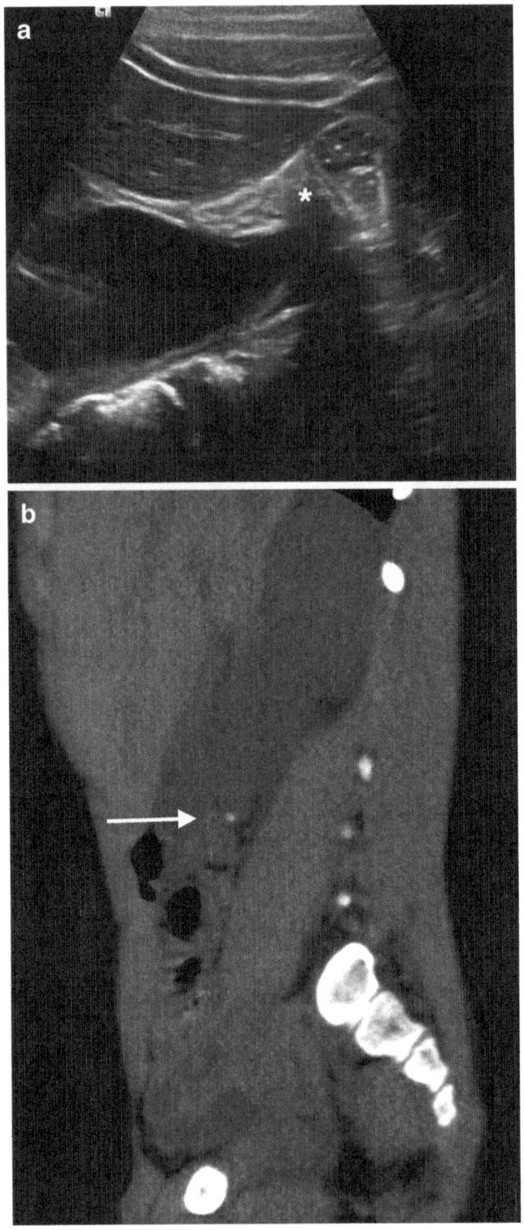

Fig. 13.8 A 5-year-old boy with right-sided abdominal pain and vomiting. (**a**) An ultrasound shows obvious obstruction with hydronephrosis. However, when attempting to look at the proximal ureter, it is obscured by bowel gas (*asterisk*). (**b**) A CT scan was performed that same day for further work-up due to a strong suspicion of stone disease. A sagittal reformation of the CT shows a dense proximal ureteral stone (*arrow*) with proximal hydroureteronephrosis

A special feature of US is the artifact created by color Doppler imaging of a rough reflective surface, known as "twinkling." Twinkling refers to the multicolor signal behind the stone simulating turbulence (Fig. 13.11). This can be used as supportive evidence when diagnosing stones by US. One study found that twinkling artifact had a 78 % positive predictive value for nephrolithiasis at subsequent CT. The true-positive rate of twinkling artifact for confirmed calculi at CT, however, was only 49 % with a 51 % false-positive rate [23]. This study used 5 mm CT sections

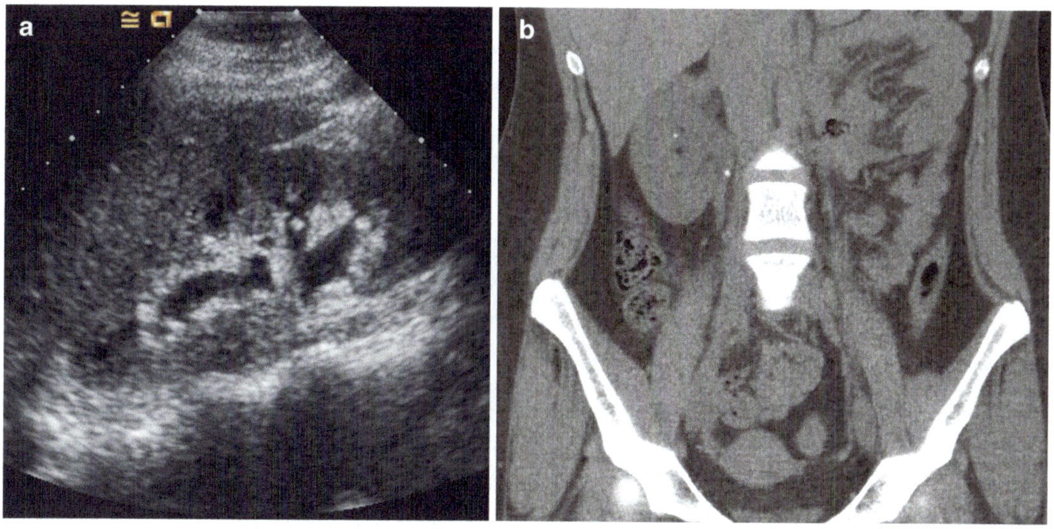

Fig. 13.9 A 16-year-old female with a history of stones presents with right-sided flank pain and nausea. (**a**) US demonstrates mild right-sided hydronephrosis without identification of a stone. Given her history and clinical picture, there was high suspicion for a stone. (**b**) Subsequent noncontrast CT that same day finds a small stone in the proximal right ureter causing obstruction, as well as a small nonobstructing stone in the right kidney

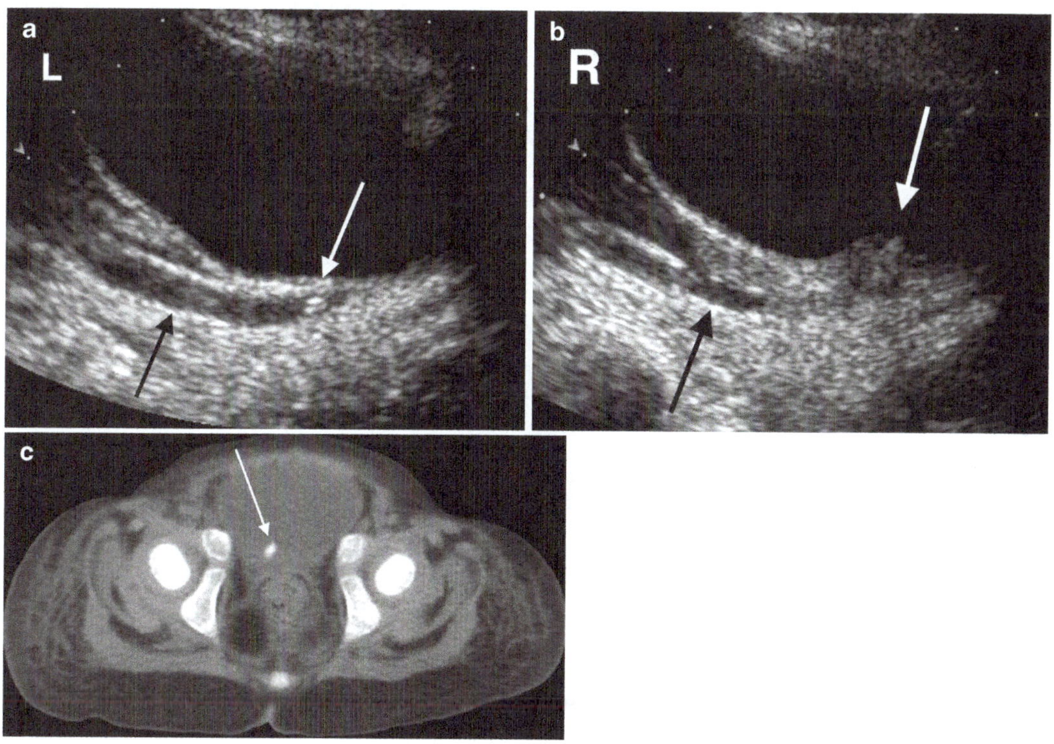

Fig. 13.10 A 28-month-old female with abdominal pain. (**a**) An initial ultrasound demonstrates a left distal ureteral stone (*white arrow*) with proximal hydroureter (*black arrow*). (**b**) There is also thickening of the right side of the bladder at the ureterovesical junction (*white arrow*) with proximal hydroureter (*black arrow*) but no definite echogenic stone or posterior acoustic shadowing. (**c**) A CT one day later demonstrates a right-sided ureterovesical junction stone (*arrow*). The left distal ureteral stone seen on US is not present on the CT, but there is residual dilation of the left ureter (not shown), suggesting the stone had passed

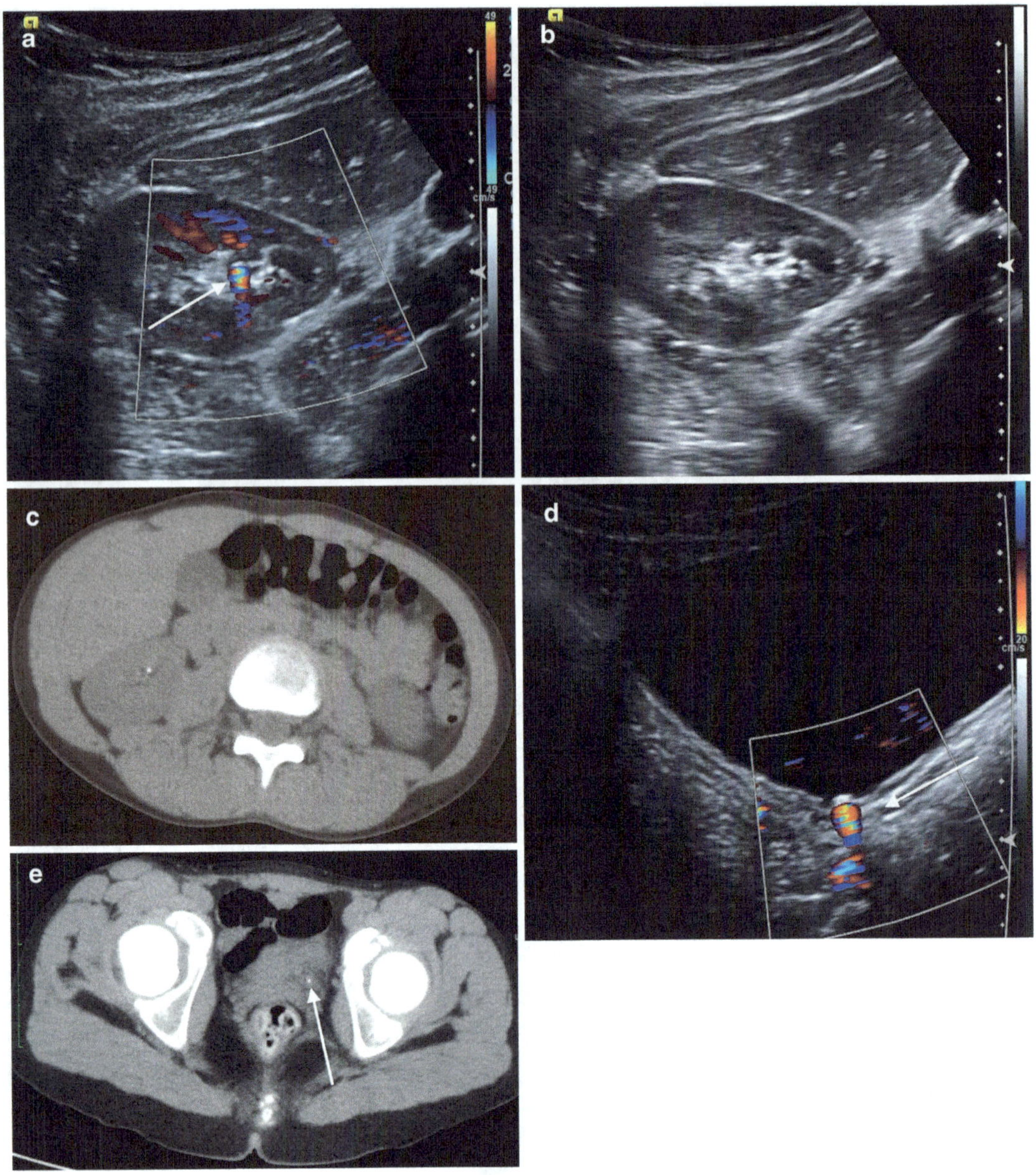

Fig. 13.11 An 11-year-old female with flank pain. (**a**) "Twinkle" is demonstrated on a color Doppler ultrasound image of the right kidney. Notice the focal multicolor signal emanating from the renal sinus (*arrow*). (**b**) The stone without the use of color Doppler is more difficult to see, particularly when surrounded by echogenic renal sinus fat. (**c**) The small renal stone is confirmed on CT imaging. (**d**) This patient also had a distal ureteral stone that demonstrates twinkle (*arrow*). (**e**) The stone is again confirmed on CT imaging (*arrow*)

to correlate with twinkle artifact, however, which may have in fact missed smaller stones that were accurately identified by twinkle artifact.

Many studies have found US to lack the sensitivity and accuracy of CT in both identifying and characterizing stones. One study by Passerotti et al. found that US had an overall sensitivity of 76 % and a specificity of 100 % in comparison to CT for urolithiasis in the kidney, ureter, or bladder [24]. Ray et al. performed a literature review and only found a 45 % pooled sensitivity for US [15]. US has been found to both miss stones averaging

2.3 mm [24] and to overestimate stones <5 mm in size by 2 mm [15]. Palmer et al. compared US and CT in symptomatic patients and found US nondiagnostic in 41 % of cases versus 5 % of cases with CT [22]. As a result, a negative US in a symptomatic patient may still require further work-up with CT imaging. Confirmatory CT is also sometimes advocated after an equivocal US and even after a positive US to evaluate stone location and burden for appropriate planning of an intervention [22]. Given the likelihood of requiring subsequent CT, some would advocate beginning with a low-dose CT to decrease the overall number of imaging exams and the burden of cost. For example, Palmer et al. advocated beginning with a CT when evaluating children >11 years old with a positive family history of stone disease [22]. This issue remains controversial, however, and the aforementioned study by Passerotti concluded that although CT is more sensitive than US for the detection of renal stones, the difference between these exams may not be clinically significant; these authors therefore recommend US as the initial imaging exam for children with suspected stones due to the potential adverse effects of ionizing radiation from CT.

As previously mentioned, the sensitivity of US can be increased if used in conjunction with abdominal radiography. Mitterberger et al. found that the combined use of radiography and native tissue harmonic imaging ultrasonography had a sensitivity and accuracy for detecting ureteric calculi of 96 % and 95 %, respectively [25]. Both modalities may be effective in following a patient with known stone disease.

While readily accessible, US is operator dependent and potentially limited by a patient's body habitus. Skeletal abnormalities such as extreme kyphosis/scoliosis may be prohibitive in visualizing the retroperitoneum with US. These factors must also be considered when choosing between US and CT.

Computed Tomography

Noncontrast computed tomography (CT) has surpassed many other imaging modalities in diagnosing and confirming stone disease; it is overall considered the gold standard imaging technique for urolithiasis. CT provides accurate information regarding the location and size of the stone and relevant surrounding anatomy [15] (Figs. 13.12, 13.13, 13.14, and 13.15). It can also be used to measure stone density to provide preliminary information regarding stone composition which may help direct therapy [18]. CT imaging has a high sensitivity and specificity independent of stone location (96–99 % sensitivity and 96–97 % specificity) [26, 27]. Using thin slice collimation of <3 mm, the sensitivity and specificity are virtually 100 % [15]. CT is typically used in the emergency setting due to its

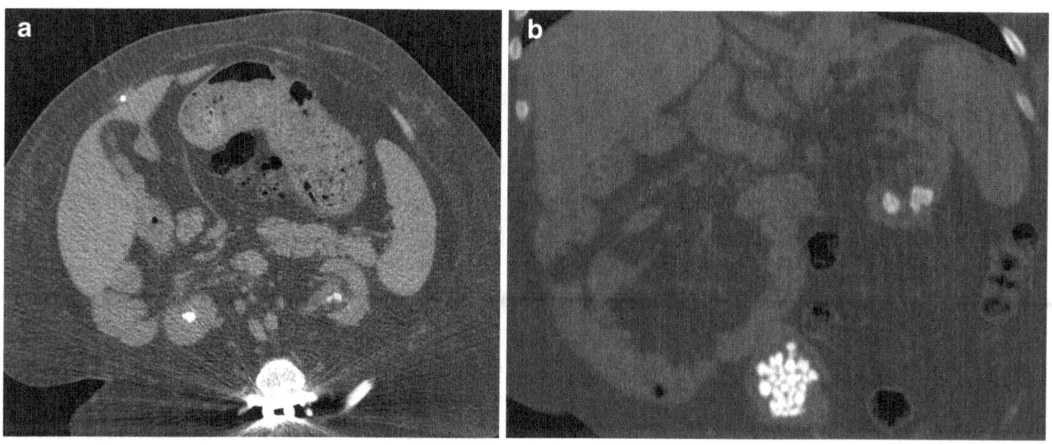

Fig. 13.12 CT imaging of stone disease. (**a**) This patient has multiple bilateral renal stones. (**b**) Coronal reformation of the same patient demonstrates bladder stones as well

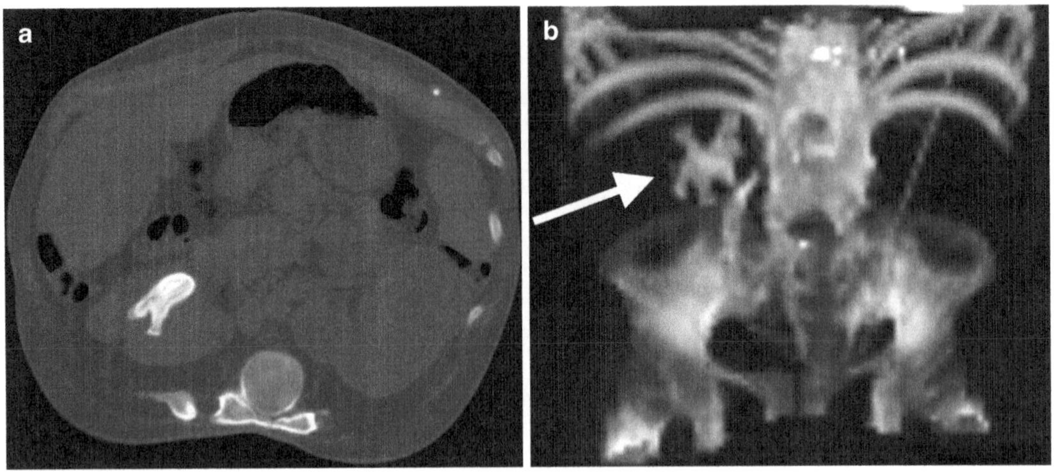

Fig. 13.13 An 18-year-old female with spina bifida, neurogenic bladder, and a history of kidney stones was found on regular follow-up to have a right-sided staghorn calculus. (**a**) This stone is demonstrated in the axial plane on noncontrast CT. Notice how the stone fills at least 2 calyces on these images. She also has a nonfunctioning left kidney. (**b**) 3D volume rendering can be used to demonstrate the full size of the staghorn calculus (*arrow*)

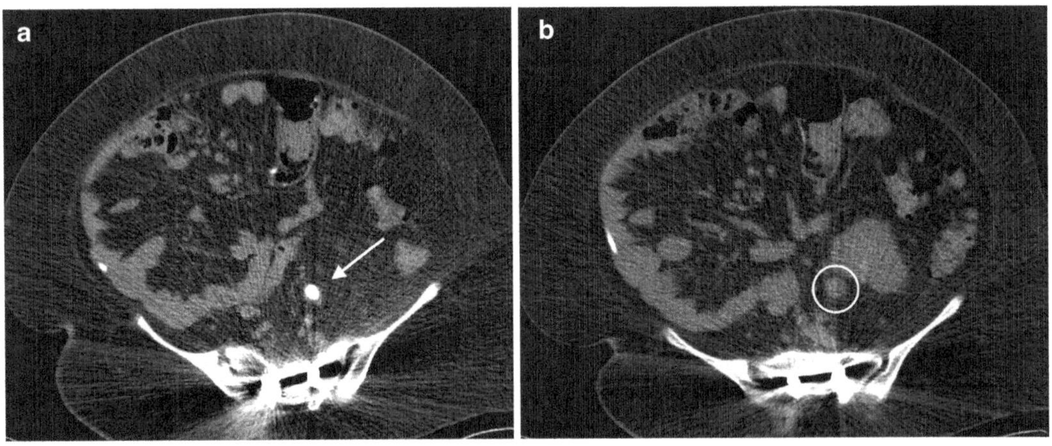

Fig. 13.14 A 14-year-old boy with spina bifida and a neurogenic bladder status post bladder augmentation, Mitrofanoff catheterizable stoma, and bladder neck closure who has a history of kidney and bladder stones. (**a**) A CT demonstrates an obstructing left ureteral stone (*arrow*). Notice the soft tissue density around the stone representing the edematous ureter. (**b**) Proximal left ureteral dilation is seen (*circle*)

speed and high sensitivity/specificity as well as its ability to rule out other pathology. CT for the evaluation of renal stones does not require IV contrast, and in fact, contrast enhancement of the renal parenchyma and excretion of contrast into the collecting system may obscure small stones. Stones which are radiolucent or too small to be seen on abdominal radiographs can generally be seen on CT.

Secondary signs of ureteral stones can also be seen on CT, such as hydronephrosis, proximal ureteral dilatation, unilateral renal enlargement, decreased renal attenuation due to edema, and perinephric or periureteral edema (Figs. 13.16, 13.17, 13.18, and 13.19). In the event that no stone is seen on the CT scan, these secondary signs can suggest recent passage of a stone. A method to distinguish a ureteral stone from a phlebolith is to look for the "rim sign" – circumferential soft tissue density representing the ureter encircling the stone, which is not found with a phlebolith (Fig. 13.20). If the obstructing

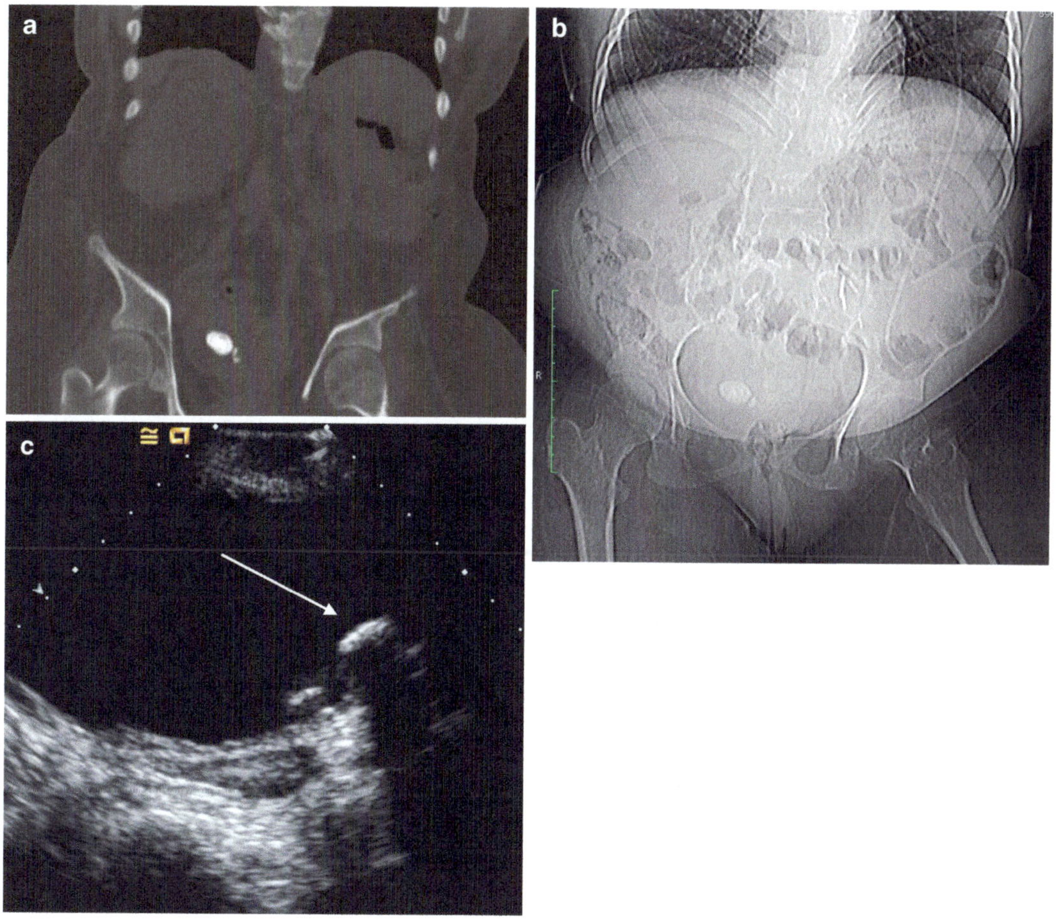

Fig. 13.15 This is a series of the same bladder stones as seen on various imaging modalities. (**a**) The stones as they appear on CT bone window. (**b**) The largest stone was big enough to be seen on the scout radiograph for the CT. (**c**) A view of the stones on US (*arrow*)

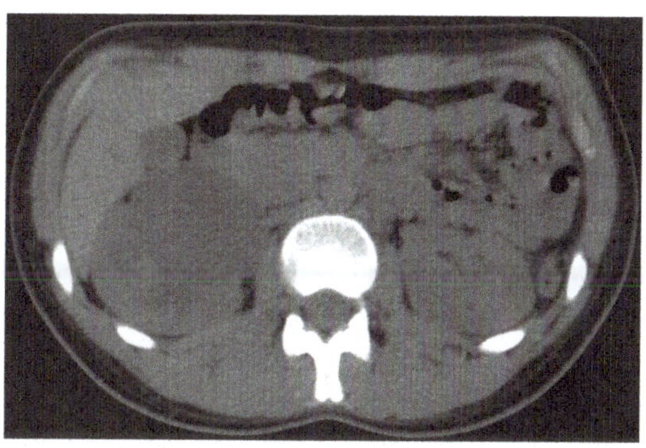

Fig. 13.16 Noncontrast CT demonstrates severe hydronephrosis of the right kidney

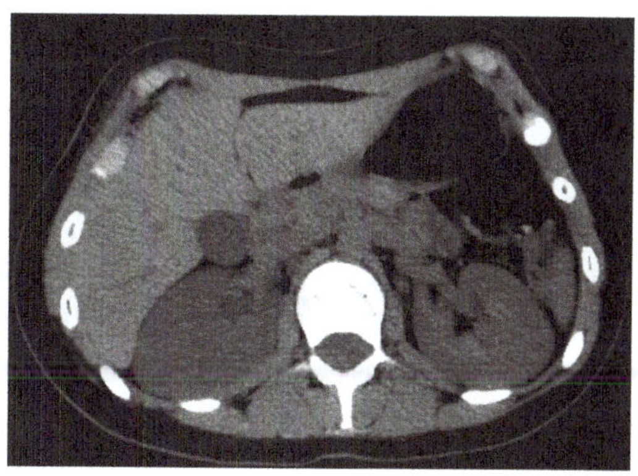

Fig. 13.17 Noncontrast CT demonstrates decreased attenuation of the right kidney as compared with the left kidney, consistent with edema. The right kidney also demonstrates mild hydronephrosis

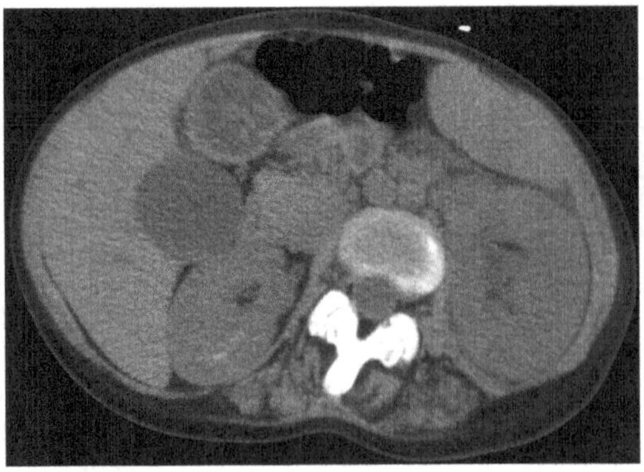

Fig. 13.18 Noncontrast CT demonstrates left-sided perinephric stranding with renal edema and enlargement

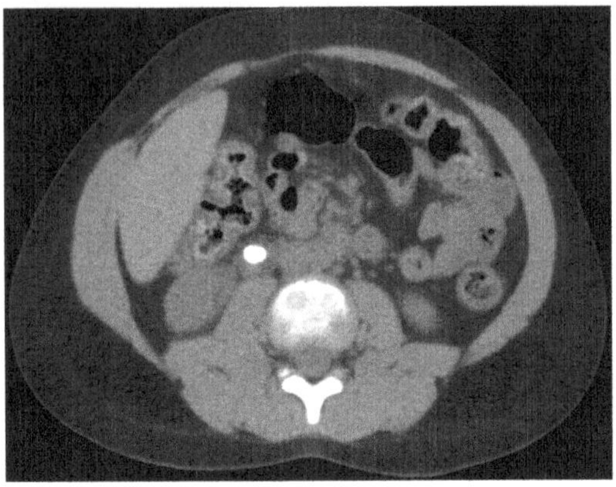

Fig. 13.19 Right-sided periureteral edema around a ureteral stone

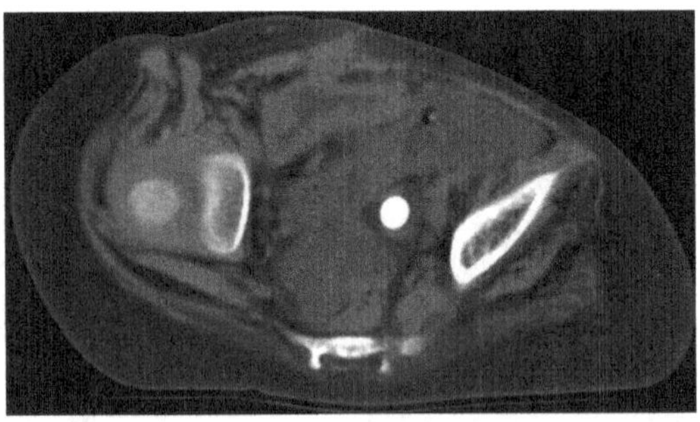

Fig. 13.20 The "rim sign" can be seen around this ureteral stone. It can be used to distinguish a stone from a phlebolith

stone is associated with infection, pyelonephritis and ureteritis can also be demonstrated using contrast-enhanced CT (Fig. 13.21).

Despite all the advantages of CT imaging, a major concern is its use of ionizing radiation, particularly as it pertains to the pediatric patient. CT utilizes significantly more ionizing radiation than the other imaging modalities: the effective dose of an abdominal/pelvic CT is 4.3–8.5 mSv as compared to an abdominal radiograph which is 0.2–0.7 mSv and MRI or US which is 0 mSv [18]. To put it further in perspective, the effective dose of a single noncontrast CT (stone protocol) for a child is about 1–2 years worth of background radiation (3 mSv) [12]. As a result, it is not necessarily the automatic first choice of imaging in the pediatric population and should be thoughtfully used in these patients who may require multiple imaging procedures in the future.

As a result, there has been keen interest in low-dose CT imaging techniques to try to reduce the amount of radiation to which the patient is exposed without affecting its diagnostic capability. Newer CT protocols have been shown to decrease the radiation-measured entrance dose by 60–90 % [28], with published effective doses for a low-dose CT of 0.98–1.5 mSv as compared to 4.3–8.5 mSv for a standard abdominal/pelvic CT [18]. Techniques such as tube current modulation, low voltage protocols, and other adjustments to alter image acquisition and reconstruction can significantly reduce patient radiation exposure [18, 29]. In a model looking at effective dose and lifetime risk of cancer, low-dose imaging (40 mA, 10 ms, 125 kVp) as compared to standard dose (80 mA, 25 ms, 125 kVp) decreased the lifetime attributable risk of cancer from 23–144 cases per 100,000 to 5–31 cases per 100,000 [30]. Diagnostic accuracy has been shown to be maintained with low-dose protocols. Karmazyn et al. found that reducing the dose of radiation did not significantly reduce the detection of ureteral or kidney stones in children weighing <50 kg [31].

It is important to remember that even with lower-dose imaging techniques, there is no threshold under which radiation is safe. A study from the Netherlands found a linear-no-threshold model for the induction of chromosomal damage induced by ionizing radiation, seeing an induction

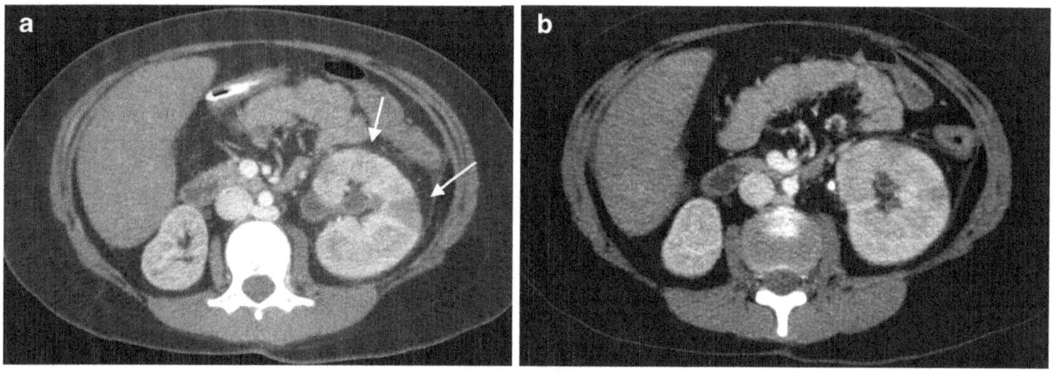

Fig. 13.21 This is a patient presenting with fever and abdominal pain. (**a**) Contrast-enhanced CT shows wedge-shaped areas of hypoenhancement suggesting infection or pyelonephritis (*arrows*). There is also hyperenhancement of the urothelium signifying infection. (**b**) The obstructing stone can be seen in the proximal ureter on a more inferior slice

of micronuclei in human fibroblasts in doses as low as 20 mGy. The damage was increased if cells were exposed during the S-phase of the cell cycle [32]. The only way to most effectively decrease the amount of radiation to which a patient is exposed is to choose nonionizing studies when possible (i.e., US). If CT has to be used, use it sparingly and limit the scan to only the area of interest [13].

Magnetic Resonance Imaging

Magnetic resonance imaging (MRI) is a very good modality for imaging the anatomy and function of the genitourinary tract using MR urography protocols and has the added benefit of lacking ionizing radiation. Its use in patients with urolithiasis, however, is limited [33]. MRI is unable to directly visualize stones; stones present instead as signal voids. It is also expensive, requires sedation for most young children, and is limited in its availability, especially in the emergent setting and at night [18].

Nuclear Scintigraphy

Nuclear medicine imaging, as MR, has no primary role in the acute evaluation of stone disease. It is only useful to distinguish obstructive hydronephrosis from nonobstructive urinary tract dilation in a pediatric patient with a possibly obstructing stone or to confirm a concomitant anatomical anomaly such as ureteropelvic junction obstruction [34]. It can also determine relative kidney function which may help guide management (i.e., remove a stone versus remove the kidney).

Fluoroscopy

Fluoroscopy is used during the time of stone intervention. It can be used alone to localize a radiopaque stone or in conjunction with retrograde contrast injection (retrograde pyelography) to visualize a radiolucent stone and/or evaluate ureteral and renal pelvic anatomy (Fig. 13.22). Fluoroscopy allows real-time stone detection, size determination, and localization to enable retrograde or percutaneous access of the urinary tract. It also enables targeted SWL and intraoperative evaluation of treatment efficacy. Fluoroscopy emits ionizing radiation and thus should be used judiciously.

Urostasis and Special Anatomical Considerations

Urostasis can predispose patients to stone formation – whether by infection leading to stone disease or simply by precipitation of solutes.

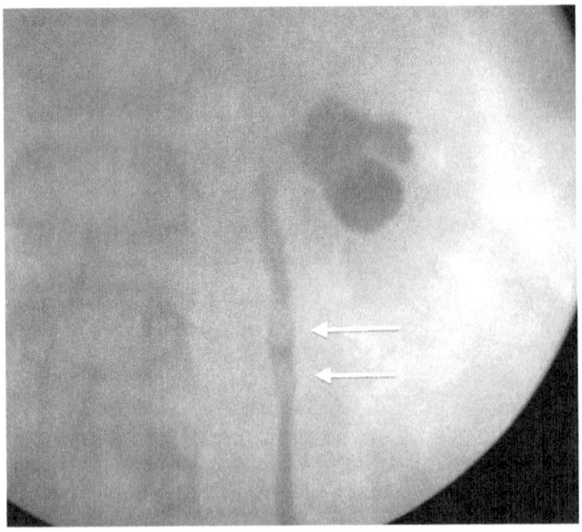

Fig. 13.22 A 17-year-old boy with history of kidney stones who was found to have an impacted left ureteral stone on work-up for intractable left-sided flank pain. Retrograde pyelography demonstrates ureteral filling defects (*arrows*)

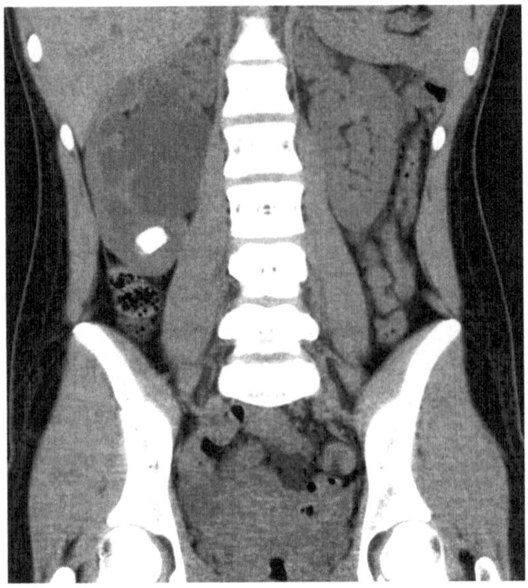

Fig. 13.23 Noncontrast CT showing severe hydronephrosis. This patient did not have a dilated ureter, classic for a UPJ obstruction. A lower pole renal stone can be seen as well, likely a result of urostasis

Urostasis can be a result of anatomic or neurologic abnormalities that interfere with urinary drainage. Anatomic anomalies may be congenital in origin or postsurgical after urinary reconstruction. Congenital abnormalities often cause obstruction of urine flow, whereas postsurgical issues can be a result of urine retention due to a reconfiguration using bowel to augment bladder capacity. Neurologic abnormalities that cause a neurogenic bladder specifically impair bladder emptying efficiency.

Congenital Genitourinary Tract Abnormalities

While metabolic abnormalities are the most common etiology for pediatric stone formation, abnormal anatomy can facilitate stone formation. There are various congenital anatomical malformations that can predispose to poor urinary drainage or cause frank obstruction. As a result, stones are found in conjunction with these congenital abnormalities: 9–34 % of urolithiasis cases are associated with an upper tract anomaly [35].

Known congenital abnormalities of the urinary system associated with stone disease include ureteropelvic junction (UPJ) obstruction (Fig. 13.23), megaureter (Fig. 13.24), ureterocele (Fig. 13.25), calyceal diverticula, multicystic dysplastic kidney (MCDK) (Fig. 13.26), horseshoe kidney, and immaturity or maldevelopment of the ureterovesical junction resulting in vesicoureteral reflux. Each of these anomalies results in either direct obstruction of the urinary tract (UPJ obstruction, ureterocele, calyceal diverticulum) or urostasis due to poor urinary drainage (megaureter, vesicoureteral reflux). In the case of horseshoe kidney, the high inserting ureter results in UPJ obstruction [36]. Despite the anatomical issues related to stone formation, usually there is an element of a concurrent metabolic disorder. For example, studies evaluating stone disease in children with UPJ obstruction often find a supporting metabolic anomaly in addition to their known obstruction [37].

In UPJ obstruction and MCDK, the majority of stones are in the kidney, and thus US and abdominal radiography (if the stone is radiopaque)

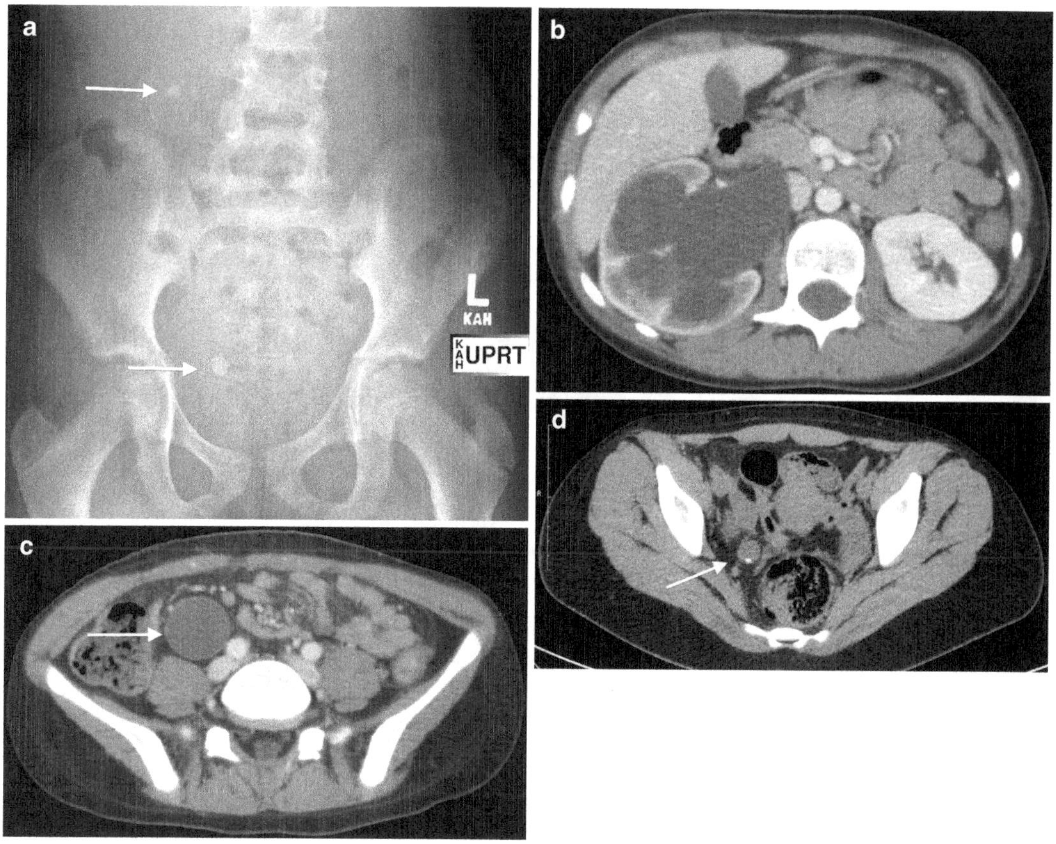

Fig. 13.24 This 12-year-old presented with urinary tract infections. (**a**) An abdominal radiograph demonstrates a right renal stone and a right distal ureteral stone (*arrows*). (**b**) Contrast-enhanced CT shows severe hydronephrosis as well as marked parenchymal thinning of the right kidney. (**c**) A markedly dilated right ureter is seen (*arrow*). (**d**) Even after laser lithotripsy to remove the stone and obstruction, the ureter remains dilated as a primary megaureter. A small postoperative fragment of stone lies dependently along the wall of the ureter but is nonobstructing (*arrow*)

should be sufficient for stone diagnosis and evaluation. In patients with megaureter and ureterocele, bladder ultrasound and abdominal radiography may also be adequate to diagnose stone disease given the distal location. In general, however, CT is to be the imaging modality of choice when evaluating anomalous anatomy to determine the location and number of stones and to clearly delineate the associated anatomy when planning for surgery [38–40]. Nuclear medicine imaging plays an important role in the evaluation of overall renal function to determine salvageability of the kidney. It can also be used to confirm obstruction.

Medullary Sponge Kidney (Nephrocalcinosis Versus Nephrolithiasis)

Medullary sponge kidney, or ectasia of the renal collecting ducts, is a congenital disorder of the kidney and is associated with nephrocalcinosis and nephrolithiasis due to hypercalciuria and hypocitraturia. Nephrocalcinosis is the diffuse deposition of calcium in the kidneys with the greatest concentration found at the tips of the pyramids; nephrolithiasis, on the other hand, refers to discrete stone formation in the collecting system [41]. While nephrocalcinosis can cause

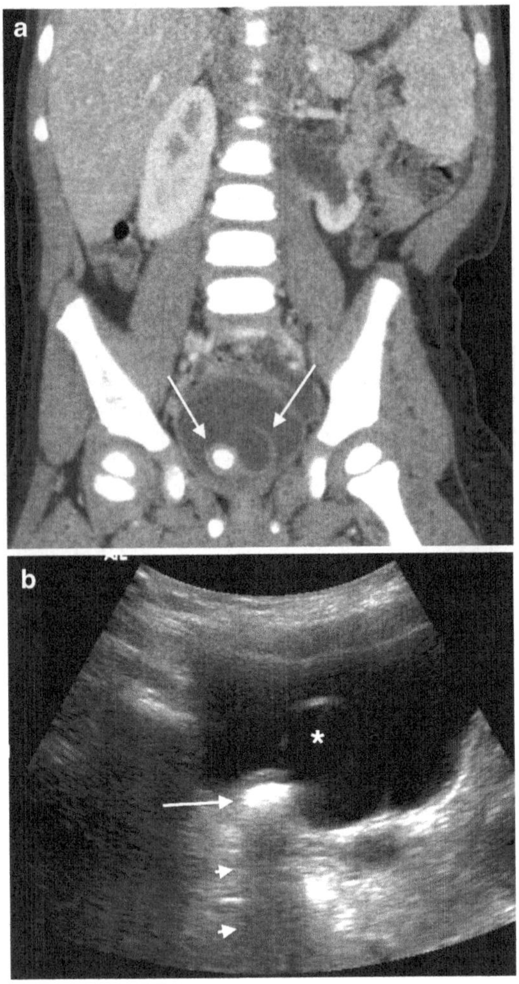

Fig. 13.25 A 20-month-old child who presented with recurrent urinary tract infections. (**a**) Bilateral ureteroceles (*arrows*) can be seen on coronal reformation of a contrast-enhanced CT. The right ureterocele contains a stone. (**b**) US showing both ureteroceles. The left ureterocele (*asterisk*) does not contain a stone. The right ureterocele stone is echogenic (*arrow*) and causes posterior acoustic shadowing (*arrowheads*)

microscopic or gross hematuria, sterile leukocyturia, and pain [16, 41], it is generally asymptomatic [16, 42]. Nephrocalcinosis is believed to share the same pathophysiology as nephrolithiasis and can lead to nephrolithiasis when calcium aggregates form and become large enough to perforate the calyceal epithelium, resulting in a nidus for stone formation in the renal collecting system. It is unclear why one patient develops one entity, the other, or both [42].

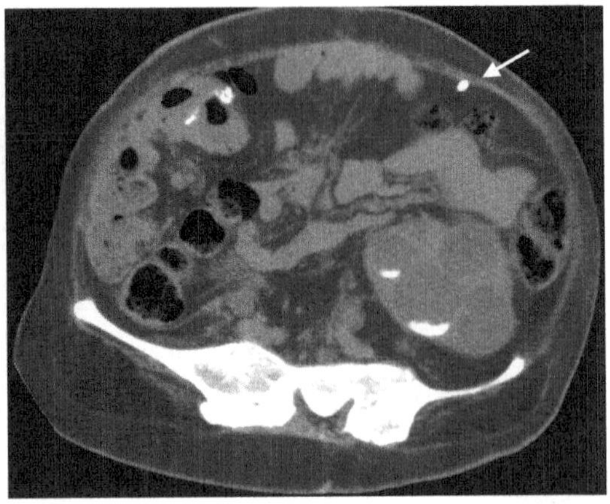

Fig. 13.26 This patient has renal stones in her multicystic dysplastic kidney due to urinary stasis. The other hyperdensity represents her ventriculoperitoneal shunt (*arrow*)

In nephrocalcinosis, calcium salts can deposit in renal tubules, tubular epithelium, and/or interstitial tissue. It is best viewed with high-resolution US [16] and thus classified by anatomic location of calcium deposition: medullary, cortical, or diffuse (with three subtypes according to degree of echogenicity) [5, 16]. In medullary nephrocalcinosis, there is increased echogenicity in the area of the medulla with posterior acoustic shadowing; this is in contrast to normal renal pyramids which are hypoechoic as compared to cortex [16] (Fig. 13.27).

The Reconstructed Genitourinary Tract

Surgical urinary reconstructions are at risk of stone formation due to poor bladder emptying and urostasis as well as technical and metabolic reasons. Often urinary stasis is a purposeful outcome of trying to correct a prior issue with continence or bladder storage. Complex reconstructions often require the use of bowel segments intermixed with the urinary system which can cause metabolic and infectious alterations contributing to stone formation. The technique utilized can significantly affect the risk of stone formation, particularly if a nidus such as a stitch or staple is

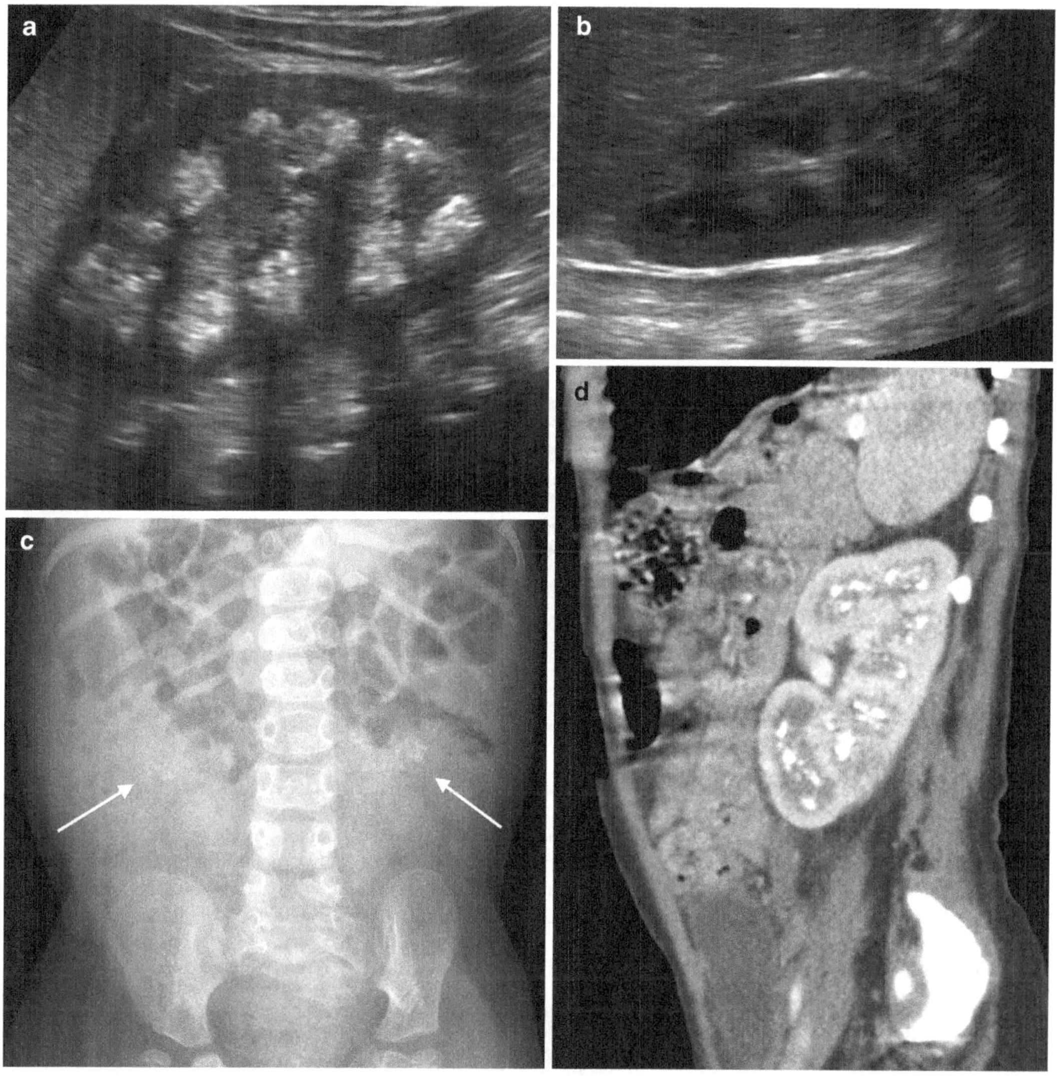

Fig. 13.27 This patient has a history of tethered cord, bony abnormalities, and nephrocalcinosis. (**a**) Ultrasound demonstrates nicely her nephrocalcinosis. The medullary pyramids are echogenic with posterior acoustic shadowing. (**b**) For comparison, this is a normal kidney ultrasound of a child of the same age. Notice that the normal medullary pyramids are hypoechoic (*dark*) as compared to the cortex. (**c**) The calcifications in the child with nephrocalcinosis can even be seen bilaterally on abdominal radiograph (*arrows*). (**d**) While nephrocalcinosis is well seen on US, a CT of this same patient nicely demonstrates the extensive calcifications. Despite this being a contrast-enhanced CT, the renal pyramid calcifications can be seen during the nephrographic phase in this sagittal reformation

left in contact with the urinary tract enabling stone formation.

Stone disease is a known complication of bladder augmentation and continent urinary diversions, with an incidence of 10–52.5 % [43–46] and 4.5–20 % [47–49], respectively (Figs. 13.28 and 13.29). It is also seen after surgical reconstruction in patients with bladder exstrophy and cloacal malformation (Fig. 13.30). Given the prevalence of infection and bacteriuria, the majority of stones are infectious but can also be calcium containing [50]. Although infection plays a significant role in stone formation for these patients, other causative factors include incomplete bladder emptying, abnormal alterations of urinary pH due to the use of intestinal segments, and possibly mucus buildup [46, 50, 51]. Catheterization alone has been found to increase the risk of stone formation due to incomplete emptying and is particularly prevalent in a nondependent catheterizable channel such as an abdominal wall stoma [52, 53] (Fig. 13.31).

A combination of US and abdominal radiography is usually adequate for diagnostic purposes; however, CT plays an important role in preoperative surgical planning. These patients will probably require a surgical procedure for stone removal.

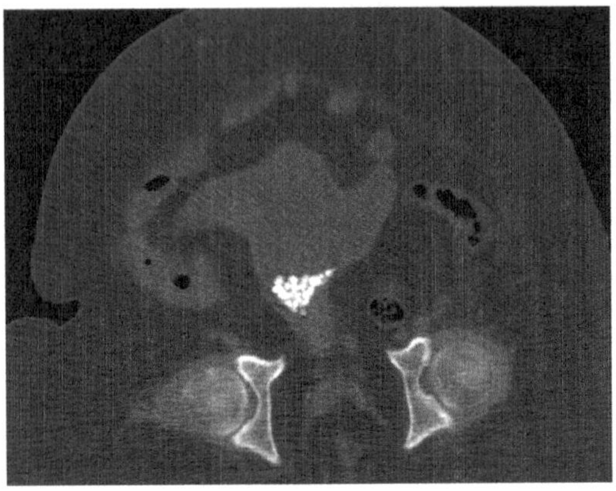

Fig. 13.28 This child has a history of spina bifida and neurogenic bladder status post bladder augmentation with chronic bladder stones. Multiple small bladder stones can be seen on this CT. Notice the irregular shape of his bladder due to bladder augmentation

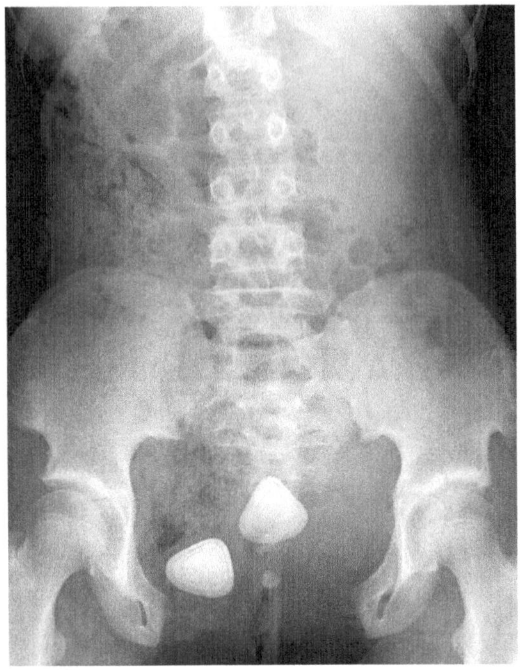

Fig. 13.30 The bladder stones in this 14-year-old girl with a history of reconstruction for bladder exstrophy are well demonstrated on this abdominal radiograph. She has had recurrent issues with bladder stones after her ileal augmentation cystoplasty

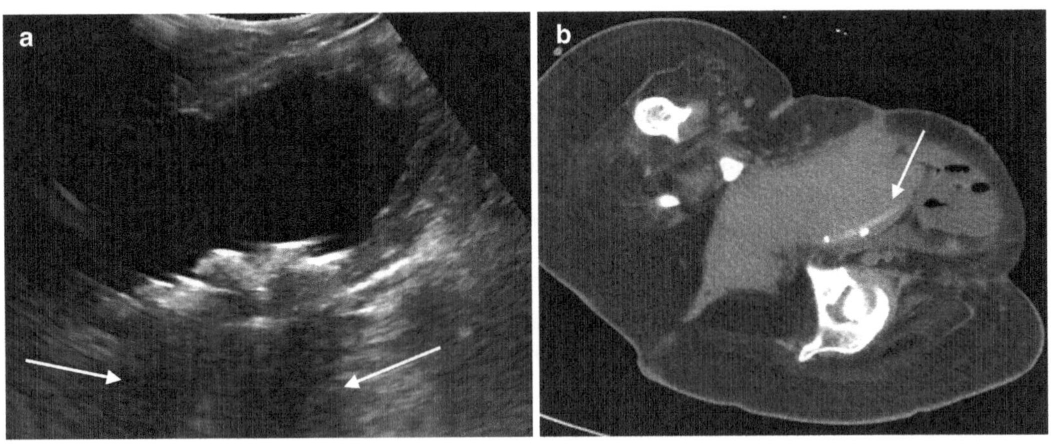

Fig. 13.29 This patient has a history of spina bifida and neurogenic bladder status post bladder augmentation, Mitrofanoff, and pubovaginal sling. She has had chronic bladder stones. (**a**) The bladder stones, echogenic, can be seen on ultrasound with posterior shadowing (*arrows*). (**b**) CT demonstrates two small stones sitting beside a suprapubic catheter (*arrow*)

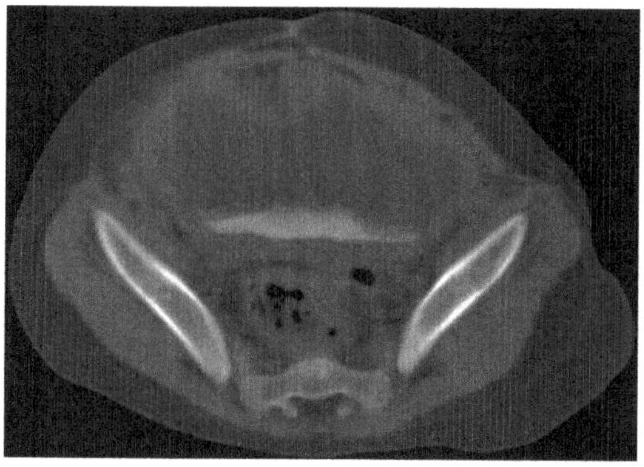

Fig. 13.31 A 10-year-old girl with a history of cloacal malformation who underwent bladder reconstruction with a bladder augmentation, bladder neck closure, and Monti. She self-catheterizes through a nondependent stoma and can be seen here to have calcific sediment in her bladder on noncontrast CT. This sediment is seen well using bone windows. Note the irregular shape of the bladder as a result of her bladder augmentation

Conclusion

Pediatric stone disease necessitates imaging for diagnosis and, in some instances, to rule out other pathology for pain in the acute setting. It is also valuable in the management and follow-up of the disease. Imaging must be used wisely in this young population to be both effective and safe.

Key Points

1. The prevalence of pediatric urolithiasis has increased over the past decade.
2. More than half of pediatric patients with stone disease have an associated metabolic abnormality, meaning these patients are faced with lifelong repeated imaging in the management of this chronic condition.
3. The pediatric population is particularly sensitive to ionizing radiation, and thus certain imaging modalities such as CT and fluoroscopy should be used with caution.
4. Imaging can be used to make the initial diagnosis of stone disease. It can also be used to follow patients over time: monitoring stone burden, evaluating success of intervention, and checking for recurrence.
5. Stone composition and location determine success of specific imaging modalities.
6. Radiography and ultrasound are important imaging tools in the pediatric population to minimize exposure to ionizing radiation.
7. Low-dose computed tomography (CT) techniques also help decrease exposure to ionizing radiation while maintaining the high sensitivity and specificity of CT imaging.
8. Congenital anomalies and genitourinary reconstruction may coexist with metabolic abnormalities causing stone disease.

References

1. Routh JC, Graham DA, Nelson CP. Epidemiological trends in pediatric urolithiasis at United States freestanding pediatric hospitals. J Urol. 2010;184:1100–10.
2. Valentini RP, Lakshmanan Y. Nephrolithiasis in children. Adv Chronic Kidney Dis. 2011;18(5):370–5.
3. Alon US. Medical treatment of pediatric urolithiasis. Pediatr Nephrol. 2009;24(11):2129–35.
4. Jayanthi VR, Arnold PM, Koff SA. Strategies for managing upper tract calculi in young children. J Urol. 1999;162(3 Pt2):1234–7.
5. Habbig S, Beck BB, Hoppe B. Nephrocalcinosis and urolithiasis in children. Kidney Int. 2011;80(12):1278–91.
6. Gearhart JP, Herzberg GZ, Jeffs RD. Childhood urolithiasis: experiences and advances. Pediatrics. 1991;87(4):445–50.
7. Manohar P, McCahy P. Repeated radiological radiation exposure in patients undergoing surgery for urinary tract stone disease in Victoria, Australia. BJU Int. 2011;108 Suppl 2:34–7.
8. Ferrandino MN, Bagrodia A, Pierre SA, Scales Jr CD, Rampersaud E, Pearle MS, Preminger GM. Radiation exposure in the acute and short-term management of urolithiasis at 2 academic centers. J Urol. 2009;181(2):668–72.
9. Fulgham PF, Assimos DG, Peare MS, Preminger GM. Clinical effectiveness protocols for imaging in the management of ureteral calculous disease: AUA technology assessment. J Urol. 2013;189(4):1203–13.
10. Pearce MS, Salotti JA, Little MP, McHugh K, Lee C, Kim KP, Howe NL, Ronckers CM, Rajaraman P, Sir Craft AW, Parker L, de Gonzalez AB. Radiation exposure from CT scans in childhood and subsequent risk of leukaemia and brain tumors: a retrospective cohort study. Lancet. 2012;380(9840):499–505.
11. Tanaka ST, Pope JC. Pediatric stone disease. Curr Urol Rep. 2009;10(2):138–43.
12. Kuhns LR, Oliver WJ, Christodoulou E, Goodsitt MM. The predicted increased cancer risk associated

with a single computed tomography examination for calculus detection in pediatric patients compared with the natural cancer incidence. Pediatr Emerg Care. 2011;27(4):345–50.

13. Goske MJ, Applegate KE, Boylan J, Butler PF, Callahan MJ, Coley BD, Farley S, Frush DP, Hernanz-Schulman M, Jaramillo D, Johnson ND, Kaste SC, Morrison G, Strauss KJ, Tuggle N. The image gently campaign: working together to change practice. AJR Am J Roentgenol. 2008;190(2):273–4.
14. VanDervoort K, Wiesen J, Frank R, Vento S, Crosby V, Chandra M, Trachtman H. Urolithiasis in pediatric patients: a single center study of incidence, clinical presentation, and outcome. J Urol. 2007;177(6): 2300–5.
15. Ray AA, Ghiculete D, Pace KT, Honey RJ. Limitations to ultrasound in the detection and measurement of urinary tract calculi. Urology. 2010;76(2):295–300.
16. Hoppe B, Kemper MJ. Diagnostic examination of the child with urolithiasis or nephrocalcinosis. Pediatr Nephrol. 2010;25(3):403–13.
17. Fulgham PF, Bishoff JT. Urinary tract imaging: basic principles. In: Wein AJ, Kavoussi LR, Partin AW, Novick AC, Peters CP, editors. Campbell-Walsh urology, vol. 1. 10th ed. Philadelphia: Elsevier Saunders; 2012.
18. Hyams ES, Shah O. Evaluation and follow-up of patients with urinary lithiasis: minimizing radiation exposure. Curr Urol Rep. 2010;11:80–6.
19. Schissel BL, Johnson BK. Renal stones: evolving epidemiology and management. Pediatr Emerg Care. 2011;27(7):676–81.
20. Raj GV, Auge BK, Assimos D, Preminger GM. Metabolic abnormalities associated with renal calculi in patients with horseshoe kidneys. J Endourol. 2004;18(2):157–61.
21. Ost M, Schneck FX. Surgical management of pediatric stone disease. In: Wein AJ, Kavoussi LR, Partin AW, Novick AC, Peters CP, editors. Campbell-Walsh urology, vol. 4. 10th ed. Philadelphia: Elsevier Saunders; 2012.
22. Palmer JS, Donaher ER, O'Riordan MA, Dell KM. Diagnosis of pediatric urolithiasis: role of ultrasound and computerized tomography. J Urol. 2005;174 (4 Pt1):1413–16.
23. Dillman JR, Kappil M, Weadock WJ, Rubin JM, Platt JF, DiPietro MA, Bude RO. Sonographic twinkling artifact for renal calculus detection: correlation with CT. Radiology. 2011;259(3):911–16.
24. Passerotti C, Chow JS, Silva A, Schoettler CL, Rosoklija I, Perez-Rossello J, Cendron M, Cilento BG, Lee RS, Nelson CP, Estrada CR, Bauer SB, Borer JG, Diamond DA, Retik AB, Nguyen HT. Ultrasound versus computerized tomography for evaluating urolithiasis. J Urol. 2009;182(4 Suppl):1829–34.
25. Mitterberger M, Pinggera GM, Pallwein L, Gradl J, Feuchtner G, Plattner R, Neururer R, Bartsch G, Strasser H, Frauscher F. Plain abdominal radiography with transabdominal native tissue harmonic imaging ultrasonography vs unenhanced computed tomography in renal colic. BJU Int. 2007;100(4):887–90.
26. Smith RC, Verga M, McCarthy S, Rosenfield AT. Diagnosis of acute flank pain: value of unenhanced helical CT. AJR Am J Roentgenol. 1996;166(1): 97–101.
27. Hamm M, Wawroschek F, Weckermann D, Knofle E, Hackel T, Hauser H, Krawczak G, Harzmann R. Unenhanced helical computed tomography in the evaluation of acute flank pain. Eur Urol. 2001;39(4): 460–5.
28. Cody DD, Moxley DM, Krugh KT, O'Daniel JC, Wagner LK, Eftekhari F. Strategies for formulating appropriate MDCT techniques when imaging the chest, abdomen, and pelvis in pediatric patients. AJR Am J Roentgenol. 2004;182(4):849–59.
29. Alzen G, Benz-Bohm G. Radiation protection in pediatric radiology. Dtsch Arztebl Int. 2011;108(24):407–14.
30. Kim S, Yoshizumi TT, Frush DP, Toncheva G, Yin FF. Radiation dose from cone beam CT in pediatric phantom: risk estimation of cancer incidence. AJR Am J Roentgenol. 2010;194(1):186–90.
31. Karmazyn B, Frush DP, Applegate KE, Maxfield C, Cohen MD, Jones RP. CT with a computer-simulated dose reduction technique for detection of pediatric nephroureterolithiasis: comparison of standard and reduced radiation doses. AJR Am J Roentgenol. 2009;192(1):143–9.
32. Boei JJ, Vermeulen S, Skubakova MM, Meijers M, Loenen WA, Wolterbeek R, Mullenders LH, Vrieling H, Giphart-Gassler M. No threshold for induction of chromosomal damage at clinically relevant low doses of X rays. Radiat Res. 2012;177(5):602–13.
33. Cerwinka WH, Kirsch AJ. MRU in pediatric urology. Curr Opin Urol. 2010;20(4):323–9.
34. Canning PA, Lambert SM. Evaluation of the pediatric urology patient. In: Wein AJ, Kavoussi LR, Partin AW, Novick AC, Peters CP, editors. Campbell-Walsh urology, vol. 4. 10th ed. Philadelphia: Elsevier Saunders; 2012
35. Chahed J, Jouini R, Krichene I, Maazoun K, Brahim MB, Nouri A. Urinary lithiasis and urinary tract malformations in children: a retrospective study of 34 cases. Afr J Paediatr Surg. 2011;8(2):168–71.
36. Stein RJ, Desai MM. Management of urolithiasis in the congenitally abnormal kidney (horseshoe and ectopic). Curr Opin Urol. 2007;17(2):127–31.
37. Tekin A, Tekgul S, Atsu N, Ergen A, Kendi S. Ureteropelvic junction obstruction and coexisting renal calculi in children: role in metabolic abnormalities. Urology. 2001;57(3):545–6.
38. Gross AJ, Fisher M. Management of stones in patients with anomalously sited kidneys. Curr Opin Urol. 2006;16(2):100–5.
39. Abdeldaeim HM, Hamdy SA, Mokhless IA. Percutaneous nephrolithotomy for the management of stones in anomalous kidneys in children. J Pediatr Urol. 2011;7(3):239–43.

40. Obrien J, Buckley O, Doody O, Ward E, Persaud T, Torreggiani W. Imaging of horseshoe kidneys and their complications. J Med Imaging Radiat Oncol. 2008;52(3):216–26.
41. Moxey-Mims MM, Stapleton FB. Hypercalciuria and nephrocalcinosis in children. Curr Opin Pediatr. 1993;5(2):186–90.
42. Alon US. Nephrocalcinosis. Curr Opin Pediatr. 1997;9(2):160–5.
43. Lopez Pereira P, Moreno Valle JA, Espinosa L, Alonso Dorrego JM, Burgos Lucena L, Martinez Urrutia MJ, Lobato Romera R, Luz Picazo M, Viguer JM, Jaureguizar ME. Enterocystoplasty in children with neuropathic bladders: long-term follow-up. J Pediatr Urol. 2008;4(1):27–31.
44. Escudero RM, Patino GE, Fernandez ER, Gil MJ, Garcia EL, Alonso AH, Pinies GO, Sanchez JP, Fernandez CH. Bladder augmentation using the gastrointestinal tract. Indication, follow-up and complications. Arch Esp Urol. 2011;64(10):953–9.
45. Rubenwolf PC, Beissert A, Gerharz EW, Riedmiller H. 15 years of continent urinary diversion and enterocystoplasty in children and adolescents: the Wurzburg experience. BJU Int. 2010;105(5):698–705.
46. Woodhouse CR, Robertson WG. Urolithiasis in enterocystoplasties. World J Urol. 2004;22(3):215–21.
47. Terai A, Ueda T, Kakehi Y, Terachi T, Arai Y, Okada Y, Yoshida O. Urinary calculi as a late complication of the Indiana continent urinary diversion: comparison with the Kock pouch procedure. J Urol. 1996;155(1):66–8.
48. Ashken MH. Stomas continent and incontinent. Br J Urol. 1987;59(3):203–7.
49. Abdol-Enein H, Ghoneim MA. Functional results of orthotopic ileal neobladder with serous-lined extramural ureteral reimplantation: experience with 450 patients. J Urol. 2001;165(5):1247–432.
50. Robertson WG, Woodhouse CR. Metabolic factors in the causation of urinary tract stones in patients with enterocystoplasties. Urol Res. 2006;34(4):231–8.
51. Hamid R, Robertsn WG, Woodhouse CR. Comparison of biochemistry and diet in patients with enterocystoplasty who do and do not form stones. BJU Int. 2008;101(11):1427–32.
52. Kaefer M, Tobin MS, Hendren WH, Bauer SB, Peters CA, Atala A, Colodny AH, Mandell J, Retik AB. Continent urinary diversion: the Children's Hospital experience. J Urol. 1997;157(4):1394–9.
53. Kaefer M, Hendren WH, Bauer SB, Goldenblatt P, Peters CA, Atala A, Retik AB. Reservoir calculi: a comparison of reservoirs constructed from stomach and other enteric segments. J Urol. 1998;160(6 Pt1):2187–90.

Bladder and Ureteral Imaging

14

Duong D. Tu, Jeanne S. Chow, and Carlos R. Estrada Jr.

The purpose of this chapter is to discuss the pathogenesis, clinical presentation, imaging, and treatment of common developmental abnormalities of the bladder and ureter in children. The abnormalities discussed in the first bladder section are bladder duplication, urachal anomalies, bladder diverticula, and neurogenic bladder. The second section related to the ureter includes retrocaval ureter, ureteral polyps, ureteral duplication, ureterocele, ectopic ureters, megaureter, and vesicoureteral reflux. This is, by no means, an exhaustive list of bladder and ureteral pathology but serves as an overview of many of the clinical entities that can be encountered in a pediatric urology practice, ordered from the relatively less to the most common. Some obvious omissions are imaging of the fetus, urolithiasis, trauma of the bladder and/or ureter, and the syndromes, such as prune belly and exstrophy. These are discussed in their respective chapters found elsewhere in this textbook.

The initial and most common imaging modality for all of the entities described is ultrasound. Ultrasound is a noninvasive, highly available, and relatively inexpensive examination, which is excellent for evaluation of the kidneys (as the origin of ureteral abnormalities), bladder, and dilated ureter. Children are naturally suited to being evaluated by ultrasound. Their smaller habitus is well penetrated by the ultrasound beams. Unlike fluoroscopy, intravenous pyelograms (IVPs), computed tomography (CT), and nuclear medicine studies, ultrasound emits no ionizing radiation and thus poses no radiation risks.

The bladder is best evaluated when full (Fig. 14.1). Normally distended ureters are easily seen near the renal pelvis, and behind the full urinary bladder, but can be challenging to follow in between. However, dilated ureters can be followed in their entire course. In addition to the commonly used transabdominal approach, transperineal imaging may show the location of an ectopic ureter and abnormalities of the bladder base (Fig. 14.2).

Although CT is commonly used in adults to evaluate the genitourinary tract, its emission of ionizing radiation makes it less attractive in children. CT scans without contrast are commonly used in the evaluation of urinary tract stones. CT scans with contrast are used to evaluate masses (parenchymal phase) and the collecting system (excretory phase).

D.D. Tu, MD • C.R. Estrada Jr., MD (✉)
Department of Urology, Harvard Medical School, Boston Children's Hospital, 300 Longwood Ave., HUNN 390, Boston, MA 02115, USA
e-mail: duong.tu@childrens.harvard.edu; carlos.estrada@childrens.harvard.edu

J.S. Chow, MD
Department of Urology, Harvard Medical School, 300 Longwood Ave., HUNN 390, Boston, MA 02115, USA

Department of Radiology, Boston Children's Hospital, 300 Longwood Ave., HUNN 390, Boston, MA 02115, USA
e-mail: jeanne.chow@childrens.harvard.edu

L.S. Palmer, J.S. Palmer (eds.), *Pediatric and Adolescent Urologic Imaging*, DOI 10.1007/978-1-4614-8654-1_14, © Springer Science+Business Media New York 2014

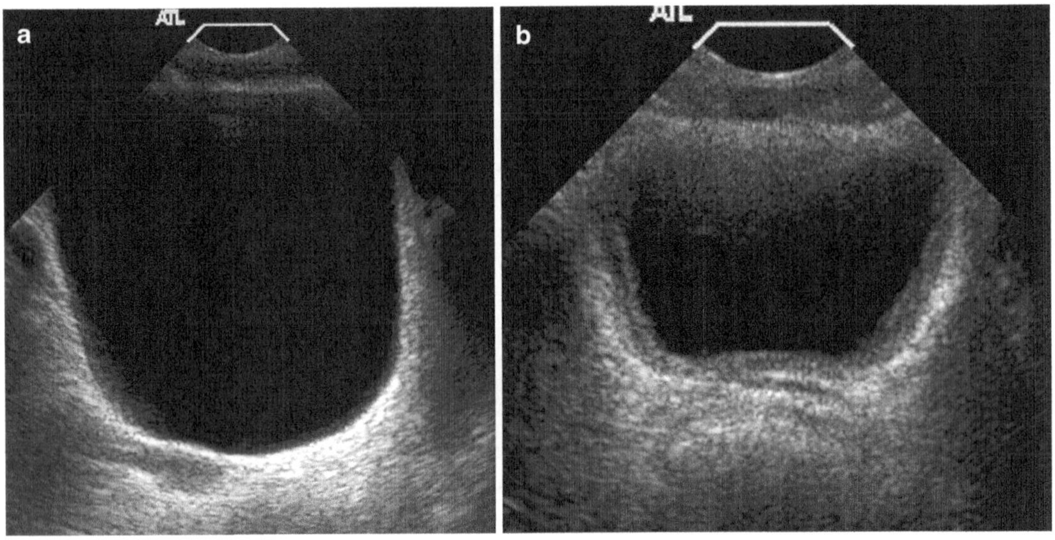

Fig. 14.1 Normal bladder. Normal bladder full and after voiding: transverse views of the bladder before (**a**) and after voiding (**b**) demonstrate the normal appearance of the bladder. Notice how the normal bladder wall when decompressed appears thicker. This demonstrates how it is normal for the degree of distention of the bladder to influence wall thickness

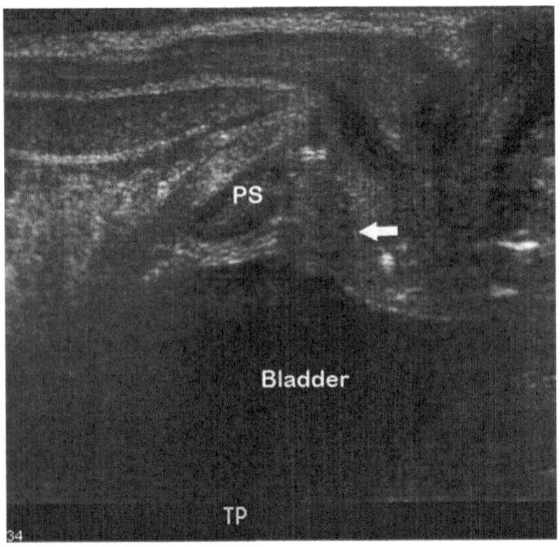

Fig. 14.2 Transperineal ultrasound. This transperineal ultrasound, performed with the transducer on the perineum in the sagittal plane, demonstrates the bladder, posterior urethra (*arrow*) surrounded by the echogenic prostate, and pubic symphysis (*PS*), among other structures. The appearance of the bladder base and posterior urethra is normal

Magnetic resonance imaging (MRI) is inherently suited to evaluating the urinary tract as the fluid in the dilated ureter and bladder is easily distinguished from adjacent soft tissues. Contrast-enhanced MR urography is also useful in evaluating the functional contribution of each kidney. The main problems are that these examinations often take an hour or more, necessitating the use of sedation for young children, are generally less available, and more expensive than other examinations.

Nuclear medicine studies DMSA and MAG-3 each show the function of the urinary tract. The agent used for DMSA is a cortical agent that allows for the precise determination of differential renal function, renal shape, and renal position. MAG-3 uses an excretory agent to determine the speed of contrast excretion, measure the degree of urinary tract obstruction, and show the general appearance of the collecting system.

The voiding cystourethrogram (VCUG) is the most common fluoroscopic examination to evaluate the lower urinary tract. After contrast is instilled into the bladder, the appearance of the bladder and filling defects such as ureteroceles are apparent. The ureters are evaluated if reflux is present. Retrograde ureterograms and antegrade pyelograms also use contrast to opacify and evaluate the ureters. Intravenous pyelograms are used rarely but continue to provide useful information regarding the function and appearance of the urinary tract.

Normal Imaging Anatomy: Bladder

The bladder resides in the pelvis where it serves its dual functions of urinary storage and emptying. When it is decompressed, it is usually contained entirely within the pelvis below the pubic symphysis, although in young children the bladder extends superiorly to the lower abdominal region. Anterior to the bladder, there is a potential space called the prevesical or retropubic space. The median umbilical ligament, the vestigial remnant of the fetal urachus, tethers the bladder apex to the abdominal wall as it attaches to the umbilicus (Fig. 14.3). The bladder is an extraperitoneal structure with the visceral peritoneum covering its superior-lateral aspects.

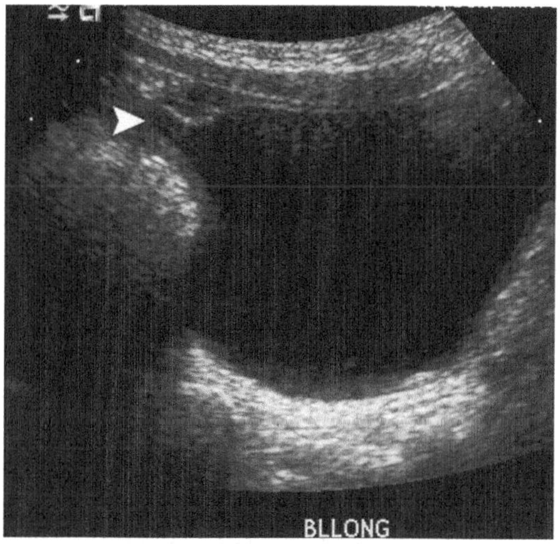

Fig. 14.3 Normal urachal remnant. This sagittal view of the bladder demonstrates a normal diverticular outpouching (*arrow*) at the anterior dome of the bladder, which is a normal urachal remnant

In boys, two seminal vesicles and the ampullae of the vasa deferentia lie posteriorly at the base of the bladder in the rectovesical space. In girls, this rectovesical space is occupied by the vagina and the uterus, which rests on the bladder dome (Fig. 14.4). The ureters enter the bladder at its base, posterior-laterally inserting into the trigone. The bladder neck rests directly on the pelvic floor muscles. However, in boys, the prostate gland lies between the bladder neck and the pelvic floor.

The wall of the bladder consists of layers of perivesical fat, serosa, smooth muscle (i.e., detrusor muscle), and mucosa (urothelium). As the bladder distends, the detrusor muscle is stretched, and the mucosa, which normally has folds, flattens causing the bladder wall to appear thinner.

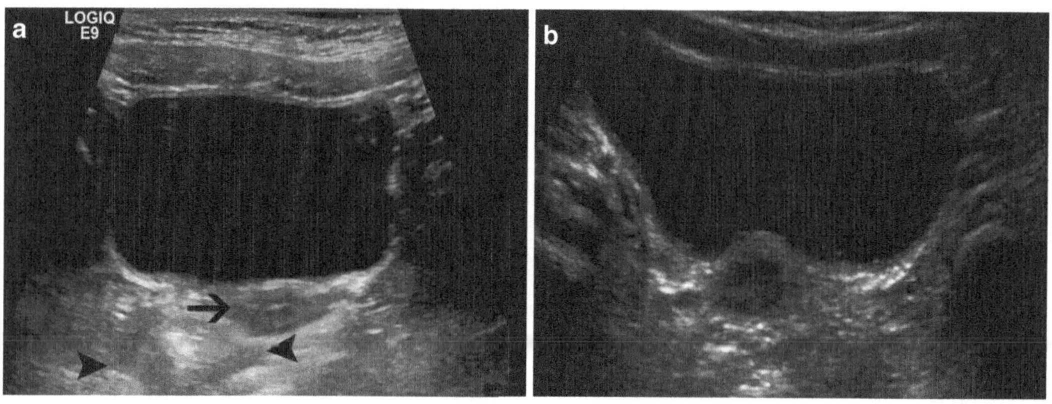

Fig. 14.4 Normal bladder: These images demonstrate the normal appearance of the bladder in girls. (**a**) The normal hypoechoic uterus is adjacent to the posterior wall of the bladder (*arrow*). The rectum is filled with gas and stool and has a variable appearance depending on its contents (*arrowhead*). (**b**) The hypoechoic uterus often indents the posterior wall of the bladder and should not be confused for a mass

Bladder Duplication

Pathogenesis

Bladder duplication is a rare clinical entity with few cases reported in the literature. When it does occur, the degree of septation of the bladder may be partial or complete and in either the coronal or sagittal plane. Complete duplication in the sagittal plane has been reported as the most common combination [1]. In complete duplication, the two resulting bladders can be functionally independent with their own respective ureter and urethras [2]. However, one bladder may not have a urethra, resulting in obstruction of its corresponding kidney, ultimately causing renal dysplasia [3]. The luminal compartments of incomplete or partially duplicated bladders are shared at some point above the bladder neck and therefore drain into a single urethra.

Duplication should be distinguished from septation, in which the bladder is divided into two separate (complete) or almost separate (partial) compartments that share a common wall (the septum). As with duplication, complete septation may form a compartment with no outlet, leading to an abnormal ipsilateral kidney.

Embryologically, the cause of duplication is unclear, although some have postulated that it may represent a defect in cloacal septation with the urorectal fold [4] or even partial twinning of the early embryo, a theory taken from its occasional association with duplication of the bowel or spine [5].

Clinical Presentation

In accordance with the variability of the abnormality in bladder duplication, the presentation and diagnosis of the disorder are equally variable. Early discovery usually arises from outward manifestations of duplication, i.e., duplicated external genitalia or spine. In the absence of symptoms such as recurrent urinary tract infections or urinary incontinence, some children are diagnosed incidentally when they are imaged radiographically for other clinical reasons.

Bladder duplication is often associated with other abnormalities related to the genitourinary system such as the genital duplication noted above [6], spinal duplication, and a variety of gastrointestinal tract anomalies, including fistulous communication with the urogenital tract and lower intestinal tract duplication [7].

Imaging

Complete understanding of the patient's anatomy is crucial to management and often requires a combination of imaging studies. Ultrasound is the initial imaging modality, which helps to define the presence of two kidneys, a solitary bladder separated by a septum, or two separate bladders (Fig. 14.5). Transperineal scanning may give further definition of urethral anatomy. Voiding cystourethrograms in combination with retrograde urethrograms, in which the suspected urethral orifices are catheterized and further defined by instillation of contrast, can also be useful to define the appearance of the urethra(s), blind channels, and bladder(s). Studies such as CT urography (CTU), MR urography (MRU), and IVP can also define the functional and anatomical relationships between kidney(s), ureters, and bladder(s). Unlike CT and IVP, MR has the benefit of the lack of ionizing radiation which needs to be weighed against the cost of the examination and potential need for sedation in younger children. Renal scans and MRU can both estimate renal function. Video-urodynamics will give much of the same information as a VCUG and will also provide functional information.

Treatment

Obstruction of a kidney should be relieved surgically to prevent infection and preserve renal function. Patients with the associated abnormalities discussed above will have individualized

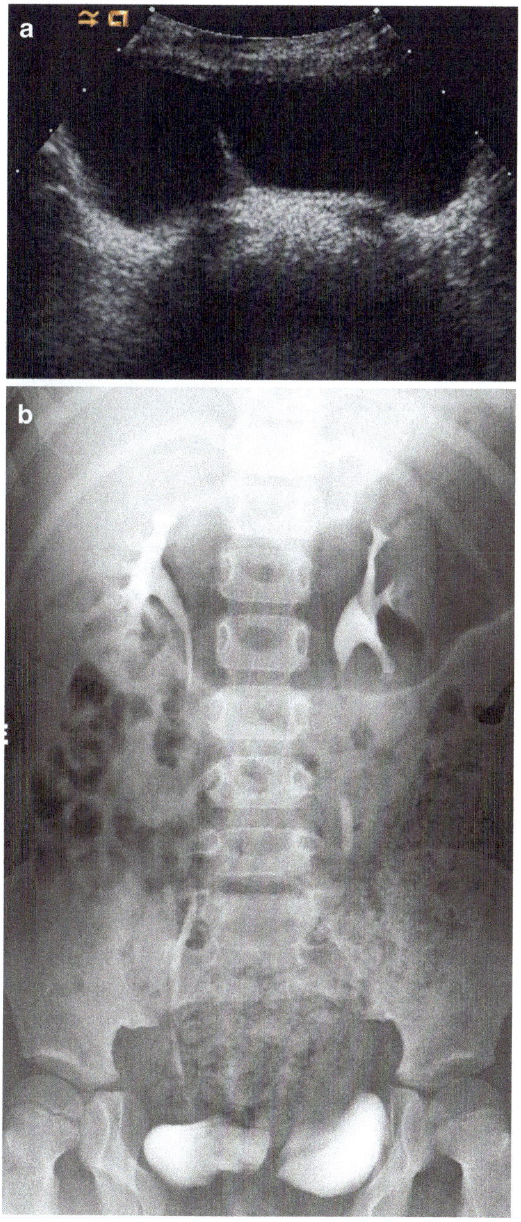

Fig. 14.5 Bladder duplication. A transverse view of the bladder (**a**) demonstrates complete bladder duplication with a septation dividing each bladder lumen. The IVP (**b**) demonstrates that each bladder is supplied by its own ureter and kidney

treatment based on their disease pattern. Long-term goals include urinary continence and functional genital reconstruction.

Urachal Anomalies

Pathogenesis

The allantoic stalk serves as the epithelial-lined conduit between the bladder and the umbilical cord in fetal life. As the bladder descends and matures, the allantois narrows and thickens into the urachus. The lumen of the urachus normally obliterates and becomes the median umbilical ligament [8]. However, by mechanisms still unclear, a portion or the entire urachus can remain patent.

Clinical Presentation

The most common symptomatic urachal anomaly is the entirely patent urachus, accounting for more than half of all disorders of the urachus. In the patent urachus, urine freely passes from the bladder and out of the umbilicus, and the child usually presents with persistent leakage. Leakage may be exacerbated with voiding or in situations of increased abdominal pressure such as with crying or straining. Symptoms can also include abdominal pain, umbilical mass, or dysuria [9].

Occasionally, the urachus can partially obliterate with varying features depending on which portion of the urachus remains open. When the patent end is distal, 15 % of cases, it is labeled as an umbilical-urachal sinus. This can also present with umbilical discharge, but since there is no communication with the bladder, it is less copious. When the patency lies at the proximal end, communicating with the apex of the bladder, it is referred to as a vesico-urachal diverticulum. Usually these do not cause any clinical symptoms since it is widely open to the bladder.

Thirty percent of urachal anomalies consist of a urachal cyst, where the urachus is patent along its middle portion and there is no communication with the umbilicus or bladder. However, sometimes these cysts can drain intermittently. The diagnosis of these may be delayed since often they are not discovered unless they become infected or are discovered incidentally during abdominal imaging or surgery. Some reports have suggested that there may be an increased incidence of vesicoureteral reflux associated with urachal anomalies [10].

Imaging

Imaging for a suspected urachal abnormality typically occurs during the newborn period. Ultrasound is the initial study for urachal anomalies [11]. Ideally, imaging should be performed when the bladder is full to better show the close relationship between the dome of the bladder, umbilicus, and urachal remnant. A patent urachus can be seen on ultrasound located at the dome of the bladder, as a fluid-filled tubular structure when viewed in the longitudinal plane. This should be distinguished from a patent vitelline, or omphalomesenteric, duct which may have a similar appearance. Urachal cysts can also be demonstrated with ultrasound with features of any cyst of the body, hypoechogenicity with variable degrees of debris, and noncommunication with the umbilicus or bladder. Vesico-urachal diverticula appear as protruding fluid-filled sacs not in continuity with the umbilicus [12]. An obliterated urachal remnant is a common finding in newborn children and warrants no further evaluation or treatment [13, 14].

A VCUG is indicated in patients who have fluid draining from their umbilicus, and a patent urachus needs to be distinguished from a urachal sinus. Contrast can be seen flowing through a patent urachus when the bladder is full (Fig. 14.6), whereas a urachal sinus will not demonstrate communication from the bladder to the umbilicus. If a patient has periumbilical drainage, a retrograde fistulogram can also determine the diagnosis of either a patent urachus or urachal sinus [9]. Retrograde injection of the contrast will demonstrate either filling of the bladder in a patent urachus or opacification of just the sinus tract in the case of the urachal sinus. If it is a patent vitelline duct, contrast will fill loops of bowel.

Urachal remnants are more common in patients with certain abnormalities. Children with prune belly syndrome often have urachal diverticula.

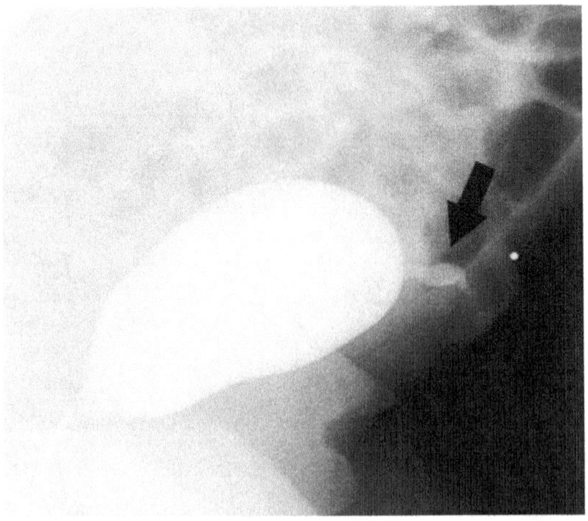

Fig. 14.6 Patent urachus. This newborn boy had clear leakage per urethra. This lateral view during a VCUG shows contrast flowing from the patent urachus at the dome of the bladder (*arrow*)

When wide mouthed, these are asymptomatic and appear as large diverticula at the dome of the bladder. Urachal diverticula can also be found during the evaluation of recurrent cystitis. Infected urachal cysts can present with fever and abdominal pain, mimic abdominal infections such as appendicitis, and be found during radiological evaluations for more common causes of abdominal pain (Fig. 14.7). These cystic structures in the pelvis can be distinguished from other cysts, e.g., enteric duplication cysts and ovarian abnormalities, by its location near the dome of the bladder.

Treatment

A patent urachus or umbilical-urachal sinus should be excised surgically. If a preceding infection is present, antibiotics and drainage if appropriate should be undertaken prior to surgery. There is a risk of malignant transformation of the urachus, so it should be removed in its entirety with a cuff of bladder [15–19]. Observation is an option in the case of the asymptomatic urachal cyst [20–22] or vesico-urachal diverticulum. However, if resolution does not occur or if symptoms arise, complete excision, cyst and tract, should be considered. In a large series from the Mayo clinic, urachal carcinoma appeared in a large proportion of the adults (51 %), with

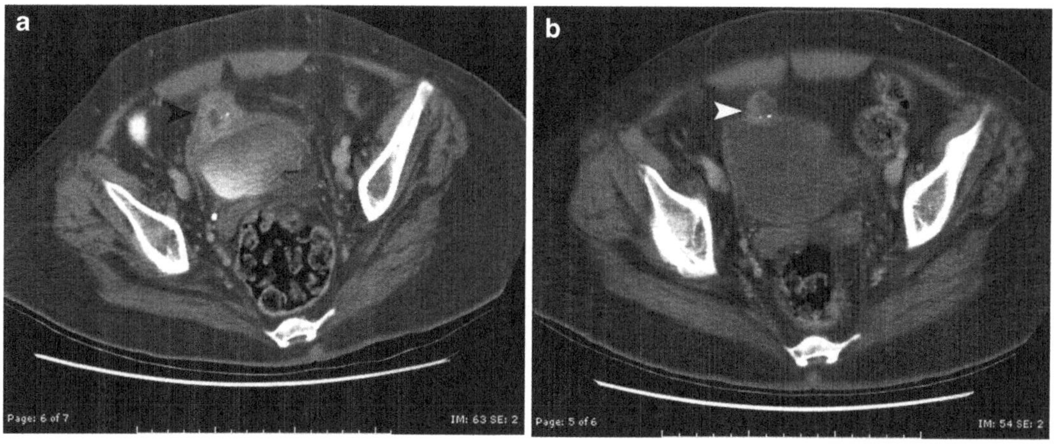

Fig. 14.7 Infected urachal cyst. This boy presented with right lower quadrant pain and fever and was thought to have appendicitis. (**a**) Axial contrast-enhanced CT scan demonstrates an irregular thick-walled circular structure adjacent to the dome of the bladder (*black arrowhead*). (**b**) After treatment with antibiotics, the appearance of the wall is smoother due to decreased inflammation (*white arrowhead*). Surgery confirmed a urachal diverticulum

the majority of them having urachal cysts. Traditionally, the prognosis for urachal cancer is abysmal with low survival rates, leading most surgeons to recommend complete excision of all urachal anomalies in childhood [19].

Bladder Diverticulum

Pathogenesis

In the adult, most bladder diverticula are secondary processes stemming from bladder outlet obstruction. In children the cause is congenital, and these mucosal outpouchings herniate through weak areas of the muscle wall of the bladder. The reported incidence is 1.7 % in a pediatric population undergoing radiologic evaluation for symptoms [23]. Diverticula can occur around the bladder's natural defects, namely, the ureters. Hutch described in 1961 two kinds of paraureteral diverticula: primary and secondary [24].

Primary or congenital diverticula occur in isolation in what is otherwise a normal appearing bladder with an absence of bladder outlet obstruction. The mucosal herniation occurs through a deficient portion of the bladder wall between the intravesical ureter and the roof of the hiatus where the ureter enters the bladder [25, 26]. As the diverticulum grows larger, the ureterovesical junction is distorted, causing either reflux [27, 28] or, worse yet, obstruction [28, 29]. Primary diverticula have been reported in children with connective tissue diseases such as Ehlers-Danlos, Menkes' kinky hair syndrome, and Williams syndrome (Fig. 14.8) [23, 30].

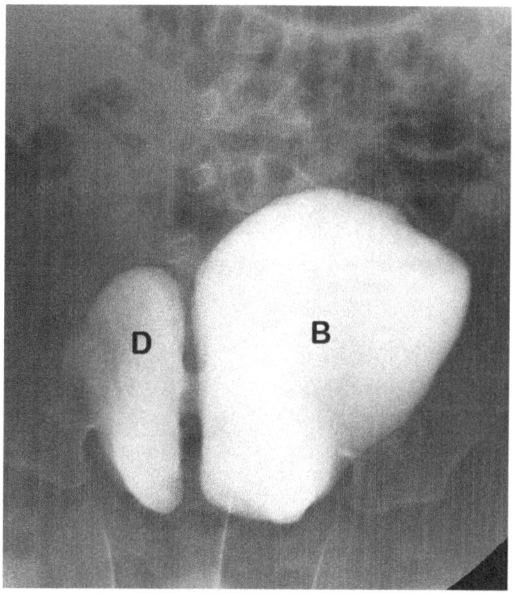

Fig. 14.8 Bladder diverticulum in a patient with Menkes disease. This 6-year-old boy has seizure disorder and red hair and a diagnosis of Menkes disease. This VCUG shows a large right-sided bladder diverticulum (*D*) communicating with the lumen of the bladder (*B*). Patients with Menkes disease, Ehlers-Danlos syndrome, and Williams syndrome frequently have multiple bladder diverticula

Secondary diverticula are acquired as a result of bladder outlet obstruction as in posterior urethral valves, detrusor sphincter dyssynergia, or neurogenic bladder. The increased intravesical pressure causes the bladder mucosa to bulge between hypertrophic muscle fibers. Diverticula that occur following bladder surgery also fall within this category.

Clinical Presentation

Presenting symptoms are varied dependent on the size and location of the diverticulum. Urinary stasis can lead to infection, the most common presenting complaint [31–33]; inflamed mucosa can cause hematuria; and mass effect can cause obstruction of the ureter or, if large enough, the bladder [32, 34–37].

In rare instances, a large bladder diverticulum can cause extrinsic compression on the intestines, and patients can have severe constipation or mechanical bowel obstruction. This has been reported in adult patients [38–41].

Imaging

A bladder diverticulum is typically found incidentally, often during the evaluation of a child with a urinary tract infection. Large bladder diverticula can be detected by ultrasound (Fig. 14.9) [42]. The bladder has to be adequately filled to allow for sonographic determination. The diverticulum typically fills during bladder distention and can enlarge further with voiding. Using 3-dimensional ultrasound, the mouth of the diverticulum can be seen [43]. If the diverticular neck is narrow, bladder air/CO_2 contrast sonography has been shown to aid in the differentiation of a diverticulum with other cystic pelvic structures by demonstrating communication [44]. Also, color Doppler can be used to demonstrate alternating, bidirectional, "jet-like" flow between the diverticulum and the bladder [45]. After voiding, residual urine is often seen within the diverticulum. Primary diverticula can appear intermittently on evaluation. If the bladder appears trabeculated, the patient is likely to have secondary diverticula and underlying causes

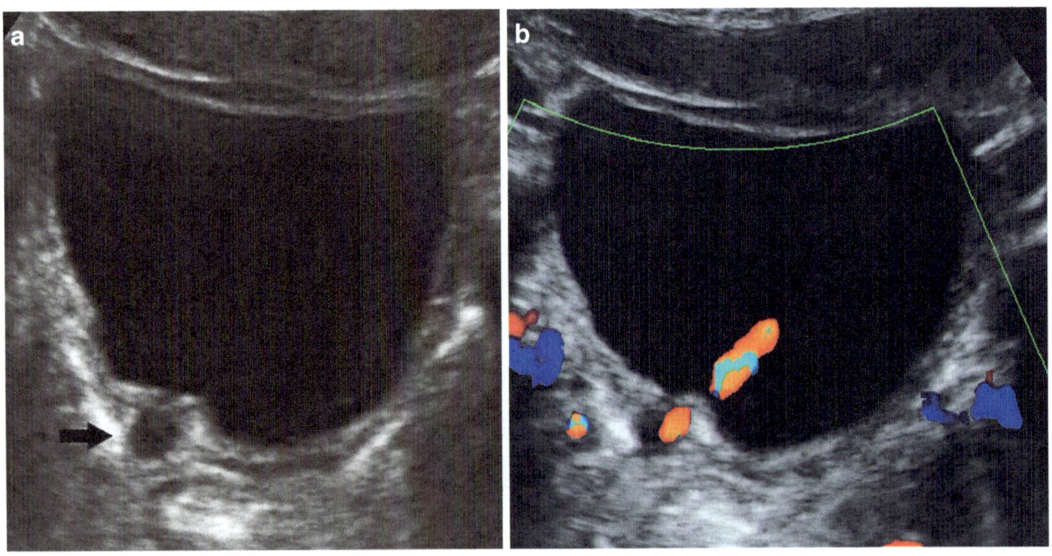

Fig. 14.9 Bladder diverticulum. This patient initially presented with recurrent urinary tract infections. (**a**) Transverse view of the bladder demonstrates an anechoic circular structure adjacent to the right posterolateral bladder wall (*arrow*). (**b**) A ureteral jet of flowing urine is present adjacent to the paraureteral diverticulum or so-called Hutch diverticulum

should be sought out (e.g., posterior urethral valves, neurogenic bladder). Large bladder diverticula may also be seen by CT and MRI.

Voiding cystourethrogram is probably the sensitive test for finding bladder diverticula because the bladder is visualized dynamically during filling and voiding. Changes in intravesical pressure are more likely to elicit the intermittently filling diverticula. The study not only demonstrates the diverticulum but also reveals associated vesicoureteral reflux when the diverticulum is located near the ureterovesical junction [44, 46, 47]. Meticulous technique is important when performing a VCUG including beginning the study with an empty bladder, real-time fluoroscopic monitoring with oblique and lateral views, and visualization during and immediately post-void [46]. This is done since the appearance of diverticula may vary with the phases of voiding and may not be present on the same study at different times. Therefore, a repeat VCUG may be warranted if clinical suspicion remains after previous negative studies.

Treatment

Symptomatic diverticula should be excised with ipsilateral ureteral reimplantation if the ureter is nearby or involved. Many surgeons correct paraureteral diverticula if it is associated with VUR. Otherwise, if the diverticulum is small, found incidentally without symptoms, or is not accompanied by VUR, observation is reasonable. In the case of secondary diverticula, bladder outlet obstruction should be remedied first, since direct treatment for the diverticulum may become unnecessary.

Bladder Rhabdomyosarcoma

Pathogenesis

Rhabdomyosarcoma (RMS) is the most common soft tissue sarcoma in children, with 20 % arising from the genitourinary (GU) tract. The most common GU sites are prostate, bladder, and paratesticular. With a bimodal age distribution, peak incidence of the disease occurs in the first 2 years of life and again in adolescence. Children under the age of 6 years comprise the majority of cases. There is a high association with certain syndromes such as Li-Fraumeni syndrome and neurofibromatosis, and the subtypes of RMS (embryonal vs. alveolar) have been shown to have distinct cytogenetic abnormalities. These abnormalities (loss of heterozygosity on chromosome 11, translocation between chromosomes 1 or 2 and 13, etc.) may not only be involved in the pathogenesis but may also have prognostic implications. Most GU RMS are of the embryonal variety and when they occur in hollow organs, such as the bladder or vagina, they present as sarcoma botryoides. Fortunately, the botryoid variants portend a more favorable prognosis.

Clinical Presentation

Presentation is dependent on the site of the primary tumor. When found in the bladder, patients often present with urinary retention and hematuria. Urinary retention, in turn, causes abdominal pain and distention and urinary tract infection. Irritative voiding symptoms such as dysuria and frequency can also occur. In a thin child, a palpable abdominal mass can sometimes be found on physical exam either from the mass itself or from a distended bladder.

Imaging

The imaging features of RMS of the bladder are nonspecific, and tumor diagnosis is via direct biopsy and tissue confirmation with cystoscopy. Intravenous urography was the imaging modality of choice even well into the late 1970s, with images of pelvic masses causing mass effect on nearby pelvic structures [48]. Filling of the bladder with contrast will reveal an irregular filling defect if the mass is indeed in the bladder.

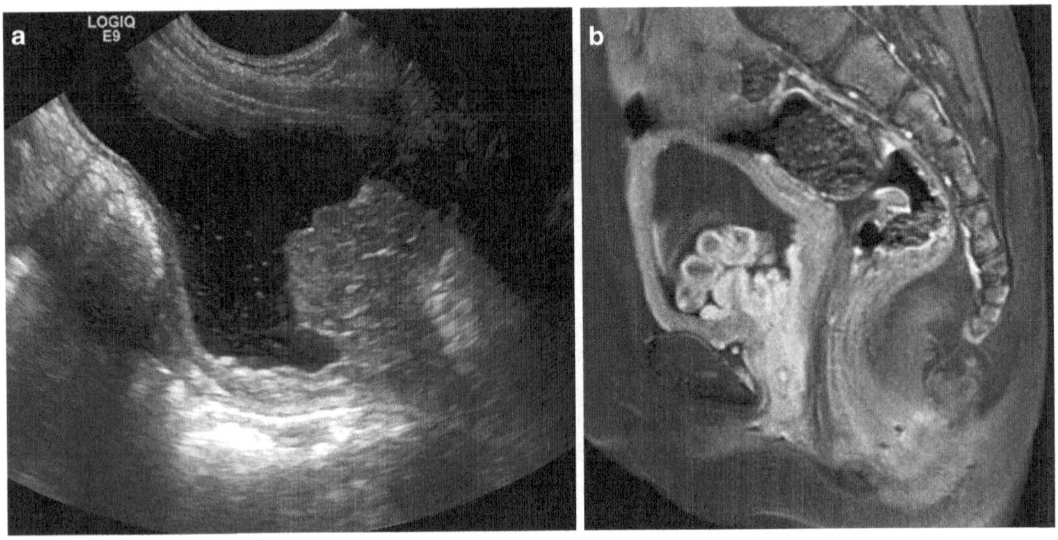

Fig. 14.10 Rhabdomyosarcoma. This 3-year-old female presented with bloody underwear and frond-like soft tissue within her perineum. (**a**) Sagittal US view of the bladder shows an echogenic lobulated mass extending from the posterior wall of the bladder to the bladder base and into the urethra. (**b**) Sagittal T1 FS postcontrast MRI demonstrates the enhancing bladder mass has multiple lobules and extends into the urethra. These appearances are classic for sarcoma botryoides

Otherwise, cystography can show extrinsic compression of the bladder from an adjacent RMS. However, this has been supplanted by sonography, CT, and MRI [49].

Ultrasonography is the screening study of choice for abdominopelvic masses. This usually demonstrates a large, heterogeneous, solid mass within the lumen [50] (Fig. 14.10a). The botryoid variant will appear as a cluster of "grapes" with its polypoid configuration. Hypoechoic foci can be seen within the mass representing hemorrhage or necrosis [49]. Spatial relationships with adjacent pelvic structures can be determined. In girls who have RMS arising from the uterus or vagina, one can visualize a pelvic mass that displaces the bladder, and invasion into the bladder wall can sometimes be seen on ultrasound. If the mass is sufficiently large, obstruction of the ureter(s) may cause hydroureter detected on US. One has to be wary for other disease processes that can mimic RMS such as inflammatory masses, such as inflammatory pseudotumor or post surgical masses. If history, laboratory values, and comparison to prior studies do not reveal the cause, cystoscopy and biopsy may be needed to distinguish these entities.

After ultrasound, MRI is the best imaging modality to assess the site of origin for a pelvic rhabdomyosarcoma and the sites of local invasion. Tumors which involve the bladder may actually have arisen from adjacent organs such as the prostate or vagina. MRI is superior to CT in tissue contrast and distinguishing the mass from adjacent organs (Fig. 14.10b).

Both CT and MRI are useful in the evaluation for enlargement of the pelvic and retroperitoneal lymph nodes and metastases. Contrast enhancement for either study is necessary for best visualization.

Treatment

Treatment of RMS has shifted from radical cystectomy to bladder preservation. Unfortunately, those tumors arising from the bladder trigone are not amenable to partial cystectomy as are those located at the dome or sides of the bladder. For those children, neoadjuvant chemotherapy and radiation can sufficiently shrink the tumor enough to allow for partial cystectomy. This approach has allowed for an increased rate of bladder function with reasonable overall survival (78 %) [51, 52]. A caveat is that patients with residual disease can have relapse of their disease, which has shown to have high mortality [52]. Also, patients who received radiation therapy have compromised functional bladder capacity and abnormal voiding patterns [53]. To address this dilemma, one group recommends a risk-based approach, taking into account the relative response of the tumor to chemotherapy for risk stratification and reserving radiation for relapse in low-risk patients (high-risk patients undergo radical cystectomy) [54].

Urinary diversion is needed following cystectomy, and these come in the form of conduits or continent reconstructions. Early reconstruction, however, should be performed when no further local therapy is required.

Neurogenic Bladder

Pathogenesis

Neurogenic bladder incorporates a rather wide range of clinical manifestations dependent on the level and extent of the lesion along the pathway between the brain and sacral spinal cord. Indeed, even similar neural injuries at the same location may result in different types of dysfunction. The complexity of diagnosis of the neurogenic or neuropathic bladder depends on a complete history and physical/neurologic examination. Radiographic studies, including video-urodynamics, are to provide a complete picture of the functional deficit.

In general, lesions above the sacral cord produce a low-capacity, high-pressure, and overactive bladder. This is demonstrated with urodynamic studies as well as anatomic studies such as VCUG and US. Lesions of this nature are usually from trauma, spinal dysraphism such as spina bifida, cerebral vascular accidents, Parkinson's disease, multiple sclerosis, infection, or tumor. Associated effects from this bladder dysfunction can include VUR from the increased bladder pressures, ureteral obstruction due to the thickened and hypertrophic bladder wall, or progressive renal insufficiency from lower urinary tract dysfunction. These effects are the result of the derangement of the neural control of urinary storage and emptying. Specifically, detrusor sphincter dyssynergia, or discoordination between the bladder and the external urethral sphincter, is thought to be the most deleterious factor.

Lesions at or below the sacral spinal cord typically result in a large capacity, areflexic, and low-pressure bladder. Not only can this dysfunction occur from direct spinal cord lesions, it can also occur from other medical conditions such as diabetes mellitus and pernicious anemia. The underlying pathology is often a deficit in sensory input to the bladder.

Clinical Presentation

Returning to the broad categorization above, patients with suprasacral injuries can present with urinary incontinence, irritative symptoms such as urgency or frequency, recurrent urinary tract infection, or upper tract changes. Patients with sacral lesions often have urinary retention and overflow incontinence.

Imaging

Since neurogenic bladder dysfunction is often a progressive disorder, initial radiologic evaluation includes an assessment of baseline renal and bladder anatomy and structure with ultrasound. The imaging findings of patients with neurogenic bladder depend on the level of the spinal cord abnormality. Abnormalities which lead to a small-capacity high-pressure bladder result in a thick-walled, trabeculated bladder. The combination of a hypertrophied bladder wall and high-pressure voiding may cause hydroureteronephrosis due to ureterovesical junction obstruction, reflux, or both. Patients with large areflexic bladders have smooth-walled bladders with greater than expected capacity for age. These patients may also have hydroureteronephrosis.

The redundant undulating mucosa and hypertrophied muscularis seen in patients with thick

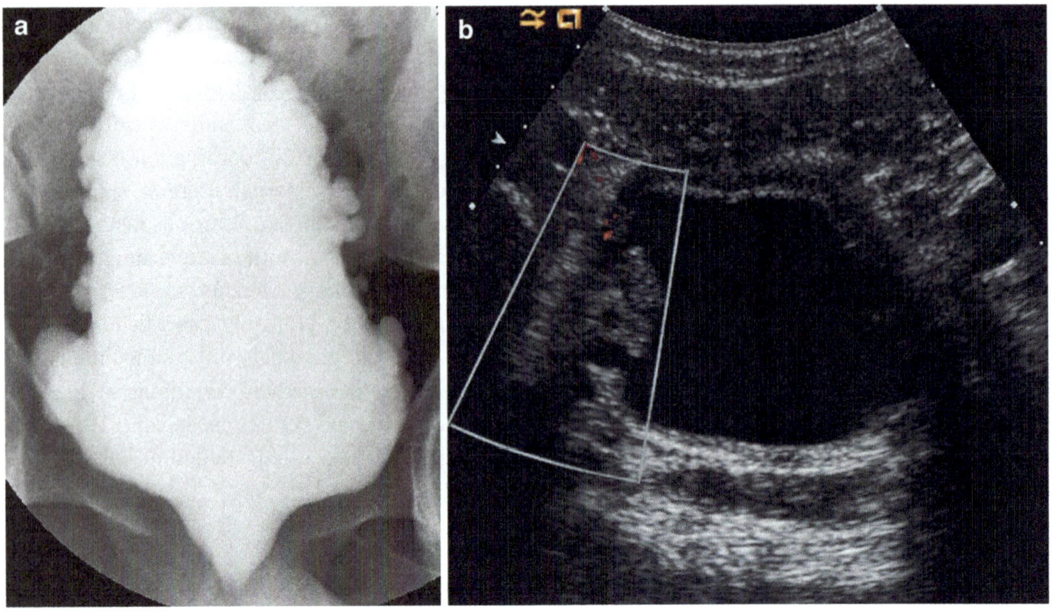

Fig. 14.11 Neurogenic bladder. This boy was born with a terminal lipomyelomeningocele and had previously undergone cord detethering. He has persistent incontinence. (**a**) AP supine image of the bladder during a VCUG demonstrating the typical "Christmas tree appearance" of a neurogenic bladder, characterized by hypertrophied muscularis and contrast-filling multiple large saccules. The trabeculation spares the bladder base. (**b**) Ultrasound image demonstrates a thick-walled bladder and multiple diverticula in this patient with a neurogenic bladder

bladder walls can be visualized by all imaging modalities, but the most common imaging study to evaluate the bladder is ultrasound (Fig. 14.11). One measure for the degree of bladder wall hypertrophy is AP bladder wall thickness. However, the thickness of the bladder varies by the degree of bladder distension and location of measurement. Tanaka et al. determined that bladder wall thickness of greater than 3.3 mm correlated with a higher risk for unfavorable urodynamic (UDS) risk patterns (i.e., parameters most likely to lead to upper urinary tract deterioration) among patients with neurogenic bladder from spina bifida. Specificity for the diagnosis of unfavorable UDS was 75 % and sensitivity was 95.1 % [55]. Leonardo et al. demonstrated that bladder wall thickness was the only sonographic parameter that was a marginal risk factor ($p=0.07$) for the finding of renal scarring on DMSA renal scan in neurogenic and nonneurogenic bladder dysfunction [56]. Some groups have advocated for routine baseline DMSA scans in patients with neurogenic bladder dysfunction given their high risk of renal function deterioration.

UDS has been an integral component of the evaluation of children with NGB, as it allows for identification of those at high risk for urinary tract deterioration. If implemented early, aggressive treatment can be initiated for preventive, renal preservation measures [57, 58].

VCUG is important as the incidence of VUR has been reported as high as 50 % in children with spina bifida [59, 60] which may lead to renal deterioration in the presence of high-pressure voiding [61]. In general, we reserve VCUG for patients with poor bladder dynamics, patients with DSD, and/or hydro- or hydroureteronephrosis. DeLair et al. identified high-grade VUR as an independent risk factor for cortical loss, especially in girls [62]. Shiroyanagi et al. demonstrated, in their small cohort of myelodysplastic patients, that all of their patients with an abnormal DMSA scan had a history of VUR [63]. The technique of VCUG and UDS can be combined in video-urodynamics (V-UDS) so that the patients are subjected to one invasive procedure rather than two. However, UDS, much less V-UDS, does not have widespread availability, and some have proposed a modified VCUG to give anatomic as well as functional data [64, 65]. This technique entails an in-depth understanding to bladder physiology/dynamics.

Since neurogenic bladder dysfunction can be progressive, ultrasonography should be performed on a regular basis, with the addition of VCUG if there is new hydroureteronephrosis or febrile UTI. The frequency of UDS varies according to patient age and clinical status.

It should be noted that the optimum position for UDS is in the sitting position if the patient is able to tolerate it. Lorenzo et al. reported that although there were no differences in maximum cystometric capacity, detrusor leak point pressure, or pressure-specific volumes at 20 and 30 cm water, based on patient positioning (supine vs. sitting), volume of first sensation and detection of detrusor overactivity was significantly lower in the sitting position. Incontinence was also detected more readily in the sitting position [66].

Treatment

As with diagnosis, treatment is individualized to the patient depending on the nature and severity of his/her dysfunction. Goals of therapy are directed towards preservation of renal function and alleviation of symptoms. Maneuvers should be done to simulate the normal functions of the bladder, namely, low-pressure storage of urine and complete emptying of urine. This is normally accomplished by the use of anticholinergic medication to lower intravesical pressure and decrease overactive contractions and clean intermittent catheterization (CIC) for bladder emptying. Early implementation of these treatment regimens in patients at risk is associated with more favorable outcomes [57, 58, 62, 63].

Normal Imaging Anatomy: Ureter

The ureter stretches from the renal pelvis of the kidney to the bladder for a length of about 25–30 cm. Along its course, there are 3 areas of relative narrowing: the ureteropelvic junction (UPJ), where the ureter crosses the iliac vessels as it dips into the pelvis, and the ureterovesical junction (UVJ). These areas are important as they are the locations where urinary calculi can become lodged. Both proximal ureters run along the psoas muscles. They are initially lateral to the gonadal vessels but switch positions just prior to the bifurcation of the aorta and vena cava as the gonadal vessels cross the ureter anteriorly. In the pelvis, the ureters course medially as they enter the bladder.

The ureter has a robust muscular layer of circular and longitudinal muscle fibers that are responsible for peristaltic propulsion of urine. Since imaging techniques are snapshots in time, relative dilations and constrictions as a result of propulsion of the bolus of urine can be misconstrued as pathologic.

Preureteral Vena Cava (Retrocaval/Circumcaval Ureter)

Pathogenesis

The normal course of the right ureter is lateral to the inferior vena cava (IVC). However, in certain circumstances (estimated 1 in 1,100) [67], the ureter takes an anomalous course, wrapping around the vena cava posteriorly, exiting between the IVC and aorta, and proceeding caudad to cross the iliac vessels anteriorly as it enters the pelvis to insert into the normal position in the bladder. This occurs because of a divergence of the normal embryologic development of the IVC. The IVC develops through a series of fusion events between multiple inchoate venous drainage systems of the 6th–8th-week embryo. Those segments that do not fuse to form the IVC selectively degenerate. One such drainage system is the posterior cardinal veins which drain the inferior portion of the embryo. The right posterior cardinal vein lies anterior to the developing ureter and with renal ascent becomes situated lateral to them. The subcardinal veins, situated medial to the ureter, are the venous segment that fuses to normally become the renal segment of the IVC. However, if the right posterior cardinal vein does not degenerate, it forms the renal segment of the IVC, and its anterior and lateral position to the ureter persists. In this conformation, the ureter may become obstructed by the overlying vena cava. Since the condition is due to a disorder of vascular development and not ureteral development, it has been suggested that it be referred to as “preureteral vena cava.”

Clinical Presentation

If the ureter becomes obstructed, patients typically present with symptoms indicative of ureteral obstruction. Symptoms may be intermittent or may not surface until a diuretic event occurs, as with the ingestion of caffeinated or alcoholic beverages. Given this, the condition is often not diagnosed until early adulthood. These symptoms may very well exist in the pediatric population, but the similarities with symptoms of gastrointestinal origin probably delays diagnosis. Conversely, the diagnosis is sometimes made incidentally during radiographic evaluation of other disorders.

The signs and symptoms are of typical renal colic, usually abdominal or flank pain and nausea and vomiting. Urinary stasis can predispose to urinary tract infections or pyelonephritis, which will prompt evaluation and intervention. Hydronephrosis can also result in gross hematuria. Urinary calculi formation and deterioration of renal function are also other presentations that lead to evaluation and diagnosis.

Imaging

Retrocaval ureters can exhibit two clinical types [68, 69]: Type 1, the more common one, is the classical obstructed ureter with hydronephrosis. Type 2 has minimal to absent hydronephrosis, suggesting a non-obstructive pattern. The diagnosis of either type of retrocaval ureter is made radiographically. However, given the sometimes absence of symptoms, early diagnosis is contingent on high clinical suspicion. In the past, as was the case in many urologic maladies of the upper tract, initial evaluation was with intravenous pyelography (IVP). One would typically see right-sided hydronephrosis tapering to a “sickle”- or “fish-hook”-shaped ureter just proximal to the IVC (Type 1). The ureter is medially deviated, and the point of obstruction appears to occur at the edge of the iliopsoas muscle, typically around the transverse process of the third lumbar vertebrae. As it arises from under the IVC, distally, the ureter may have incomplete opacification. With retrograde pyelography, one can see the above findings, except the distal ureter is more clearly opacified. Of note, mid-ureteral valves, another exceedingly rare congenital entity, can masquerade as a retrocaval ureter with similar radiographic findings due to obstruction.

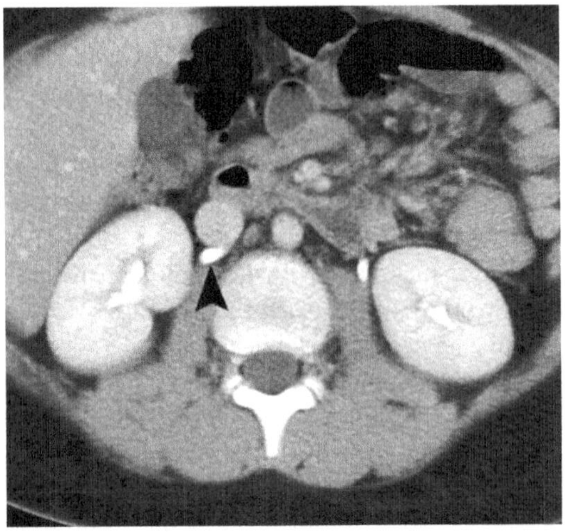

Fig. 14.12 Retrocaval ureter. This CT scan performed for trauma demonstrates that the right ureter is posterior to the inferior vena cava (*arrowhead*). This retrocaval ureter or preureteral vena cava configuration was not associated with obstruction or hydronephrosis

The contemporary modality for diagnosis is contrast-enhanced CT (Fig. 14.12) since the ureter and IVC can be visualized simultaneously, thus clinching the diagnosis [70–74]. As expected, the retrocaval ureter passes posterior and medial to the IVC, and if the ureter is obstructed, like on IVP, the distal ureter may not fill with contrast. However, the anatomical advantage of CT clearly delineates the necessary spatial relationship of the two structures for diagnosis.

The use of MRI has been also reported, in which multiplanar reconstruction images can map out the entire course of the retrocaval ureter with the same findings as in CT imaging [75, 76]. The advantage of lack of radiation or iodinated contrast medium makes MRI an attractive alternative for older children, who do not require sedation.

Treatment

If ureteral obstruction is present, intervention is warranted. Open ureteroureterostomy [77] has largely been replaced by laparoscopic reconstruction given its decreased postoperative convalescence and relative technical ease [78–88]. The retroperitoneal laparoscopic approach [89–95] as well as robotic-assisted laparoscopic approach have also been reported in the literature [96–101]. Regardless of the modality, the basic steps of the reconstruction are the same: division of the ureter on either side of the IVC, repositioning of the ureteral ends lateral to the IVC, and reanastomosis to restore continuity.

Ureteral Polyps

Pathogenesis

Fibroepithelial polyps (FEP) have unclear etiology. As the name implies, these benign soft tissue masses consist of mainly fibrous stromal tissue, vasculature, and normal urothelium. Inflammation is usually not present. They may develop anywhere along the urothelial-lined urinary tract. These polyps can be obstructive, but the combination of ureteral peristalsis and urine flow produces persistent traction causing the peduncle of the mass to grow and elongate. When they are situated proximally (most common) and have not undergone significant longitudinal growth, they are a rare cause of ureteropelvic junction (UPJ) obstruction.

Clinical Presentation

Fibroepithelial polyps are uncommon in children. In one large series of all UPJ cases requiring pyeloplasty in a 35-year period, fibroepithelial polyps occurred 0.5 % of the time [102]. Cassar Delia et al. performed a literature review of polyps causing UPJ obstruction in children showing that the ratio of boys to girls was 13.5:1. The left side was involved in 67 % of cases and bilateral occurrence was 7 % [103]. Abdominal or flank pain was the presenting symptom in 86 % of cases. These polyps can be quite long, even prolapsing into the bladder or urethra. They may also present clinically with hematuria or as an incidental finding after workup for hydronephrosis. Reports of metachronous FEPs have also been reported after excision and pyeloplasty [104]. There has been one report of FEP causing complete obstruction and leading to complete loss of renal function [105].

Imaging

A recent series of 35 children with confirmed fibroepithelial polyps reported a 62 % accuracy rate of establishing the diagnosis on ultrasonography, as well as inferior accuracy with intravenous pyelography (IVP) (24 %) [106]. Younger and thinner children were examined with higher frequency transducers (L5-12, 5–8 MHz) while lower frequency transducers (C8-5, 5–8 MHz) were utilized in older and larger children. Echogenic non-shadowing, well-defined masses were discovered with distention of the renal pelvis. If the mass is obstructing, hydronephrosis or hydroureter is present. Doppler detected blood flow [106].

In a review of the literature, Cassar Delia et al. found that a filling defect is only discovered 36 % of the time on IVP (Fig. 14.13) but 70 % of retrograde pyelograms (RPG) [103]. Consequently, preoperative recognition of these polyps is uncommon in the absence of RPG. The ureter usually appears narrow at the point of attachment of the polyp stalk with hydroureter distally

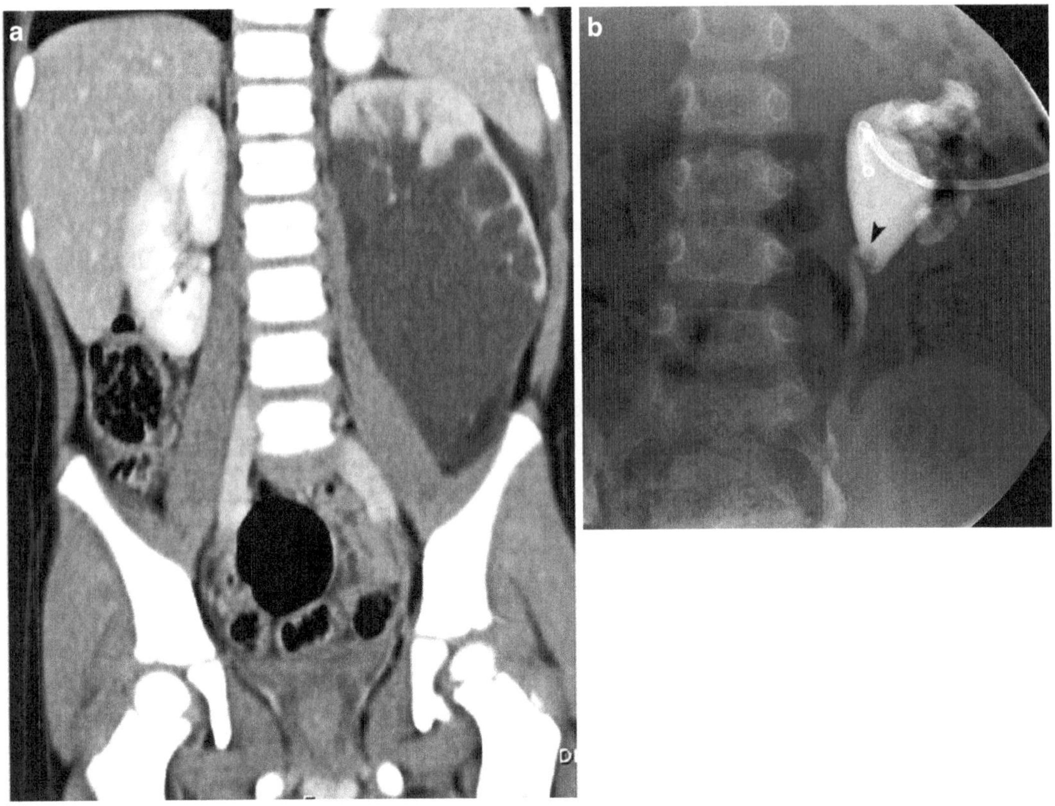

Fig. 14.13 Ureteral polyp. (**a**) This coronal contrast-enhanced CT scan performed for flank pain demonstrates severe hydronephrosis of the left lower pole. The right kidney is normal. (**b**) After a nephrostomy tube was placed, antegrade nephrostogram demonstrates a circular filling defect at the ureteropelvic junction (*arrowhead*), a ureteral polyp, which was causing the ureteropelvic junction obstruction

around the body of the polyp secondary to partial obstruction. The mass presents as a long, slender filling defect with surrounding contrast. These filling defects can be mistaken for radiolucent urinary calculi or blood clots, especially in patients with a history of hematuria.

On computed tomography (CT), FEPs appear as a soft tissue mass in a dilated system with contrast surrounding it circumferentially [107, 108]. Polyps can appear as either a long, pedunculated, smooth-walled soft tissue mass or a short mass with multiple, polypoid projections [109]. CT ureteroscopy is a method of CT imaging using special surface-rendering techniques and endoscopic software that has been reportedly used to diagnose FEP [110]. An obvious disadvantage is the increase in radiation exposure associated with CT-based imaging.

Magnetic resonance imaging (MRI) characterization of FEP has been described as a ureteral lesion hyperintense to the skeletal muscle on T2-weighted images and hypointense (to muscle) on T1-weighted images. There is intense post-gadolinium enhancement (T1), and its lower signal intensity relative to high-intensity urine on T2-weighted images allows for visualization in a dilated collecting system [111, 112]. Short of the lack of radiation, this imaging modality does not appear to garner additional useful information compared to the "simpler" methods described above, especially given its added expense.

Treatment

Management is dependent on location of the polyp. Since the majority of the polyps are located around the UPJ, and preoperative diagnosis of FEP is relatively uncommon, a significant proportion are discovered and treated while undergoing open [109, 113–115] or laparoscopic and robotic-assisted laparoscopic pyeloplasty [104, 116–118]. Historically, nephroureterectomy was performed when polyps were mistaken for malignancy. Since then, different open surgical options have also be described, including ureterotomy [119–123] or pyelotomy with excision [124]. However, in the contemporary literature, numerous reports describe successful endoscopic treatment with ureteroscopy [125–137] or percutaneous nephroscopy [131] for lesions at the UPJ. Recurrence should be on the differential diagnosis for patients who have had a previous FEP and have reappearance of symptoms [104].

Ureteral Duplication

Pathogenesis

Embryologically, abnormalities of the ureteric bud, sprouting off the caudal end of the mesonephric ducts to interact with the metanephric blastema, can lead to ureteral duplication. It is a relatively common congenital malformation, occurring in approximately 1 in 125 based on autopsy studies. It is found slightly more often in girls and unilaterally. When two separate ureteric buds sprout from the mesonephric duct, each induces different portions of the metanephric mesenchyme, dividing the eventual kidney into upper and lower poles. When the separate buds incorporate into the bladder, the more cranial bud (serving the upper 1/3 of the kidney) terminates in a location more caudal and medial than expected. Conversely, the most caudal bud (which will drain the lower pole of the kidney) ends more cranial and lateral. This phenomenon is known as the Weigert-Meyer rule and holds true in all but the rarest exceptions. The lower pole ureter tends to have a shorter course within in the bladder wall due to its lateral positioning, predisposing it to vesicoureteral reflux (VUR), whereas the upper pole ureter with a long course within the bladder wall is more often associated with obstruction or ureterocele (see next section). Partial duplications will have convergence of the ureters into a single system prior to its entry into the bladder (ureterovesical junction, UVJ). These duplications, a result of branching of the ureteric bud prior to interaction with the metanephric blastema, often are associated with normal renal systems.

Clinical Presentation

Patients with partial duplication most often are asymptomatic and are diagnosed incidentally. However, lower pole ureteropelvic junction obstruction (UPJO) can be associated with partial duplications and would present similarly to single-system UPJO, i.e., hydronephrosis on antenatal imaging or intermittent flank pain in an older child. Clinical presentation of complete duplications is dependent on the associated pathology. Upper pole ureteral ectopia can result in incontinence or acute or recurrent urinary tract infections. If a ureterocele is present, UTI or sepsis can occur along with a palpable abdominal mass (severe hydronephrosis). If it is large enough to prolapse from the urethra, it can present as a vaginal mass and even cause bladder outlet obstruction. Urinary incontinence and hematuria can also be clinical symptoms. VUR to the lower pole is similar to single-system VUR in presentation, i.e., UTI and pyelonephritis.

Imaging

Ureteral duplications may be detected by various imaging modalities. Many are seen on antenatal ultrasound with nonspecific hydronephrosis (Fig. 14.14). Sonographically, duplicated systems will have an intervening bar of renal parenchyma separating the upper and lower poles. This parenchyma is more evident in the presence of hydronephrosis. The hydronephrosis can be due to obstruction (upper pole ureterocele/ectopia, lower pole UPJO) or VUR (lower pole). Upper pole renal moieties, since they are often obstructed, may have varying degrees of dysplasia represented as hyperechoic parenchyma and smaller relative size with varying degrees of

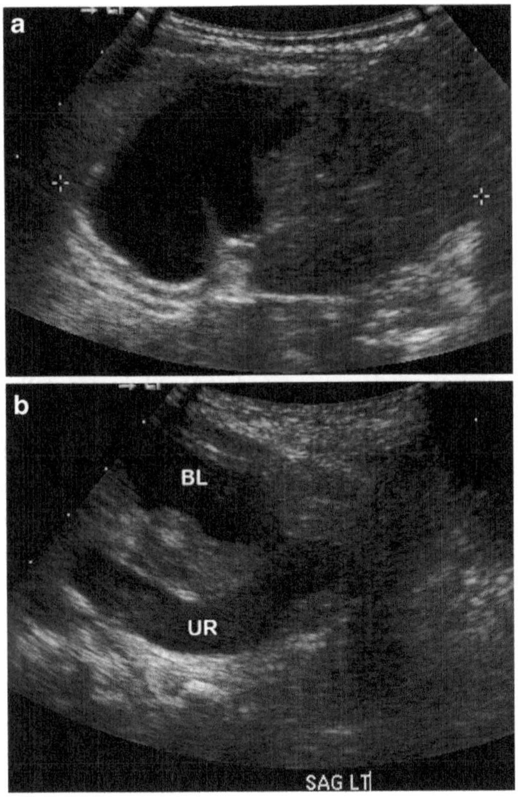

Fig. 14.14 Ureteral duplication (ultrasound). This patient had prenatal hydronephrosis. (**a**) A sagittal image of the left kidney demonstrates a duplex kidney with hydronephrosis of the upper pole. (**b**) A sagittal view of the deep pelvis demonstrates the dilated upper pole ureter (*UR*) extending below the bladder base (*BL*). These two images demonstrate the Weigert-Meyer rule of duplex kidneys in which when there is complete ureteral duplication, the upper pole ureter is ectopic

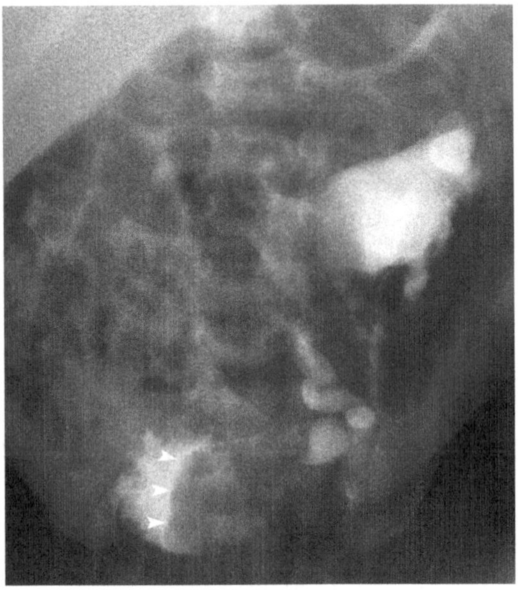

Fig. 14.15 Complete ureteral duplication. This VCUG demonstrates left lower pole reflux. The axis of the calyces is towards the ipsilateral shoulder, with the appearance of the calyces resembling a "drooping lily." The round filling defect (*arrowheads*) within the bladder is the ureterocele associated with the ectopic upper pole ureter

thickness. Ureters may show dilation, and if present on ultrasound, it is important to note the site of insertion of the distal ureter to evaluate for an ectopic location. Ureteroceles (see next section) will reveal a thin-walled cystic structure on the posterior wall of the bladder. The sonographer must ensure that the bladder is not too distended because an effaced ureterocele may avoid detection. Conversely, if the bladder is too empty, the ureterocele can easily be lost among the folds of the bladder wall. If the ureterocele is particularly large, enough to obstruct the contralateral ureteral orifice, bilateral hydronephrosis can be seen.

Ureteral ectopia, in the absence of a ureterocele, can be delineated with intravenous pyelography (IVP). When the upper pole hydronephrosis displaces the lower pole downward and outward, the renal pelvis and calyces appear as a "drooping lily" (see Fig. 14.15). The ureter can be followed down to its ectopic insertion.

UPJO presents with significant hydronephrosis on US. MAG-3 renography is used to confirm obstruction, as in single-system UPJO.

VUR is not typically diagnosed with renal ultrasound, but hydronephrosis with or without hydroureter may be seen. Since duplication is often associated with VUR, a voiding cystourethrogram (VCUG) is often performed. VUR into a lower pole ureter may present itself with the "drooping lily" sign, as in the IVP (described above) (Fig. 14.15).

Treatment

After determining the patient's anatomy, management is dictated by what anomalies are present, e.g., VUR, ectopic ureter, ureterocele, and

UPJO. Duplication in of itself does not require specific treatment unless there is concomitant pathology. Please refer to those specific sections for management.

Ureterocele

Pathogenesis

Ureteroceles are cystic dilations of the terminal ureter on the posterior wall of the bladder. They do not always confine themselves to within the bladder but can extend into the bladder neck or into the urethra. Since these structures are variations of the ectopic ureter, they can be found in single renal systems but generally affect the upper pole in duplex systems (80 %). There is ipsilateral lower pole vesicoureteral reflux (VUR) 40–60 % of the time [138, 139], and contralateral VUR may also be present [139, 140]. Single-system ureteroceles, found more commonly in boys, are usually orthotopic and are less prone to being obstructed or be associated with renal dysplasia. There are multiple classification systems for ureteroceles, based on the predominant location, i.e., intravesical versus extravesical, descriptive characteristics (cecoureterocele, stenotic, sphincteric, sphinctero-stenotic, etc.) [141], or location of the orifice (ectopic vs. orthotopic). A clinical/functional classification system is based on the degree of risk to renal units (upper pole, entire kidney, contralateral kidney) a ureterocele poses [142, 143] and is useful in directing management.

There are multiple theories for the etiology of ureteroceles, the oldest of which is the theory of persistence of a bilayered membrane of the distal ureter, called the Chwalla membrane, which separates it from the urogenital sinus in early embryologic development [144]. Other theories have focused on abnormal muscular development of the terminal ureter [145], ureteral bud malpositioning on the mesonephric duct [146], or embryologic stimuli responsible for bladder expansion also affecting the distal ureter [141]. Recent evidence based on observations in murine models have increased the understanding of interactions of the maturing ureteral bud with the bladder, although the mechanisms have yet to be fully elucidated [147].

Clinical Presentation

Ureteroceles are 4 times more common in girls and are found almost exclusively in Caucasians [148, 149]. The increased utilization of prenatal ultrasonography has led to the increased prenatal diagnosis of ureteroceles. However, many children are still diagnosed clinically [143, 150]. The most common presentation is urinary tract infection and, in extreme cases, urosepsis. Physical exam revealed a palpable abdominal mass indicative of a severely hydronephrotic kidney or an interlabial mass representing the prolapsed ureterocele from the urethral meatus. Large ectopic ureteroceles in the bladder neck or urethra can cause bladder outlet obstruction or incontinence from disruption of normal sphincter function. Longstanding obstruction and urinary stasis increases risk of urolithiasis. In infants, the only symptom may be failure to thrive.

Imaging

The bladder should always be evaluated when a sonographic survey of the kidneys is performed (Fig. 14.16). Since ureteroceles are most commonly associated with duplicated collecting systems, a duplex kidney (seen as two separate renal collecting systems separated by a bar of renal

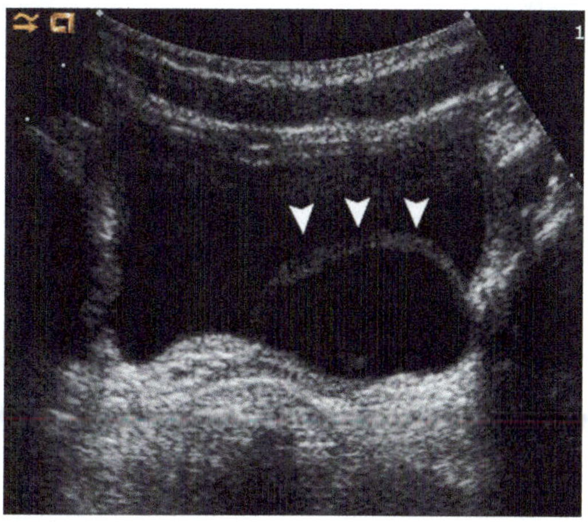

Fig. 14.16 Ureterocele. This transverse view of the bladder demonstrates the thin wall (*arrowheads*) outlines the anterior margin of a ureterocele. The ureter was dilated (not shown)

parenchyma) with a hydronephrotic upper pole and hydroureter should prompt a detailed look for bladder pathology with a suspicion for ureterocele. The robustness (or lack thereof) and echogenicity of the rim of parenchyma surrounding the upper pole hydronephrosis can give a rough estimate of function, but this must never be relied upon solely, given its variability. The ipsilateral lower pole can also be hydronephrotic if vesicoureteral reflux is present or a severely dilated upper pole collecting system impedes drainage of the lower system. In the bladder, a ureterocele appears as a thin-walled cystic structure on the posterior wall of the bladder. Potential pitfalls for the ultrasonographer are ensuring that the bladder is not too distended as an effaced ureterocele may avoid detection. Conversely, an empty bladder with its folded mucosa can mask a ureterocele, or if large the ureterocele can be mistaken for the bladder itself. One has to be cautious of misinterpreting a dilated distal ureter pressing on the bladder wall for a ureterocele, i.e., "pseudoureterocele" [151–154]. The discriminating feature is the thickness of the wall of the cystic dilation, e.g., thin-walled for a true ureterocele and thicker bilaminar bladder wall for a pseudoureterocele (Fig. 14.17). In addition, a ureterocele that is associated with a non-hydronephrotic dysplastic upper pole, referred to as a non-obstructive ectopic ureterocele [155] or ureterocele disproportion [156], can easily be overlooked.

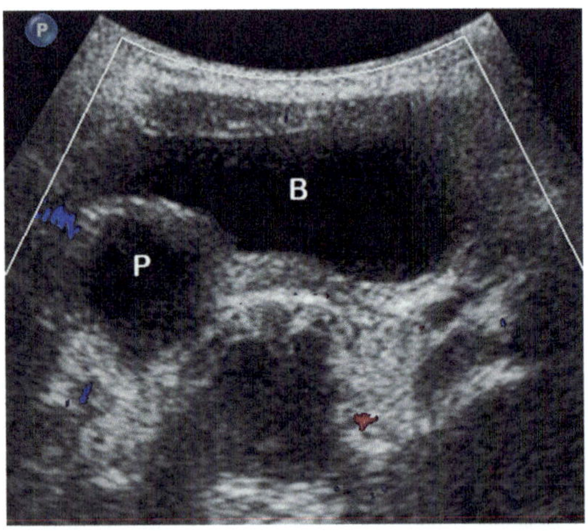

Fig. 14.17 Pseudoureterocele. Transverse view of the bladder demonstrates a round structure posterior to the right base of the bladder which is the pseudoureterocele (*P*). There is a thick-wall interface between this structure and the lumen of the bladder (*B*), distinguishing this pseudoureterocele from a ureterocele

Intravenous pyelography (IVP) has been largely replaced by VCUG (anatomic) and nuclear renography (functional). Contrast drainage from the affected upper pole may give a suggestion of the level of retained function of that moiety. The upper pole will be laterally deviated with delayed or no excretion of contrast. This pushes the lower pole to cause it to deviate laterally and inferiorly, giving it the "drooping lily" appearance. The corresponding lower pole ureter can appear tortuous and notched due to impingement of the dilated upper pole ureter. If the upper pole is non- or poorly functional, only the lower pole may be seen, so the kidney appears to have a decreased number of calyces. If the upper pole unit is functional, contrast can fill the ureterocele in the bladder and produce the "cobra-head" sign.

The VCUG provides details of the bladder, distal ureters, and urethra (voiding phase). It can distinguish ureteroceles from pseudoureteroceles and evaluates the dynamic nature of the ureterocele. They are best seen early in the study, during the filling phase, since if the bladder is too full, the ureterocele can be effaced. It typically appears as a large, smooth, filling defect on the posterior wall/trigone. VUR to the lower pole moiety can be demonstrated also. Once the bladder is full, the ureterocele may evert to look like a diverticulum with its location at the bladder base the only indication of being a ureterocele. Finally, during the voiding phase, prolapse of a large ureterocele can be demonstrated with movement of it into the urethra. Dimercaptosuccinic acid (DMSA) radionuclide scans are useful to evaluate for the degree of function of the upper pole moiety. The presence of function is to determine the salvageability of the renal unit but there are no objective criteria for what level of function deserves saving.

There are proponents of magnetic resonance urography due to its ability to provide both high-definition anatomical detail and functional data. The fact that the study requires sedation and is more costly has limited its use to equivocal cases where the anatomy is unclear. Since there is no ionizing radiation, MRI has been effective in its use for prenatal evaluation, especially in cases of oligohydramnios where ultrasonography is limited. It has been found to be accurate in diagnosing genitourinary abnormalities such as ureterocele [157–159].

Treatment

Due to the anatomic and physiologic variation of the disorder, management for each child should be individualized. Even in situations where surgical intervention is warranted, no specific surgery will remedy all cases. However, it is generally agreed upon that all children with a ureterocele should be on prophylactic antibiotics to prevent UTI/urosepsis [160]. The treatment for a child with a ureterocele and sepsis, unresponsive to antibiotics, is urgent endoscopic decompression via transurethral incision (TUI). When this method was first described [161, 162], subsequent high rates of VUR and consequently, need for secondary surgery, relegated it to be reserved for septic children as an emergency decompressing procedure. However, advances in both the technology and technique of the procedure have expanded its applicability as an initial treatment option. Nevertheless, a recent meta-analysis confirms that the relative risk for reoperation was higher when VUR was present and if the ureterocele was extravesical [163].

Ultimately, renal preservation, in the absence of obstruction and VUR, and urinary continence (in the case of ectopic ureteroceles) are primary goals. However, the majority of affected upper pole moieties do not contribute much to overall renal function and are often removed. This fact is independent of whether the ureterocele was diagnosed antenatally or postnatally [164]. Removal of these units are based on accounts of increased risk for UTI and histological evaluation that indicate dysplastic, nonreversible changes [165]. For the less common single-system ureterocele, there are two treatment options: (1) endoscopic decompression or (2) excision of ureterocele with ureteral reimplant. A recent meta-analysis of the literature suggests endoscopic decompression as the treatment of choice in single-system ureteroceles [163].

For duplex systems, surgery is more complex and there are differences in opinion as to which approach is best. The "upper tract" approach consists of upper pole nephrectomy and partial/total ureterectomy (for a nonfunctional upper pole) or ipsilateral ureteropyelostomy or proximal ureteroureterostomy (for salvageable moiety). This approach avoids a second operation in up to 80 % of patients [166, 167]. The belief is with decompression of the ureterocele and subsequent less distortion of the trigone, some cases of lower pole VUR resolves. The "lower tract" approach entails ureterocele excision with common sheath reimplantation of both upper and lower pole ureters. This approach, obviously, is only feasible if the upper pole has salvageable function. Some surgeons advocate the "combined" approach which treats VUR or ectopic ureteroceles with excision and reimplantation and the nonfunctional upper pole with nephroureterectomy. This approach necessitates 2 incisions but in one series, only 14 % required a second operation for persistent VUR, making it an attractive option [148].

Some have advocated expectant (nonsurgical) management in specific subsets of patients, e.g., nonfunctional upper pole moiety, non-obstructed lower pole, or lower pole with low-grade VUR [168–171].

Ectopic Ureters

Pathogenesis

Ectopic ureters, or ureters that do not insert normally into the bladder trigone [172], are usually associated with ureteral duplication. However, 20 % are associated with single system kidneys, and in boys, most drain single systems. The embryologic mechanism of ureteral duplication, as discussed in the respective section, entails abnormal sprouting of the ureteric buds from the mesonephric duct. When the bud originates in a more cranial position than expected, its incorporation into the posterior wall of the bladder causes the orifice to assume a more caudal and medial position, such as the bladder neck or, most commonly, the urethra. It is believed that the more cranial the budding position on the mesonephric duct, the more ectopic the position of the orifice. Too cranial of a position may actually preclude incorporation into the bladder wall and force termination of the ureter into various derivatives of the common mesonephric duct or mesonephric duct remnants. In boys, ureters may therefore insert into a prostatic utricle, seminal vesicles, vas deferens, or epididymis. In girls, ureters can terminate into the vagina, uterus, fallopian tubes, and Gartner's duct. The abnormal budding may fail to appropriately induce differentiation of the metanephric mesenchyme, resulting in its frequent association with a hypoplastic or dysplastic renal unit. The more remote the location of the ureteral orifice, the greater the degree of renal maldevelopment.

Clinical Presentation

Given the widespread use of antenatal ultrasonography, ectopic ureters may be discovered prior to birth if they are associated with hydroureteronephrosis. However, in cases where hydronephrosis is not present, ectopic ureters may not be suspected until later in childhood when other clinical issues may arise. Because mesonephric duct derivatives are all proximal to the external urethral sphincter (EUS) in boys, these children are invariably continent. However, insertion into the urethra can induce sensations of urinary urgency and frequency. Ectopic ureters can be obstructed leading to hydroureteronephrosis, or have reflux, presenting with a febrile urinary tract infection. Drainage into the epididymis, vas deferens, or seminal vesicles can cause a chemical epididymitis. In girls, in whom ureteral ectopia is at least twice as common, the clinical presentation may be urinary incontinence and constant dribbling despite normal voiding habits, due to the insertion of the ureters into mesonephric duct remnant derivatives that are distal to the EUS or outside the urethra (such as vagina or uterus). Before the period of toilet training, infants may have failure to thrive, recurrent UTI, or persistent vaginal discharge.

Imaging

In cases where an ectopic ureter is suspected, radiological evaluation begins with a renal and bladder ultrasound (US). The greater the degree of ureteral dilation, the easier it is to determine the site of ectopic insertion. In cases of single-system ectopic ureters, the corresponding renal unit may be difficult to find because these may be dysplastic, small, and/or ectopic. Most commonly, hydronephrosis of the upper pole of a duplex kidney with a normal bladder is noted. These upper renal moieties can have hyperechoic parenchyma and thinning as a result of the hydronephrosis and high association with renal dysplasia. A severely dilated ureter can give the appearance of a "pseudoureterocele" (see ureterocele section – Fig. 14.17), which if not careful can be mistaken for and treated as a ureterocele. Traditionally, intravenous pyelography (IVP) was used to diagnose an ectopic ureter. As discussed in the previous section on ureteral duplication, upper pole hydronephrosis can displace the lower pole inferiorly, giving it the "drooping lily" sign. Since ectopic ureters may drain renal moieties with decreased or minimal function, the upper pole may not show excretion, and the altered axis of the lower pole (pointing towards the ipsilateral shoulder) as well as the appearance of a decreased number of calyces provide evidence of the renal duplicity. The ureter can sometimes be followed down to its ectopic insertion with filling of the space with contrast, such as the vagina in a girl.

VCUG can not only demonstrate vesicoureteral reflux (VUR) to the lower pole of a duplex system, but if reflux were to occur into the ectopic ureter itself, it can give the examiner an estimation of the location of the orifice. Reflux visualized during the filling or voiding phase occurs with insertions proximal to the bladder neck. Insertions into the urethra (distal to bladder neck) demonstrate reflux only with voiding. This finding may require several cycles of voiding under fluoroscopy, referred to as cyclic VCUG [173].

If US is unable to show the dysplastic upper pole of a duplex kidney or the dysplastic ectopic kidney, then any contrast-enhanced study, CT or MRI, can be useful. MRI has been advocated by some as the imaging study of choice for this situation or when location of the orifice is in question [174–177]. Several reports state superiority of MRI in evaluating the distal ureter compared to US and IVP [178, 179]. No contrast is needed and ionizing radiation is absent. T2-weighted images are excellent at delineating fluid-filled structures such as an ectopic ureter [180]. In addition, MRI is excellent in showing the location of the orifice [175, 181–184], especially with sagittal views. However, despite accounts of successful MRI without sedation [180], most institutions utilizing MRI for young children have required sedation in some form for optimal imaging. This fact, along with the increased cost, has limited MRI to equivocal cases in need of definition of anatomy rather than as a screening modality.

Despite the ability for MRI to offer renal functional data, dimercaptosuccinic acid (DMSA) radionuclide scans remain the gold standard. The presence of function may determine salvageability, and guide surgical plan, but there are no objective criteria for what level of function deserves saving.

Treatment

Since many ectopic ureters drain minimally functioning moieties, partial nephrectomy to remove the affected unit is often carried out. Finding the location of the ectopic ureteral insertion is not crucial if nephrectomy or partial nephrectomy is planned. This has been done with a variety of approaches, i.e., open, laparoscopic, and robotic assisted. If the offending ureter also has VUR, a second lower incision is made to remove it in its entirety. However, if the moiety has salvageable function, two approaches are feasible: uretero-ureterostomy (high anastomosis of upper pole ureter with lower pole ureter) or ureteral reimplantation of the ectopic ureter. Treatment of single-system ectopic ureters is similar, with total nephrectomy for a non-salvageable renal moiety and also ureterectomy if there is concomitant VUR. There have been reports of successful renal embolization for single-system kidneys with scant function [185, 186]. With salvageable kidneys, ureteral reimplantation of the single system is performed.

Megaureter

Pathogenesis

The term megaureter is purely a descriptive term for any ureter >7 mm in diameter [187] and does not imply a particular pathology. There are four main classifications of megaureter [188, 189]:

1. Obstructed: adynamic/aperistaltic segment of distal ureter
2. Refluxing: pressure transmission to ureter during bladder cycling and filling
3. Non-obstructed and non-refluxing (most common): possible delay in normal maturation of the distal ureter or disease states that produce excessive polyuria that overwhelms a normal UVJ
4. Refluxing and obstructed (least common): disrupted valve mechanism and also ineffective peristalsis of distal ureteral segment

This classification is contingent on an abnormality inherent to the ureterovesical junction, termed primary megaureter. Secondary megaureter, on the other hand, occurs due to abnormalities involving the bladder or urethra that lead to functional or mechanical obstruction.

Clinical Presentation

Primary megaureter is usually asymptomatic and commonly presents with hydroureter on antenatal ultrasound. Less commonly it can be diagnosed later in life on evaluation for UTI, abdominal pain, or hematuria.

Imaging

Working through the classification described above, the radiographic evaluation for megaureter follows an orderly progression (Fig. 14.18).

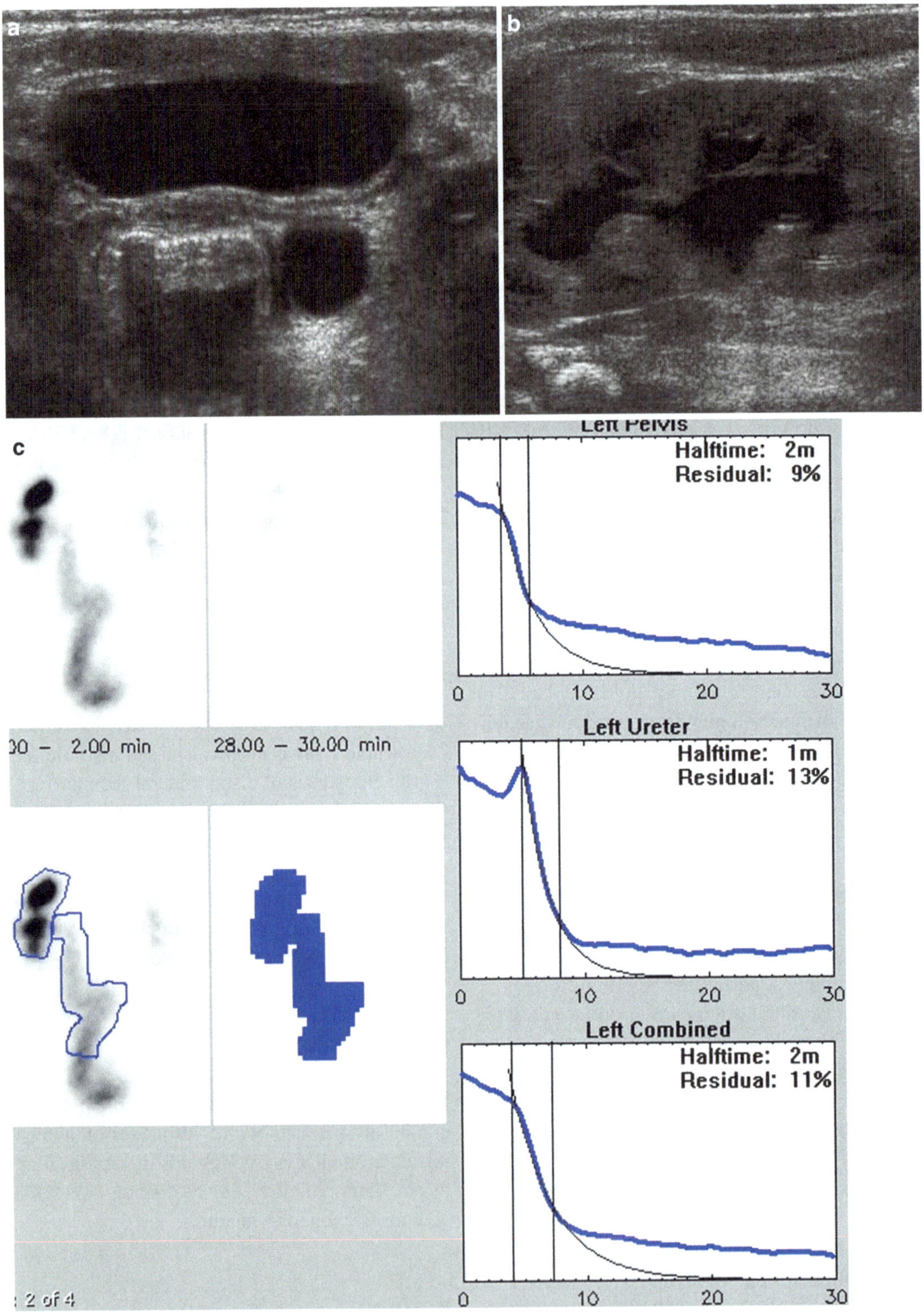

Fig. 14.18 Megaureter. This infant was evaluated for prenatal hydronephrosis. (**a**) Transverse view of the bladder demonstrates a dilated hypoechoic structure posterior and to the left of the bladder. This structure elongated and was the dilated ureter. (**b**) Sagittal views of the left kidney demonstrate moderate hydronephrosis. (**c**) Tc99 MAG3 demonstrates mildly retained contrast within the moderately dilated left renal pelvis and ureter without obstructive parameters after the administration of furosemide

Since the majority are diagnosed with antenatal US, it is logical to use the same imaging modality for confirmation of persistence of dilation postnatally. Findings on US, which is mainly a descriptive study, can be suggestive of the etiology of the dilation. Characteristically, the dilation of the distal ureter is often of higher magnitude compared to the upper ureter and collecting system. The distal aperistaltic segment can also be elucidated on US with the ureter immediately above the lesion actually exhibiting hyperperistalsis [190]. Ultrasound can also be useful to evaluate the bladder and urethra for pathology that may indicate a secondary cause for megaureter, although urethral anatomy is often difficult to discern. If the postnatal US confirms the condition (hydroureteronephrosis), then a VCUG is performed to exclude vesicoureteral reflux (VUR) and provide more anatomical detail of the bladder and urethra [191]. VUR and obstruction, as paradoxical as it sounds, can coexist in a small proportion of patients and is suggested if a delayed film is obtained following the VCUG [192]. However, clinical suspicion is instrumental, since, despite the ability of delayed films for both VCUG and RNC to diagnose reflux and obstruction, delayed films are not standard.

In the absence of VUR, assessment is made with diuretic renography (DR) for obstruction. The two most commonly used agents are 99 m Tc-diethylenetriaminepentaacetic acid (DTPA) and 99 m Tc-mercaptoacetyltriglycine (MAG-3). MAG-3 is the standard agent for infants due to improved imaging in immature or poorly functioning systems [191, 193]. DR should be deferred in very young infants since the relatively low neonatal glomerular filtration rate produces a blunted response to diuretics [192]. This fact and urinary stasis due to the inherent nature of a dilated system can give a falsely elevated half-time ($T_{1/2}$). To counteract this and since furosemide reaches its maximal effect after 15–18 min, a modification to the standard DR, known as furosemide-15 (F-15), entails administration of the diuretic 15 min prior to injection of the radiotracer in order to maximize urinary flow rates at the beginning of the study [194]. Since many variables can affect the outcome of DR, the "well-tempered" renogram has been proposed for uniformity of method

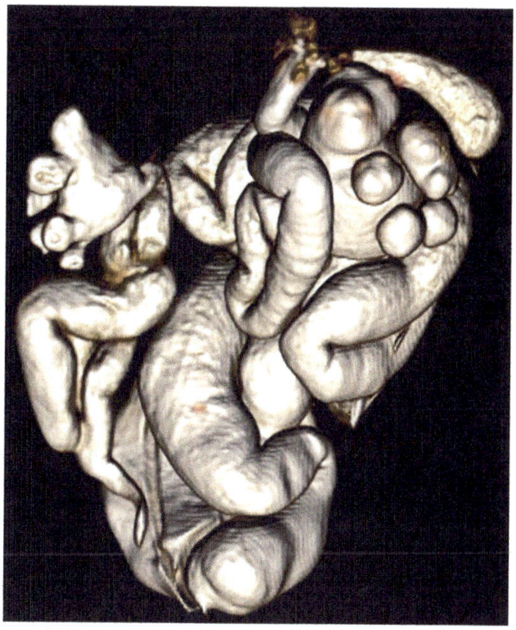

Fig. 14.19 MRU of severe bilateral megaureter. This 3D rendering of an MRU demonstrates severely dilated and tortuous ureters bilaterally. This patient had bilateral obstructed megaureters

[195]. It has three main components: appropriate patient preparation (pre-study hydration and bladder catheterization for the duration of the study), DR technique (type of radiopharmaceutical, timing, dosage, and data acquisition), and data analysis (curve patterns, differential function, measuring diuretic response).

Magnetic resonance urography has been recently proposed as an alternative to renal scintigraphy due to comparable ability to detect renal obstruction and superior anatomic and functional data acquisition. It also has the added advantage of not exposing children to ionizing radiation. However, this modality has only been described at certain specialized centers and requires a level of expertise not widely available [196–200]. This, coupled with the fact that sedation is required for an optimal study, has limited widespread use (Fig. 14.19).

Treatment

Many cases of antenatally diagnosed primary nonrefluxing megaureter will resolve spontaneously

[201–205]. Surgical correction is often indicated for increasing dilation or persistence, worsening renal function, or infections. Since non-obstructed and non-refluxing megaureters most commonly resolve without intervention and do not cause renal compromise, the main goal is to distinguish this type of megaureter from the more dangerous obstructed megaureter; one is treated with observation/serial imaging and prophylactic antibiotics, the other with surgery (ureteral reimplantation ± ureteral tapering). Primary refluxing megaureter is treated like vesicoureteral reflux as discussed above. Even after correction, some degree of residual dilation of the ureter usually persists.

In the case of duplicated ureters, management is dependent on renal function. If function is salvageable, ureteroureterostomy or common sheath reimplantation is performed. In a non-salvageable kidney, heminephrectomy and megaureter excision can be done.

Vesicoureteral Reflux (VUR)

Pathogenesis

Vesicoureteral reflux (VUR) can be classified as primary and secondary. Primary VUR is caused by an intrinsic deficiency of the UVJ with a normal bladder and ureter. The ureteral segment that traverses the wall of the bladder (intramural ureter) serves as a valve mechanism when the bladder contracts to prevent retrograde flow of urine [206]. To prevent VUR, the intramural length and the width of the ureter require a ratio of approximately 5:1. If the intramural length is too short or if the ureteral diameter is too large, the normal ureteral valve mechanism is incompetent and reflux can occur [207].

Secondary VUR is caused by processes that overwhelm the normal UVJ with abnormally high bladder filling and voiding pressures, such as voiding dysfunction or mechanical obstruction from posterior urethral valves or a prolapsing ureterocele. In addition, a paraureteral diverticulum can disrupt the normal architecture of the UVJ leading to VUR.

Regardless of the cause, the end result is a retrograde flow of urine from the bladder up to the ureter and in more severe cases to the renal pelvicalyceal system. Although not a risk factor for urinary tract infection itself, it can facilitate pyelonephritis. In turn, repeated bouts of pyelonephritis can lead to renal scarring and eventual dysfunction.

Clinical Presentation

Indications for imaging of VUR is controversial. Usually VUR is diagnosed during an evaluation for a history of prenatal hydronephrosis or after a child develops a febrile urinary tract infection. In general, for patients with a history of moderate or greater prenatal hydronephrosis, a VCUG is warranted. Thirty to 50 % of children with a febrile UTI are found to have VUR, and the rate can be as high as 70 % in those less than 1 year old [208]. In all children presenting with a febrile UTI or any male child with a UTI (febrile or not), further workup with a VCUG should be considered. There appears to be a genetic basis for some cases of VUR as there is a 27 % incidence of VUR among siblings of children with VUR and a 100 % concordance among identical twins. In addition, the incidence of VUR in offspring of a parent with a history of VUR is 36 % [209–212]. Given this increased risk for VUR, both the European Association of Urology (EUA) and the American Urological Association (AUA) recommend screening siblings, even if asymptomatic [211, 213, 214]. However, this is controversial, and the authors of this chapter have largely abandoned screening in asymptomatic siblings. Voiding cystourethrogram (VCUG) is used to assess the severity of VUR according to the International Reflux Study Committee (IRSC) grading system.

Imaging

The two primary gold standard studies for the detection of reflux are the VCUG and the radionuclide cystogram (RNC) (Figs. 14.20 and 14.21). Both require urethral catheterization,

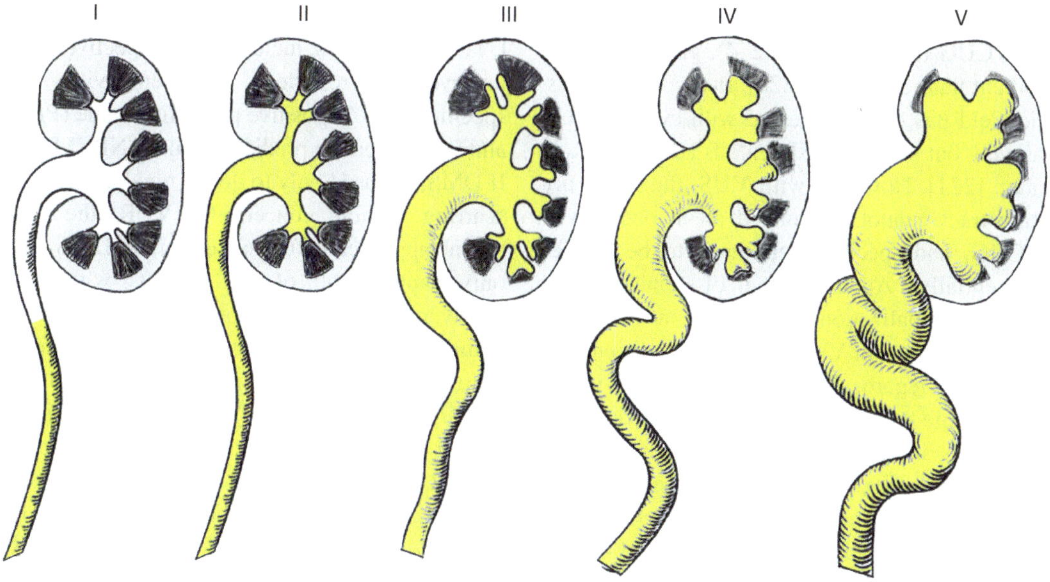

Fig. 14.20 International reflux grading system. This diagram shows representative images of the five grades of reflux as determined by voiding cystourethrogram studies. Please note that the grading system by radionuclide cystograms is done in a scale from 1 to 3

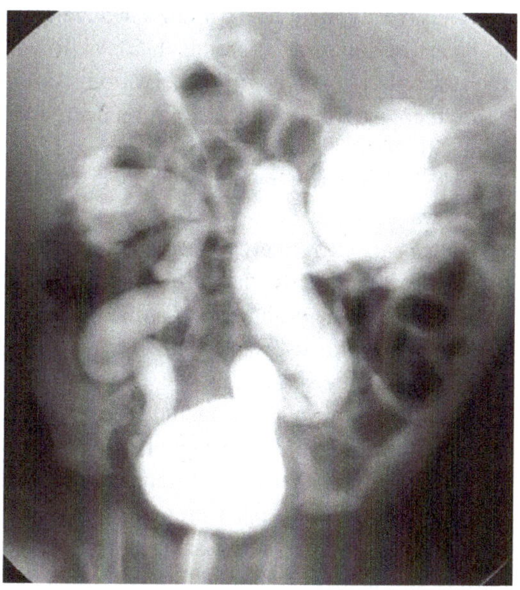

Fig. 14.21 Bilateral high-grade reflux. This VCUG image during voiding demonstrates right reflux, grade 4, and left reflux, grade 5

instillation of contrast, and voiding. RNC has been found to be more sensitive in detecting VUR than VCUG, but due to the decreased resolution of RNC, the grading scale is necessarily simpler with only three grades. Given this inability to discern anatomic detail, RNC is usually reserved for the monitoring of already established VUR and to observe for resolution (spontaneous or postsurgical).

In the constant pursuit to limit ionizing radiation in children, multiple studies in the literature advocate considering ultrasound for VUR screening, especially in the screening for sibling reflux [215]. To improve the "resolution" of sonographic detection, the use of ultrasound contrast agents have been developed and are currently in use in several European countries [216–218]. The contrast agent, however, has not been FDA approved and therefore is not available for clinical use in the United States. Contrast-enhanced voiding urosonography (VUS) requires intravesical instillation of the contrast agent, via a urethral catheter, and specialized software to visualize it. In the literature, diagnostic accuracy has ranged from 78 to 96 %. When compared with VCUG, the difference in the reflux detection rate was not significant, and missed cases were typically grade 1 [219]. Also, the dynamic nature of ultrasonography accounts for the cases of VUR detected on VUS but missed on VCUG (usually grades 2–4), given the intermittent nature of VUR [220]. Increased diagnostic yield has been suggested with cyclic VCUG as well, but this obviously entails additional radiation [221]. However, with VUS, the entire urinary tract cannot be imaged all at once, as in VCUG, and specific areas have to be imaged sequentially. Another area of contention is whether visualization and evaluation of the urethra is adequate in VUS. Reports have been variable in this regard, although more recent evidence is favorable for VUS [222–224]. For obvious reasons, this imaging modality requires a skillful ultrasonographer, and currently, the procedure has not been standardized. As such, VCUG remains the first-line study for urethral evaluation and, consequently, as the first examination for boys [225]. For instances of follow-up, screening of high-risk patients, and first examination in girls, VUS appears to be a viable alternative where available, with the above limitations [216, 219].

There are also advocates of evaluating the kidneys with a dimercaptosuccinic acid (DMSA) renal scan with a child's first febrile UTI to detect pyelonephritic changes and renal scarring before performing invasive studies such as VCUG [226]. Deemed the "top-down" approach, the idea is that if a child with her/his first febrile UTI has a normal DMSA scan, then the likelihood that the child has significant VUR is low which obviates the need for a VCUG [226–229]. Proponents of this approach aim to limit catheterization in children, a procedure considered to be painful and invasive. However, with a skilled team, VCUG can be well tolerated without the need for sedation [230]. Disadvantages of the "top-down" approach include increased imaging cost and radiation doses (compared to VCUG/US) [231], the need for intravenous administration of the radiotracer, variability in how DMSA scans are performed [232], increased length of the study (3–4 h), and the potential to need sedation for infants [226]. A recent retrospective study [233] and a meta-analysis [234] reported low sensitivity (79 %) and specificity (53 %) in detecting VUR and did not recommend DMSA as a replacement for VCUG after the first febrile UTI. Other studies, including a prospective study, however, have reported a 96 % sensitivity, 72 % specificity, 83 % positive predictive value (PPV), and 92 % negative predictive value (NPV) [229]. If DMSA is used only to detect renal infection or scarring without concern for VUR, the "top-down" approach is further supported. DMSA not only captures all of the patients with renal involvement with VUR, but also those with no demonstrative VUR but still at risk for further scarring. Therefore, patients that are missed with DMSA are those with VUR that is clinically insignificant, i.e., has not resulted in renal injury [228, 235, 236].

Ultimately, there is no consensus as to whether a "top-down" or "bottom-up" approach should be used for initial imaging of VUR.

Treatment

Management options for VUR are dependent on its severity and the patient's age. Eighty to 85 % of low-grade (grades 1–2) VUR will spontaneously resolve with observation. As the grade increases, the rate of resolution decreases, with 50 % of grade 3 VUR resolving and only 25 % or fewer resolving with grade 4–5 (high-grade) VUR.

VUR is also less likely to resolve if diagnosed at an older age. VUR diagnosed during sibling screening or in the evaluation of a history of prenatal hydronephrosis is more likely to resolve and rarely require surgery.

The treatment options include observation, with or without antibiotic prophylaxis, or surgical management either via endoscopic bulking of the ureteral orifice or open ureteral reimplantation. Management is individualized based on a variety of factors including family preference, clinical variables, and ability to tolerate repeated invasive diagnostic testing. The use of antibiotic prophylaxis is controversial, and reports have shown benefit and lack thereof [237–240]. Further studies are necessary to clarify this important question. The success rate for surgical correction (ureteral reimplantation) is very high

(100 % for low grade and 90–95 % for high grade), whereas success rates for endoscopic injection are more variable (50–94 %) among studies, with increasing grades of VUR negatively affecting success [241–243].

Indications for anti-reflux surgery include breakthrough UTI, new renal scarring, high-grade VUR with evidence of scarring or renal compromise, associated congenital abnormalities of the ureterovesical junction that may affect the rate of resolution, failure of renal growth or worsening function, persistent VUR in females at puberty, and noncompliance with or non-tolerance of medical management.

References

1. Abrahamson J. Double bladder and related anomalies: clinical and embryological aspects and a case report. Br J Urol. 1961;33:195–214.
2. Esham W, Holt HA. Complete duplication of bladder and urethra: a case report. J Urol. 1980;123(5):773–5.
3. Cheng EY, Maizels M. Complete duplication of the bladder and urethra in the coronal plane: case report. J Urol. 1996;155(4):1414–15.
4. Bellagha I, Chaouachi B, Hammou A, Dhaoui R, Kaabar N, Aloulou T, et al. [An exceptional combined malformation: duplication of the lower urinary tract, the vulva and the posterior intestine]. Ann Urol (Paris). 1993;27(2):101–5.
5. Ravitch MM, Scott WW. Duplication of the entire colon, bladder, and urethra. Surgery. 1953;34(5): 843–58.
6. Kossow JH, Morales PA. Duplication of bladder and urethra and associated anomalies. Urology. 1973;1(1):71–3.
7. Berrocal T, Lopez-Pereira P, Arjonilla A, Gutierrez J. Anomalies of the distal ureter, bladder, and urethra in children: embryologic, radiologic, and pathologic features. Radiographics. 2002;22(5):1139–64.
8. Nix JT, Menville JG, Albert M, Wendt DL. Congenital patent urachus. J Urol. 1958;79(2): 264–73.
9. Cilento Jr BG, Bauer SB, Retik AB, Peters CA, Atala A. Urachal anomalies: defining the best diagnostic modality. Urology. 1998;52(1):120–2.
10. Fox JA, McGee SM, Routh JC, Granberg CF, Ashley RA, Hutcheson JC, et al. Vesicoureteral reflux in children with urachal anomalies. J Pediatr Urol. 2011;7(6):632–5.
11. Yapo BR, Gerges B, Holland AJ. Investigation and management of suspected urachal anomalies in children. Pediatr Surg Int. 2008;24(5):589–92.
12. Yu JS, Kim KW, Lee HJ, Lee YJ, Yoon CS, Kim MJ. Urachal remnant diseases: spectrum of CT and US findings. Radiographics. 2001;21(2):451–61.
13. Cacciarelli AA, Kass EJ, Yang SS. Urachal remnants: sonographic demonstration in children. Radiology. 1990;174(2):473–5.
14. Zieger B, Sokol B, Rohrschneider WK, Darge K, Troger J. Sonomorphology and involution of the normal urachus in asymptomatic newborns. Pediatr Radiol. 1998;28(3):156–61.
15. Sheldon CA, Clayman RV, Gonzalez R, Williams RD, Fraley EE. Malignant urachal lesions. J Urol. 1984;131(1):1–8.
16. Upadhyay V, Kukkady A. Urachal remnants: an enigma. Eur J Pediatr Surg. 2003;13(6):372–6.
17. Scabini S, Rimini E, Romairone E, Scordamaglia R, Vallarino L, Giasotto V, et al. Urachal tumour: case report of a poorly understood carcinoma. World J Surg Oncol. 2009;7:82.
18. Fancher TT, Dudrick SJ, Palesty JA. Papillary adenocarcinoma of the urachus presenting as an umbilical mass. Conn Med. 2010;74(6):325–7.
19. Ashley RA, Inman BA, Routh JC, Rohlinger AL, Husmann DA, Kramer SA. Urachal anomalies: a longitudinal study of urachal remnants in children and adults. J Urol. 2007;178(4 Pt 2):1615–18.
20. Lipskar AM, Glick RD, Rosen NG, Layliev J, Hong AR, Dolgin SE, et al. Nonoperative management of symptomatic urachal anomalies. J Pediatr Surg. 2010;45(5):1016–19.
21. Ueno T, Hashimoto H, Yokoyama H, Ito M, Kouda K, Kanamaru H. Urachal anomalies: ultrasonography and management. J Pediatr Surg. 2003;38(8):1203–7.
22. Ozbek SS, Pourbagher MA, Pourbagher A. Urachal remnants in asymptomatic children: gray-scale and color Doppler sonographic findings. J Clin Ultrasound. 2001;29(4):218–22.
23. Blane CE, Zerin JM, Bloom DA. Bladder diverticula in children. Radiology. 1994;190(3):695–7.
24. Hutch JA. Saccule formation at the ureterovesical junction in smooth walled bladders. J Urol. 1961;86:390–9.
25. Stephens FD. The vesicoureteral hiatus and paraureteral diverticula. J Urol. 1979;121(6):786–91.
26. Mackellar A, Stephens FD. Vesical diverticula in children. Aust N Z J Surg. 1960;30:20–31.
27. Amar AD. Vesicoureteral reflux associated with congenital bladder diverticulum in boys and young men. J Urol. 1972;107(6):966–8.
28. Barrett DM, Malek RS, Kelalis PP. Observations on vesical diverticulum in childhood. J Urol. 1976;116(2):234–6.
29. Livne PM, Gonzales Jr ET. Congenital bladder diverticula causing ureteral obstruction. Urology. 1985;25(3):273–6.
30. Harcke Jr HT, Capitanio MA, Grover WD, Valdes-Dapena M. Bladder diverticula and Menkes' syndrome. Radiology. 1977;124(2):459–61.
31. Bauer SB, Retik AB. Bladder diverticula in infants and children. Urology. 1974;3(6):712–15.

32. Bogdanos J, Paleodimos I, Korakianitis G, Stephanidis A, Androulakakis PA. The large bladder diverticulum in children. J Pediatr Urol. 2005;1(4):267–72.
33. Garat JM, Angerri O, Caffaratti J, Moscatiello P, Villavicencio H. Primary congenital bladder diverticula in children. Urology. 2007;70(5):984–8.
34. Bhat A, Bothra R, Bhat MP, Chaudhary GR, Saran RK, Saxena G. Congenital bladder diverticulum presenting as bladder outlet obstruction in infants and children. J Pediatr Urol. 2012;8(4):348–53.
35. Shukla AR, Bellah RA, Canning DA, Carr MC, Snyder HM, Zderic SA. Giant bladder diverticula causing bladder outlet obstruction in children. J Urol. 2004;172(5 Pt 1):1977–9.
36. Verghese M, Belman AB. Urinary retention secondary to congenital bladder diverticula in infants. J Urol. 1984;132(6):1186–8.
37. Oge O, Gemalmaz H, Ozeren B. Acute urinary retention in a child caused by a congenital bladder diverticulum. J Pediatr Surg. 2002;37(6):926–7.
38. Akbulut S, Cakabay B, Sezgin A, Isen K, Senol A. Giant vesical diverticulum: a rare cause of defecation disturbance. World J Gastroenterol. 2009;15(31):3957–9.
39. Kaufman JJ, Mills H. Giant diverticulum of the bladder with gastrointestinal manifestations. Calif Med. 1957;86(5):331–3.
40. Mirow L, Brugge A, Fischer F, Roblick UJ, Durek C, Burk C, et al. Giant bladder diverticulum as a rare cause of intestinal obstruction: report of a case. Surg Today. 2007;37(8):702–3.
41. Shaked G, Czeiger D. Distended urinary bladder and diverticulum-a rare cause of large-bowel obstruction. Am J Surg. 2009;197(2):e23–4.
42. Maynor CH, Kliewer MA, Hertzberg BS, Paulson EK, Keogan MT, Carroll BA. Urinary bladder diverticula: sonographic diagnosis and interpretive pitfalls. J Ultrasound Med. 1996;15(3):189–94.
43. Mahran MA, Sayed AT, Hashad AM, Fattah IH, Rashed A. The place of ultrasound in urogynaecology clinic. Arch Gynecol Obstet. 2010;281(1):5–10.
44. Schneider K, Fendel H, Kohn MM. Differential diagnosis of intra- and perivesical abnormalities using bladder air/CO_2 contrast sonography. Pediatr Radiol. 1986;16(4):309–12.
45. Weingardt JP, Nemcek Jr AA, Miljkovic SC. The diverticular jet effect: color Doppler differentiation of bladder diverticula from other pelvic fluid collections. J Clin Ultrasound. 1994;22(6):397–400.
46. Boechat MI, Lebowitz RL. Diverticula of the bladder in children. Pediatr Radiol. 1978;7(1):22–8.
47. Lebowitz RL, Colodny AH, Crissey M. Neonatal hydronephrosis caused by vesical diverticula. Urology. 1979;13(3):335–41.
48. Tannous WN, Azouz EM, Homsy YL, Kiruluta HG, Grattan-Smith D. CT and ultrasound imaging of pelvic rhabdomyosarcoma in children. A review of 56 patients. Pediatr Radiol. 1989;19(8):530–4.
49. Agrons GA, Wagner BJ, Lonergan GJ, Dickey GE, Kaufman MS. From the archives of the AFIP. Genitourinary rhabdomyosarcoma in children: radiologic-pathologic correlation. Radiographics. 1997;17(4):919–37.
50. Poggiani C, Teani M, Auriemma A, Bianchi P, Sadou Y. Sonographic detection of rhabdomyosarcoma of the urinary bladder. Eur J Ultrasound. 2001;13(1):35–9.
51. Hays DM, Raney RB, Wharam MD, Wiener E, Lobe TE, Andrassy RJ, et al. Children with vesical rhabdomyosarcoma (RMS) treated by partial cystectomy with neoadjuvant or adjuvant chemotherapy, with or without radiotherapy. A report from the Intergroup Rhabdomyosarcoma Study (IRS) Committee. J Pediatr Hematol Oncol. 1995;17(1):46–52.
52. Hays DM, Lawrence Jr W, Crist WM, Wiener E, Raney Jr RB, Ragab A, et al. Partial cystectomy in the management of rhabdomyosarcoma of the bladder: a report from the Intergroup Rhabdomyosarcoma Study. J Pediatr Surg. 1990;25(7):719–23.
53. Yeung CK, Ward HC, Ransley PG, Duffy PG, Pritchard J. Bladder and kidney function after cure of pelvic rhabdomyosarcoma in childhood. Br J Cancer. 1994;70(5):1000–3.
54. El-Sherbiny MT, El-Mekresh MH, El-Baz MA, Ghoneim MA. Paediatric lower urinary tract rhabdomyosarcoma: a single-centre experience of 30 patients. BJU Int. 2000;86(3):260–7.
55. Tanaka H, Matsuda M, Moriya K, Mitsui T, Kitta T, Nonomura K. Ultrasonographic measurement of bladder wall thickness as a risk factor for upper urinary tract deterioration in children with myelodysplasia. J Urol. 2008;180(1):312–16; discussion 6.
56. Leonardo CR, Filgueiras MF, Vasconcelos MM, Vasconcelos R, Marino VP, Pires C, et al. Risk factors for renal scarring in children and adolescents with lower urinary tract dysfunction. Pediatr Nephrol. 2007;22(11):1891–6.
57. Edelstein RA, Bauer SB, Kelly MD, Darbey MM, Peters CA, Atala A, et al. The long-term urological response of neonates with myelodysplasia treated proactively with intermittent catheterization and anticholinergic therapy. J Urol. 1995;154(4):1500–4.
58. Dik P, Klijn AJ, de Jong-de Vos van Steenwijk CC, de Jong TP. Early start to therapy preserves kidney function in spina bifida patients. Eur Urol. 2006;49(5):908–13.
59. Flood HD, Ritchey ML, Bloom DA, Huang C, McGuire EJ. Outcome of reflux in children with myelodysplasia managed by bladder pressure monitoring. J Urol. 1994;152(5 Pt 1):1574–7.
60. Sidi AA, Peng W, Gonzalez R. Vesicoureteral reflux in children with myelodysplasia: natural history and results of treatment. J Urol. 1986;136(1 Pt 2):329–31.
61. Bauer SB, Hallett M, Khoshbin S, Lebowitz RL, Winston KR, Gibson S, et al. Predictive value of urodynamic evaluation in newborns with myelodysplasia. JAMA. 1984;252(5):650–2.

62. DeLair SM, Eandi J, White MJ, Nguyen T, Stone AR, Kurzrock EA. Renal cortical deterioration in children with spinal dysraphism: analysis of risk factors. J Spinal Cord Med. 2007;30 Suppl 1: S30–4.
63. Shiroyanagi Y, Suzuki M, Matsuno D, Yamazaki Y. The significance of 99mtechnetium dimercapto-succinic acid renal scan in children with spina bifida during long-term followup. J Urol. 2009;181(5): 2262–6; discussion 6.
64. Fotter R. Neurogenic bladder in infants and children–a new challenge for the radiologist. Abdom Imaging. 1996;21(6):534–40.
65. Fotter R, Kopp W, Klein E, Hollwarth M, Uray E. Unstable bladder in children: functional evaluation by modified voiding cystourethrography. Radiology. 1986;161(3):811–13.
66. Lorenzo AJ, Wallis MC, Cook A, Buffett-Fairen A, Bozic D, Bagli DJ, et al. What is the variability in urodynamic parameters with position change in children? Analysis of a prospectively enrolled cohort. J Urol. 2007;178(6):2567–70.
67. Nielsen PB. Retrocaval ureter; report of a case. Acta Radiol. 1959;51(3):179–88.
68. Bateson EM, Atkinson D. Circumcaval ureter: a new classification. Clin Radiol. 1969;20(2):173–7.
69. Kenawi MM, Williams DI. Circumcaval ureter: a report of four cases in children with a review of the literature and a new classification. Br J Urol. 1976; 48(3):183–92.
70. Kokubo T, Okada Y, Yashiro N, Itai Y, Iio M. CT diagnosis of retrocaval ureter associated with double inferior vena cava: report of a case. Radiat Med. 1990;8(3):96–8.
71. Lautin EM, Haramati N, Frager D, Friedman AC, Gold K, Kurtz A, et al. CT diagnosis of circumcaval ureter. AJR Am J Roentgenol. 1988;150(3): 591–4.
72. Lin WC, Wang JH, Wei CJ, Chang CY. Assessment of CT urography in the diagnosis of urinary tract abnormalities. J Chin Med Assoc. 2004;67(2):73–8.
73. Murphy BJ, Casillas J, Becerra JL. Retrocaval ureter: computed tomography and ultrasound appearance. J Comput Tomogr. 1987;11(1):89–93.
74. Pienkny AJ, Herts B, Streem SB. Contemporary diagnosis of retrocaval ureter. J Endourol. 1999; 13(10):721–2.
75. Uthappa MC, Anthony D, Allen C. Case report: retrocaval ureter: MR appearances. Br J Radiol. 2002;75(890):177–9.
76. Lin HY, Chou YH, Huang SP, Li YC, Tsai HN, Jeng HS, et al. Retrocaval ureter: report of two cases and literature review. Kaohsiung J Med Sci. 2003; 19(3):127–31.
77. Stojkovic J, Zvara V. Treatment of retrocaval ureter. Czech Med. 1986;9(1):15–22.
78. Ramalingam M, Selvarajan K. Laparoscopic transperitoneal repair of retrocaval ureter: report of two cases. J Endourol. 2003;17(2):85–7.
79. Montoya-Martinez G, Maldonado-Alcaraz E, Moreno-Palacios J, Serrano-Brambila E, Martinez-Vargas A, Torres-Mercado LO. Laparoscopic management of retrocaval ureter: case report and literature review. Cir Cir. 2011;79(4):338–42.
80. Bhandarkar DS, Lalmalani JG, Shivde S. Laparoscopic ureterolysis and reconstruction of a retrocaval ureter. Surg Endosc. 2003;17(11):1851–2.
81. Singh V, Sinha RJ. Laparoscopic dismembered pyeloplasty and pyelolithotomy in a patient with a retrocaval ureter: our experience and review of literature. Urol J. 2011;8(3):231–5.
82. Chung BI, Gill IS. Laparoscopic dismembered pyeloplasty of a retrocaval ureter: case report and review of the literature. Eur Urol. 2008;54(6):1433–6.
83. Ding GQ, Xu LW, Li XD, Li GH, Yu YL, Yu DM, et al. Pure transperitoneal laparoscopic correction of retrocaval ureter. Chin Med J (Engl). 2012; 125(13):2382–5.
84. Asimakopoulos AD, D'Orazio A, Pereira CF, Hoepffner JL, Mugnier C, Gaston R, et al. Surgery illustrated–focus on details: laparoscopic repair of obstructing retrocaval ureter. BJU Int. 2011;107(8):1330–4.
85. Autorino R, Khanna R, White MA, Haber GP, Shah G, Kaouk JH, et al. Laparoendoscopic single-site repair of retrocaval ureter: first case report. Urology. 2010;76(6):1501–5.
86. Dogan HS, Oktay B, Vuruskan H, Yavascaoglu I. Treatment of retrocaval ureter by pure laparoscopic pyelopyelostomy: experience on 4 patients. Urology. 2010;75(6):1343–7.
87. Simforoosh N, Nouri-Mahdavi K, Tabibi A. Laparoscopic pyelopyelostomy for retrocaval ureter without excision of the retrocaval segment: first report of 6 cases. J Urol. 2006;175(6):2166–9; discussion 9.
88. Fernandez-Fernandez JA, Pachano-Arenas FE. Laparoscopic-assisted correction of a retrocaval ureter. J Pediatr Surg. 2008;43(8):1560–2.
89. Li HZ, Ma X, Qi L, Shi TP, Wang BJ, Zhang X. Retroperitoneal laparoscopic ureteroureterostomy for retrocaval ureter: report of 10 cases and literature review. Urology. 2010;76(4):873–6.
90. Miyazato M, Kimura T, Ohyama C, Hatano T, Miyazato T, Ogawa Y. Retroperitoneoscopic ureteroureterostomy for retrocaval ureter. Hinyokika Kiyo. 2002;48(1):25–8.
91. Xu DF, Yao YC, Ren JZ, Liu YS, Gao Y, Che JP, et al. Retroperitoneal laparoscopic ureteroureterostomy for retrocaval ureter: report of 7 cases. Urology. 2009;74(6):1242–5.
92. Chen S, Xu B, Liu J, Ren Q, Hu X, Yang Y, et al. Retroperitoneal laparoscopic reconstruction for retrocaval ureter: experience and literature review. J Endourol. 2012;26(9):1147–52.
93. Kang N, Zhang JH, Niu YN, Wang JW, Tian XQ, Yong Y, et al. Retroperitoneal laparoendoscopic single-site surgery for the treatment of retrocaval ureter. World J Urol. 2012;31(1):205–11.

94. Chen Z, Chen X, Wu ZH, Luo YC, Li NN. Treatment of retrocaval ureter by retroperitoneal laparoscopic ureteroureterostomy: experience on 12 patients. J Laparoendosc Adv Surg Tech A. 2011;21(9):803–7.
95. Tobias-Machado M, Lasmar MT, Wroclawski ER. Retroperitoneoscopic surgery with extracorporeal uretero-ureteral anastomosis for treating retrocaval ureter. Int Braz J Urol. 2005;31(2):147–50.
96. Hemal AK, Rao R, Sharma S, Clement RG. Pure robotic retrocaval ureter repair. Int Braz J Urol. 2008;34(6):734–8.
97. Krane LS, Hemal AK. Surgeon-controlled robotic ureteral surgery. Curr Opin Urol. 2012;22(1):70–7.
98. LeRoy TJ, Thiel DD, Igel TC. Robot-assisted laparoscopic reconstruction of retrocaval ureter: description and video of technique. J Laparoendosc Adv Surg Tech A. 2011;21(4):349–51.
99. Hemal AK, Nayyar R, Gupta NP, Dorairajan LN. Experience with robot assisted laparoscopic surgery for upper and lower benign and malignant ureteral pathologies. Urology. 2010;76(6):1387–93.
100. Smith KM, Shrivastava D, Ravish IR, Nerli RB, Shukla AR. Robot-assisted laparoscopic ureteroureterostomy for proximal ureteral obstructions in children. J Pediatr Urol. 2009;5(6):475–9.
101. Gundeti MS, Duffy PG, Mushtaq I. Robotic-assisted laparoscopic correction of pediatric retrocaval ureter. J Laparoendosc Adv Surg Tech A. 2006;16(4): 422–4.
102. Adey GS, Vargas SO, Retik AB, Borer JG, Mandell J, Hendren WH, et al. Fibroepithelial polyps causing ureteropelvic junction obstruction in children. J Urol. 2003;169(5):1834–6.
103. Cassar Delia E, Joseph VT, Sherwood W. Fibroepithelial polyps causing ureteropelvic junction obstruction in children–a case report and review article. Eur J Pediatr Surg. 2007;17(2):142–6.
104. Kojima Y, Lambert SM, Steixner BL, Laryngakis N, Casale P. Multiple metachronous fibroepithelial polyps in children. J Urol. 2011;185(3):1053–7.
105. Oguzkurt P, Oz S, Oguzkurt L, Kayaselcuk F, Tercan F. An unusual cause of complete distal ureteral obstruction: giant fibroepithelial polyp. J Pediatr Surg. 2004;39(11):1733–4.
106. Wang XM, Jia LQ, Wang Y, Wang N. Utilizing ultrasonography in the diagnosis of pediatric fibroepithelial polyps causing ureteropelvic junction obstruction. Pediatr Radiol. 2012;42(9):1107–11.
107. Bellin MF, Springer O, Mourey-Gerosa I, Coumbaras J, Chartier-Kastler E, Delcourt A, et al. CT diagnosis of ureteral fibroepithelial polyps. Eur Radiol. 2002;12(1):125–8.
108. Oesterling JE, Liu HY, Fishman EK. Real-time, multiplanar computerized tomography: a new diagnostic modality used in the detection and endoscopic removal of a distal ureteral fibroepithelial polyp and adjacent calculus. J Urol. 1989;142(6):1563–6.
109. Liddell RM, Weinberger E, Schofield DE, Pelman RS. Fibroepithelial polyp of the ureter in a child. AJR Am J Roentgenol. 1991;157(6):1273–4.
110. Chou CP, Wu TT, Levenson RB, Huang JS, Pan HB. Ureteral fibroepithelial polyp diagnosed preoperatively on virtual CT ureteroscopy. Abdom Imaging. 2007;32(3):421–3.
111. Patheyar V, Venkatesh SK, Siew EP, Consiglieri DT, Putti T. MR imaging features of fibroepithelial ureteral polyp in a patient with duplicated upper urinary tract. Singapore Med J. 2011;52(3):e45–7.
112. Lai TK, Chung CH, Chin AC, Szeto PS, Wong WC, Chan RY, et al. Magnetic resonance imaging for ureteral fibroepithelial polyp. Hong Kong Med J. 2008;14(5):408–10.
113. Li WM, Wu WJ, Ke HL, Chai CY, Chou YH, Huang CH. Fibroepithelial polyps causing ureteropelvic junction obstruction in a child. Kaohsiung J Med Sci. 2005;21(6):282–5.
114. Zeman L, Dusek M, Lisy J, Moravek J, Rygl M, Stejskal J, et al. Multiple fibroepithelial polyps of the upper ureter in a 17-year-old boy–case report and review of the literature. Eur J Pediatr Surg. 2004;14(5):358–61.
115. Karaca I, Sencan A, Mir E, Sayan A, Ortac R. Ureteral fibroepithelial polyps in children. Pediatr Surg Int. 1997;12(8):603–4.
116. Jin XB, Meng HL, Zhang YD, Jiang SB, Wang HB, Wang J. Laparoscopic treatment of a massive fibroepithelial polyp accompanied by ureteral intussusception. Chin Med J (Engl). 2011;124(20):3436–9.
117. Iwatsuki S, Kojima Y, Mizuno K, Tozawa K, Kohri K, Hayashi Y. Laparoscopic management for fibroepithelial polyp causing ureteropelvic junction obstruction in a child. Urology. 2010;76(1):146–8.
118. Kijvikai K, Maynes LJ, Herrell SD. Laparoscopic management of large ureteral fibroepithelial polyp. Urology. 2007;70(2):373.e4–7.
119. Cooper CS, Hawtrey CE. Fibroepithelial polyp of the ureter. Urology. 1997;50(2):280–1.
120. Debruyne FM, Moonen WA, Daenekindt AA, Delaere KP. Fibroepithelial polyp of ureter. Urology. 1980;16(4):355–9.
121. Mydlo J, Reda E, Gill B, Kogan SJ, Ziprkowski MN, Weiss R, et al. Fibroepithelial polyp in a child. Urology. 1988;31(4):318–20.
122. Bartone FF, Johansson SL, Markin RJ, Imray TJ. Bilateral fibroepithelial polyps of ureter in a child. Urology. 1990;35(6):519–22.
123. Schiotz HA. Fibroepithelial polyp of the ureter. A case history and discussion. Acta Obstet Gynecol Scand. 1990;69(3):267–8.
124. Zisman A, Tieder M, Alon H, Eidelman A. Benign fibroepithelial polyps of the ureter and renal pelvis in childhood. Two case reports. Scand J Urol Nephrol. 1994;28(2):191–3.
125. Childs MA, Umbreit EC, Krambeck AE, Sebo TJ, Patterson DE, Gettman MT. Fibroepithelial polyps of the ureter: a single-institutional experience. J Endourol. 2009;23(9):1415–19.
126. Coloma del Peso A, Bocardo Fajardo G, Teba del Pino F, Fernandez Gonzalez I, Brime Menendez R, Fernandez Borrell A, et al. Endoscopic treatment of

a giant fibroepithelial polyp of the ureter. Arch Esp Urol. 2010;63(4):305–8.
127. Sun Y, Xu C, Wen X, Ren S, Ye H, Gao X. Is endoscopic management suitable for long ureteral fibroepithelial polyps? J Endourol. 2008;22(7):1459–62.
128. Baltogiannis D, Kafetsoulis A, Giannakis D, Saito M, Miyagawa I, Sofikitis N. Fibroepithelial polyp of distal ureter with periodic prolapse into bladder. Urol Int. 2008;80(3):338–40.
129. Kumar A, Das SK, Trivedi S, Dwivedi US, Singh PB. Genito-urinary polyps: summary of the 10-year experiences of a single institute. Int Urol Nephrol. 2008;40(4):901–7.
130. Carey RI, Bird VG. Endoscopic management of 10 separate fibroepithelial polyps arising in a single ureter. Urology. 2006;67(2):413–15.
131. Lam JS, Bingham JB, Gupta M. Endoscopic treatment of fibroepithelial polyps of the renal pelvis and ureter. Urology. 2003;62(5):810–13.
132. Yagi S, Kawano Y, Gotanda T, Kitagawa T, Kawahara M, Nakagawa M, et al. Endoscopic treatment of a long fibroepithelial ureteral polyp. Int J Urol. 2001;8(8):467–9.
133. Faerber GJ, Ahmed MM, Marcovich R, Crisco CP, Belville WD. Contemporary diagnosis and treatment of fibroepithelial ureteral polyp. J Endourol. 1997;11(5):349–51.
134. Kim H, Kim DK, Lee SJ, Chang SG. Fibroepithelial ureteral polyp–a case report; endoscopic removal of large ureteral polyp. J Korean Med Sci. 1996;11(1): 80–3.
135. Bolton D, Stoller ML, Irby 3rd P. Fibroepithelial ureteral polyps and urolithiasis. Urology. 1994;44(4):582–7.
136. Muslumanoglu AY, Karaman MI, Ergenekon E, Semercioz A, Sakiz D. A distal ureteral fibrous polyp and the role of ureteroscopic resection in its management. J Endourol. 1994;8(3):199–201.
137. Minevich E, Defoor W, Reddy P, Nishinaka K, Wacksman J, Sheldon C, et al. Ureteroscopy is safe and effective in prepubertal children. J Urol. 2005;174(1):276–9; discussion 9.
138. Shekarriz B, Upadhyay J, Fleming P, Gonzalez R, Barthold JS. Long-term outcome based on the initial surgical approach to ureterocele. J Urol. 1999;162(3 Pt 2):1072–6.
139. Pfister C, Ravasse P, Barret E, Petit T, Mitrofanoff P. The value of endoscopic treatment for ureteroceles during the neonatal period. J Urol. 1998;159(3): 1006–9.
140. Monfort G, Guys JM, Coquet M, Roth K, Louis C, Bocciardi A. Surgical management of duplex ureteroceles. J Pediatr Surg. 1992;27(5):634–8.
141. Stephens D. Caecoureterocele and concepts on the embryology and aetiology of ureteroceles. Aust N Z J Surg. 1971;40(3):239–48.
142. Churchill BM, Sheldon CA, McLorie GA. The ectopic ureterocele: a proposed practical classification based on renal unit jeopardy. J Pediatr Surg. 1992;27(4):497–500.
143. DeFoor W, Minevich E, Tackett L, Yasar U, Wacksman J, Sheldon C. Ectopic ureterocele: clinical application of classification based on renal unit jeopardy. J Urol. 2003;169(3):1092–4.
144. Chwalle R. The process of formation of cystic dilations of the vesical end of the ureter, and of diverticula at the ureteral ostium. Urol Cutan Rev. 1927;31:499.
145. Tokunaka S, Gotoh T, Koyanagi T, Tsuji I. Morphological study of the ureterocele: a possible clue to its embryogenesis as evidenced by a locally arrested myogenesis. J Urol. 1981;126(6): 726–9.
146. Tanagho EA. Embryologic basis for lower ureteral anomalies: a hypothesis. Urology. 1976;7(5):451–64.
147. Mendelsohn C. Using mouse models to understand normal and abnormal urogenital tract development. Organogenesis. 2009;5(1):306–14.
148. Scherz HC, Kaplan GW, Packer MG, Brock WA. Ectopic ureteroceles: surgical management with preservation of continence–review of 60 cases. J Urol. 1989;142(2 Pt 2):538–41; discussion 42–3.
149. Brock WA, Kaplan GW. Ectopic ureteroceles in children. J Urol. 1978;119(6):800–3.
150. Coplen DE, Duckett JW. The modern approach to ureteroceles. J Urol. 1995;153(1):166–71.
151. Sumfest JM, Burns MW, Mitchell ME. Pseudoureterocele: potential for misdiagnosis of an ectopic ureter as a ureterocele. Br J Urol. 1995;75(3):401–5.
152. Mitty HA, Schapira HE. Ureterocele and pseudoureterocele: cobra versus cancer. J Urol. 1977;117(5): 557–61.
153. Vinson RK, Silver TM, Thornbury JR. Pseudoureterocele: a uroradiologic entity. Urology. 1977;10(5):482–5.
154. Diard F, Chateil JF, Bondonny JM, Nicolau A, de Lambilly C. [Pseudo-ureteroceles resulting from the impression of a loop of a megaureter with an ectopic subvesical orifice]. J Radiol. 1987;68(3):177–84.
155. Bauer SB, Retik AB. The non-obstructive ectopic ureterocele. J Urol. 1978;119(6):804–7.
156. Share JC, Lebowitz RL. Ectopic ureterocele without ureteral and calyceal dilatation (ureterocele disproportion): findings on urography and sonography. AJR Am J Roentgenol. 1989;152(3):567–71.
157. Caire JT, Ramus RM, Magee KP, Fullington BK, Ewalt DH, Twickler DM. MRI of fetal genitourinary anomalies. AJR Am J Roentgenol. 2003;181(5): 1381–5.
158. Kajbafzadeh AM, Payabvash S, Sadeghi Z, Elmi A, Jamal A, Hantoshzadeh Z, et al. Comparison of magnetic resonance urography with ultrasound studies in detection of fetal urogenital anomalies. J Pediatr Urol. 2008;4(1):32–9.
159. Payabvash S, Kajbafzadeh AM, Saeedi P, Sadeghi Z, Elmi A, Mehdizadeh M. Application of magnetic resonance urography in diagnosis of congenital urogenital anomalies in children. Pediatr Surg Int. 2008;24(9):979–86.

160. Husmann DA, Ewalt DH, Glenski WJ, Bernier PA. Ureterocele associated with ureteral duplication and a nonfunctioning upper pole segment: management by partial nephroureterectomy alone. J Urol. 1995;154(2 Pt 2):723–6.
161. Tank ES. Experience with endoscopic incision and open unroofing of ureteroceles. J Urol. 1986;136 (1 Pt 2):241–2.
162. Wines RD, O'Flynn JD. Transurethral treatment of ureteroceles. A report on 45 cases mostly treated by transurethral resection. Br J Urol. 1972;44(2):207–16.
163. Byun E, Merguerian PA. A meta-analysis of surgical practice patterns in the endoscopic management of ureteroceles. J Urol. 2006;176(4 Pt 2):1871–7; discussion 7.
164. Upadhyay J, Bolduc S, Braga L, Farhat W, Bagli DJ, McLorie GA, et al. Impact of prenatal diagnosis on the morbidity associated with ureterocele management. J Urol. 2002;167(6):2560–5.
165. Arena F, Nicotina A, Cruccetti A, Centonze A, Arena S, Romeo G. Can histologic changes of the upper pole justify a conservative approach in neonatal duplex ectopic ureterocele? Pediatr Surg Int. 2002;18(8):681–4.
166. Mandell J, Colodny AH, Lebowitz R, Bauer SB, Retik AB. Ureteroceles in infants and children. J Urol. 1980;123(6):921–6.
167. Caldamone AA, Snyder 3rd HM, Duckett JW. Ureteroceles in children: followup of management with upper tract approach. J Urol. 1984;131(6):1130–2.
168. Shankar KR, Vishwanath N, Rickwood AM. Outcome of patients with prenatally detected duplex system ureterocele; natural history of those managed expectantly. J Urol. 2001;165(4):1226–8.
169. Coplen DE, Austin PF. Outcome analysis of prenatally detected ureteroceles associated with multicystic dysplasia. J Urol. 2004;172(4 Pt 2):1637–9; discussion 9.
170. Han MY, Gibbons MD, Belman AB, Pohl HG, Majd M, Rushton HG. Indications for nonoperative management of ureteroceles. J Urol. 2005;174(4 Pt 2):1652–5; discussion 5–6.
171. Direnna T, Leonard MP. Watchful waiting for prenatally detected ureteroceles. J Urol. 2006;175(4): 1493–5; discussion 5.
172. Glassberg KI, Braren V, Duckett JW, Jacobs EC, King LR, Lebowitz RL, et al. Suggested terminology for duplex systems, ectopic ureters and ureteroceles. J Urol. 1984;132(6):1153–4.
173. Wyly JB, Lebowitz RL. Refluxing urethral ectopic ureters: recognition by the cyclic voiding cystourethrogram. AJR Am J Roentgenol. 1984;142(6):1263–7.
174. Gylys-Morin VM, Minevich E, Tackett LD, Reichard E, Wacksman J, Sheldon CA. Magnetic resonance imaging of the dysplastic renal moiety and ectopic ureter. J Urol. 2000;164(6):2034–9.
175. Krishnan A, Baskin LS. Identification of ectopic ureter in incontinent girl using magnetic resonance imaging. Urology. 2005;65(5):1002.
176. Ehammer T, Riccabona M, Maier E. High resolution MR for evaluation of lower urogenital tract malformations in infants and children: feasibility and preliminary experiences. Eur J Radiol. 2011;78(3): 388–93.
177. Joshi M, Parelkar S, Shah H, Sanghvi B, Agrawal A, Mishra P. Role of magnetic resonance urography in the diagnosis of single-system ureteral ectopia with congenital renal dysplasia: a tertiary care center experience in India. J Pediatr Surg. 2009;44(10): 1984–7.
178. Avni FE, Nicaise N, Hall M, Janssens F, Collier F, Matos C, et al. The role of MR imaging for the assessment of complicated duplex kidneys in children: preliminary report. Pediatr Radiol. 2001;31(4): 215–23.
179. Riccabona M, Simbrunner J, Ring E, Ruppert-Kohlmayr A, Ebner F, Fotter R. Feasibility of MR urography in neonates and infants with anomalies of the upper urinary tract. Eur Radiol. 2002;12(6):1442–50.
180. Staatz G, Rohrmann D, Nolte-Ernsting CC, Stollbrink C, Haage P, Schmidt T, et al. Magnetic resonance urography in children: evaluation of suspected ureteral ectopia in duplex systems. J Urol. 2001;166(6):2346–50.
181. Kibar Y, Avci A, Akay O, Dayanc M. Dribbling of urine due to ectopic vaginal insertion of an upper pole ureter diagnosed by magnetic resonance urography. Int Urol Nephrol. 2005;37(4):695–7.
182. Wille S, von Knobloch R, Klose KJ, Heidenreich A, Hofmann R. Magnetic resonance urography in pediatric urology. Scand J Urol Nephrol. 2003;37(1): 16–21.
183. Damry N, Hall M, Avni F. Ectopic vaginal insertion of a duplicated ureter: demonstration by magnetic resonance imaging (MRI). JBR-BTR. 2001;84(6):270.
184. Duong DT, Shortliffe LM. A case of ectopic dysplastic kidney and ectopic ureter diagnosed by MRI. Nat Clin Pract Urol. 2008;5(11):632–6.
185. Solinas A, De Giorgi F, Frongia M. Embolization of a hypoplastic kidney with a vaginal ectopic ureter in a case of pseudo-incontinence. Arch Ital Urol Androl. 2004;76(3):117–18.
186. Kudoh K, Kadota M, Nakayama Y, Imuta M, Yasuda T, Yamashita Y, et al. Transcatheter arterial embolization therapy for a hypoplastic pelvic kidney with a single vaginal ectopic ureter to control incontinence: the usefulness of three-dimensional CT angiography using multidetector-row helical CT. Cardiovasc Intervent Radiol. 2003;26(5):479–81.
187. Hellstrom M, Hjalmas K, Jacobsson B, Jodal U, Oden A. Normal ureteral diameter in infancy and childhood. Acta Radiol Diagn (Stockh). 1985;26(4):433–9.
188. King LR. Megaloureter: definition, diagnosis and management. J Urol. 1980;123(2):222–3.
189. Pfister RC, Hendren WH. Primary megaureter in children and adults. Clinical and pathophysiologic

features of 150 ureters. Urology. 1978;12(2): 160–76.
190. Wood BP, Ben-Ami T, Teele RL, Rabinowitz R. Ureterovesical obstruction and megaloureter: diagnosis by real-time US. Radiology. 1985;156(1):79–81.
191. Khoury AE, Bagli DJ. Reflux and megaureter. In: Campbell MF, Wein AJ, Kavoussi LR, editors. Campbell-Walsh urology. 9th ed. Philadelphia: W.B. Saunders; 2007.
192. Shokeir AA, Nijman RJ. Primary megaureter: current trends in diagnosis and treatment. BJU Int. 2000;86(7):861–8.
193. Hodges SJ, Werle D, McLorie G, Atala A. Megaureter. ScientificWorldJournal. 2010;10:603–12.
194. English PJ, Testa HJ, Lawson RS, Carroll RN, Edwards EC. Modified method of diuresis renography for the assessment of equivocal pelviureteric junction obstruction. Br J Urol. 1987;59(1):10–4.
195. Conway JJ, Maizels M. The "well tempered" diuretic renogram: a standard method to examine the asymptomatic neonate with hydronephrosis or hydroureteronephrosis. A report from combined meetings of The Society for Fetal Urology and members of The Pediatric Nuclear Medicine Council – The Society of Nuclear Medicine. J Nucl Med. 1992;33(11):2047–51.
196. Grattan-Smith JD, Jones RA. MR urography in children. Pediatr Radiol. 2006;36(11):1119–32; quiz 228–9.
197. Grattan-Smith JD, Perez-Bayfield MR, Jones RA, Little S, Broecker B, Smith EA, et al. MR imaging of kidneys: functional evaluation using F-15 perfusion imaging. Pediatr Radiol. 2003;33(5):293–304.
198. Kirsch AJ, Grattan-Smith JD, Molitierno Jr JA. The role of magnetic resonance imaging in pediatric urology. Curr Opin Urol. 2006;16(4):283–90.
199. Perez-Brayfield MR, Kirsch AJ, Jones RA, Grattan-Smith JD. A prospective study comparing ultrasound, nuclear scintigraphy and dynamic contrast enhanced magnetic resonance imaging in the evaluation of hydronephrosis. J Urol. 2003;170(4 Pt 1):1330–4.
200. Rodriguez LV, Spielman D, Herfkens RJ, Shortliffe LD. Magnetic resonance imaging for the evaluation of hydronephrosis, reflux and renal scarring in children. J Urol. 2001;166(3):1023–7.
201. McLellan DL, Retik AB, Bauer SB, Diamond DA, Atala A, Mandell J, et al. Rate and predictors of spontaneous resolution of prenatally diagnosed primary nonrefluxing megaureter. J Urol. 2002;168(5):2177–80; discussion 80.
202. Arena S, Magno C, Montalto AS, Russo T, Mami C, Baldari S, et al. Long-term follow-up of neonatally diagnosed primary megaureter: rate and predictors of spontaneous resolution. Scand J Urol Nephrol. 2012;46(3):201–7.
203. Baskin LS, Zderic SA, Snyder HM, Duckett JW. Primary dilated megaureter: long-term followup. J Urol. 1994;152(2 Pt 2):618–21.
204. Keating MA, Escala J, Snyder 3rd HM, Heyman S, Duckett JW. Changing concepts in management of primary obstructive megaureter. J Urol. 1989;142(2 Pt 2):636–40; discussion 67–8.
205. Liu HY, Dhillon HK, Yeung CK, Diamond DA, Duffy PG, Ransley PG. Clinical outcome and management of prenatally diagnosed primary megaureters. J Urol. 1994;152(2 Pt 2):614–17.
206. Elbadawi A. Anatomy and function of the ureteral sheath. J Urol. 1972;107(2):224–9.
207. Paquin Jr AJ. Ureterovesical anastomosis: the description and evaluation of a technique. J Urol. 1959;82:573–83.
208. Baker R, Maxted W, Maylath J, Shuman I. Relation of age, sex, and infection to reflux: data indicating high spontaneous cure rate in pediatric patients. J Urol. 1966;95(1):27–32.
209. Skoog SJ, Peters CA, Arant Jr BS, Copp HL, Elder JS, Hudson RG, et al. Pediatric Vesicoureteral Reflux Guidelines Panel summary report: clinical practice guidelines for screening siblings of children with vesicoureteral reflux and neonates/infants with prenatal hydronephrosis. J Urol. 2010;184(3): 1145–51.
210. Hollowell JG, Greenfield SP. Screening siblings for vesicoureteral reflux. J Urol. 2002;168(5):2138–41.
211. Noe HN. The long-term results of prospective sibling reflux screening. J Urol. 1992;148(5 Pt 2):1739–42.
212. Giannotti G, Menezes M, Hunziker M, Puri P. Sibling vesicoureteral reflux in twins. Pediatr Surg Int. 2011;27(5):513–15.
213. Riedmiller H, Androulakakis P, Beurton D, Kocvara R, Gerharz E. EAU guidelines on paediatric urology. Eur Urol. 2001;40(5):589–99.
214. Ferrer FA, McKenna PH, Hochman HI, Herndon A. Results of a vesicoureteral reflux practice pattern survey among American Academy of Pediatrics, Section on Pediatric Urology members. J Urol. 1998;160(3 Pt 2):1031–7.
215. Giel DW, Noe HN, Williams MA. Ultrasound screening of asymptomatic siblings of children with vesicoureteral reflux: a long-term followup study. J Urol. 2005;174(4 Pt 2):1602–4; discussion 4–5.
216. Darge K, Ghods S, Zieger B, Rohrschneider W, Troeger J. Reduction in voiding cystourethrographies after the introduction of contrast enhanced sonographic reflux diagnosis. Pediatr Radiol. 2001;31(11):790–5.
217. Novljan G, Levart TK, Kljucevsek D, Kenig A, Kenda RB. Ultrasound detection of vesicoureteral reflux in children. J Urol. 2010;184(1):319–24.
218. Zimbaro G, Ascenti G, Visalli C, Bottari A, Zimbaro F, Martino N, et al. Contrast-enhanced ultrasonography (voiding urosonography) of vesicoureteral reflux: state of the art. Radiol Med. 2007;112(8):1211–24.
219. Darge K. Voiding urosonography with US contrast agents for the diagnosis of vesicoureteric reflux in children. II. Comparison with radiological examina-

tions. Pediatr Radiol. 2008;38(1):54–63; quiz 126–7.
220. McCarville MB. Contrast-enhanced sonography in pediatrics. Pediatr Radiol. 2011;41 Suppl 1:S238–42.
221. Gelfand MJ, Koch BL, Elgazzar AH, Gylys-Morin VM, Gartside PS, Torgerson CL. Cyclic cystography: diagnostic yield in selected pediatric populations. Radiology. 1999;213(1):118–20.
222. Berrocal T, Gaya F, Arjonilla A. Vesicoureteral reflux: can the urethra be adequately assessed by using contrast-enhanced voiding US of the bladder? Radiology. 2005;234(1):235–41.
223. Riccabona M, Fotter R. Urinary tract infection in infants and children: an update with special regard to the changing role of reflux. Eur Radiol. 2004;14 Suppl 4:L78–88.
224. Duran C, Valera A, Alguersuari A, Ballesteros E, Riera L, Martin C, et al. Voiding urosonography: the study of the urethra is no longer a limitation of the technique. Pediatr Radiol. 2009;39(2):124–31.
225. Darge K. Voiding urosonography with US contrast agent for the diagnosis of vesicoureteric reflux in children: an update. Pediatr Radiol. 2010;40(6):956–62.
226. Hardy RD, Austin JC. DMSA renal scans and the top-down approach to urinary tract infection. Pediatr Infect Dis J. 2008;27(5):476–7.
227. Tseng MH, Lin WJ, Lo WT, Wang SR, Chu ML, Wang CC. Does a normal DMSA obviate the performance of voiding cystourethrography in evaluation of young children after their first urinary tract infection? J Pediatr. 2007;150(1):96–9.
228. Preda I, Jodal U, Sixt R, Stokland E, Hansson S. Normal dimercaptosuccinic acid scintigraphy makes voiding cystourethrography unnecessary after urinary tract infection. J Pediatr. 2007;151(6):581–4, 4 e1.
229. Herz D, Merguerian P, McQuiston L, Danielson C, Gheen M, Brenfleck L. 5-year prospective results of dimercapto-succinic acid imaging in children with febrile urinary tract infection: proof that the top-down approach works. J Urol. 2010;184 (4 Suppl):1703–9.
230. Sandy NS, Nguyen HT, Ziniel SI, Minnillo BJ, Penna FJ, Franceschi AM, et al. Assessment of parental satisfaction in children undergoing voiding cystourethrography without sedation. J Urol. 2011;185(2):658–62.
231. Routh JC, Grant FD, Kokorowski PJ, Nelson CP, Fahey FH, Treves ST, et al. Economic and radiation costs of initial imaging approaches after a child's first febrile urinary tract infection. Clin Pediatr (Phila). 2012;51(1):23–30.
232. Ziessman HA, Majd M. Importance of methodology on (99m)technetium dimercapto-succinic acid scintigraphic image quality: imaging pilot study for RIVUR (Randomized Intervention for Children With Vesicoureteral Reflux) multicenter investigation. J Urol. 2009;182(1):272–9.
233. Fouzas S, Krikelli E, Vassilakos P, Gkentzi D, Papanastasiou DA, Salakos C. DMSA scan for revealing vesicoureteral reflux in young children with urinary tract infection. Pediatrics. 2010;126(3):e513–19.
234. Mantadakis E, Vouloumanou EK, Georgantzi GG, Tsalkidis A, Chatzimichael A, Falagas ME. Acute Tc-99m DMSA scan for identifying dilating vesicoureteral reflux in children: a meta-analysis. Pediatrics. 2011;128(1):e169–79.
235. Pohl HG, Belman AB. The "top-down" approach to the evaluation of children with febrile urinary tract infection. Adv Urol. 2009:783409.
236. Hansson S, Dhamey M, Sigstrom O, Sixt R, Stokland E, Wennerstrom M, et al. Dimercapto-succinic acid scintigraphy instead of voiding cystourethrography for infants with urinary tract infection. J Urol. 2004;172(3):1071–3; discussion 3–4.
237. Craig JC, Simpson JM, Williams GJ, Lowe A, Reynolds GJ, McTaggart SJ, et al. Antibiotic prophylaxis and recurrent urinary tract infection in children. N Engl J Med. 2009;361(18):1748–59.
238. Williams G, Craig JC. Long-term antibiotics for preventing recurrent urinary tract infection in children. Cochrane Database Syst Rev. 2011;3: CD001534.
239. Brandstrom P, Esbjorner E, Herthelius M, Swerkersson S, Jodal U, Hansson S. The Swedish reflux trial in children: III. Urinary tract infection pattern. J Urol. 2010;184(1):286–91.
240. Roberts KB. Urinary tract infection: clinical practice guideline for the diagnosis and management of the initial UTI in febrile infants and children 2 to 24 months. Pediatrics. 2011;128(3):595–610.
241. Dave S, Lorenzo AJ, Khoury AE, Braga LH, Skeldon SJ, Suoub M, et al. Learning from the learning curve: factors associated with successful endoscopic correction of vesicoureteral reflux using dextranomer/hyaluronic acid copolymer. J Urol. 2008;180 (4 Suppl):1594–9; discussion 9–600.
242. Routh JC, Inman BA, Reinberg Y. Dextranomer/hyaluronic acid for pediatric vesicoureteral reflux: systematic review. Pediatrics. 2010;125(5): 1010–19.
243. Kirsch AJ, Perez-Brayfield M, Smith EA, Scherz HC. The modified sting procedure to correct vesicoureteral reflux: improved results with submucosal implantation within the intramural ureter. J Urol. 2004;171(6 Pt 1):2413–16.

15 Urethral Imaging

Martin Kathrins, Dana A. Weiss, Kavita Gupta, Douglas A. Canning, and Richard D. Bellah

Imaging of the pediatric and adolescent urethra is largely the purview of dynamic fluoroscopy. However, recent advances have led to the use of ultrasound and MR imaging in an attempt to reduce the traditionally invasive nature of urethral imaging.

Normal Anatomy (Fig. 15.1)

The male urethra is composed of an anterior segment and a posterior segment. The anterior urethra is distal to the urogenital diaphragm and includes the bulbar and pendulous (penile) urethra. The posterior urethra is composed of the membranous (sphincteric) and prostatic urethra. The one constant landmark in fluoroscopic imaging of the urethra is the verumontanum, which is seen as an indentation in the membranous urethra. On oblique urethrogram, narrowing of the urethra may be seen as it traverses the urogenital diaphragm. The most distal aspect of the penile urethra is the fossa navicularis (the histologic convergence of urothelium and distal squamous epithelium) which is visualized as a slightly narrowed segment just proximal to the meatus.

The female urethra extends from bladder neck to introitus. The striated sphincter complex encompasses the distal two-thirds of the urethra. Dynamic contraction of the complex leads to urethral narrowing and has been mistaken for meatal stenosis in the past. Reflux into the vagina is frequently seen after voiding on urethrograms.

M. Kathrins, MD
Division of Urology, Department of Urology, Children's Hospital of Philadelphia, Philadelphia, PA, USA

Division of Urology, Department of Surgery, University of Pennsylvania Health System, Philadelphia, PA, USA

D.A. Weiss, MD
Division of Urology, Department of Surgery, The Children's Hospital of Philadelphia, 34th Street and Civic Center Blvd, 3rd Floor – Wood Center, Philadelphia, PA 19104-4399, USA
e-mail: weissd1@email.chop.edu

K. Gupta, BA, MD
Division of Urology, Department of Surgery, The Children's Hospital of Philadelphia, 34th Street and Civic Center Blvd, 3rd Floor – Wood Center, Philadelphia, PA 19104-4399, USA
e-mail: kgupta77@gwmail.gwu.edu

D.A. Canning, MD (✉)
Division of Urology, Department of Surgery, The Children's Hospital of Philadelphia, 34th Street and Civic Center Blvd, 3rd Floor – Wood Center, Philadelphia, PA 19104-4399, USA

Division of Urology, Department of Surgery, Perelman School of Medicine, University of Pennsylvania, Philadelphia, PA, USA
e-mail: canning@email.chop.edu

R.D. Bellah, MD
Perelman School of Medicine, University of Pennsylvania, Philadelphia, PA, USA

Department of Radiology, The Children's Hospital of Philadelphia, 34th Street and Civic Center Blvd, Philadelphia, PA 19104, USA
e-mail: bellah@email.chop.edu

L.S. Palmer, J.S. Palmer (eds.), *Pediatric and Adolescent Urologic Imaging*, DOI 10.1007/978-1-4614-8654-1_15,

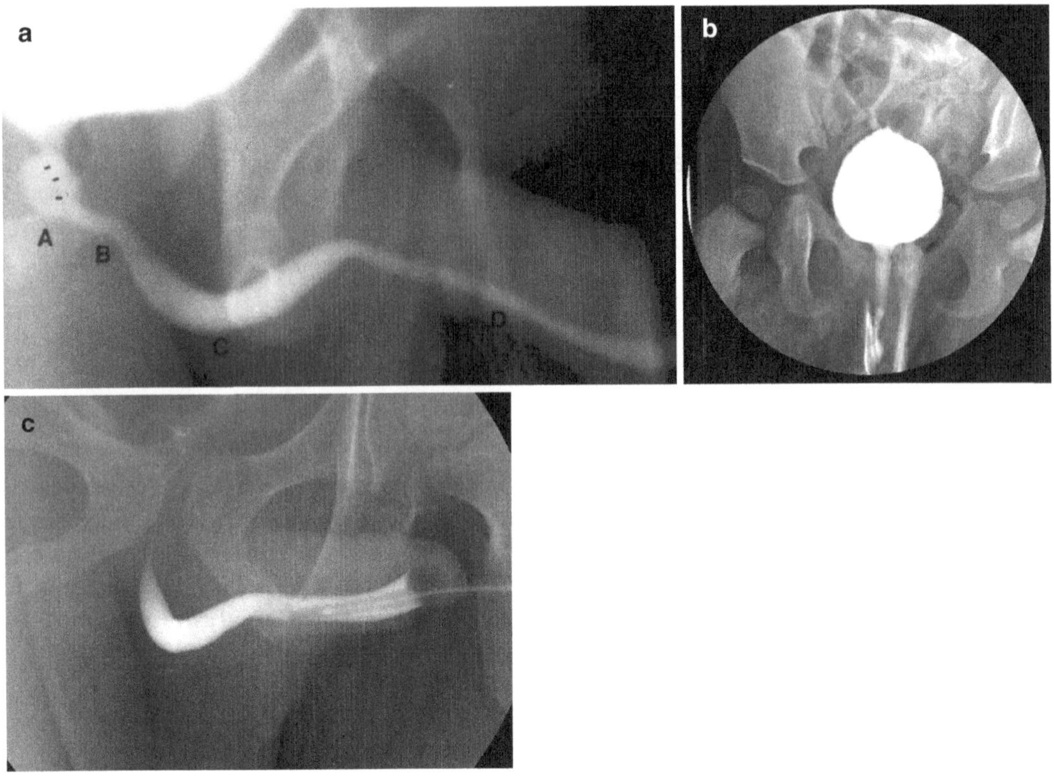

Fig. 15.1 (**a**) Normal male VCUG. *A* prostatic urethra; *B* membranous urethra; *C* pendulous urethra; *D* penile urethra. (**b**) Normal female urethra on VCUG. (**c**) Normal male RUG

Voiding Cystourethrogram

The voiding cystourethrogram (VCUG) is the most effective method to dynamically image the urethra. Clinicians also use the VCUG to evaluate the upper tracts in cases where vesicoureteral reflux exists. A "cyclic" VCUG where the bladder empties multiple times is helpful to identify vesicoureteral reflux (VUR) in duplicated systems. An anterior-posterior scout fluoroscopic image is first performed to evaluate for radiopaque stones and bony abnormalities, such as pelvic diastasis. It is our practice to use periprocedural antibiotics with gram-negative coverage and to obtain urinalysis and urine culture in select children prior to imaging.

An appropriately sized catheter is inserted into the bladder through the urethra or an indwelling suprapubic tube, without inflation of the catheter balloon. The bladder is drained and a urine culture obtained.

In males, the patient is placed supine with the penis laterally displaced for oblique images, while females remain supine for AP images. Iodinated contrast of an age and weight appropriate volume is instilled to opacify the bladder. Filling the bladder beyond predicted age and weight capacity may overestimate vesicoureteral reflux. The child then voids while monitoring with intermittent fluoroscopy. The voiding component evaluates the bladder neck for funneling and radiographic bladder emptying several minutes post-void. The appearance of the sphincter is monitored as the bladder neck begins to open at the initiation of voiding.

The VCUG provides essential imaging of the posterior urethra. Anterior-posterior images are obtained to evaluate the bladder and lateral/oblique images for the bladder neck and the urethra. Close communication between dedicated consistent radiology and urology staff is important for the best outcomes. Interobserver reliability may be poor, specifically when evaluating obstruction at the bladder neck and in the prostatic urethra in retrospective series [1].

Retrograde Urethrogram

The retrograde urethrogram—without voiding phase—is the preferred study to evaluate the anterior urethra, particularly in the male. For this study, a catheter is inserted into the fossa navicularis and the balloon partially inflated and placed on gentle traction to occlude the distal urethra. With the child in the lateral decubitus position, contrast is gently injected with slow steady pressure under fluoroscopy to overcome resistance of the external sphincter opacifying the posterior urethra as much as possible. In attempting to diagnose a suspected stricture to facilitate surgical planning, we try to opacify flanking aspects of the normal urethra by rotating the child or the fluoroscopy unit. To perform an adequate retrograde urethrogram in the shorter female urethra, a "double-balloon" catheter is sometimes used in adults to occlude both the meatus and bladder neck; this is not commonly used in children.

Newer Modalities

Magnetic resonance imaging (MRI) is used more commonly to image the upper urinary tract in children. Despite the use of triple-phased contrast-enhanced imaging (MR urogram) for functional imaging of the upper urinary tracts, a regular role for urethral imaging is yet to be identified.

Voiding enhanced urosonography is a newer imaging modality that reduces radiation exposure. This technique is under active investigation but has not yet been widely used [2]. Researchers have used it most often as an alternative to VCUG in children with suspected VUR. Nonlinear imaging techniques are used to differentiate anatomic structures from contrast-enhanced bubbles (galactose-palmitic acid) in this technique [3]. Transperineal imaging is used for males with a full bladder and normal micturition. Alternatively, the transpubic approach may be used to diagnose males with inability to control micturition and in females to better examine the bladder neck. Isolated reports describe the use of transpubic ultrasound to identify posterior urethral valves in two patients, and a dilated prostatic utricle and anterior urethral diverticulum were also diagnosed in two patients [4]. In a prospective comparison of VCUG and contrast-enhanced ultrasonography in patients with suspected urethral pathology, ultrasonography accurately diagnosed posterior urethral valves, anterior valves, urethral stenosis, and detrusor sphincter dyssynergia in all. Two patients with syringocele were not identified with ultrasound but were diagnosed with VCUG [5].

While ultrasonography is useful for studying stricture length and depth in adults with anterior urethral strictures, we use it less in children. One study examined differences in echogenicity, luminal narrowing, and changes in periurethral tissue in non-contrast-enhanced ultrasound to diagnose anterior urethral stricture. The authors estimated the degree of urethral distention to determine stricture length. According to the authors, the use of perioperative ultrasound led to a change in planned surgical approach in 58 % of patients [6]. However, VCUG remains the study of choice for diagnosis of posterior urethral pathology.

Imaging of Acquired and Congenital Defects

Adequate imaging of the urethra is important for proper diagnosis of both acquired and congenital urological abnormalities. A wide range of congenital anomalies affects the urethra and requires urgent and repeated imaging. These include posterior urethral valves (PUV), prune belly syndrome, megalourethra, anterior urethral diverticula, anterior urethral valves, and urethral duplication. Acquired conditions may include trauma, strictures, diverticula, infections, urethrorrhagia, and sources of obstruction such as polyps or stones.

Congenital Urethral Anomalies

Congenital Urethral Polyps

Congenital urethral polyps arise from the verumontanum. They may result in bladder outlet obstruction in boys. Boys may complain of discomfort and straining to void. The diagnosis is usually made by VCUG, but polyps may be seen on ultrasound as well. The diagnosis is confirmed and the polyp is managed with cystoscopy and transurethral resection [7].

Posterior Urethral Valves (Fig. 15.2)

PUV are the most common congenital cause of bladder outlet obstruction in children. A defect in the developing Wolffian duct folds is thought to be causative, and the valves become obstructive at variable times after the 8th week of development [8]. PUV are often diagnosed before birth—with ultrasound, with as many as 45 % of cases identified in utero [9]. Findings include a distended bladder often with bilateral hydronephrosis and a variable finding of oligohydramnios, depending on the severity of the obstruction and degree of renal injury. Postnatal renal bladder ultrasound (RBUS) and VCUG confirm the diagnosis. The sensitivity of RBUS in detection of valves is 95 % [10]. Findings of RBUS include a dilated, thick walled bladder often with diverticula/cellules, dilated upper tracts, and a dilated posterior

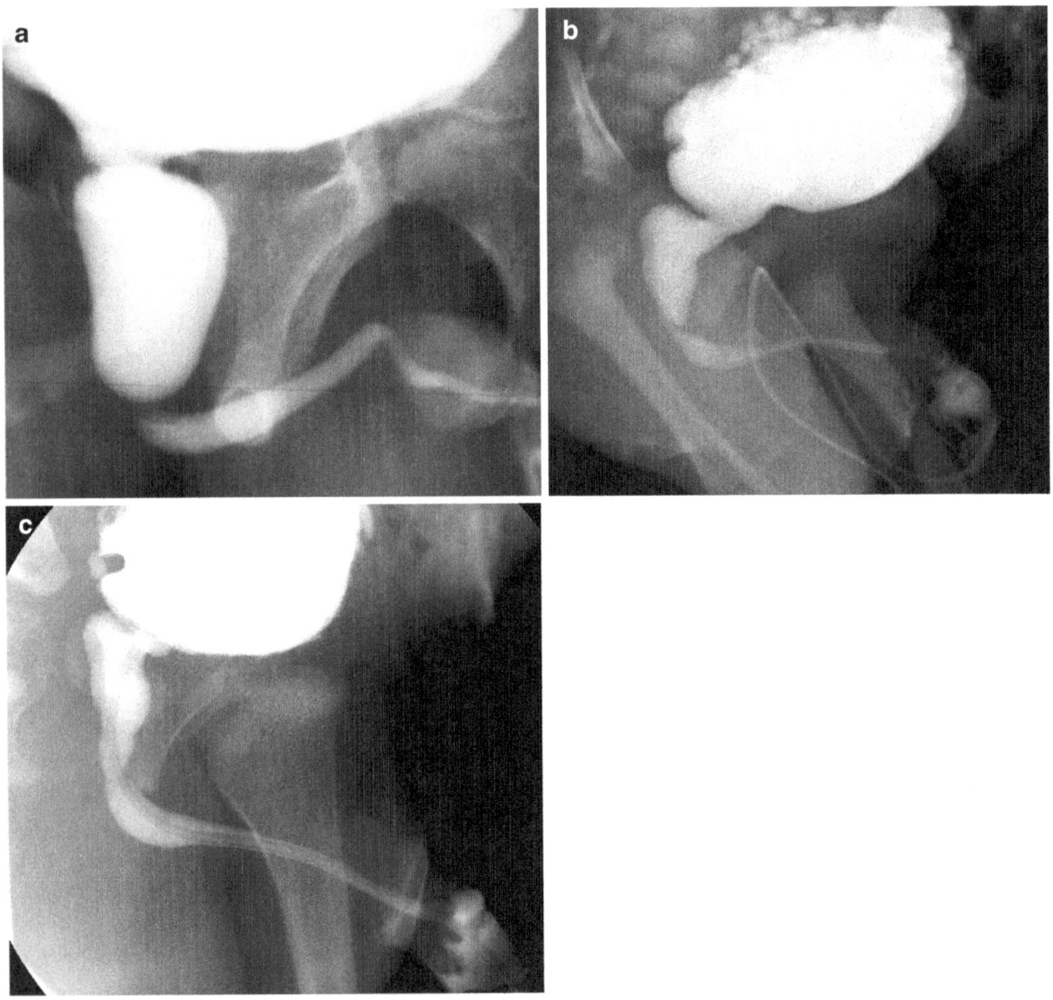

Fig. 15.2 Posterior urethral valves. (**a**) PUV showing dilated and elongated urethra. (**b**) PUV showing dilated and elongated urethra and multiple bladder diverticula. (**c**) PUV after valve ablation showing smooth transition across posterior urethra

urethra, the "key-hole" appearance. Urethral catheterization is the initial treatment prompted either by retention and/or ultrasound imaging.

VCUG/RUG is performed via urethral catheter or suprapubic tube, if present. The voiding phase is critical for differentiation from other forms of bladder outlet obstruction. While removal of the urethral catheter during the voiding phase is not always necessary, as it does not obscure the identification of the valves [11], our practice does remove the catheter unless contraindicated. Pathognomonic findings include the appearance of the valve which may be seen as an indentation on lateral imaging along with a dilated and elongated posterior urethra. Incomplete bladder emptying is also present. VUR is present in the majority of cases. After valve ablation, a follow-up imaging study is recommended in 4–6 weeks to assess decompression. If the degree of dilation of ureters and kidneys does not improved despite a decompressed bladder, a repeat VCUG could be performed to rule out residual obstruction.

Prune Belly Syndrome

Prune belly (Fig. 15.3) or triad syndrome (PBS) describes a triad of laxity of abdominal musculature, bilateral undescended testicles, and GU tract abnormalities, which include hydronephrosis, renal dysplasia, and urethral dilation. Variations of PBS may occur along a spectrum of these three clinical characteristics—so-called pseudo-prune belly syndrome [12]. Urethral dilation in PBS may arise from one of three etiologies. The first, urethral obstruction, occurs early in gestation and is believed to occur in 20 % of cases, from urethral atresia, urethral valves, or urethral diverticulum. Alternatively, the urethral dilation may be related to a functional abnormality of bladder emptying without obstruction. In the absence of an obstructive lesion, the dilation may result from prostatic hypoplasia. VCUG in PBS shows tapering of the dilated posterior urethra to the membranous urethra. A prostatic utricle is often present [13, 14].

Congenital Anterior Urethral Obstruction

At least 260 reports have described cases of congenital anterior urethral obstruction, either congenital anterior urethral diverticula or anterior valves. Astute clinicians will suspect diverticula in boys with ventral penile swelling, post-void dribbling, dysuria, and recurrent urinary tract infection. When the diverticulum fills during voiding, it may progress to obstruction. Two forms of diverticula have been identified—saccular (Fig. 15.4) and globular. Diverticula are differentiated radiographically from congenital

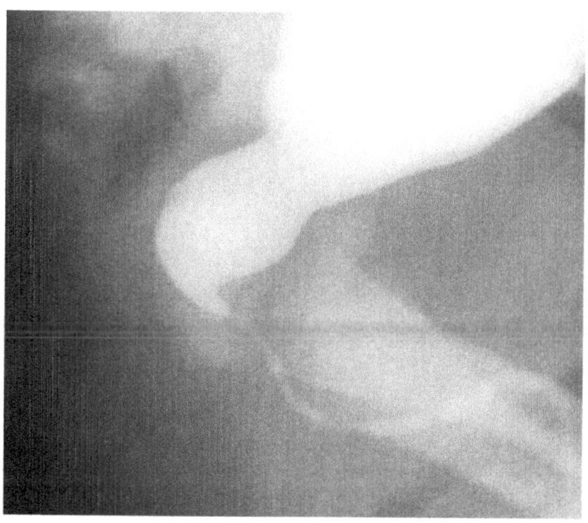

Fig. 15.3 Prune belly with wide open bladder neck, dilated but short posterior urethra

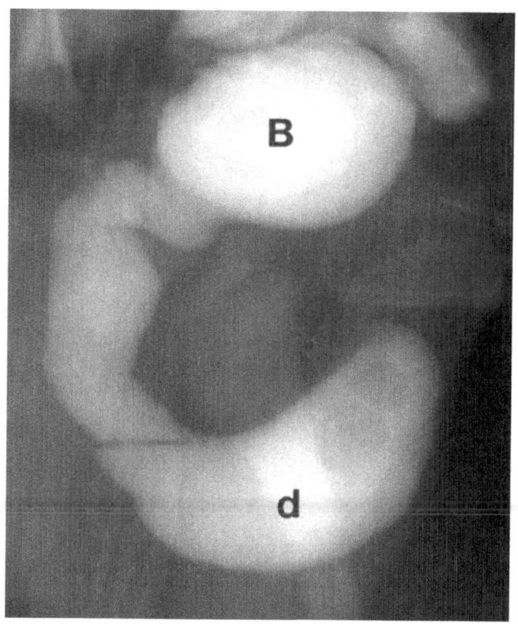

Fig. 15.4 Image from a VCUG of a boy with a saccular anterior urethral diverticulum. The bladder (*B*) is nearly empty, and contrast is seen in the posterior urethra and then filling the diverticulum (*D*)

anterior valves by the presence of an acute angle between the proximal parts of the dilated urethra, which is not present with valves [15]. Iatrogenic anterior urethral diverticula may also develop after hypospadias repair due to distal obstruction and after repair of anorectal malformation if the rectourethral fistula is not trimmed close to the urethra. Diagnosis is made by VCUG/RUG.

Anterior urethral valves are a rare, obstructing condition of unclear embryologic origin. The valves originate close to the penoscrotal junction or bulbar urethra. They arise from the ventral portion of the urethra and obstruct urine flow during voiding. Many believe that valves are part of the spectrum of congenital urethral diverticula. Indeed, valves may develop into diverticula secondary to outflow obstruction. However, pathologic findings indicate that congenital valves are always bordered by the corpus spongiosum and true congenital urethral diverticula develop outside the corpus spongiosum [16]. The gold-standard diagnostic study remains VCUG/RUG; however, contrast-enhanced ultrasonography has been used to make this diagnosis.

Urethral Duplication (Fig. 15.5)

Urethral duplication more commonly occurs in the sagittal axis rather than the coronal according the aggregate of case reports. The duplication develops from misalignment of the cloacal membrane, the genital tubercle, and the urogenital sinus. Dorsal duplication may occur with a single normal meatus, dorsal penile curvature, and a second epispadiac meatus. The dorsal urethra may communicate with the more normal, ventral urethra. Ventral duplicated urethra, which is less common is also known as "Y-type duplication," splits at the prostatic urethra. The duplicated ventral urethra may track to the rectum or perineum [17]. Urethral duplication is most easily diagnosed with VCUG/RUG. In some cases, additional retrograde urethrogram of a small, accessory urethra is necessary to fully image the aberrant duplicated urethra.

Cowper's Syringocele (Fig. 15.6)

Cowper's syringocele is a condition resulting from a rare, cystic dilation of Cowper's duct. The Cowper's glands are located in the deep perineal pouch within the urogenital diaphragm and are involved in secretion of pre-ejaculate fluid. Cowper's syringocele may be open to the urethra or closed. Either may present with pain. Closed syringocele may also present with obstructive voiding symptoms due to passive expansion and mass effect. Open syringocele may present with post-void dribbling, urethral discharge, and recurrent urinary tract infection. It may also obstruct

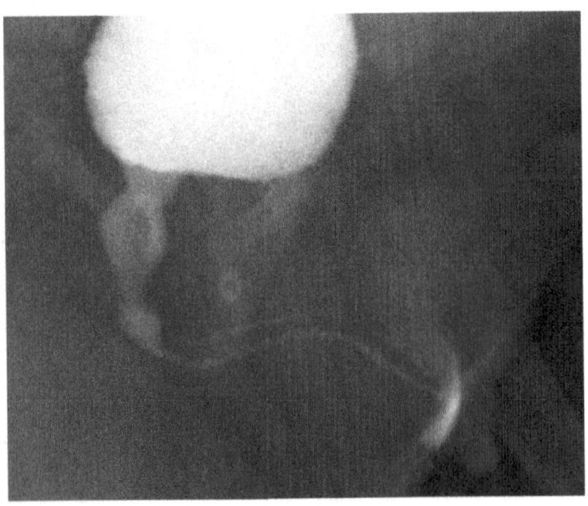

Fig. 15.5 Urethral duplication. The ventral urethra is of normal caliber while the dorsal one is narrow but does emanate from the bladder and terminate on the glans penis

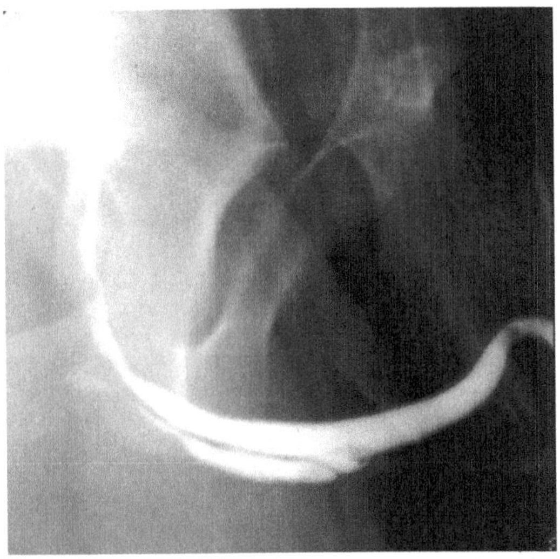

Fig. 15.6 Cowper's syringoceles. They are oblong contrast-filled spaces running parallel to the urethra starting from the bulbous urethra

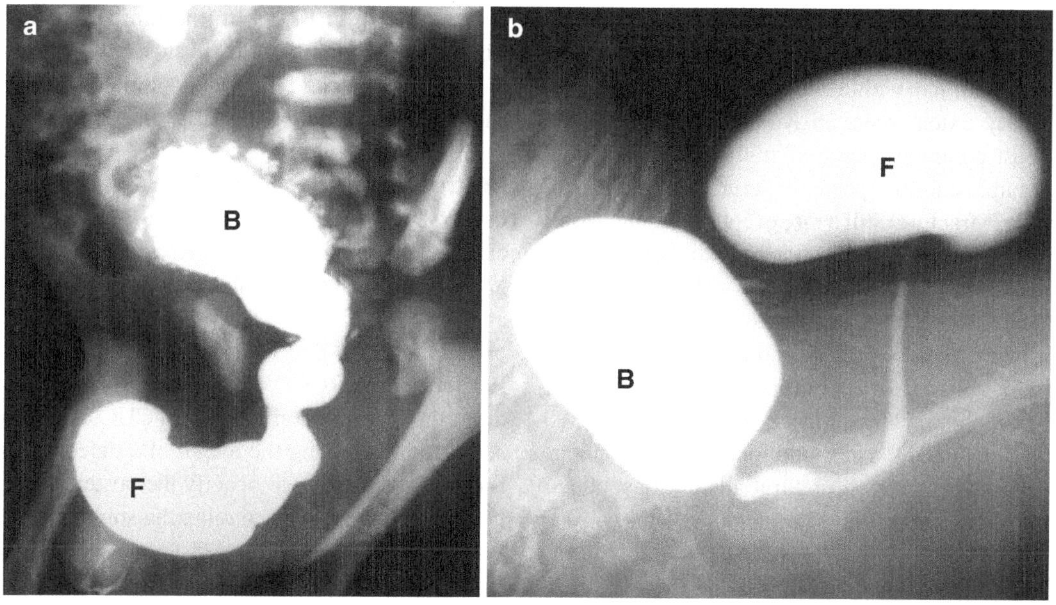

Fig. 15.7 Scaphoid (**a**) and fusiform (**b**) megalourethrae are seen demonstrating the billowing out of the urethra during voiding. The entire urethra is affected in the fusiform type while only a segment of the urethra is affected in the scaphoid type. *B* bladder; *F* megalourethra

urethral flow in some cases. Either transrectal or transperineal ultrasound may reveal a cystic structure (closed) or, in one case report, an open syringocele [18]. Retrograde urethrogram or VCUG will aid diagnosis. Cystoscopy with careful attention to the proximal bulbar urethra is diagnostic.

Congenital Megalourethra (Fig. 15.7)

Megalourethra is a congenital, non-obstructive dilation of the anterior urethra. It presents with an enlarged, deformed phallus with distention during voiding. It is more commonly seen in patients with PBS than in other syndromes. Two forms are recognized: fusiform and scaphoid. Fusiform megalourethra is secondary to a deficiency of the corpus cavernosum. On VCUG, the entire urethra dilates with voiding. Scaphoid megalourethra is caused by a deficiency of the corpus spongiosum. Only the ventral urethra dilates with voiding in these cases. Catheterization of these patients may be difficult and may require urethroscopy.

Urethral Fistula

Urethral-enteric fistulae may develop secondary to congenital anorectal malformations. Eighty percent of boys with anorectal malformations have uro-enteric fistula, most often associated with imperforate anus. An initial VCUG/RUG as a screening test is diagnostic [19]. Alternatively, MR imaging in the initial evaluation may provide a noninvasive alternative [20]. However, diagnosis of the fistula is often made in the operating room during colostomy creation or distal colostogram performed prior to definitive pull-through procedure. Congenital urethral cutaneous fistula is extremely rare. They may be associated with penile curvature or hypospadias. We have seen at least two of these associated with anorectal anomalies. One case report cites a congenital urethro-perineal cutaneous fistula in a 12-year-old male [21]. The appearance of the VCUG/RUG appears similar to urethral duplication; however, the dorsal channel is invariably functional. Clinically, boys with congenital fistulae may present with recurrent UTI, pneumaturia, or perineal dribbling.

Urethral Trauma (Fig. 15.8)

Urethral trauma is far more common in males than in females but can be devastating in both.

Male urethral trauma has been divided into anterior and posterior disruption [22] and has been subclassified within these groups based on the injury extent seen on RUG. In pediatrics, the most common source of trauma is blunt pelvic trauma causing posterior urethral injury from pelvic fracture (still a rare event occurring in only 0.47–4.2 % of pelvic fractures and pelvic fractures have an incidence of only 2.4–4.6 %). Because the developing prostate is more prone to rupture than in adults and due to the relative intra-abdominal location of the bladder in children, blunt pelvic trauma poses an increased risk to the bladder neck and penopubic ligaments [23, 24]. Anterior urethral disruptions due to straddle injuries have an incidence of 0.6–10 % [25]. Radiologic grading of male urethral injuries varies by the location of injury.

In boys, the initial imaging in the trauma setting remains a RUG; however, caution is warranted because imaging that indicates a complete disruption does not rule out a partial tear [26] (Fig. 15.8). Opacification of a periurethral urinoma proximal to urethral defect may be mistaken for the lumen of the posterior urethra after a complete disruption injury. The use of several oblique angles during urethrography may avoid this misinterpretation. In girls, due to the limitations of a RUG in the shorter urethra, a cystoscopy and vaginoscopy is superior to any radiographic imaging and is indicated if clinical suspicion is present.

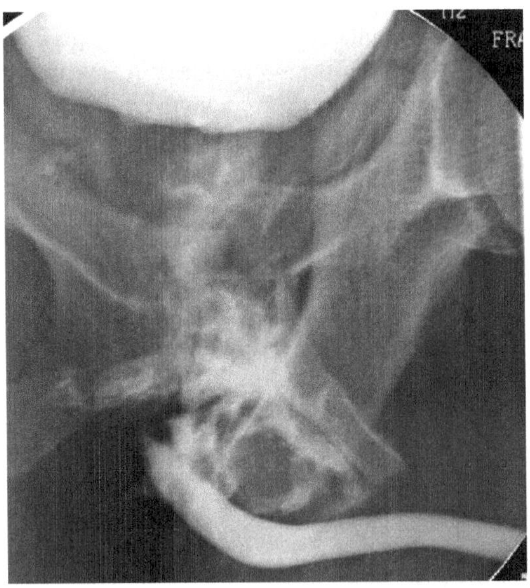

Fig. 15.8 RUG showing complete disruption of posterior urethra

Urethral Strictures (Fig. 15.9)

Urethral strictures may be due to infection (especially C. trachomatis in adolescent males and gonococcal urethritis, which can be seen at any age), iatrogenic injury such as instrumentation, or trauma [27]. The gold standard for imaging strictures is a RUG/VCUG. However, in children, the combination of RUG/VCUG is not as accurate in assessing the length of a defect. This is due to an inability to opacify the posterior urethra due to an inability to relax the sphincter [8]. A static cystogram performed via an indwelling suprapubic tube that shows opacification of the posterior urethra may indicate the presence of an incompetent bladder neck. Overestimation or underestimation of the defect may lead to a suboptimal surgical approach between the options of transpubic or perineal [9].

Sonourethrography, with sterile lubricating jelly instilled retrograde has become a common adjunct to RUG in order to guide treatment planning and help estimate length of stricture. While MR urethrography has been evaluated in adults for stricture disease, it has still not been widely accepted. In adults, comparisons have indicated equal or better accuracy compared with RUG, with improved anatomic detail of associated soft tissue injury provided [28, 29].

Postoperative strictures from hypospadias repairs are often evaluated functionally rather than by a specific appearance, so there are fewer data on the optimal imaging in this setting. At our institution, children are evaluated with noninvasive urine flow when they present with complaint of difficulty voiding. If there is diminished flow, we consider RUG and more commonly surgical exploration and reconstruction.

While rarer in young boys than adults, lichen sclerosis (LS) may contribute to stricture formation. LS causes genital scarring with possible voiding and sexual consequences [30]. The incidence is confused by a historical failure to identify and diagnose this condition. LS can lead to

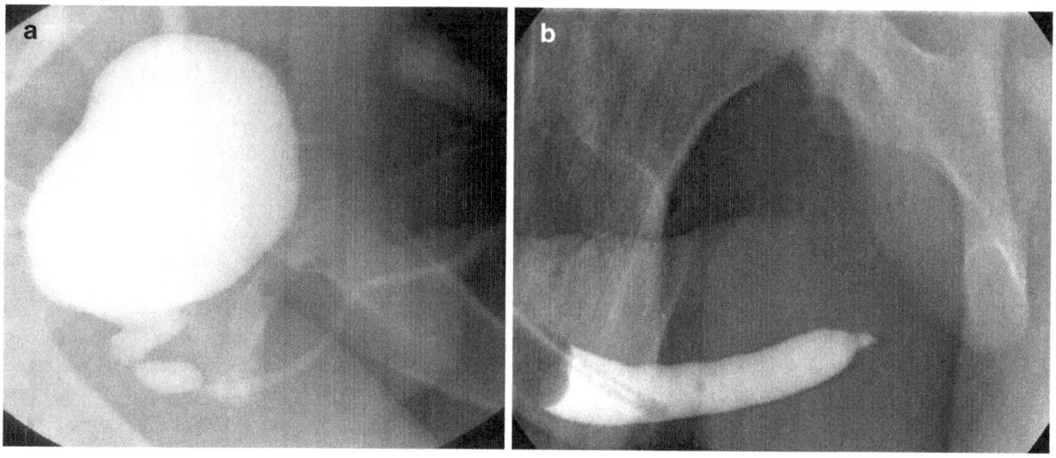

Fig. 15.9 (**a**) VCUG of bulbar urethral stricture. (**b**) RUG of urethral stricture

true stricture formation in 2–40 % of cases. LS may also develop after failed hypospadias repair with distal urethral obstruction and can progress to cause severe pan-urethral stricture disease. Notable findings include development of squamous metaplasia involving the ducts of periurethral glands that stiffen and open. RUG/VCUG is used to evaluate the urethra and may even demonstrate these open periurethral glands [31].

The myriad of pediatric urethral conditions may be effectively diagnosed with a RUG and VCUG. Newer technologies have at times been found to be equally effective but have yet to achieve the proliferation and practiced results of the traditional fluoroscopic urethrography. Facility with these techniques and their interpretation is essential for any pediatric urologist.

References

1. de Kort LM, Uiterwaal CS, Beek EJ, Jan Nievelstein RA, Klijn AJ, de Jong TP. Reliability of voiding cystourethrography to detect urethral obstruction in boys. Urology. 2004;63:967–71. discussion 971–962.
2. Renjen P, Bellah R, Hellinger JC, Darge K. Advances in uroradiologic imaging in children. Radiol Clin North Am. 2012;50:207–18.
3. Bosio M. Cystosonography with echocontrast: a new imaging modality to detect vesicoureteric reflux in children. Pediatr Radiol. 1998;28:250–5.
4. Duran C, Valera A, Alguersuari A, Ballesteros E, Riera L, Martin C, Puig J. Voiding urosonography: the study of the urethra is no longer a limitation of the technique. Pediatr Radiol. 2009;39:124–31.
5. Berrocal T, Rivas S, Jaureguizar E, Gomez-Leon N, Lobato R, Martinez-Urrutia MJ, Lopez-Pereira P. Contrast-enhanced sonourethrography versus conventional miction cystourethrography in the assessment of the urethra: preliminary study. Cir Pediatr. 2004;17:58–60.
6. Gong EM, Arellano CM, Chow JS, Lee RS. Sonourethrogram to manage adolescent anterior urethral stricture. J Urol. 2010;184:1699–702.
7. Jain P, Shah H, Parelkar SV, Borwankar SS. Posterior urethral polyps and review of literature. Indian J Urol. 2007;23:206–7.
8. Mitchell ME, Close CE. Early primary valve ablation for posterior urethral valves. Semin Pediatr Surg. 1996;5:66–71.
9. Dinneen MD, Dhillon HK, Ward HC, Duffy PG, Ransley PG. Antenatal diagnosis of posterior urethral valves. Br J Urol. 1993;72:364–9.
10. Williams CR, Perez LM, Joseph DB. Accuracy of renal-bladder ultrasonography as a screening method to suggest posterior urethral valves. J Urol. 2001;165: 2245–7.
11. Ditchfield MR, Grattan-Smith JD, de Campo JF, Hutson JM. Voiding cystourethrography in boys: does the presence of the catheter obscure the diagnosis of posterior urethral valves? AJR Am J Roentgenol. 1995;164:1233–5.
12. Bellah RD, States LJ, Duckett JW. Pseudoprune-Belly syndrome: imaging findings and clinical outcome. AJR Am J Roentgenol. 1996;167:1389–93.
13. Berrocal T, Lopez-Pereira P, Arjonilla A, Gutierrez J. Anomalies of the distal ureter, bladder, and urethra in children: embryologic, radiologic, and pathologic features. Radiographics. 2002;22:1139–64.
14. Reinberg Y, Chelimsky G, Gonzalez R. Urethral atresia and the prune belly syndrome. Report of 6 cases. Br J Urol. 1993;72:112–14.
15. Kadian YS, Rattan KN, Singh M, Kajal P. Congenital anterior urethral diverticulum in children: a case report and review. ISRN Surg. 2011;2011:120307.

16. Paulhac P, Fourcade L, Lesaux N, Alain JL, Colombeau P. Anterior urethral valves and diverticula. BJU Int. 2003;92:506–9.
17. Coleman RA, Winkle DC, Borzi PA. Urethral duplication: cases of ventral and dorsal complete duplication and review of the literature. J Pediatr Urol. 2010;6:188–91.
18. Melquist J, Sharma V, Sciullo D, McCaffrey H, Khan SA. Current diagnosis and management of syringocele: a review. Int Braz J Urol. 2010;36:3–9.
19. Hong AR, Acuna MF, Pena A, Chaves L, Rodriguez G. Urologic injuries associated with repair of anorectal malformations in male patients. J Pediatr Surg. 2002;37:339–44.
20. Le Bayon AG, Carpentier E, Boscq M, Lardy H, Sirinelli D. Imaging of anorectal malformations in the neonatal period. J Radiol. 2010;91:475–83.
21. Ghadimi-Mahani M, Dillman JR, Pai D, Park J, DiPietro M. MRI of congenital urethroperineal fistula. Pediatr Radiol. 2010;40 Suppl 1:S1–5.
22. Colapinto V, McCallum RW. Injury to the male posterior urethra in fractured pelvis: a new classification. J Urol. 1977;118:575–80.
23. Ranjan P, Ansari MS, Singh M, Chipde SS, Singh R, Kapoor R. Post-traumatic urethral strictures in children: what have we learned over the years? J Pediatr Urol. 2012;8:234–9.
24. Koraitim MM. Posttraumatic posterior urethral strictures in children: a 20-year experience. J Urol. 1997; 157:641–5.
25. Voelzke BB, Breyer BN, McAninch JW. Blunt pediatric anterior and posterior urethral trauma: 32-year experience and outcomes. J Pediatr Urol. 2012;8: 258–63.
26. Kotkin L, Koch MO. Impotence and incontinence after immediate realignment of posterior urethral trauma: result of injury or management? J Urol. 1996;155:1600–3.
27. Kawashima A, Sandler CM, Wasserman NF, LeRoy AJ, King Jr BF, Goldman SM. Imaging of urethral disease: a pictorial review. Radiographics. 2004;24 Suppl 1:S195–216.
28. Oh MM, Jin MH, Sung DJ, Yoon DK, Kim JJ, du Moon G. Magnetic resonance urethrography to assess obliterative posterior urethral stricture: comparison to conventional retrograde urethrography with voiding cystourethrography. J Urol. 2010;183:603–7.
29. Osman Y, El-Ghar MA, Mansour O, Refaie H, El-Diasty T. Magnetic resonance urethrography in comparison to retrograde urethrography in diagnosis of male urethral strictures: is it clinically relevant? Eur Urol. 2006;50:587–93. discussion 594.
30. Kulkarni S, Barbagli G, Kirpekar D, Mirri F, Lazzeri M. Lichen sclerosus of the male genitalia and urethra: surgical options and results in a multicenter international experience with 215 patients. Eur Urol. 2009;55:945–54.
31. Becker K. Lichen sclerosus in boys. Dtsch Arztebl Int. 2011;108:53–8.

16 Adrenal Gland Imaging

Jessica T. Casey, Earl Y. Cheng,
and James S. Donaldson

Abbreviations

ACTH	Adrenocorticotropic hormone
AIDS	Acquired immunodeficiency syndrome
CAH	Congenital adrenal hyperplasia
CT	Computed tomography
DOPA	Dihydroxyphenylalanine
EBV	Epstein-Barr virus
FDG	Fluorodeoxyglucose
HVA	Homovanillic acid
INSS	International Neuroblastoma Staging System
MDP	Methylene diphosphonate
MEN	Multiple endocrine neoplasia
MIBG	Metaiodobenzylguanidine
MR	Magnetic resonance imaging
17-OHP	17-hydroxyprogesterone
PET	Positron emission tomography
US	Ultrasonography
VIP	Vasoactive intestinal peptide
VMA	Vanillylmandelic acid

J.T. Casey, MS, MD
Department of Urology,
Northwestern University Feinberg School of Medicine,
303 E Chicago Avenue, Tarry 16-703,
Chicago, IL 60611, USA
e-mail: jtcasey@fsm.northwestern.edu

E.Y. Cheng, MD (✉)
Division of Urology, Ann and Robert H. Lurie
Children's Hospital of Chicago,
Northwestern University Feinberg
School of Medicine, 225 E Chicago Avenue,
Chicago, IL 60611, USA
e-mail: echeng@luriechildrens.org

J.S. Donaldson, MD
Radiology, Department of Medical Imaging,
Ann and Robert H. Lurie Children's Hospital of Chicago,
Northwestern University Feinberg School of Medicine,
225 E Chicago Avenue, Chicago, IL 60611, USA
e-mail: jdonaldson@luriechildrens.org

Normal Anatomy, Physiology, and Embryology

The adrenal glands are paired retroperitoneal organs consisting of an outer cortex derived from the intermediate mesoderm of the urogenital ridge and an inner medulla derived from neural crest cells [1]. The crescent-shaped left adrenal gland is located anteromedially to the superior pole of the left kidney and lateral to the aorta [1]. The triangular right adrenal gland is located on the superior pole of the right kidney slightly behind the inferior vena cava [1]. Three separate arteries supply the adrenal glands: superior adrenal artery (originates from the inferior phrenic artery), middle adrenal artery (originates from the aorta at the level of the celiac plexus), and inferior adrenal artery (originates from the main renal artery) [1]. One adrenal vein drains each adrenal gland: the right adrenal vein drains directly into the inferior vena cava, and the left adrenal vein drains into the left renal vein; however, variants in adrenal vein drainage have been described [1, 2].

The cortex of the adrenal gland is composed of three zones: the outermost zona glomerulosa

L.S. Palmer, J.S. Palmer (eds.), *Pediatric and Adolescent Urologic Imaging*,
DOI 10.1007/978-1-4614-8654-1_16, © Springer Science+Business Media New York 2014

which produces mineralocorticoids (primarily aldosterone), the middle zona fasciculata which produces glucocorticoids (such as cortisol), and the innermost zona reticularis which produces sex steroids (such as adrenal androgens and estrogens) [3]. Hormone synthesis from the adrenal cortex is controlled by the hypothalamic-pituitary-adrenal axis via corticotrophin-releasing hormone (from the hypothalamus) and adrenocorticotropic hormone (ACTH, from the pituitary) [3]. The adrenal medulla, which encompasses less than 10 % of adrenal mass, releases catecholamines (epinephrine, norepinephrine, and dopamine) as part of the autonomic nervous system [4].

At birth, the fetal adrenal gland is twice the weight of an adult adrenal gland and about one-third the size of the kidney due to the presence of the fetal adrenal cortex, which initially composes 80 % of the adrenal gland mass [3, 5]. The adrenal gland's large size at birth makes them easily visualized by ultrasonography (US) during the neonatal period [1, 3]. Atrophy of the fetal cortex begins after birth and is resorbed completely by 12 months of age [3, 6]. During this time, the zona glomerulosa and fasciculata of the adult adrenal cortex begin to develop; however, the zona reticularis does not completely differentiate until 3 years of age [7, 8].

General Concepts of Normal Adrenal Imaging

As early as the second trimester of pregnancy, the adrenal glands can be visualized by antenatal US. Given the relatively large size of the neonatal adrenal gland due to the presence of fetal adrenal cortex, US can easily visualize the adrenal glands during the neonatal period [1]. After the fetal cortex has involuted, US cannot reliably discern anatomic details of the adrenal glands. Thus, computed tomography (CT) and magnetic resonance imaging (MR) are best employed for imaging the adrenal glands in children and older infants [1].

On US, the normal appearance of the adrenal gland is two separate zones of echogenicity: a core consisting of a thin, central hyperechoic stripe (representing the central veins, the connective tissue, and the relatively small neonatal medulla) and a surrounding rim of thicker hypoechoic tissue (representing the fetal and peripheral adult adrenal cortex) (Fig. 16.1) [5]. In some neonates, the thin, central hyperechoic core is replaced by a broader band of echogenicity, likely representing congested sinusoids resulting from hemorrhagic necrosis of the involuting fetal adrenal cortex in addition to the neonatal medulla and central veins [5]. The surface of a normal neonatal adrenal gland is smooth to slightly

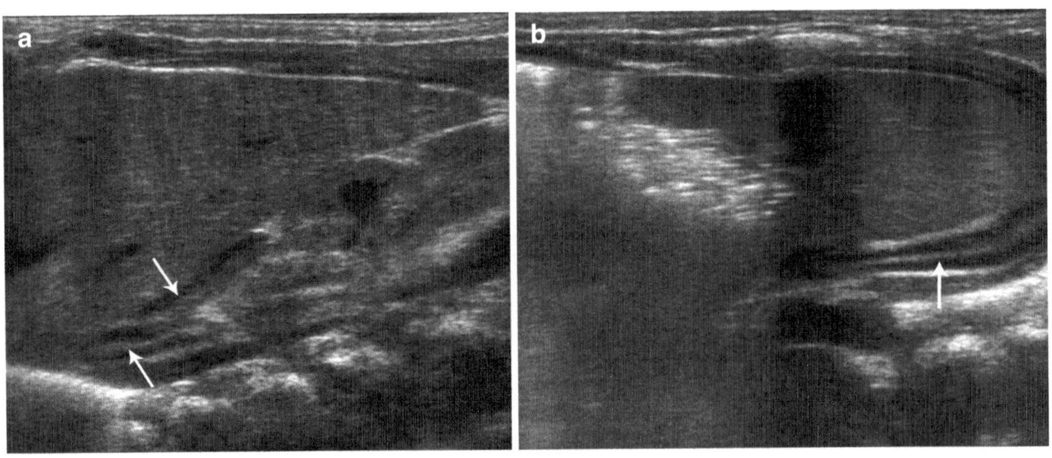

Fig. 16.1 Normal infant adrenal gland – US. Longitudinal ultrasound image of the right adrenal gland (**a**) and transverse ultrasound image of the left adrenal gland (**b**) in a 2-month-old girl illustrate the normal appearance (*arrows*) with hypoechoic adrenal cortex surrounding the central echogenic adrenal medulla creating an "Oreo cookie" appearance

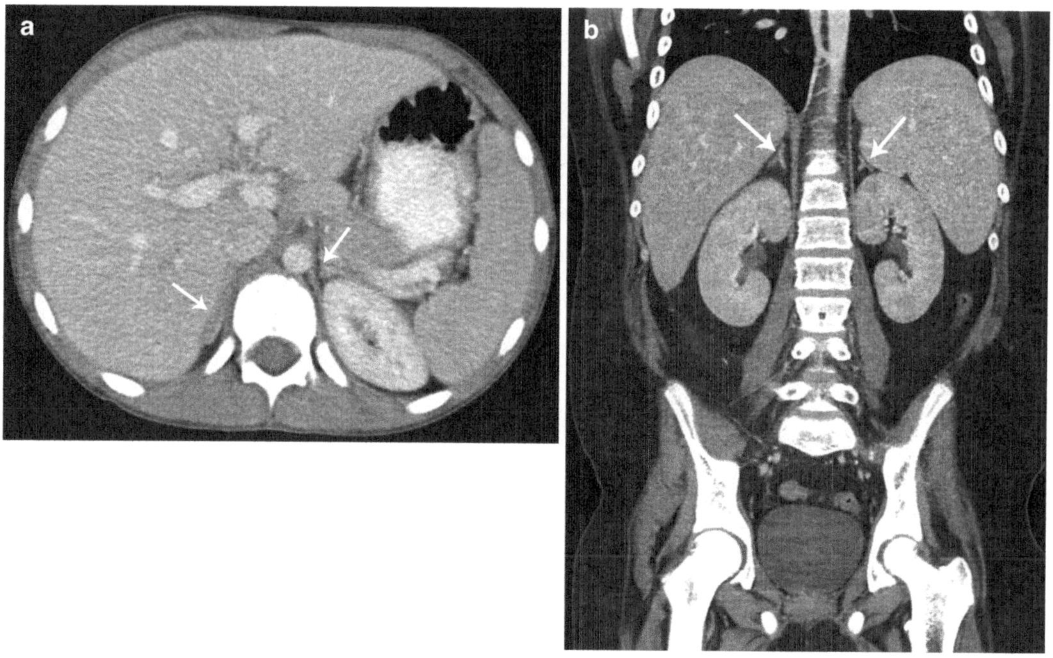

Fig. 16.2 Normal adrenal gland – CT. Axial contrast-enhanced CT image in a 12-year-old girl (**a**) and coronal contrast-enhanced CT image in a 14-year-old boy (**b**) show normal size and appearance of the adrenal glands (*arrows*) which are isodense to the liver

undulating, without nodular protuberances [3, 5]. In normal adrenal glands, limbs should be uniform in length, and their width should be less than 4 mm [5, 9]. The adult appearance of the adrenal gland is formed between 1 and 3 years of age, and they may be seen as very thin, linear, hypoechoic structures isoechoic to the liver [10].

The adrenal glands can be visualized anteromedial to the upper pole of the ipsilateral kidney at all ages on both CT and MR [1]. The right adrenal gland lies medial to the right lobe of the liver, lateral to the right crus of the diaphragm, and posterior to the inferior vena cava [1]. The left adrenal gland lies medial to the spleen, lateral to the aorta and left crus of the diaphragm, and posterior to the pancreatic tail and stomach [1]. To estimate normal adrenal size, the adrenal glands should be thinner than the adjacent diaphragmatic crura on axial images [1]. CT and MR can similarly demonstrate detailed information on adrenal anatomy; though, in determining the modality of choice, their respective risks and benefits should be considered (e.g., radiation exposure from CT and the risk of sedation during MR). On CT, the adrenal gland's soft tissue attenuation is similar to the liver (Fig. 16.2) [11]. For MR, on spin-echo T1-weighted images, adrenal glands have intermediate signal intensity (less than fat and similar to the liver); on T2-weighted and fat-suppressed images, adrenal glands are much brighter than fat and slightly brighter than the liver (Fig. 16.3) [11].

Anomalies of Shape and Position of the Adrenal Gland

As adrenal development and renal development are separate processes, adrenal glands will develop in their normal position within the retroperitoneum despite ipsilateral renal agenesis, malrotation, or ectopia [12]. However, in these cases, they are often flattened or discoid in shape, as well as slightly longer and thicker (referred to as a "straight adrenal gland") (Fig. 16.4) [5, 6, 11, 13]. This straight adrenal gland is not seen after nephrectomy or acquired renal atrophy [5].

Anomalies of the adrenal glands are exceedingly rare. The two most common fusion anomalies are

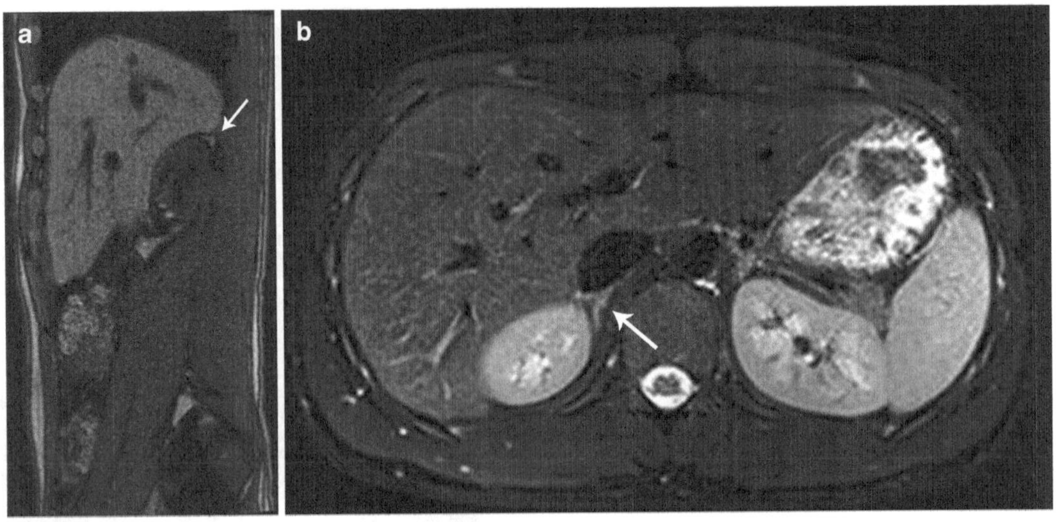

Fig. 16.3 Normal adrenal gland – MR. MR images in a 13-year-old boy reveal normal adrenal gland. On sagittal T1 images (**a**) the adrenal gland (*arrows*) is intermediate signal intensity similar to the liver. On axial T2 fat-suppressed images (**b**) the right adrenal gland (*arrow*) is intermediate signal intensity and brighter than the adjacent liver

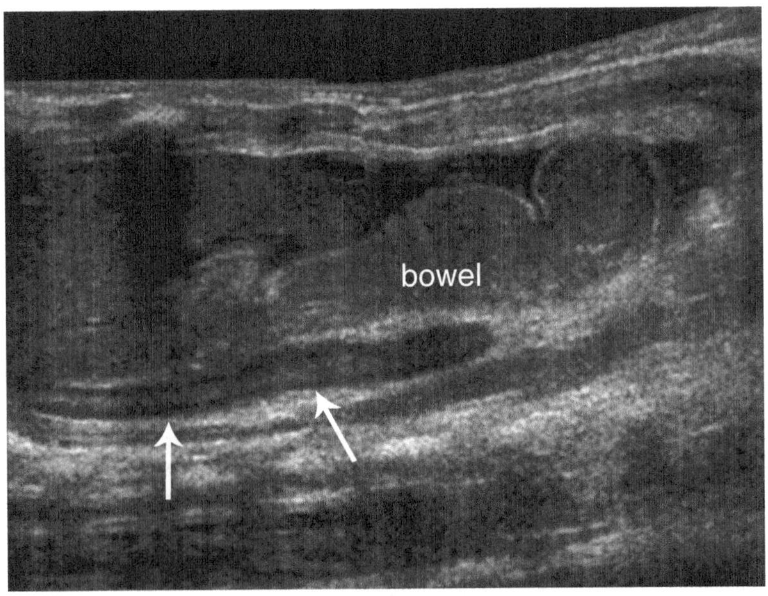

Fig. 16.4 Renal agenesis. Longitudinal ultrasound image of the left upper quadrant in a neonate with left renal agenesis. Bowel loops fill the left renal fossa with a straight, discoid left adrenal gland (*arrows*) seen

the circumrenal adrenal and the horseshoe adrenal [3, 14]. In the circumrenal adrenal, the fused limbs fuse around the upper pole of the ipsilateral kidney [3, 14]. Horseshoe adrenal describes fusion of the right and left adrenal glands in the midline anterior to the spine and posterior to the aorta [3, 14]. Horseshoe adrenals are often associated with renal anomalies (horseshoe kidney, renal agenesis), central nervous system anomalies such as neural tube defects, and asplenia with visceral heterotaxy [3, 14]. The isthmus of the horseshoe adrenal usually passes posterior to the aorta, but in association with asplenia the isthmus passes anterior [14].

Adrenal rests, or accessory adrenal glands, are mainly composed of cortical tissue, with the occasional presence of medullary tissue. They can be found anywhere along the path of gonadal descent in the retroperitoneum. Most commonly they are located near the celiac plexus, but can also be seen along the course of the gonadal veins and within the broad ligament, ovary, inguinal canal, testes, and epididymis [3]. Adrenal rests typically atrophy with time; therefore, although they can be found in up to 50 % of neonates, they are found in only 1 % of adults [7]. Males with congenital adrenal hyperplasia have a high prevalence of persistent adrenal rests in the testes [15].

Anomalies of Size of the Adrenal Gland

Congenital Adrenal Hyperplasia

Congenital adrenal hyperplasia (CAH) is collection of autosomal recessive disorders characterized by low cortisol production, potential aldosterone deficiency, and androgen excess due to an enzymatic defect in the cholesterol-steroid biosynthesis pathway [5]. Over 95 % of cases are due to a deficiency in the enzyme 21-hydroxylase [5]. Androgen excess leads to virilized genitalia in female infants and early virilization in male infants [11]. In the most severe form, concomitant aldosterone deficiency leads a salt-losing crisis in either sex during the newborn period [5]. Diagnosis can be made by a very high concentration of 17-hydroxyprogesterone (17-OHP) after three days of life [16].

Most neonates with CAH have enlargement of the adrenal glands with a width measurement of >4 mm and a length measurement of >20 mm [17]. Additional signs which may be seen on US include a cerebriform appearance of the surface of the adrenal gland and a stippled central adrenal echogenicity [18, 19]. In a series by Al-Alwan et al., US in the immediate neonatal period had a sensitivity of 92 % and a specificity of 100 % for the diagnosis of CAH and may be employed before conclusive 17-OHP levels are available [18]. Diagnosis of CAH can be made by the demonstration of two of three sonographic signs: (1) adrenal limb width of >4 mm, (2) cerebriform or crenated appearance of the surface of the adrenal gland, and (3) replacement of the central hyperechoic stripe with a diffusely stippled pattern of echogenicity or a diffuse thickened band of echogenicity (Fig. 16.5) [18].

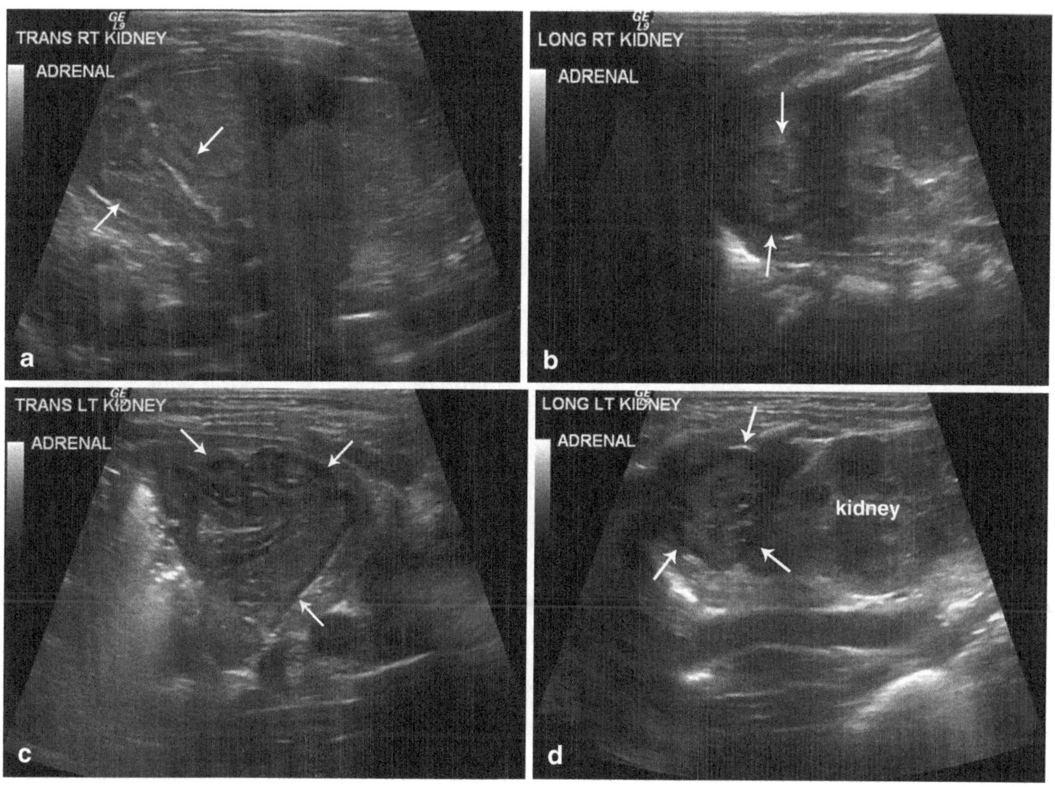

Fig. 16.5 Congenital adrenal hyperplasia. Retroperitoneal ultrasound images from both flanks (**a**–**d**) performed on a newborn girl with ambiguous genitalia due to congenital adrenal hyperplasia reveal enlarged adrenal glands with a cerebriform contour (*arrows*)

Case reports suggest that CAH due to deficiencies in 11β-hydroxylase or 3β-hydroxysteroid dehydrogenase leads to similar changes on adrenal US [20]. Lipoid adrenal hyperplasia is a rare form of CAH due to cholesterol desmolase deficiency, and adrenal glands appear enlarged with echogenicity or attenuation similar to fat due to accumulation of cholesterol and its esters [21].

Adrenal Hyperplasia

When adrenocortical hyperplasia presents in older children, it is classified as primary or secondary [1]. Primary adrenocortical hyperplasia results in either Cushing syndrome or, less commonly, primary hyperaldosteronism (Conn syndrome) [1]. Secondary adrenocortical hyperplasia is due to excess ACTH: either endogenous in those with Cushing disease or ectopic ACTH production or exogenous in those receiving ACTH administration (e.g., for infantile spasms) [1]. Clinical features of Cushing syndrome include central obesity, moon facies, buffalo hump, proximal muscle weakness, easy bruisability, abdominal striae, hypertension, dyslipidemia, insulin resistance, and elevated 24-h urinary cortisol and 17-hydroxycorticoids [22]. Clinical manifestations of Conn syndrome include muscle weakness, hypokalemia, and hypertension [23].

Adrenal glands are not normally visible by US in older children; therefore, if they are visible, the diagnosis of adrenal hyperplasia should be entertained [1]. CT and MR may be used to visualize the adrenals in older children with adrenal hyperplasia. Hyperplastic adrenal glands in these cases will be bilaterally, symmetrically, and evenly enlarged with increased relative enhancement [1]. Alternatively, in some cases of adrenal hyperplasia, adrenal glands may be normal in size, demonstrate uneven enlargement, or contain small nodular areas (Fig. 16.6) [1].

Cushing syndrome and Conn syndrome can also be associated with adrenal adenomas. Benign adrenal adenomas cannot be reliably distinguished from adrenal carcinomas based on histopathology, clinical features, or imaging [24]. However, in general, adrenal adenomas are smaller (<6 cm) compared to adrenal carcinoma and have less heterogeneity on US, CT, and MR. Adrenal carcinomas can have a similar appearance to adrenal adenomas, but tend to be larger and more complex [24]. The only definitive signs of malignancy are hematogenous metastases or venous spread [24].

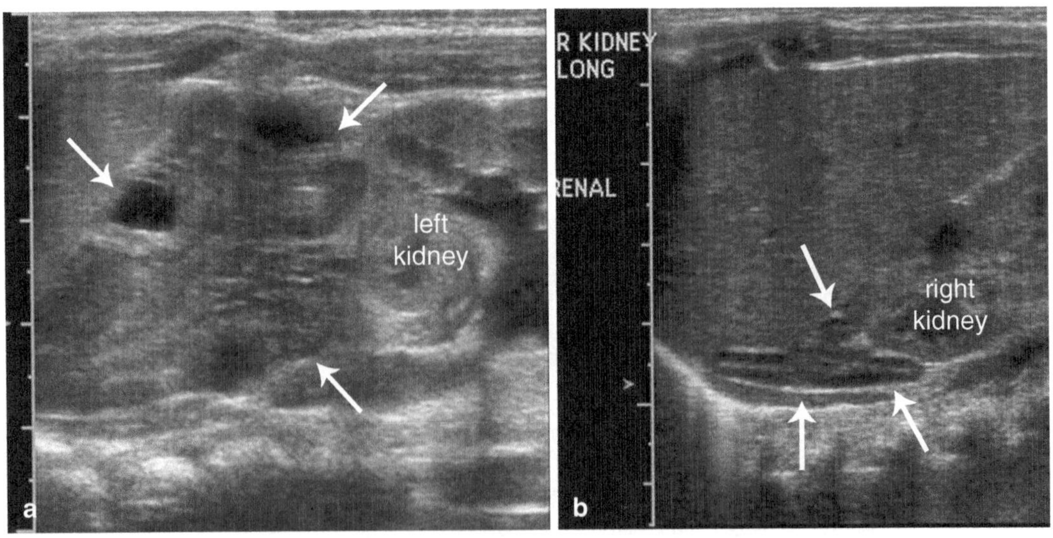

Fig. 16.6 Atypical congenital hyperplasia. US images from the left flank (**a**) reveal an enlarged adrenal gland with a cerebriform contour (*arrows*) and an anatomically normal-appearing adrenal gland from the right flank (**b**)

Primary pigmented nodular adrenocortical disease is a rare form of Cushing syndrome and is associated with Carney complex (Sertoli cell tumors of the testis, cardiac myxomas, soft tissue myxomas, and skin pigmentation) [25]. On imaging, the adrenal gland has multiple, <2 mm cortical-secreting adenomas with atrophic cortex between the nodules [25].

Wolman Disease

Wolman disease, a rare disorder, is an inherited deficiency of lysosomal acid lipase leading to the accumulation of cholesterol esters and triglycerides in many organs, especially in the adrenals [3]. Wolman disease presents in the first few weeks of life with hepatosplenomegaly with abdominal distension, jaundice, vomiting, diarrhea, steatorrhea, anemia, and growth failure and is rapidly progressive leading to death in the first year [3, 5]. On US, the adrenals appear markedly enlarged with calcifications appearing as a long, linear echogenic band with posterior acoustic shadowing [5]. On CT, the adrenals also appear enlarged with a cortical distribution of calcification [5]. Plain film will also demonstrate the densely calcified adrenal gland (Fig. 16.7) [5]. Imaging of adrenals in Wolman disease can look similar to resolving adrenal hemorrhage; however, in adrenal hemorrhage the adrenals are smaller and have globular calcifications [5, 26, 27].

Adrenal Masses

Adrenal masses in children and neonates may be attributable to hemorrhage, neoplasms, cysts, or abscesses [5]. The age and clinical presentation of the child, in conjunction with the imaging features of the mass, will allow one to develop an appropriate list of diagnostic considerations.

In the neonate with an adrenal mass lesion, the most likely entities include adrenal hemorrhage, neuroblastoma, and rarely extralobar pulmonary sequestration. In children less than 5 years of age, neural crest tumors including neuroblastoma and ganglioneuroblastoma are more likely than adrenal hemorrhage and adrenocortical neoplasms except when the child is exhibiting signs and symptoms of a hormonally active tumor. In older children and adolescents, adrenal masses may be related to neural crest tumors (more frequently the mature ganglioneuromas as opposed to neuroblastoma or ganglioneuroblastoma), as well as other tumors including pheochromocytomas and adrenocortical neoplasms. Other rarely seen adrenal masses in children include rhabdoid tumors, myelolipomas, and smooth muscle adrenal tumors [28].

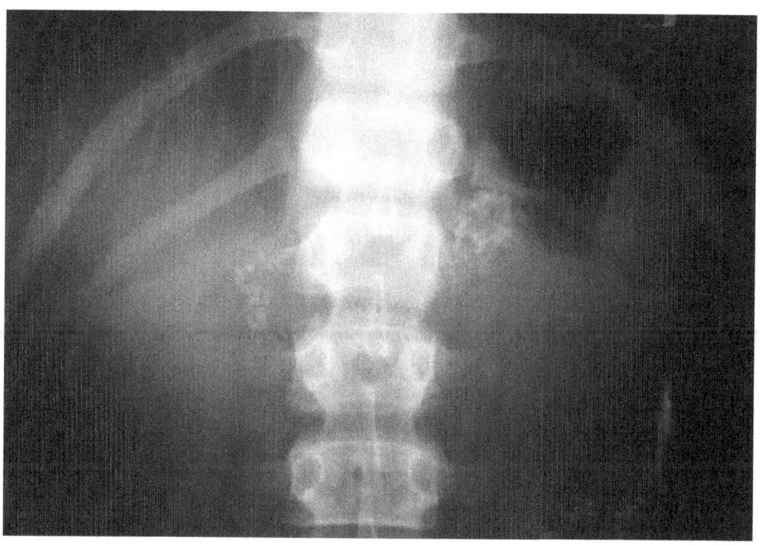

Fig. 16.7 Wolman disease. Abdominal radiograph in a 6-month-old boy reveals calcifications outlining the enlarged adrenal glands, findings typical of Wolman disease

Adrenal Hemorrhage

Adrenal hemorrhage in the perinatal period can occur in response to perinatal stress (such as difficult or traumatic delivery, hypoxia, or sepsis) or bleeding disorders [29]. Large babies such as those of diabetic mothers or with Beckwith-Wiedemann syndrome have a higher predisposition [30]. Associated clinical signs may include palpable flank mass, anemia, jaundice, or rarely hypovolemic shock. However, there is normally no associated adrenal insufficiency in the immediate phase or long-term as the major insult is to the regressing fetal cortex [5]. Beyond the neonatal period, adrenal hemorrhage is frequently seen in the setting of trauma but has also been documented to occur in older children with overwhelming sepsis (specifically *Neisseria meningitidis*), steroid therapy, anticoagulation therapy, and after liver transplantation [5, 11].

Adrenal hemorrhage more often occurs on the right (70 %), and in only 10 % of cases does it occur bilaterally [5]. Hemorrhage size can vary from as small as a few centimeters and up to several centimeters [5]. With conservative management, the natural course of adrenal hemorrhage is central liquefaction with resorption of blood leading to eventual decrease in size to the normal shape and a residual focus of calcification [5].

US is the modality of choice for initial imaging of adrenal masses in neonates as well as for follow-up assessment [31, 32]. On initial US, adrenal hemorrhages have a varied appearance depending on the duration of the hemorrhage. They usually have complex echogenicity with echogenic and echo-free areas but can also appear evenly echogenic, hypoechoic, or anechoic [5]. Smaller hemorrhages may be focal or retain the shape of the adrenal (triangular or crescent-shaped), and adjacent normal adrenal tissue can be identified. Larger adrenal hemorrhages are usually round in shape, and normal unaffected adrenal tissue can be hard to identify (Figs. 16.8a, b) [5]. Large hemorrhages may encompass the upper pole of the kidney (with the appearance of a perinephric hemorrhage) and may track down the retroperitoneum. Clinically, this can lead to scrotal swelling and hematoma, which may mimic testicular torsion [5, 33]. Occasionally, there may be associated ipsilateral renal vein thrombosis, especially on the left since the adrenal vein drains into the left renal vein [5]. To help differentiate adrenal hemorrhage (which is avascular) from neuroblastoma or other adrenal neoplasms, evaluation with color and spectral Doppler assessment should be performed (Fig. 16.8c). Additionally, ultrasound examination should include evaluation of the liver to assess for the presence of hepatic metastases and evaluation of the remainder of the abdomen and pelvis to look for metastatic lymphadenopathy, which can be seen in association with adrenal tumors.

Because of the varied imaging characteristics of adrenal hemorrhage in the acute phase, it may be difficult initially to distinguish from neuroblastoma [34, 35]. Thus, follow-up US imaging is of utmost importance in differentiating a resolving adrenal hemorrhage from a neuroblastoma. Masses due to adrenal hemorrhage decrease in size over several weeks as the hemorrhage liquefies and resorbs and become more hypoechoic or anechoic (Fig. 16.9) [36], whereas in contrast, the size of a neuroblastoma is unlikely to decrease. In cases where the diagnosis is uncertain, a short delay with serial US imaging is not harmful as neonatal neuroblastoma has a relatively good prognosis [11].

In some instances adrenal calcification may be incidentally seen on imaging (plain film, CT, MR) on older children. If the calcification is confined to adrenals of normal size and without evidence for a soft tissue mass, it is assumed to have resulted from previous adrenal hemorrhage in the neonatal period and is of no clinical significance (Fig. 16.10) [5].

In neonates with a suprarenal retroperitoneal mass, the possibility of an intra-abdominal extralobar pulmonary sequestration must also be considered in addition to adrenal hemorrhage and neuroblastoma [3]. Intra-abdominal extralobar pulmonary sequestrations occur more commonly on the left than the right, are usually hyperechoic, and can contain cysts related to coexistent congenital pulmonary airway malformation (Fig. 16.11) [28, 37]. As imaging with US, CT, and MR is rarely diagnostic, surgical diagnosis and treatment is often necessary [38].

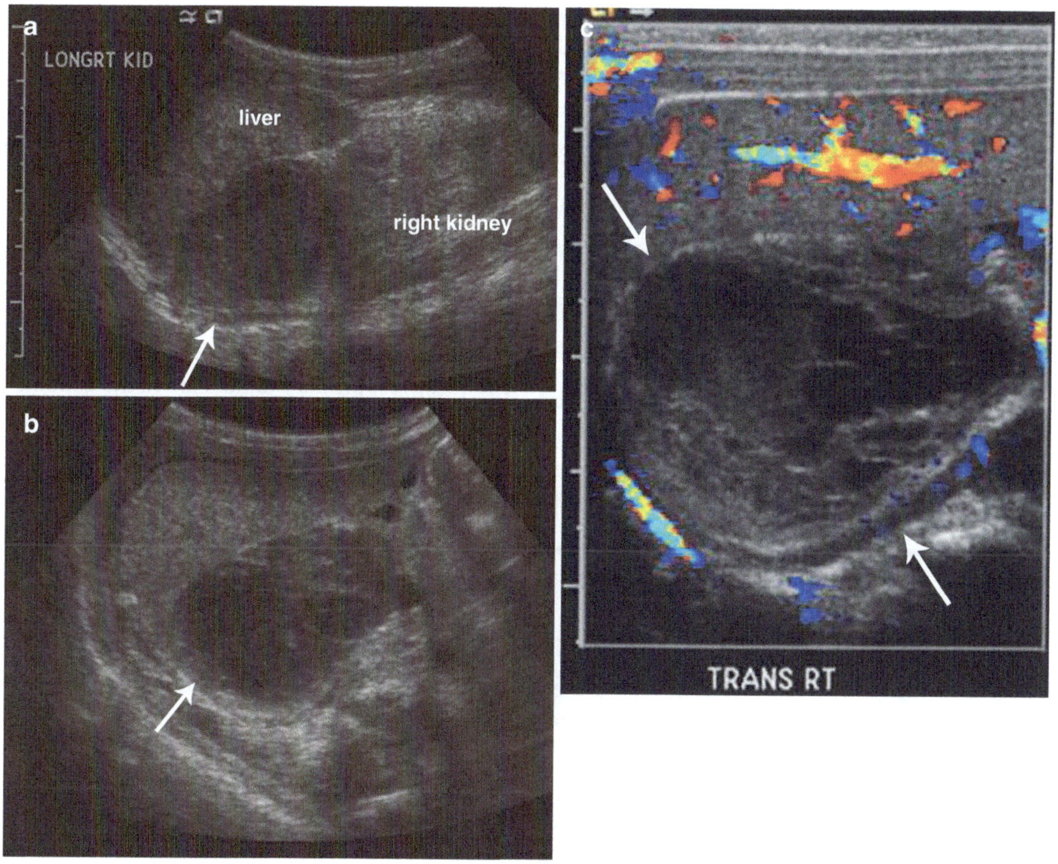

Fig. 16.8 Adrenal hemorrhage. Longitudinal (**a**) and transverse (**b**) ultrasound images in a 2-week-old boy with right adrenal hemorrhage reveal a rounded heterogeneously hypoechoic right adrenal mass (*arrow*). Color Doppler ultrasound image (**c**) shows that the right adrenal mass is avascular (*arrows*) and suggestive of an adrenal hemorrhage

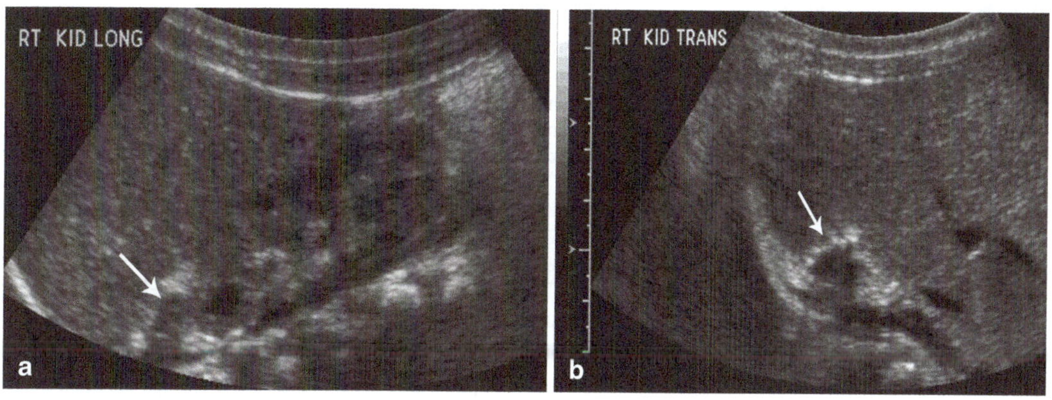

Fig. 16.9 Resolving adrenal hemorrhage. Follow-up longitudinal (**a**) and transverse (**b**) ultrasound images (obtained 2 weeks after the images shown in Fig. 16.8) reveal diminution in the size of the right adrenal gland (*arrows*) and increased peripheral echogenicity (likely early calcification) consistent with a resolving adrenal hemorrhage

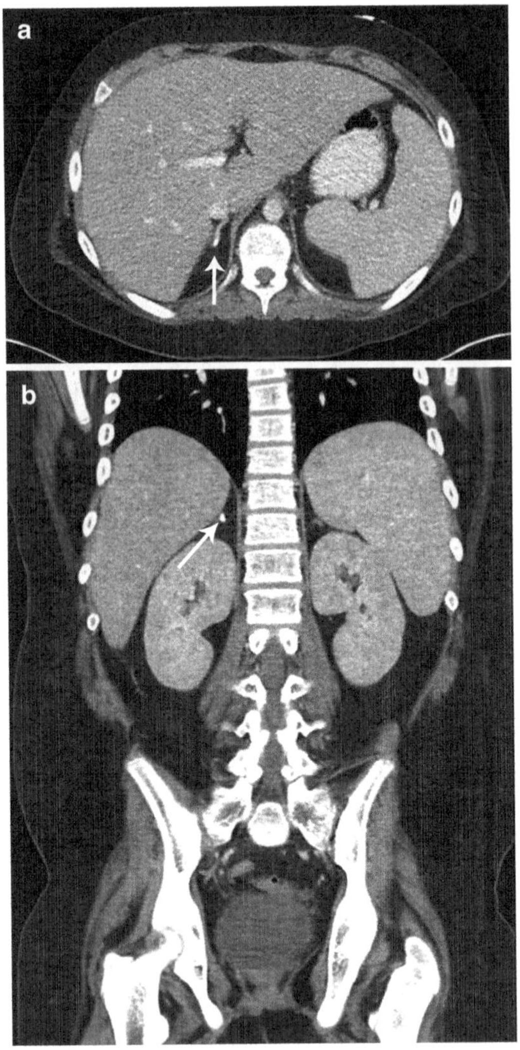

Fig. 16.10 Old adrenal hemorrhage. Axial (**a**) and coronal (**b**) contrast-enhanced CT images of the abdomen in a 10-year-old boy reveal a small focus of calcification in the right adrenal gland (*arrows*) with no associated soft tissue mass, presumed the sequela of prior adrenal hemorrhage

Medullary Neoplasms

Medullary adrenal neoplasms include the neuroblastoma, ganglioneuroblastoma, ganglioneuroma, and pheochromocytoma. These can occur within the medulla of the adrenal gland but also along the sympathetic nervous chain [1].

Neuroblastoma

Neuroblastoma, ganglioneuroblastoma, and ganglioneuroma are tumors which arise from the neural crest cells of the sympathetic nervous system [39]. Neuroblastomas are malignant tumors composed of immature neuroblasts. Ganglioneuroblastomas are composed of both immature and mature cells and have malignant potential. Ganglioneuromas composed entirely of mature gangliocytes and mature stroma are benign [39].

Neuroblastoma represents 8–10 % of all childhood cancers making it the most common extracranial solid tumor of childhood [39–41]. The median age of neuroblastoma diagnosis is 19 months, most present between 1 and 5 years of age [3]. Most primary tumors are in the abdomen (65 %), although children have a higher frequency of adrenal tumors than infants (40 % vs. 25 %). The remaining abdominal and pelvic tumors mostly originate in the paravertebral sympathetic ganglia or in the presacral area from the organ of Zuckerkandl [3].

Most children present with abdominal pain or a palpable mass, but others are identified by manifestations of their metastatic disease, as up to 70 % of patients have metastases at presentation [3]. Patterns of metastases vary with age at presentation, and locations can include lymph nodes, liver, skeleton, bone marrow, and skin [3]. Neonates and younger infants more commonly have cutaneous lesions (blueberry muffin syndrome) and extensive hepatic involvement (however, hepatic metastases can occur at any age), whereas older infants and children more commonly have skeletal metastases [3]. Additionally, patients may present with paraneoplastic syndromes. Serum or urinary levels of catecholamines or their metabolites (vanillylmandelic acid (VMA), homovanillic acid (HVA)) are increased in 90 % of children with neuroblastoma [42]; however, secretion of catecholamines rarely leads to symptoms such as those seen in pheochromocytoma: paroxysmal hypertension, palpitations, flushing, and headaches. Secretion of catecholamines or vasoactive intestinal peptide (VIP) may lead to severe watery diarrhea, hypokalemia, and acidosis [43]. Additionally, one can present with acute myoclonic encephalopathy comprised of myoclonus, opsoclonus (rapid multidirectional eye movements), and cerebellar ataxia; this is thought to be due to an immune response to the primary tumor leading to production of anti-neural antibodies that cross-react with cerebellar tissue [44].

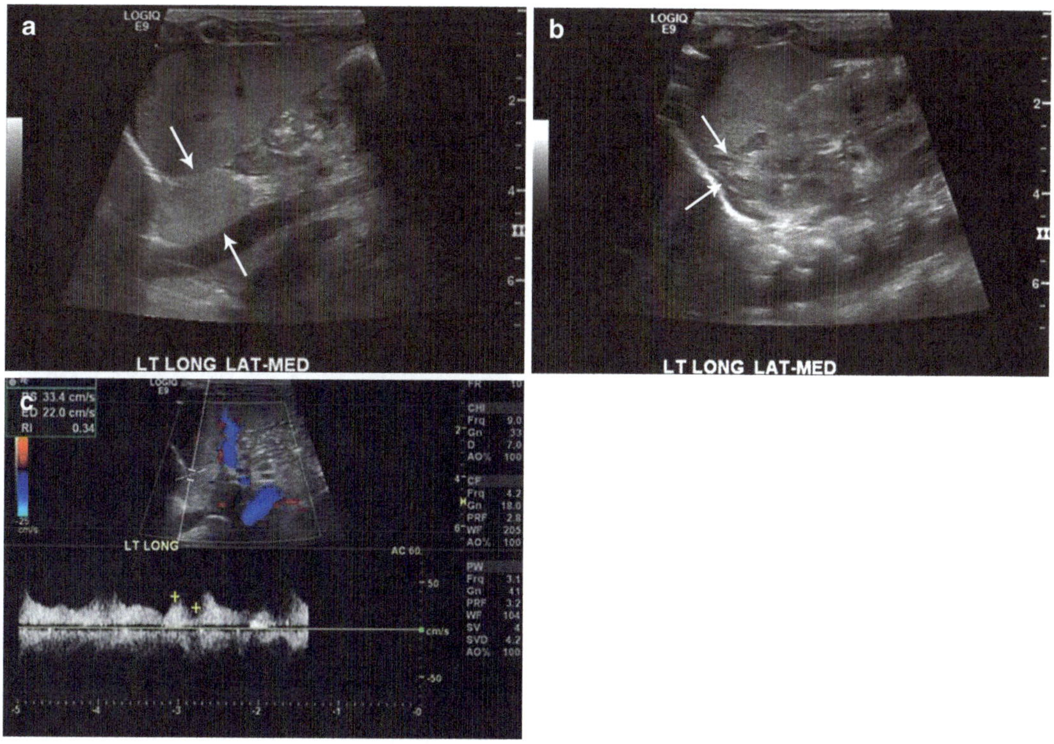

Fig. 16.11 Retroperitoneal extralobar pulmonary sequestration. Longitudinal ultrasound images of the left upper abdomen (**a**) in an 11-day-old boy with prenatally diagnosed mass reveal an echogenic mass medially (*arrows*) and a normal-appearing adrenal gland laterally (**b**). Doppler assessment confirmed internal blood flow (**c**) with large systemic artery typical for an extralobar pulmonary sequestration

Table 16.1 International neuroblastoma staging system

Stage	Description
1	Localized tumor with complete gross excision, with or without microscopic residual disease; representative ipsilateral lymph nodes negative for tumor microscopically
2A	Localized tumor with incomplete gross excision; representative ipsilateral nonadherent lymph nodes negative for tumor microscopically
2B	Localized tumor with or without complete gross excision, with ipsilateral nonadherent lymph nodes positive for tumor. Enlarged contralateral lymph nodes must be negative microscopically
3	Unresectable unilateral tumor infiltrating across the midline, with or without regional lymph node involvement; localized unilateral tumor with contralateral regional lymph node involvement; or midline tumor with bilateral extension by infiltration (unresectable) or by lymph node involvement. The midline is defined as the vertebral column. Tumors originating on one side and crossing the midline must infiltrate to or beyond the opposite side of the vertebral column
4	Any primary tumor with dissemination to distant lymph nodes, bone, bone marrow, liver, skin, and/or other organs, except as defined for stage 4S
4S	Localized primary tumor, as defined for stage 1, 2A, or 2B, with dissemination limited to skin, liver, and/or bone marrow (limited to infants younger than 1 year). Marrow involvement should be minimal (i.e., <10 % of total nucleated cells identified as malignant by bone biopsy or by bone marrow aspirate). More extensive bone marrow involvement would be considered stage 4 disease. The results of the metaiodobenzylguanidine (MIBG) scan, if performed, should be negative for disease in the bone marrow

Adapted from Brodeur et al. [45]

The prognosis of neuroblastoma is related to age, stage at presentation (see Table 16.1), and tumor site [1]. According to the International Neuroblastoma Staging System (INSS), the distribution at presentation is as follows: stage 1, 17 %; stage 2A/2B, 16 %; stage 3, 16 %; stage 4,

44 %; and stage 4S, 7 % [41]. However, newer staging systems based on imaging, instead of surgical, findings are in development [46]. Favorable prognosis occurs in patients <1 year of age, low-stage disease at presentation, and tumors arising from extra-abdominal sites. For example, 2-year survival is 80 % in patients with localized disease, whereas it is less than 5 % for patients with skeletal metastases [11]. Additionally, poor prognostic signs are N-myc amplification (>10 copies), allelic loss of chromosome 1p, and diploid karyotype, whereas favorable prognostic factors are unamplified N-myc oncogene, absence of abnormalities on chromosome 1p, triploid karyotype, and well-differentiated stroma on histology [39].

Treatment consists of a combination of surgery, chemotherapy, and radiation depending on the stage at presentation. Primary surgical resection is used for more localized tumors and chemotherapy for unresectable lesions or in a neoadjuvant setting to shrink lesions sufficiently for delayed surgical resection [39].

Neuroblastomas (and ganglioneuroblastoma) have varied appearance by US [3, 39]. They appear either as a suprarenal or paraspinal masses with the retroperitoneal location evident by anterior displacement of the inferior vena cava or aorta or displacement of retroperitoneal organs [3]. On US, neuroblastomas may be homogeneous or heterogeneous in echogenicity with hyperechoic areas of calcification (often without acoustic shadowing) and hypoechoic areas due to a combination of hemorrhage, necrosis, and cystic change (Fig. 16.12) [39]. In newborns, neuroblastomas may instead be hypoechoic or mainly cystic [11]. Doppler US may be used to confirm the presence of blood flow in the mass and to evaluate patency of encased vessels [39, 40].

Cross-sectional imaging for staging of neuroblastoma is needed in order to assess the organ of origin, extent of the tumor, local invasion, vascular encasement or displacement, calcification, lymphadenopathy, and metastases [24, 47]. On CT, neuroblastoma lesions have attenuation similar or less than that of the muscle [1]. Calcification is present in up to 85 % of cases and may be finely stippled, curvilinear, coarse, or globular [1]. With intravenous contrast, neuroblastoma lesions enhance heterogeneously demonstrating

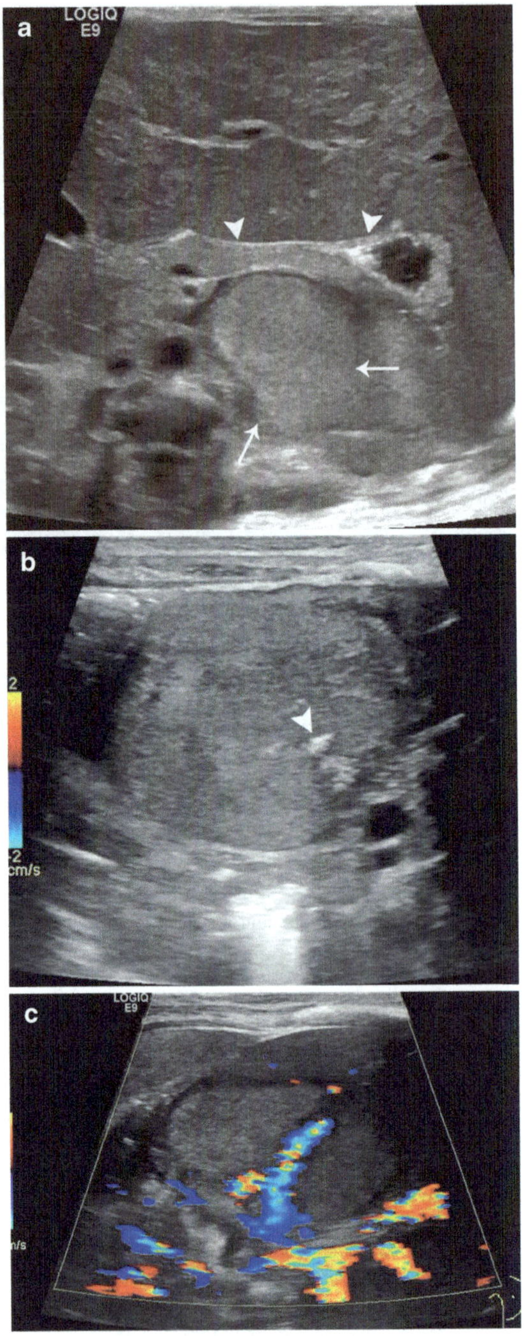

Fig. 16.12 Neuroblastoma – *US*. Transverse ultrasound image of the upper abdomen (**a**) in this neonate reveals a solid-appearing mass arising from the left adrenal gland (*arrows*) which displaces the pancreas (*arrowhead*) anteriorly. On focused ultrasound image (**b**) the left adrenal mass contains echogenic foci (*arrowheads*) due to calcifications. Color Doppler image of the left adrenal mass (**c**) demonstrates internal vascularity (*arrow*) unlike the appearance of an adrenal hemorrhage (See Fig. 16.8)

areas of vascularity and low attenuation regions up to 4 cm in diameter representing necrosis or hemorrhage (Fig. 16.13) [1]. On MR, neuroblastomas are often heterogeneous with variable enhancement. On T1-weighted images, lesions have low to intermediate signal intensity and high signal intensity on T2-weighted and fat-suppressed images [1]. Cysts and areas of necrosis are hypointense on T1-weighted images and hyperintense on T2-weighted images; these areas do not demonstrate enhancement with gadolinium. Areas of calcification demonstrate hypointensity on all MR sequences (Fig. 16.14) [11].

CT or MR should also be used to determine the full extent of the tumor within the abdomen. Vascular encasement and compression can be seen of the inferior vena cava, aorta, celiac artery, superior mesenteric artery, renal vessels, and splenic vein; hypertension may result from renal vascular compression (Fig. 16.13) [39]. Renal hilar, porta hepatis, and retroperitoneal lymphadenopathy may be demonstrated [39].

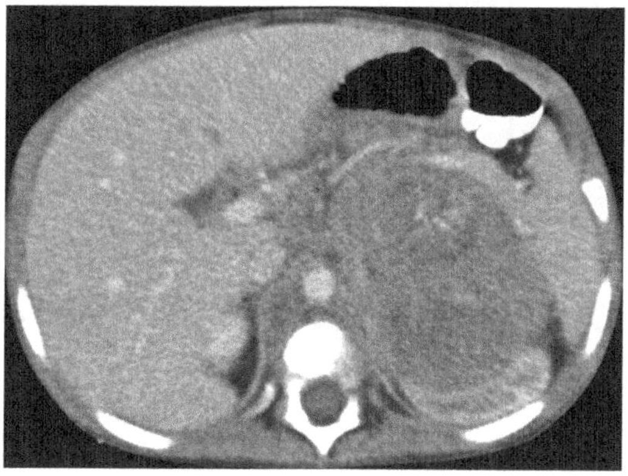

Fig. 16.13 Neuroblastoma – *CT.* Contrast-enhanced axial CT images in an 18-month-old boy with an adrenal gland origin neuroblastoma compressing and displacing the adjacent kidney

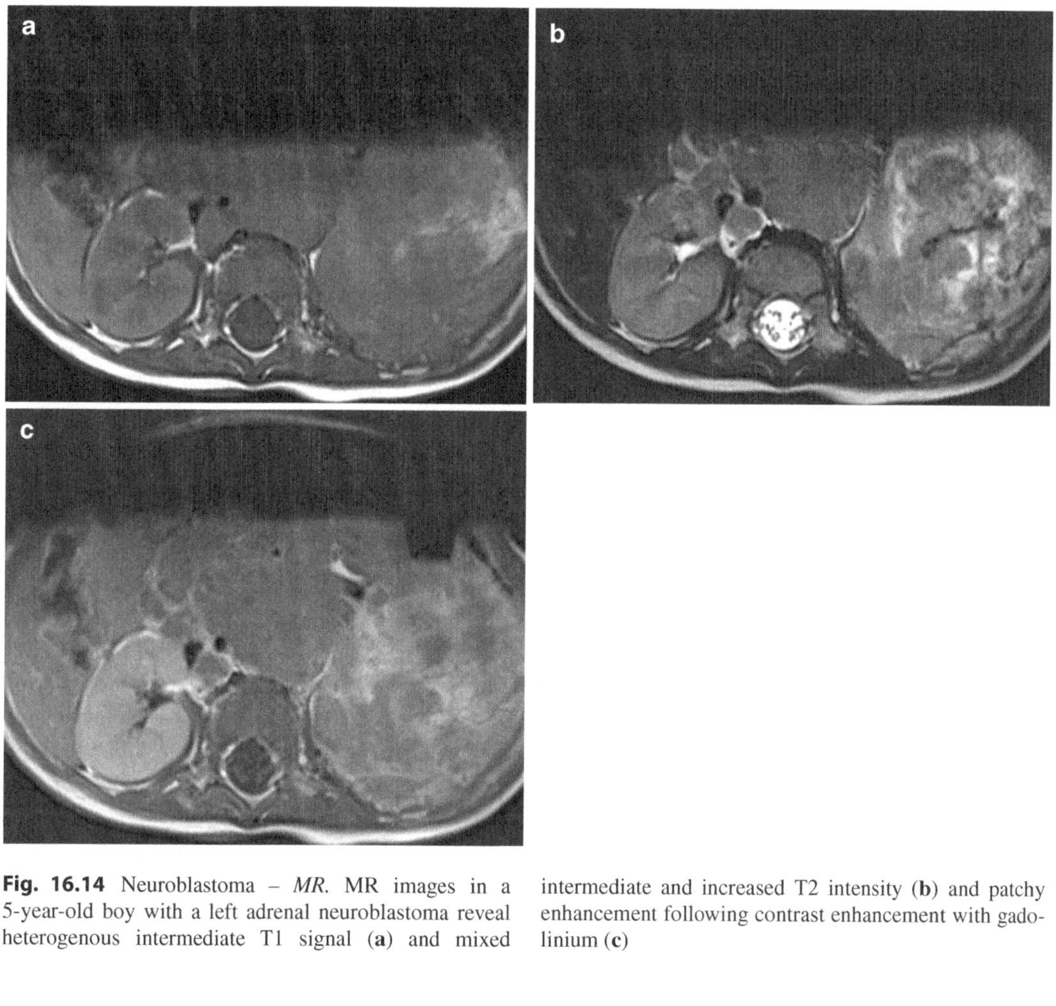

Fig. 16.14 Neuroblastoma – *MR.* MR images in a 5-year-old boy with a left adrenal neuroblastoma reveal heterogenous intermediate T1 signal (**a**) and mixed intermediate and increased T2 intensity (**b**) and patchy enhancement following contrast enhancement with gadolinium (**c**)

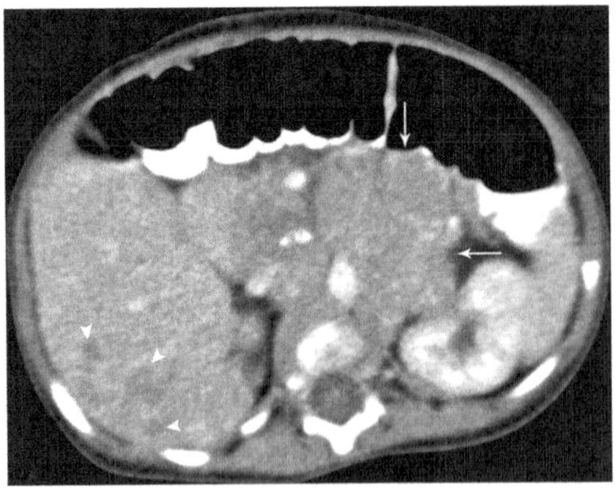

Fig. 16.15 Neuroblastoma. Contrast-enhanced axial CT images in a 5-month-old girl with stage 4S Neuroblastoma (*arrows*). CT image reveals a heterogeneously enhancing left adrenal mass (*arrows*) and multiple low attenuation liver metastases (*arrowheads*)

Metastases into the liver, lung, lymph nodes, and brain can be demonstrated by both CT and MR (Fig. 16.15) [39]. Imaging should be assessed for direct invasion into the kidneys, liver, psoas, paraspinal muscles, and epidural space; MR may more easily demonstrate locoregional invasion (Fig. 16.16) [39]. MR is superior to CT for visualization of the intraspinal tumor extension and bone marrow infiltration (Fig. 16.16) [39, 48].

In addition to cross-sectional imaging, patients with neuroblastomas and ganglioneuroblastomas routinely undergo metaiodobenzylguanidine (MIBG) scans to evaluate for sites of metastatic disease. MIBG is taken up by catecholamine-producing tumors including neuroblastomas, ganglioneuroblastomas, and ganglioneuromas [39]. Greater than 90 % of neuroblastomas are MIBG avid [49]. Other tumors which are typically MIBG avid include pheochromocytomas, carcinoid tumors, and medullary thyroid carcinomas [39]. MIBG scintigraphy is highly sensitive for the detection of metastatic bone disease, allowing visualization of both cortical and bone marrow metastatic disease [39]. Alternatively, Tc-99m methylene diphosphonate (MDP) bone scans can be used to detect bone metastases (Fig. 16.17).

Positron emission tomography (PET) with the glucose analogue ^{18}F fluorodeoxyglucose (FDG) currently has a limited role in the evaluation of neuroblastoma because MIBG is more sensitive for the detection of neuroblastoma [49]. ^{18}F-FDG PET scans may be helpful for the evaluation of MIBG-negative neuroblastomas as well as stage 1 and 2 neuroblastomas (Fig. 16.18) [50]. Additionally, ^{18}F-FDG PET scans are recommended when cross-sectional (CT and MR) imaging studies suggest greater extent of disease than seen on MIBG imaging. Another positron emitting imaging agent, ^{18}F dihydroxyphenylalanine (DOPA) which is not yet widely available, has shown promise in initial studies of patients with stage 3 and 4 neuroblastoma when compared to ^{123}I-MIBG [51].

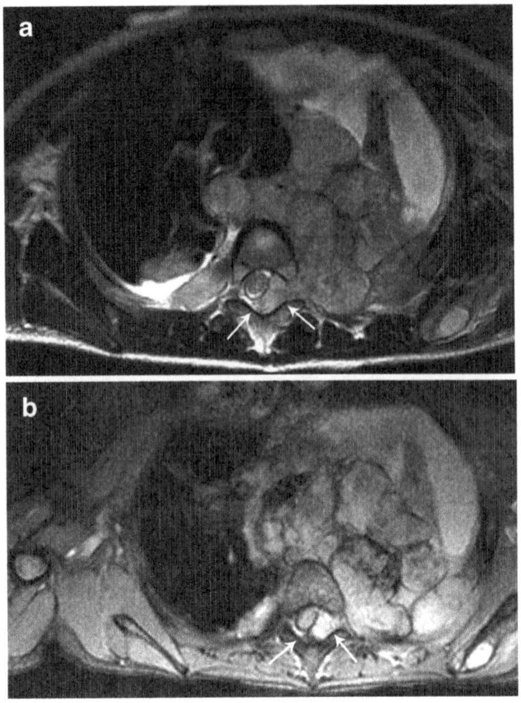

Fig. 16.16 Neuroblastoma. Axial MR images (**a**, **b**) in a 5-year-old boy with a large posterior mediastinal neuroblastoma demonstrates evidence of tumor extension into the spinal canal (*arrows*) with associated displacement and compression of the spinal cord

Ganglioneuroma

In comparison to neuroblastomas, ganglioneuromas are benign completely differentiated tumors of mature ganglion cells [11]. Ganglioneuromas may arise de novo, develop from maturing neuroblastoma or ganglioneuroblastoma, or arise from treated neuroblastoma or ganglioneuroblastoma [1]. In contrast to neuroblastoma, ganglioneuromas are more often found in asymptomatic older

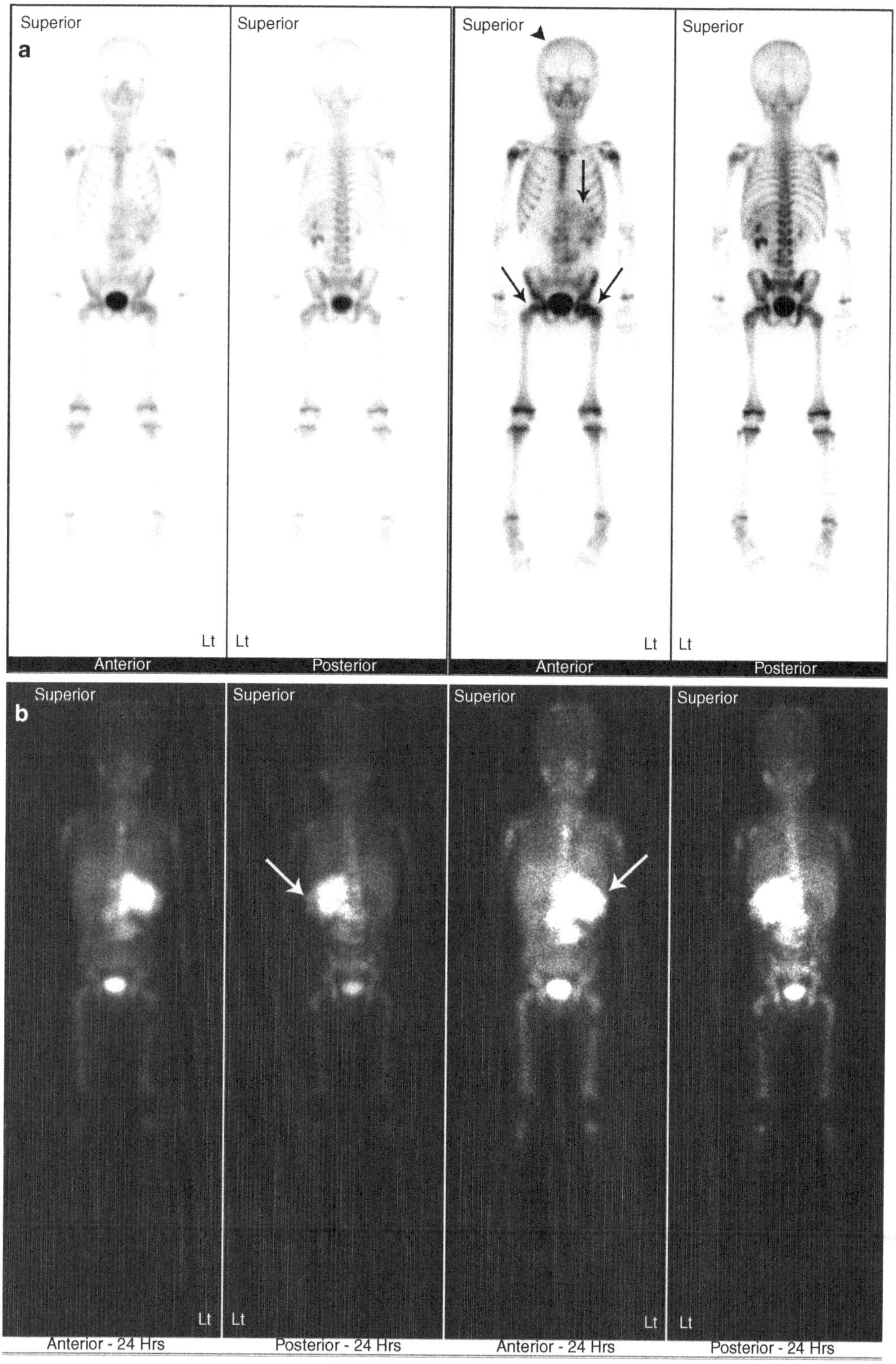

Fig. 16.17 Neuroblastoma. Bone scan (**a**) and MIBG scan (**b**) were performed in a 3-year-old boy with stage 4 neuroblastoma. Abnormally increased radiotracer localization on the bone scan (**a**) is seen in the skull (*arrowhead*), primary left retroperitoneal mass (*arrows*), and proximal femurs bilaterally (*arrows*). MIBG scan (**b**) shows evidence of extensive metastatic disease in the bone and bone marrow and in the primary left retroperitoneal tumor (*arrow*). All of the visualized skeletal activity on the MIBG scan represents sites of metastatic bone and/or bone marrow disease

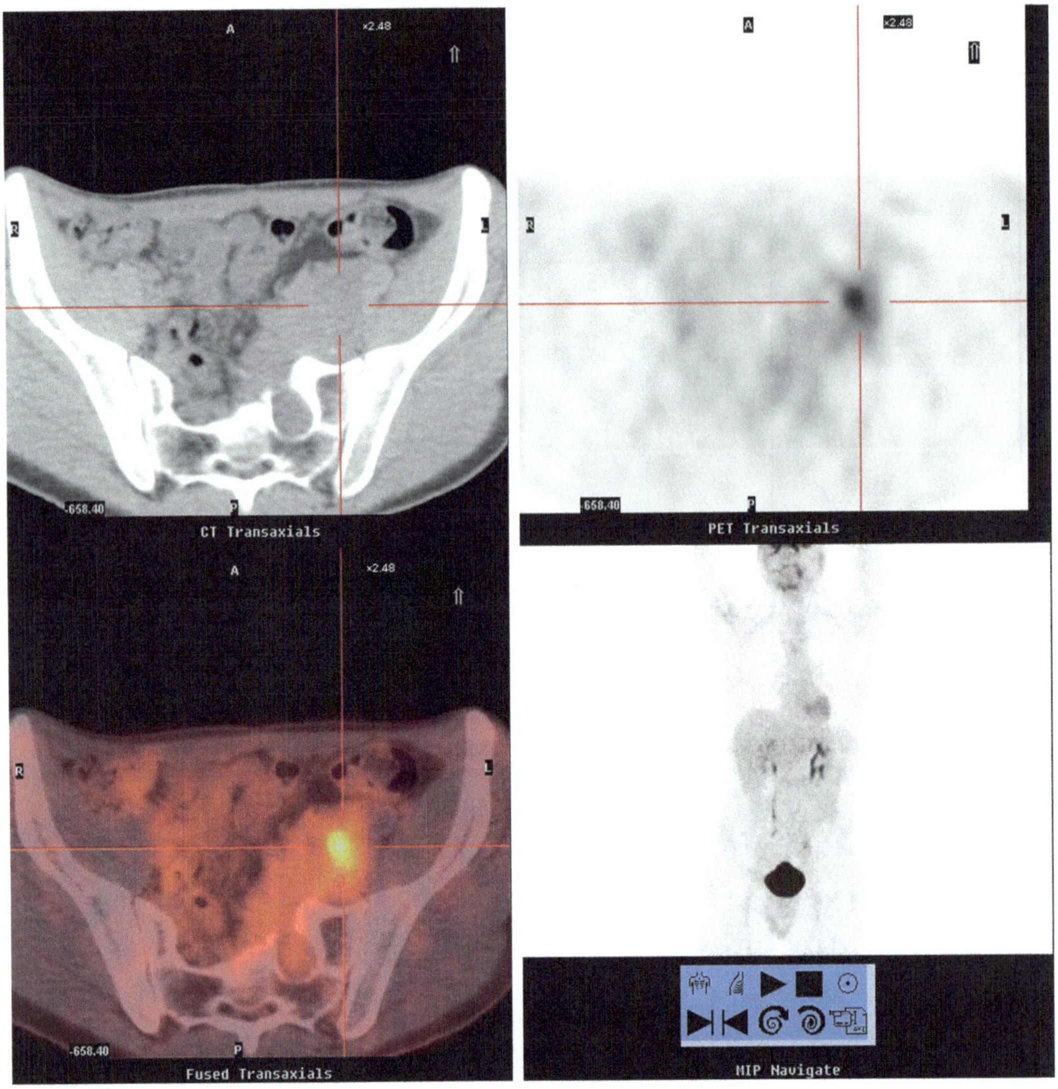

Fig. 16.18 Neuroblastoma. PET/CT scan in a 17-year-old boy with a left presacral neuroblastoma (centered in the crosshairs) on localizing noncontrast CT (labeled CT transaxials) with increased metabolic activity on the PET (labeled PET transaxials) and fused PET/CT (labeled fused transaxials) images

children (median age of 7) as an incidental finding on imaging performed for other reasons [1]. Most ganglioneuromas arise in the posterior mediastinum, and only one-third arise in the abdomen (mostly paravertebral, less frequently suprarenal) (Fig. 16.19) [1]. As ganglioneuroma appearance on imaging is similar to that of neuroblastoma, diagnosis is made by histologic examination of tumor tissue [1]. A needle biopsy is not sufficient due to sampling error and cannot reliably confirm benign histology throughout the entire lesion. Treatment consists of complete surgical resection when possible with subsequent periodic radiologic surveillance; if surgical removal is not possible (large tumors, involvement of vessels or other vital structures, or extension into the intervertebral foramina), patients should be followed for life to monitor for development of malignant peripheral nerve sheath tumors [1].

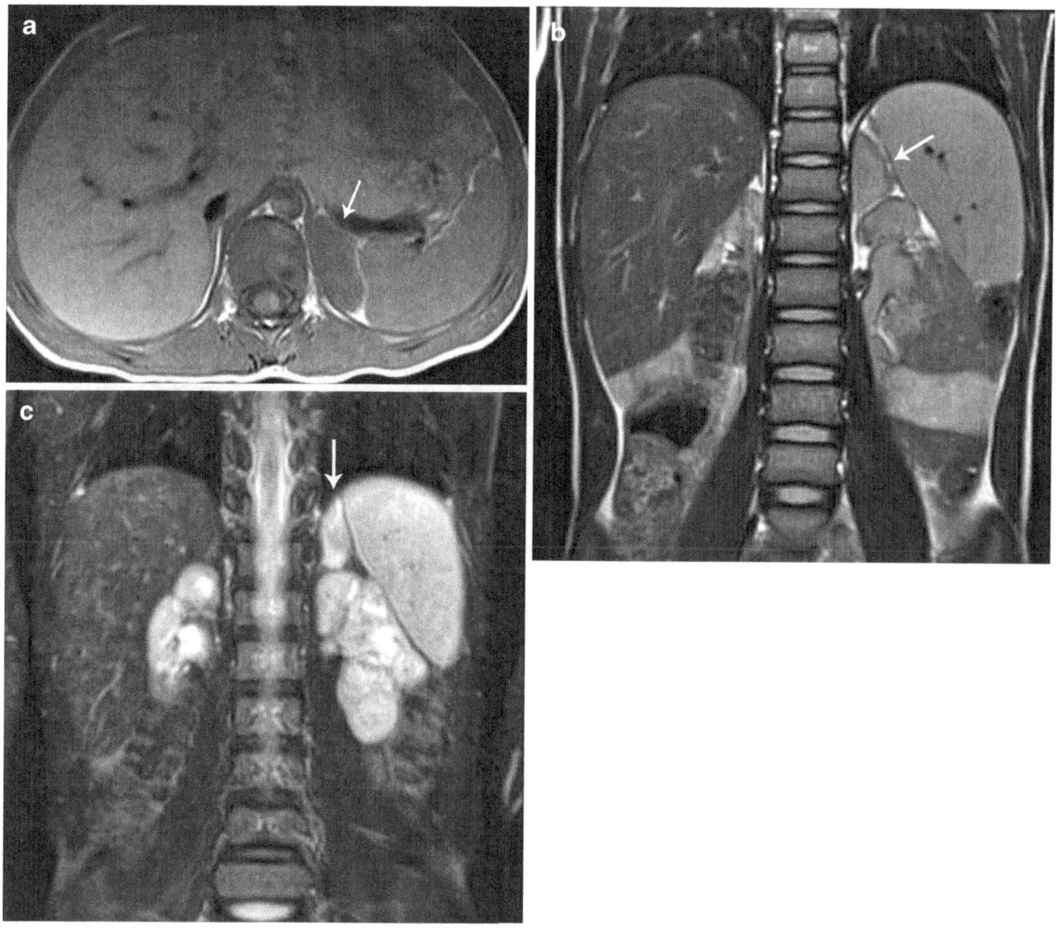

Fig. 16.19 Ganglioneuroma. MR scans ((**a**) axial T1, (**b**) coronal T1, (**c**) coronal T2) in a 5-year-old boy with history of neurogenic bladder and bilateral ureteral reflux revealed an adrenal mass (*arrows*). This proved to be a benign left adrenal ganglioneuroma

Pheochromocytoma

Pheochromocytoma is a functionally active catecholamine-secreting tumor involving chromaffin cells of the sympathetic nervous system. Most originate in the adrenal medulla; however, up to 30 % are extra-adrenal (termed paragangliomas) in locations such as the paravertebral sympathetic chain, para-aortic bodies, bladder wall, spermatic cord, or vagina [1, 3]. Pheochromocytoma is an uncommon neoplasm in children as only 5 % of all pheochromocytomas occur in children and they represent under 1 % of childhood neoplasms [1]. In children, 70 % of pheochromocytomas arise in the adrenal gland and 24 % are bilateral [1]. There is a higher incidence of pheochromocytoma (in addition to multiple and/or bilateral tumors) in patients with multiple endocrine neoplasia (MEN) type 2 (with medullary thyroid carcinoma and parathyroid hyperplasia), tuberous sclerosis, neurofibromatosis, hemihypertrophy, Sturge-Weber syndrome, and von Hippel-Lindau disease [3]. Clinical manifestations of pheochromocytomas are due to epinephrine and norepinephrine release, and include paroxysmal hypertension, tachycardia, sweating, flushing, headaches, blurred vision, papilledema, hypertensive encephalopathy, diarrhea, weight loss, and micturition syncope (in the case of bladder wall paragangliomas) [1]. Diagnosis is made with elevated levels of plasma or urinary levels of catecholamines or their metabolites (vanillylmandelic acid [VMA], homovanillic acid [HVA]) [3].

Imaging is necessary to localize the primary lesion(s) and any sites of metastatic spread to allow for treatment via surgical removal [3, 40]. Pheochromocytomas can range in size from 1 to 10 cm at presentation; however, most are between 2 and 5 cm [1]. On US, pheochromocytoma lesions can be homogeneously or heterogeneously echoic with hypoechoic areas of hemorrhage and necrosis and hyperechoic areas of hemorrhage and calcification. Smaller pheochromocytomas are more likely to be homogeneous and larger lesions heterogeneous [1, 3]. On CT, pheochromocytomas have soft tissue attenuation, and enhancement may be diffuse, heterogeneous, or rim-enhancing (Figs. 16.20a, b) [1]. On MR T1-weighted images, pheochromocytomas are

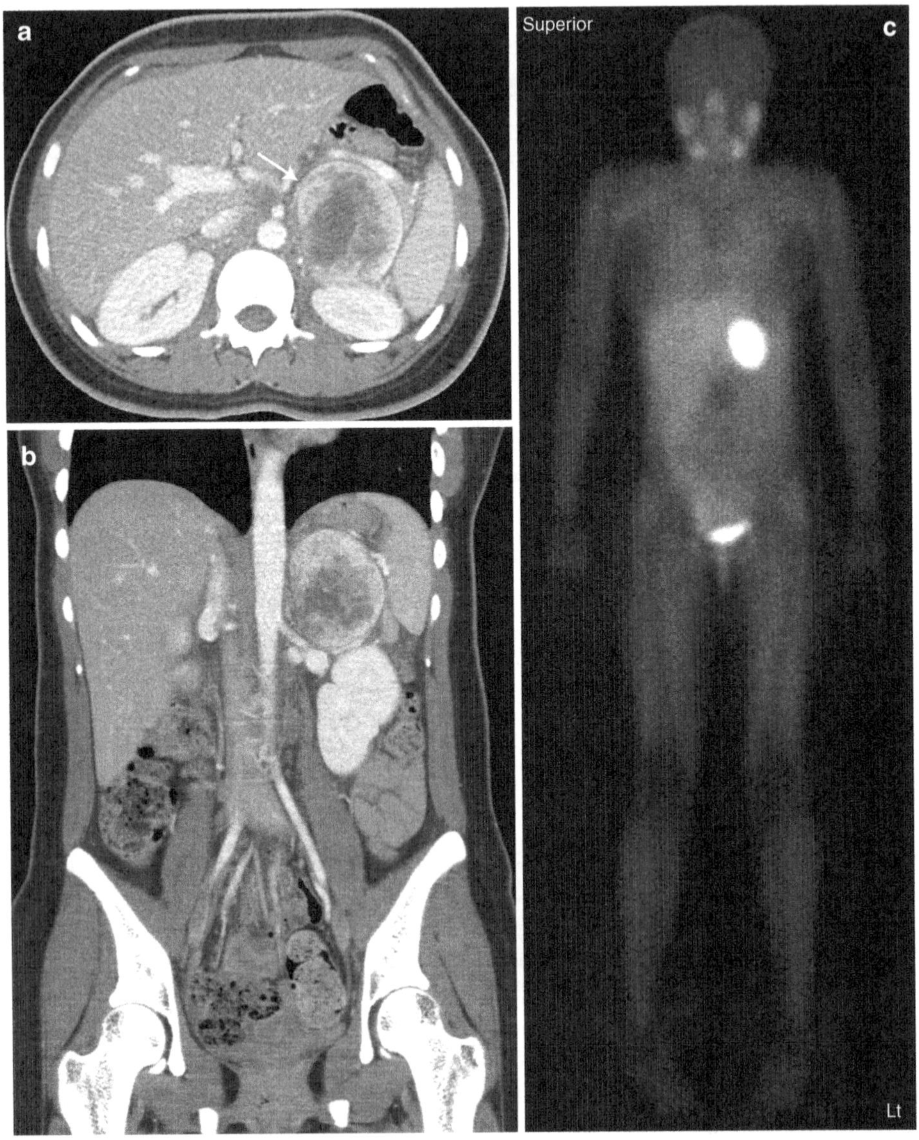

Fig. 16.20 Pheochromocytoma. Axial (**a**) and coronal (**b**) contrast-enhanced CT images and MIBG scan (**c**) performed in a teenage girl with history of tachycardia and hypertension reveal a heterogeneously enhancing left adrenal mass (*arrows*) on CT which is strongly MIBG avid on MIBG scan (**c**) and was confirmed to be a pheochromocytoma

hypointense to the liver; on T2-weighted and fat-suppressed images, pheochromocytomas are hyperintense to the liver and fat [11]. Of note, they show a higher signal intensity compared to adrenocortical tumors. After gadolinium infusion, these lesions have moderate to marked heterogeneous enhancement with a slow washout period [1, 11]. Whole body MIBG scintigraphy can also be used to localize lesions and metastatic sites (Fig. 16.20c) [1].

Adrenocortical Neoplasms

Adrenocortical tumors are not common in children. The majority of these lesions are hyperfunctioning hormone-producing tumors with the most common abnormality being the overproduction of androgens [24, 52]. Girls present with signs of virilization including facial hair, advanced pubic and axillary hair development, advanced bone age, increased muscle mass, and clitoromegaly [24]. While boys present with signs of isosexual pseudoprecocious puberty including early acne, pubic hair, and penile enlargement [24]. In the rare nonfunctioning lesions, a child may present with an abdominal mass or incidental finding on imaging. Girls are more commonly affected than boys, in a 2–3:1 ratio. Carcinomas are more common than adenomas [1, 24]. Adrenocortical neoplasms are less common than neuroblastoma but more common than pheochromocytoma [28].

Unfortunately, compared to adult tumors, pediatric adrenal adenoma and adrenal carcinoma are difficult to distinguish histopathologically [24]. In adults, adrenal adenomas have a low nuclear-to-cytoplasmic ratio with very little necrosis or hemorrhage and rare mitoses; however, in children, these tumors are more likely to show nuclear atypia, pleomorphism, necrosis, and mitotic activity [24]. In comparison, adrenal carcinomas have a wide range of morphology from normal-appearing adrenal cells to completely undifferentiated cells [24]. Multiple attempts have been made to classify adrenal adenomas vs. adrenal carcinomas based on tumor size, clinical findings, and histopathologic features. However, these two lesions cannot be reliably differentiated based on these systems [24, 52]. Only the detection of metastases can distinguish malignant tumors from benign lesions.

Adrenocortical Carcinoma

Adrenocortical carcinoma is a malignant neoplasm of the adrenal cortex and is quite rare, accounting for <1 % of all pediatric malignancies [24, 52]. Most present at a mean age of 9 years with androgen overproduction (virilization in girls, pseudoprecocious puberty in boys) as seen by elevated urinary 17-ketosteroids and normal to slightly elevated urinary cortisol levels [3]. Unusual presentations include pure Cushing syndrome, hyperaldosteronism leading to hypertension, or estrogen secretion leading to feminization on boys [24]. There is an association between adrenal cancer and hemihypertrophy, Beckwith-Wiedemann syndrome, and Li-Fraumeni syndrome [24]. As stated above, definitive diagnosis of adrenal adenoma vs. carcinoma cannot be made on imaging characteristics, biochemical criteria, or even histopathologically; however, larger or palpable lesions are more likely to be carcinoma [1]. Adrenal carcinoma may locally invade the kidney, renal vein, or inferior vena cava; distant metastases are most common in the lungs, liver, peritoneum, pleura, diaphragm, abdominal lymph nodes, and kidney [24]. Treatment consists of complete resection with adjuvant chemotherapy reserved for metastases, recurrent disease, or persistently elevated hormones after resection [24]. Survival is related to age at presentation: Lack et al. demonstrated a 13 % survival rate for children older than 5 years and 70 % for children 5 years or younger (combined adrenal carcinoma and adenoma cases) [53].

Adrenal carcinomas are normally large at presentation, mostly greater than 5 cm, but can vary in size [24, 52]. On US, larger lesions are usually heterogeneous with necrosis, hemorrhage, and calcification (in up to 40 %) leading to hypoechoic or hyperechoic areas [3]. Smaller lesions may be more homogeneous in nature (Fig. 16.21a) [3]. US Doppler imaging may be used to detect venous tumor thrombus [3]. On CT and MR, larger lesions also appear more heterogeneous

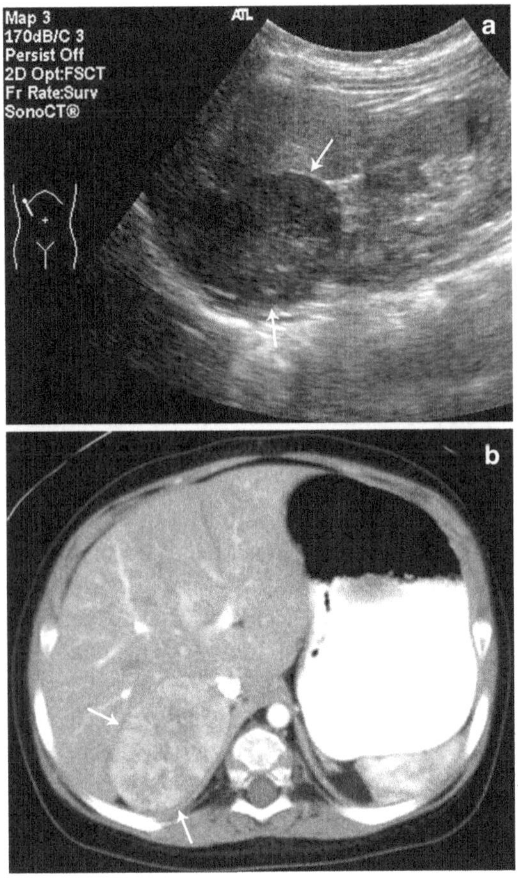

Fig. 16.21 Adrenocortical neoplasm. US (**a**) and CT (**b**) images through the upper abdomen reveal a solid soft tissue mass (*arrows*) found to be an adrenocortical neoplasm

compared to the homogeneous smaller lesions. Larger lesions may have a central scar with radiation linear bands representing areas of calcification and necrosis (Fig. 16.21b) [1]. On MR, adrenal lesions (adenomas and carcinomas) tend to be intermediate signal intensity on T1-weighted images and high signal intensity compared to the liver on T2-weighted images [24]. CT and MR are superior to US in assessing for local invasion and metastatic spread and are of paramount importance when assessing for inferior vena cava tumor thrombus which may involve a thoracoabdominal surgical approach for intrahepatic or right atrial tumor thrombus [24]. ^{18}F-FDG PET scan can be used to locate distant metastases or tumor recurrence not detected on CT or MR. Additionally, Tc-99m MDP bone scans can be used in the initial evaluation to detect bone metastases in those limited cases. As noted, the diagnosis of malignancy is characterized by local spread, invasion, and metastatic disease, not histopathology or primary mass imaging characteristics [24, 52].

Other Adrenal Neoplasms

Leiomyomas

Leiomyomas, smooth muscle tumors, have been described to occur in the adrenal glands, gastrointestinal, tracheobronchopulmonary, and hepatobiliary symptoms in pediatric acquired immunodeficiency syndrome (AIDS) in association with Epstein-Barr virus (EBV) [54]. They are usually unilateral, but can be bilateral and are thought to arise from adrenal vasculature smooth muscle [1]. Most leiomyomas within the adrenal gland are small and benign appearing by imaging (i.e., homogeneous). However, some leiomyomas are larger and more complex on US, CT, and MR, and they have inconsistent ^{18}F-FDG PET avidity; therefore, the recommendation is surgical removal for those >6 cm [55].

Myelolipoma

Myelolipomas are cortical, nonfunctioning, benign tumors that are rare, mostly unilateral, and most often found in the adrenal gland. These lesions are more common in adults (frequently in the fifth–seventh decades), but are rarely seen in children [56]. Tumors are usually small and asymptomatic and found incidentally on imaging. Myelolipomas are composed of fat and bone marrow components, and on US the fat components are highly echogenic and myeloid components are hypoechoic or isoechoic to adrenal parenchyma [3]. On CT, the fat component is easily identified by regions of low Hounsfield unit (HU) attenuation (−30 to −100 HU) [57]. MR can be used to confirm adrenal origin by defining tissue planes, and lipid-containing regions can be identified by high signal intensity on T1-weighted images, intermediate signal intensity on T2-weighed images, and loss of signal intensity on fat suppression scans [57]. Treatment is usually conservative when patients are asymptomatic.

Adrenal Cysts

Cysts in the adrenal gland can form in multiple disease states. Adrenal cysts can form during resolution of neonatal adrenal hemorrhage [5]. Additionally, neuroblastoma can present in a cystic form prenatally or in the neonate [5]. Beckwith-Wiedemann syndrome and hemihypertrophy may be associated with adrenal microcysts located in the capsule or superficial adult cortex [5]. These microcysts can undergo exaggerated development leading to macroscopic adrenal cysts at birth. Macroscopic adrenal cysts associated with Beckwith-Wiedemann syndrome are usually unilateral and large (up to several centimeters), may be multiloculated, and are usually hemorrhagic [5]. Treatment is conservative as they shrink and may disappear with time [58].

On US, adrenal cysts are round anechoic masses with well-circumscribed thin walls and through-sound transmission [3]. However, septations, fluid-fluid levels, wall calcification, and multilocular cystic masses can also occur [3]. Other suprarenal, but extra-adrenal, cysts due to bronchogenic foregut malformations, such as bronchogenic cysts, cystic adenomatoid malformation, intra-abdominal sequestration with cystic elements, and esophageal or gastric duplication cyst, may occur [59]. The extra-adrenal origin of these cysts may not be possible, but attempts to distinguish the adrenal gland from the cystic lesions with thorough US or cross-sectional imaging with MR or CT should be made.

Adrenal Abscess

Seeding of an adrenal hemorrhage in the setting of neonatal or maternal septicemia can lead to the formation of an adrenal abscess [60]. Typical organisms include *Escherichia coli,* meningococcus, group B hemolytic streptococcus, *Staphylococcus,* and *Bacteroides* [5]. On US, adrenal abscess often have a rim-like calcification, fluid filled center, echogenic debris, and increased flow and enhancement of the wall; however, the appearance is varied and may be hard to differentiate from an adrenal hemorrhage or neuroblastoma [3]. Clinical correlation of an adrenal mass in the setting of sepsis and follow-up imaging can assist with the diagnosis. Adrenal abscess complications include local extension (into the ipsilateral kidney, spleen, and pancreas), inferior vena cava compression, and rarely adrenobronchial fistula [61].

Key Points to Remember

- Given the relatively large size of the neonatal adrenal gland due to the presence of fetal adrenal cortex, ultrasound (US) can easily visualize the adrenal glands during the neonatal period.
- After the fetal cortex has involuted, ultrasound cannot reliably discern the anatomic details of the adrenal glands; therefore, computed tomography (CT) and magnetic resonance imaging (MR) are best employed for imaging the adrenal glands in children and older infants.
- On US, the normal appearance of the neonatal adrenal gland is two separate zones of echogenicity: a core consisting of a thin, central hyperechoic stripe and a surrounding rim of thicker hypoechoic tissue. The surface of a normal neonatal adrenal gland is smooth to slightly undulating, without nodular protuberances, and adrenal limbs should be uniform in length with a width of less than 4 mm.
- On CT, the adrenal gland's soft tissue attenuation is similar to the liver. On MR, on spin-echo T1-weighted images, adrenal glands have intermediate signal intensity (less than fat and similar to the liver); on T2-weighted and fat-suppressed images, adrenal glands are much brighter than fat and slightly brighter than the liver.
- Diagnosis of congenital adrenal hyperplasia can be made by the demonstration of two of three sonographic signs: (1) adrenal limb width of >4 mm, (2) cerebriform or crenated appearance of the surface of the adrenal gland, and (3) replacement of the central hyperechoic stripe with a diffusely stippled pattern of echogenicity or a diffuse thickened band of echogenicity.

- Adrenal masses in children and neonates may be attributable to hemorrhage, neoplasms, cysts, or abscesses; the age and clinical presentation of the child, in conjunction with the imaging features of the mass, will allow one to develop an appropriate list of diagnostic considerations.
- Use serial imaging to differentiate adrenal hemorrhage from neuroblastoma. Masses due to adrenal hemorrhage decrease in size over several weeks as the hemorrhage liquefies and resorbs and become more hypoechoic or anechoic, whereas in contrast, the size of a neuroblastoma is unlikely to decrease.
- Neuroblastoma has varied appearance on US, CT, and MR. Cross-sectional imaging for staging of neuroblastoma is needed in order to assess the organ of origin, extent of the tumor, local invasion, vascular encasement or displacement, calcification, lymphadenopathy, and metastases.
- Compared to adult tumors, pediatric adrenal adenoma and adrenal carcinoma are difficult to distinguish histopathologically or radiologically. Only the detection of metastases can distinguish malignant tumors from benign lesions.

Acknowledgement Ellen C. Benya, MD, Department of Medical Imaging, Ann and Robert H. Lurie Children's Hospital of Chicago for her assistance with radiological images

References

1. Daneman A, Navarro O, Haller JO. The adrenal and retroperitoneum. In: Solvis TL, editor. Caffey's pediatric diagnostic imaging. Maryland Heights: Mosby; 2007.
2. Parnaby CN, Galbraith N, O'Dwyer PJ. Experience in identifying the venous drainage of the adrenal gland during laparoscopic adrenalectomy. Clin Anat. 2008;71(7):660–5.
3. Siegel MJ, Chung EM. Adrenal glands, pancreas, and other retroperitoneal strictures. In: Siegel MJ, editor. Pediatric sonography. Philadelphia: Lippincott Williams & Wilkins; 2011.
4. Kutikov A, Crispen PL, Uzzo RG. Pathophysiology, evaluation, and medical management of adrenal disorder. In: Wein AJ, Kavoussi LR, Novick AC, Partin AW, Peters CA, editors. Campbell-Walsh urology. 10th ed. Philadelphia: Elsevier Inc; 2011.
5. Daneman A, Traubici J. The adrenal gland. In: Solvis TL, editor. Caffey's pediatric diagnostic imaging. Maryland Heights: Mosby; 2007.
6. Mitty HA. Embryology, anatomy, and anomalies of the adrenal gland. Semin Roentgenol. 1988;23(4): 271–9.
7. Barwick TD, Malhotra A, Webb JA, Savage MO, Reznek RH. Embryology of the adrenal glands and its relevance to diagnostic imaging. Clin Radiol. 2005;60(9):953–9.
8. Kempná P, Flück CE. Adrenal gland development and defects. Best Pract Res Clin Endocrinol Metab. 2008;22(1):77–93.
9. Oppenheimer DA, Carroll BA, Yousem S. Sonography of the normal neonatal adrenal gland. Radiology. 1983;146(1):157–60.
10. Kangarloo H, Diament MJ, Gold RH, Barrett C, Lippe B, Geffner M, Boechat MI, Dietrich RB, Amundson GM. Sonography of adrenal glands in neonates and children: changes in appearance with age. J Clin Ultrasound. 1986;14(1):43–7.
11. Siegel MJ, Coley B. The core curriculum: pediatric imaging. Philadelphia: Lippincott Williams & Wilkins; 2005.
12. Daneman D, Daneman A. Diagnostic imaging of the thyroid and adrenal glands in childhood. Endocrinol Metab Clin North Am. 2005;34(3):745–68.
13. Hoffman CK, Filly RA, Callen PW. The "lying down" adrenal sign: a sonographic indicator of renal agenesis or ectopia in fetuses and neonates. J Ultrasound Med. 1992;11(10):533–6.
14. Burton EM, Strange ME, Edmonds DB. Sonography of the circumrenal and horseshoe adrenal gland in the newborn. Pediatr Radiol. 1993;23(5):362–4.
15. Çakir ED, Mutlu FS, Eren E, Paşa AO, Sağlam H, Tarim O. Testicular adrenal rest tumors in patients with congenital adrenal hyperplasia. J Clin Res Pediatr Endocrinol. 2013;4(2):94–100.
16. Merke DP, Bornstein SR. Congenital adrenal hyperplasia. Lancet. 2005;365(9477):2125–36.
17. Sivit CJ, Hung W, Taylor GA, Catena LM, Brown-Jones C, Kushner DC. Sonography in neonatal congenital adrenal hyperplasia. AJR Am J Roentgenol. 1991;156(1):141–3.
18. Al-Alwan I, Navarro O, Daneman D, Daneman A. Clinical utility of adrenal ultrasonography in the diagnosis of congenital adrenal hyperplasia. J Pediatr. 1999;135(1):71–5.
19. Avni EF, Rypens F, Smet MH, Galetty E. Sonographic demonstration of congenital adrenal hyperplasia in the neonate: the cerebriform pattern. Pediatr Radiol. 1993;23(2):88–90.
20. Bentsen D, Schwartz DS, Carpenter TO. Sonography of congenital adrenal hyperplasia due to partial deficiency of 3β-hydroxysteroid dehydrogenase: a case report. Pediatr Radiol. 1997;27(7):594–5.
21. Kohda E, Yamazaki H, Hisazumi H, Tutumi Y, Ogata T, Shiraga N. Imaging of congenital lipoid adrenal hyperplasia. Radiat Med. 2006;24(3):217–19.

22. Pivonello R, De Martino MC, De Leo M, Lombardi G, Colao A. Cushing's syndrome. Endocrinol Metab Clin North Am. 2008;37(1):135–49.
23. Young Jr WF, Klee GG. Primary aldosteronism. Diagnostic evaluation. Endocrinol Metab Clin North Am. 1988;17(2):367–95.
24. Agrons GA, Lonergan GJ, Dickey GE, Perez-Monte JE. Adrenocortical neoplasms in children: radiologic-pathologic correlation. Radiographics. 1999;19(4): 989–1008.
25. Doppman JL, Travis WD, Nieman L, Miller DL, Chrousos GP, Gomez MT, Cutler Jr GB, Loriaux DL, Norton JA. Cushing syndrome due to primary pigmented nodular adrenocortical disease: findings at CT and MR imaging. Radiology. 1989;172(2):415–20.
26. Dutton RV. Wolman's disease. Ultrasound and CT diagnosis. Pediatr Radiol. 1985;15(2):144–6.
27. Ozmen MN, Aygün N, Kiliç L, Kuran L, Yalçin B, Besim A. Wolman's disease: ultrasonographic and computed tomographic findings. Pediatr Radiol. 1992;22(7):541–2.
28. Balassy C, Navarro OM, Daneman A. Adrenal masses in children. Radiol Clin North Am. 2011;49(4): 711–27.
29. Abdu AT, Kriss VM, Bada HS, Reynolds EW. Adrenal hemorrhage in a newborn. Am J Perinat. 2009;26(8):553–7.
30. Swischuk LE. Genitourinary tract and adrenal glands. In: Swischuk LE, editor. Imaging of the newborn, infant, and young child. Philadelphia: Lippincott Williams & Wilkins; 2004.
31. Heij HA, Taets van Amerongen AH, Ekkelkamp S, Vos A. Diagnosis and management of neonatal adrenal hemorrhage. Pediatr Radiol. 1989;19(6–7):391–4.
32. Mittelstaedt CA, Volberg FM, Merten DF, Brill PW. The sonographic diagnosis of neonatal adrenal hemorrhage. Radiology. 1979;131(2):453–7.
33. Miele V, Galluzzo M, Patti G, Mazzoni G, Calisti A, Valenti M. Scrotal hematoma due to neonatal adrenal hemorrhage: the value of ultrasonography in avoiding unnecessary surgery. Pediatr Radiol. 1997;27(8):672–4.
34. Calisti A, Oriolo L, Molle P, Miele V, Spagnol L. Neonatal adrenal masses: do we have reliable criteria for differential diagnosis and expectant management? Minerva Pediatr. 2012;64(3):313–18.
35. Eo H, Kim JH, Jang KM, Yoo SY, Lim GY, Kim MJ, Kim OH. Comparison of clinic-radiological features between congenital cystic neuroblastoma and neonatal adrenal hemorrhagic pseudocyst. Korean J Radiol. 2011;12(1):52–8.
36. Bergami G, Malena S, Di Mario M, Fariello G. Echography in the follow-up of neonatal adrenal hemorrhage. The presentation of fourteen cases. Radiol Med. 1990;79(5):474–8.
37. Curtis MR, Mooney DP, Vacarro TJ, Williams JC, Cendrom M, Shorter NA, Sargent SK. Prenatal ultrasound characterization of the suprarenal mas: the distinction between neuroblastoma and subdiaphragmatic extralobar pulmonary sequestration. J Ultrasound Med. 1997;16(2):75–83.
38. Franko J, Bell K, Pezzi CM. Intraabdominal pulmonary sequestration. Curr Surg. 2006;63(1):35–8.
39. Lonergan GJ, Schwab CM, Suarez ES, Carlson CL. Neuroblastoma, ganglioneuroblastoma, ganglioneuroma: radiologic-pathologic correlation. Radiographics. 2002;22(4):911–34.
40. Abramson SJ. Adrenal neoplasms in children. Radiol Clin North Am. 1997;35(6):1415–53.
41. Brodeur GM, Hogarty MD, Mosse YP, Maris JM. Neuroblastoma. In: Pizzo PA, Poplack DG, editors. Principles and practice of pediatric oncology. Philadelphia: Lippincott Williams & Wilkins; 2011.
42. Williams CM, Greer M. Homovanillic acid and vanillylmandelic acid in diagnosis of neuroblastoma. JAMA. 1963;183:836–40.
43. Cooney DR, Voorhess ML, Fisher JE, Brecher M, Karp MP, Jewett TC. Vasoactive intestinal peptide producing neuroblastoma. J Pediatr Surg. 1982;17(6): 821–5.
44. Rothenberg AB, Berdon WE, D'Angio GJ, Yamashiro DJ, Cowles RA. The association between neuroblastoma and opsoclonus-myoclonus syndrome: a historical review. Pediatr Radiol. 2009; 39(7):723–6.
45. Brodeur GM, Pritchard J, Berthold F, Carlsen NL, Castel V, Castelberry RP, De Bernardi B, Evans AE, Favrot M, Hedborg F, Kaneko M, Kemshead J, Lampert F, Lee REJ, Look AT, Pearson ADJ, Philip T, Roald B, Sawada T, Seeger RC, Tsuchida Y, Voute PA. Revisions of the international criteria for neuroblastoma diagnosis, staging, and response to treatment. J Clin Oncol. 1993;11(8):1466–77.
46. Brisse HJ, McCarville MB, Granata C, Krug KB, Wootton-Gorges SL, Kanegawa K, Giammarile F, Schmidt M, Shulkin BL, Matthay KK, Lewington VJ, Sarnacki S, Hero B, Kaneko M, London WB, Pearson AD, Cohn SL, Monclair T. Guidelines for imaging and staging of neuroblastic tumors: consensus report from the International Neuroblastoma Risk Group Project. Radiology. 2011;261(1):243–57.
47. Stark DD, Moss AA, Brasch RC, de Lorimier AA, Albin AR, London DA, Gooding CA. Neuroblastoma: diagnostic imaging and staging. Radiology. 1983; 148(1):101–5.
48. McHugh K. Renal and adrenal tumors in children. Cancer Imaging. 2007;7:41–51.
49. Sharp SE, Gelfand MJ, Shulkin BL. Pediatrics: diagnosis of neuroblastoma. Semin Nucl Med. 2011;41(5):345–53.
50. Sharp SE, Shulkin BL, Gelfand M, Salisbury S, Furman WL. 123I-MIBG scintigraphy and 18-F-FDG PET in neuroblastoma. J Nucl Med. 2009;50(8):1237–43.
51. Piccardo A, Lopa E, Conte M, Garaventa A, Foppiani L, Altrinetti V, Nanni C, Bianchi P, Cistaro A, Sorrentino S, Cabria M, Pession A, Puntoni M, Villavecchia G, Fanti S. Comparison of 18F-dopa

PET/CT and 123I-MIBG scintigraphy in stage 3 and 4 neuroblastoma: a pilot study. Eur J Nucl Mol Imaging. 2012;39:57–71.
52. Ribeiro RC, Figueiredo B. Childhood adrenocortical tumors. Eur J Cancer. 2004;40(8):1117–26.
53. Lack EE, Mulvihill JJ, Travis WD, Kozakewich HP. Adrenal cortical neoplasms in the pediatric and adolescent age group. Clinicopathological study of 30 cases with emphasis on epidemiological and prognostic factors. Pathol Annu. 1992;27(Pt 1):1–53.
54. Jimenez-Heffernan JA, Hardisson D, Palacios J, Garcia-Viera M, Gamallo C, Nistal M. Adrenal gland leiomyoma in a child with acquired immunodeficiency syndrome. Pediatr Pathol Lab Med. 1995;15(6): 923–6.
55. Lin J, Wasco MJ, Korobkin M, Doherty G, Giordano TJ. Leiomyoma of the adrenal gland presenting as a non-functioning adrenal incidentaloma: case report and review of the literature. Endocr Pathol. 2007; 18(4):239–43.
56. Ammoury RF, Heptulla RA, Tatevian N, Elenberg E. Laparoscopic adrenalectomy of an adrenal adenoma with myelolipoma relieves severe hypertension in a 16-year-old patient. Pediatr Nephrol. 2006;21(3): 433–6.
57. Guo YK, Yang ZG, Li Y, Deng YP, Ma ES, Min PQ, Zhang XC. Uncommon adrenal masses: CT and MRI features with histopathologic correlation. Eur J Radiol. 2007;62(3):359–70.
58. Ciftci AO, Salman AB, Tanyel FC, Hiçsönmez A. Bilateral multiple adrenal pseudoocysts associated with incomplete Beckwith-Wiedemann syndrome. J Pediatr Surg. 1997;32(9):1388–90.
59. Reichelt O, Grieser T, Wunderlich H, Möller A, Schubert J. Bronchogenic cyst. A rare differential diagnosis of retroperitoneal tumors. Urol Int. 2000; 64(4):216–19.
60. Steffens J, Zaubitzer T, Kirsch W, Humke U. Neonatal adrenal abscesses. Eur Urol. 1997;31(3):347–9.
61. Pointe HD, Osika E, Montagne JP, Prudent M, Tournier G, Sebbouh D. Adrenobronchial fistula complicating a neonatal adrenal abscess: treatment by percutaneous aspiration and antibiotics. Pediatr Radiol. 1997;27(2):184–5.

Scrotal Imaging

17

Ronnie G. Fine, Lee Kathleen Collins, and Lane S. Palmer

Introduction

Imaging of the scrotum is the mainstay of the workup of a patient who presents with scrotal pathology. The different imaging modalities that are utilized include ultrasound, MRI, and nuclear scintigraphy, each with different advantages and limitations. Ultrasonography is the most commonly used modality due to its noninvasive nature, high degree of accuracy, low cost, and simplicity [1, 2]. Avoiding the need for ionizing radiation and contrast material is an added benefit when there is a need to image the testes, which are exquisitely sensitive to toxins. The study is interactive, and an experienced radiologist can tailor the study to the patient's history and clinical findings. More recently, the combination of color and power Doppler ultrasound has become the most prevalent method of sonographic evaluation of the testes. It is more sensitive to low-flow states and low velocities, but lacks directionality and has poor temporal resolution [3]. This is of special importance in the pediatric population as the pre-adolescent testes have low blood flow, which may be easily missed on routine Doppler ultrasound.

Nuclear scintigraphy with technetium 99 is used in the evaluation of the acute scrotum in cases that are equivocal on ultrasound. It may be used to differentiate between cases of testicular torsion, requiring emergent surgical intervention, versus a nonsurgical pathology such as epididymitis or orchitis. The benefits of this study must be weighed against the possible delay in treatment in a case of testicular torsion. In equivocal cases, when blood flow is undetectable by color Doppler ultrasound, nuclear scintigraphy may be a powerful tool as it may detect testicular perfusion in age-appropriate low-flow states [4].

Magnetic resonance imaging is another radiographic modality to help elucidate cases that are diagnostically equivocal on ultrasound. Although ultrasound is indispensible in the evaluation of the scrotum, the MRI is an excellent second-line modality when the diagnosis is inconclusive after sonogram [5]. There are characteristics of scrotal solid masses on MRI that may assist in planning surgery and in deciding whether a scrotal mass is malignant or benign and amenable to a partial orchiectomy or nonsurgical management [6].

R.G. Fine, MD (✉)
Division of Pediatric Urology,
Cohen Children's Medical Center of New York,
New Hyde Park, NY, USA

Hofstra North Shore-LIJ School of Medicine,
New Hyde Park, NY, USA
e-mail: rog2003@gmail.com

L.K. Collins, MD
Division of Pediatric Radiology,
Department of Radiology, Long Island Jewish Hospital,
New Hyde Park, NY, USA
e-mail: leekcollins@hotmail.com

L.S. Palmer, MD, FACS, FAAP
Hofstra North Shore-LIJ School of Medicine,
New Hyde Park, NY, USA

Division of Pediatric Urology,
Cohen Children's Medical Center of New York,
Long Island, NY, USA
e-mail: lpalmermd@gmail.com

L.S. Palmer, J.S. Palmer (eds.), *Pediatric and Adolescent Urologic Imaging*,
DOI 10.1007/978-1-4614-8654-1_17, © Springer Science+Business Media New York 2014

Technique

Scrotal ultrasonography is performed with the patient positioned supine and with a support, such as a warm folded towel underneath the scrotal sac for support. The penis should be displaced superiorly or superolaterally and a towel may be draped over it. A scrotal ultrasound scan is performed with a high-frequency (7.5–15-MHz) transducer for optimal resolution. Imaging should be conducted in sequential sagittal and transverse planes, proceeding in a systematic fashion. The first images should be transverse and include both testes side by side to allow comparison of echotexture, echogenicity, size, and flow, as well as documenting the presence of two testicles. The patient should be warm and as comfortable as possible, otherwise the scrotal contents retract and the scrotal skin thickens, making evaluation challenging. Color flow and duplex Doppler are pertinent when assessing testicular perfusion and viability as well as in identifying vascular injuries. It is also important to identify infection and the vascularity of a mass. Pinggera et al. have suggested the use of resistive index as a predictor of testicular dysfunction. They found that RI >0.6 correlates with an abnormal semen analysis or subfertility [7].

Nuclear scanning of the testicle is usually reserved for cases of indeterminate findings on ultrasound performed when testicular torsion is suspected but is not diagnostic. Details regarding performance of the study were described in a previous chapter. Briefly, scrotal scintigraphy is generally performed using technetium 99 for detection of blood flow. Images are typically taken every 3–5 s for 1–2 min.

MRI of the scrotum and testes is used as a second-line radiologic modality to aid in the diagnosis of masses in the scrotum that are indeterminate on ultrasound. A 1.5T magnet is used with a 5-in. (13 cm) coil. Imaging includes a large field of view frame to include the renal vessels to assess for hernias and allow evaluation of the lymph node drainage of the testicles in the retroperitoneum. A high-resolution T2-weighted fast spin echo sequence is used in the axial, sagittal, and coronal planes to image the scrotum. A high-resolution axial T1-weighted spoiled gradient echo sequence is also used to identify hemorrhage. Gadolinium can aid in differentiating between a benign cystic lesion and a cystic neoplasm and can be used to assess for areas of absent or reduced testicular perfusion, such as in segmental testicular infarct [8].

Anatomy

The scrotum is divided into two compartments by a fibromuscular septum. The main components of each scrotal compartment are the testicle and the epididymis, which is located on the posterolateral aspect of the testicle. The epididymis is comprised of a cauda, body, and caput, with the appendix attached to the caput. The average size of the epididymis in an adult is 6–7 cm in length and the epididymal head is 1–1.2 cm in cross section. The body of the epididymis should be less than 4 mm in cross section and the 1–2 mm on average. The appendix testis is a Müllerian remnant, also known as the hydatid of Morgagni, which may be found on the upper pole of the testis. The appendix epididymis (pedunculated hydatid) is found on the caput (head) of the epididymis and is a Wolffian duct remnant.

The arterial supply to the testicle and the venous drainage from the testicle are important components of the scrotal sac, and evaluation of those is a key factor on imaging. Changes to the skin and to the layers surrounding the testicle can also be noted. The potential space between the visceral and parietal layers of the tunica vaginalis, which are a continuation of the visceral and parietal peritoneum, may be commented upon.

Testicular arterial supply includes the testicular (gonadal) artery, the vasal artery, and the cremasteric artery. The vasal artery is a branch of the internal iliac artery, the gonadal artery is a branch off of the aorta, and the cremasteric artery is a branch off of the inferior epigastric. The majority of the blood supply to the testicle is derived from the gonadal artery [9]. The venous drainage is mainly a function of the pampiniform plexus, which may be dilated and result in a finding of a varicocele. This plexus drains into the internal iliac vein bilaterally as well as the gonadal vein which empties into the renal vein on the left and the aorta on the right [10].

The adult testicle is an elliptical structure which measures on average 25 ml by orchidometer and14 ml by ultrasound. Its dimensions are 4–5 cm longitudinally and 2.5 cm across. The size of the testicle in the pediatric population according to the patient's age was measured sonographically and reported in several studies. The size of the testicle increases significantly in the first 5 months of life, from 0.27 ml to 0.44 ml. By 9 months of age the testicle is 0.31 ml on average and remains stable in size until puberty [11]. Goede et al. collected data from 932 patients age 6 months to 18 years and found that the mean testicle volume at age 1 was 0.48 ml, at age 10 it was 0.97 ml, and at age 18 it was 13.73 ml. The greatest variability was found at age 14, where the range was 1.69–19.98 [12].

The spermatic cord is also evaluated sonographically, as it may harbor pathologies such as a mass, hydrocele, hernia, or varicocele. Normally the cord is comprised of the testicular vasculature, the vas deference, as well as nerves and lymphatics that drain the testicle directly into the retroperitoneal lymph nodes.

Ultrasound is the primary imaging study of the scrotum and its contents (Fig. 17.1). The testes should have a homogenous echotexture surrounded by the tunica vaginalis which is not visible in the absence of a hydrocele. A hyperechoic stripe that is parallel to the epididymis represents the mediastinum testis. The epididymis sits superior to the testis and is normally iso- or hypoechoic to the adjacent testicle. The individual components of the spermatic cord are not discernible by ultrasound, but bidirectional flow may be discerned by Doppler. This can be challenging in the prepubertal child.

Normal testes are homogeneous in appearance on MR imaging. There is intermediate signal intensity on T1-weighted images and high signal intensity on T2-weighted images relative to skeletal muscle (Fig. 17.2). The epididymis is similar to testicular parenchyma on T1-weighted images, but low signal intensity on T2-weighted images. The tunica albuginea is low signal intensity on both T1- and T2-weighted images. The mediastinum testis will be a low-signal band posterior in the testicle on T2-weighted images. Normal testis parenchyma is

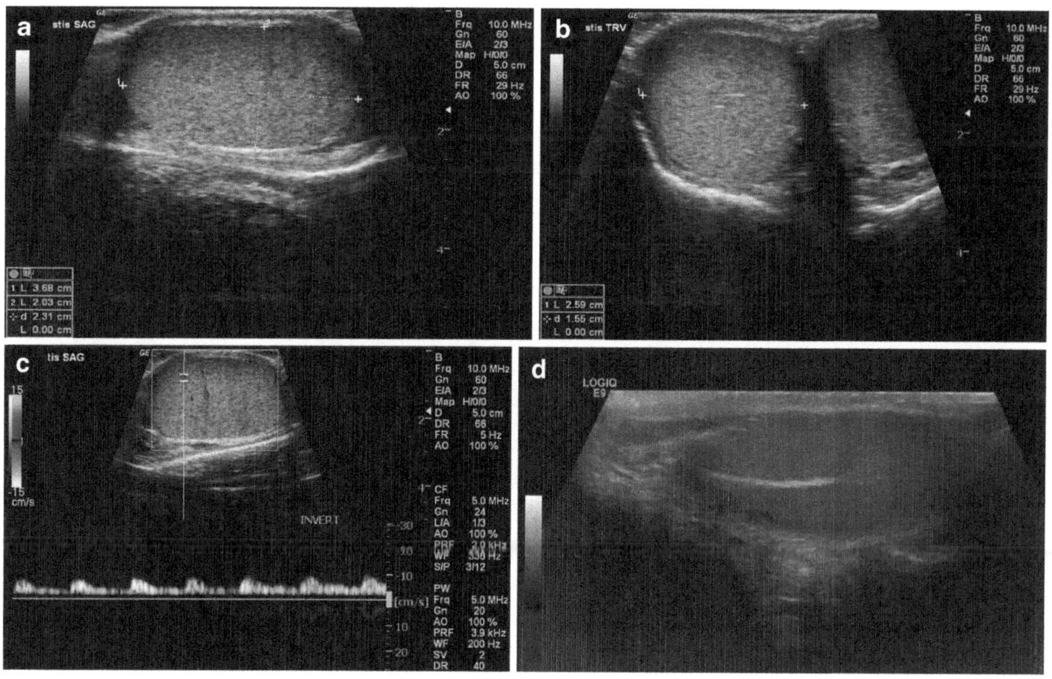

Fig. 17.1 Normal testis. Sagittal (**a**) and transverse (**b**) views of normal testes demonstrating homogeneous parenchyma. The markers take measurements of testicular size in both dimensions. Spectral Doppler tracing of a normal testis measured from a vessel noted in color Doppler (**c**). The mediastinum testis is seen as a hyperechoic stripe in the mid-testis (**d**)

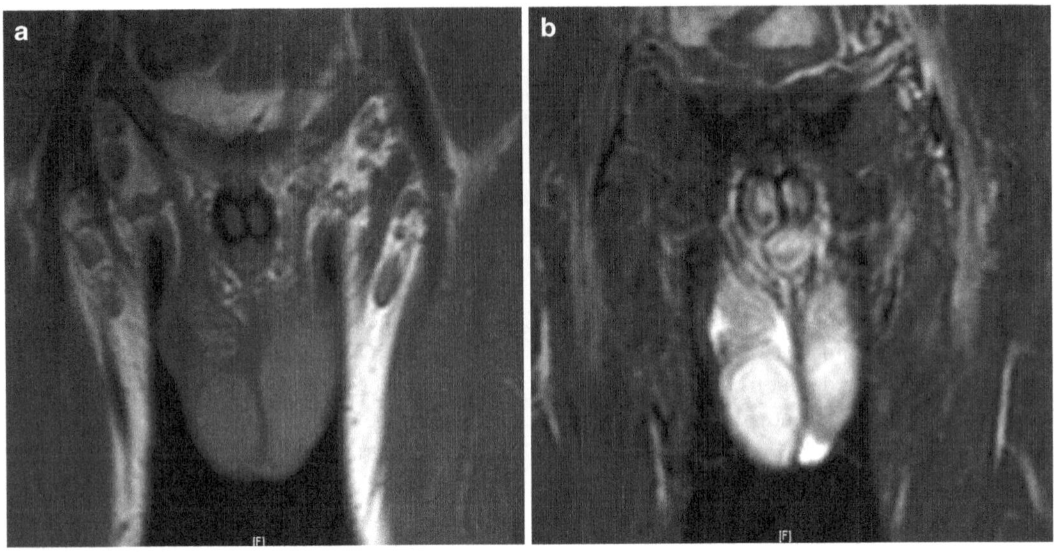

Fig. 17.2 Normal testis. MR images demonstrating the normal testes from a young teen imaged for osteomyelitis of the hip. The T1 images (**a**) demonstrate the hypointense testes in the scrotum. The T2 image (**b**) demonstrates the hyperintense ovoid structures in the scrotum. The size discrepancy reflects their position within the scrotum

homogenous in attenuation and enhancement on CT examinations. CT is not typically used to image testicle pathology, but rather to image the chest, abdomen, and pelvis for testicular cancer staging.

Acute Scrotum

The acute scrotum provides a unique radiological dilemma as interpretation of ultrasound findings relies on the clinical history. A detorsion event may present with similar findings as an epididymitis or epididymal torsion. This underscores the importance of obtaining a good history and maintaining open communication between the radiologist and the clinician.

Testicular Torsion

Testicular torsion is the single most common emergency within the realm of pediatric urology. Torsion can occur at any age but is most common in 12–18-year-old adolescents. Recovery of the testicle is most likely within the first 6 h after the event, after which testicular salvage rates drop precipitously. The etiology in the adolescent population is due to a bell-clapper deformity in which the tunica vaginalis encircles the epididymis, distal spermatic cord, and the testis rather than attaching to the posterolateral aspect of the testis. The deformity leaves the testis free to swing and rotate within the tunica vaginalis, as a clapper inside a bell.

The diagnosis of testicular torsion is primarily reliant on the clinical presentation. A typical history is a sudden onset of extreme and unremitting testicular pain that may or may not be associated with physical activity. Clinically, the patient is in severe pain, has difficulty ambulating, and may experience nausea and vomiting. The testicle is tender and in an abnormal transverse, high-riding lie, while the scrotum is erythematous. The cremasteric reflex is typically absent on the affected side and the Prehn's maneuver is negative, i.e., there is no pain relief with elevation of the testicle. Attempts at scoring systems have been made but are not yet widely used [13].

Ultrasonography has been shown as highly reliable in diagnosis of the acute scrotum in the emergency department, with a sensitivity of 94 %, specificity of 96 %, and accuracy of 95.5 % [2]. Radiographically, the appearance of the testicle changes according to the degree of torsion and the time since the onset of the event. In complete torsion (540–720° twisting), the testis may

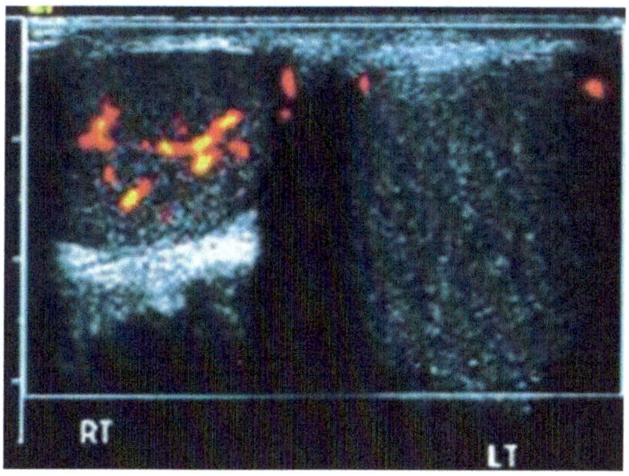

Fig. 17.3 Left testicular torsion for 5 h. Transverse images of the scrotum demonstrate the absence of flow and enlargement consistent with engorgement and edema

have normal echotexture with absent blood flow very early in the process. After 4–6 h, the testis is enlarged, the parenchyma may appear normal or have some patchy hypoechoic areas present, and the blood flow is still absent (Fig. 17.3). Additional findings include enlargement of the epididymis, thickening of the scrotal skin, as well as the presence of a reactive hydrocele. Sonographic examination of the cord may demonstrate a whirlpool sign, representing the twisted congested vessels of the cord [14]. Kalfa et al. determined that sonography of the spermatic cord is highly sensitive and specific for the diagnosis of acute torsion [15]. Decreased blood flow may be seen with a partial torsion of 180–360°, where there is a longer window of viability to the testicle.

Torsion longer than 24 h may clinically present with diminished pain due to the presence of a completely infarcted and unsalvageable testicle. Sonographically the testicle appears to have heterogeneous echotexture and absent blood flow, and it is surrounded by reactive hyperemia [16]. It may be enlarged in size and contain areas of decreased echogenicity (Fig. 17.4).

Flow velocity is evaluated by Doppler ultrasound. In the prepubertal patient, it may be challenging to detect blood flow. The addition of power Doppler increases blood flow detection rate from 80 to 90 % in that age group. The velocity scale should be set to the lowest setting in order to increase the sensitivity to flow detection. Spectral Doppler sonography allows for comparison between the two testicles and findings of asymmetry in blood flow. The diagnostic accuracy of ultrasound is equivalent to that of nuclear scanning; however, the two modalities may be complementary in cases of uncertain diagnosis.

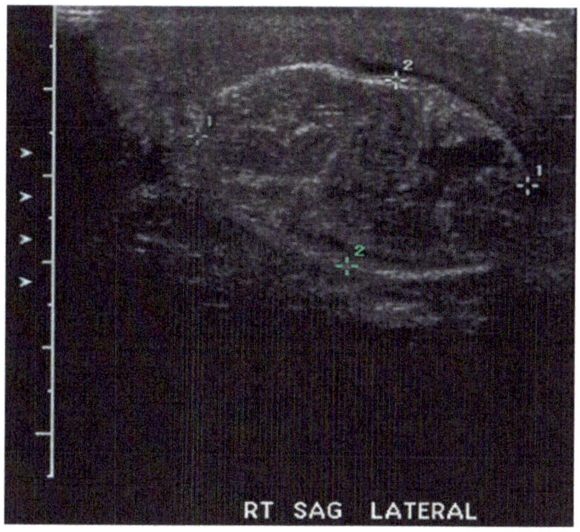

Fig. 17.4 Missed torsion. Sagittal view of the right testis on a 16-year-old male 18 h after the onset of testicular pain demonstrating heterogeneity of the parenchyma. Doppler flow was not demonstrable on the left. The left testis was normal

Scintigraphy and sonography show similar high sensitivity for the diagnosis of testicular torsion; however, in equivocal cases these modalities can complement one another to further increase the diagnostic accuracy [17, 18] (Fig. 17.5). In a multi-institutional review of 130 pediatric patients with acute scrotal pain, Baker et al. demonstrated 89 % sensitivity and 99 % specificity for color Doppler ultrasonography for differentiating testicular torsion from other nonsurgical etiologies. The mean age at the time of ultrasonography was 11 years. Seventeen patients were suspected to have testicular torsion and were emergently explored. The remainder of outcomes was obtained by clinical follow-up with outpatient sonograms. The mean length of follow-up was 1.3 years, but 23 % of patients were lost to follow-up and could not be evaluated. There were two cases of missed testicular torsion which resulted in delayed testis atrophy and one case that underwent surgical exploration for a torsed epididymal appendage [17].

These limitations were addressed by Lam et al. in a large single institution review of 626 patients

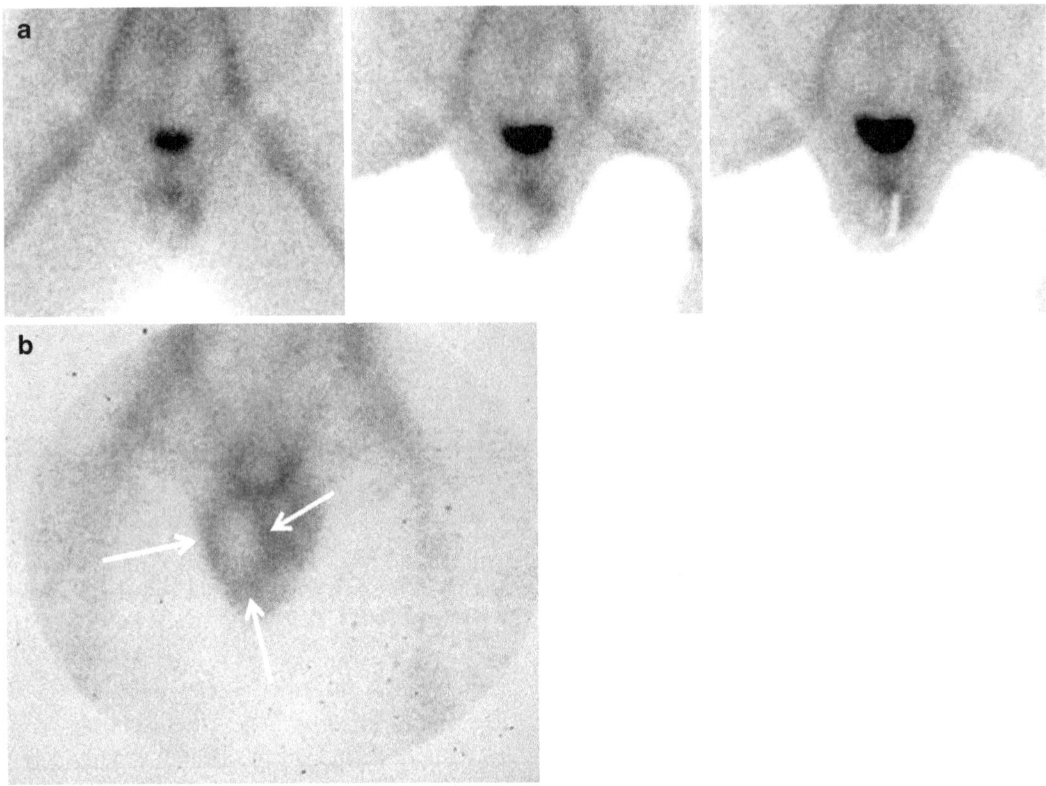

Fig. 17.5 Nuclear scintigraphy of two boys with acute onset of testicular pain. (**a**) There is a paucity of uptake of tracer in the right hemiscrotum after pain of 5 h duration (*arrow*). (**b**) There is absence of flow but surrounding hyperemia (*arrows*) on the right hemiscrotum after 24 h of pain consistent with a missed torsion

who presented with acute scrotal pain. Forty-seven percent were explored immediately, leaving 332 (53 %) who underwent initial color Doppler US at time of presentation. Mean age was 8 years, and all patients had at least 2 weeks follow-up. Nine patients showed no flow on color Doppler US, and all were confirmed as testicular torsion upon exploration. Four of 323 patients who were found to have normal or increased flow on sonogram and explored based on clinical suspicion were found to have testicular torsion. Overall, color Doppler US yielded nine true-positive results and 319 true-negative results out of 332 which computes to a sensitivity of 69 %, specificity of 100 %, and an accuracy of 98.8 % [18].

Other authors have demonstrated better sensitivity for Doppler US in older patients. Yagil et al. report their results using Doppler US as a screening tool in the ED for triage of patients with acute scrotum. The patients studied were slightly older than in prior series, with a mean age of 16 years. In this review of over 620 patients, testicular torsion was suspected by Doppler US in 20 patients and confirmed via surgical exploration in 18. There were two false positives and one false negative. The reported study sensitivity, specificity, and accuracy were 94, 96, and 95.5 %. The only false-negative exam occurred in a 3-year-old boy who had present, but slightly diminished flow in the affected testicle. Surgical exploration due to a high index of clinical suspicion revealed torsion. This outstanding diagnostic accuracy may be due in part to an older study population which may have improved the performance of Doppler US in detecting arterial flow [19].

Other authors have noted that Doppler US is often user dependent and that documenting flow in the prepubertal testis can be unreliable [20–23]. An oft-quoted report by Ingram et al. showed that in 50 normal boys ranging in age from 2 months to 13 years, blood flow could be detected by color Doppler in both testes in only 58 % of boys and 34 % had no detectable flow [21]. Albrecht et al. report similar abilities of color and power Doppler to detect testicular blood flow in normal prepubertal boys (69 % vs. 65 %), with the combination of the two marginally better at 79 % [20]. This was confirmed in a prospective comparison by Blask et al. of scintigraphy and Doppler ultrasonography in 46 children who presented with an acute scrotum in which flow was demonstrated in the asymptomatic testis in only 60 % [24].

Appendix Testis/Epididymis Torsion

Torsion of an appendix is most common in 6–12-year-old patients. The clinical presentation is acute onset of pain, limited to the superior pole of the testicle at the level of the appendix. The occasional finding of a blue dot seen through the scrotal skin is due to ischemia and necrosis of the appendage. Sonographically the epididymis and sometimes the entire testicle are inflamed, and on occasion the enlarged and avascular appendix can be seen and palpated due to swelling and hyperemia. Treatment is symptomatic relief with nonsteroidal anti-inflammatory agents and scrotal elevation.

Epididymitis/Orchitis

These entities are common causes of an acute scrotum in the pediatric population. The onset is more gradual than that of testicular or appendix torsion, and it may be accompanied by fevers. In prepubertal patients the cause is usually nonbacterial and may be related to dysfunctional voiding. In the postpubescent patient this is usually related to retrograde spread of infection or to chemical irritation of the epididymis secondary to reflux of urine. In sexually active patients, this may be associated with the spread of a sexually transmitted disease. Sonographically, the epididymis and/or testis appear hyperemic and hypervascular, enlarged, and hypoechoic (Fig. 17.6). Reactive hydroceles and scrotal edema are also

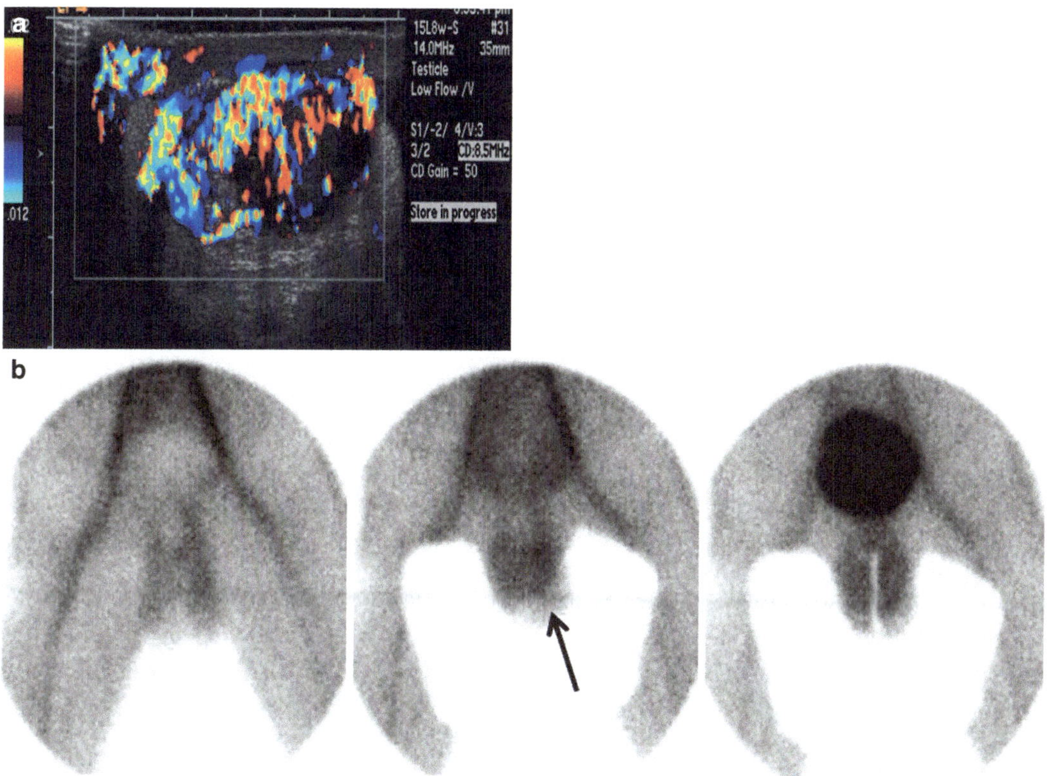

Fig. 17.6 Ultrasound (**a**) and nuclear scintigraphy (**b**) demonstrating the features of epididymo-orchitis. Increased Doppler flow is noted on ultrasound to both the testicle and epididymis when compared to the asymptomatic side. There is increased uptake of nuclear tracer to the left hemiscrotum (arrow)

common findings. Nuclear perfusion scintigraphy studies using technetium 99 rely on flow images showing abnormal increased testicular perfusion, as well as static pictures showing a "cold" defect in the area of hydrocele (Fig. 17.6). Inflammatory conditions are characterized by diffusely increased uptake of radiotracer into the affected testicle. A study by Mueller et al. found that when supplementing scintigraphy with sonography, the interpretation was changed in 14 % of cases, which spared 31 % of patients from a surgical procedure [18].

Trauma

The main objective of a sonographic evaluation is to assess whether there is presence of blood flow to the testicle and to identify whether the tunica albuginea surrounding the testicle is intact, as absence of flow or the presence of testicular rupture are indications for scrotal exploration. Indeterminate findings or high clinical suspicion is also an indication for exploration.

In testicular rupture there is extrusion of seminiferous tubules out of the testicle, and the tunica appears discontinuous. Salvage rate of testicular rupture is upwards of 90 % even after 72 h post-trauma. Buckley and McAninch reported that the finding of heterogeneous parenchyma and irregular contour had 100 % sensitivity and 93.5 % specificity for the diagnosis of testicular rupture [19] (Fig. 17.7).

Contusions can be seen as a hypoechoic area, but are not indications for scrotal exploration if the tunica albuginea is intact. A testicular fracture is a break in the parenchyma of the testis without a tear in the tunica albuginea. It will appear as a linear hypoechoic band and may be managed nonoperatively if there are no abnormalities in Doppler flow imaging.

Hematomas may occur anywhere within the scrotum following trauma. Acute injury is represented by a hyperechoic dense fluid collection whereas an older bleed will be hypoechoic and without vascularity. The fluid collection of a hematoma is usually complex and heterogeneous.

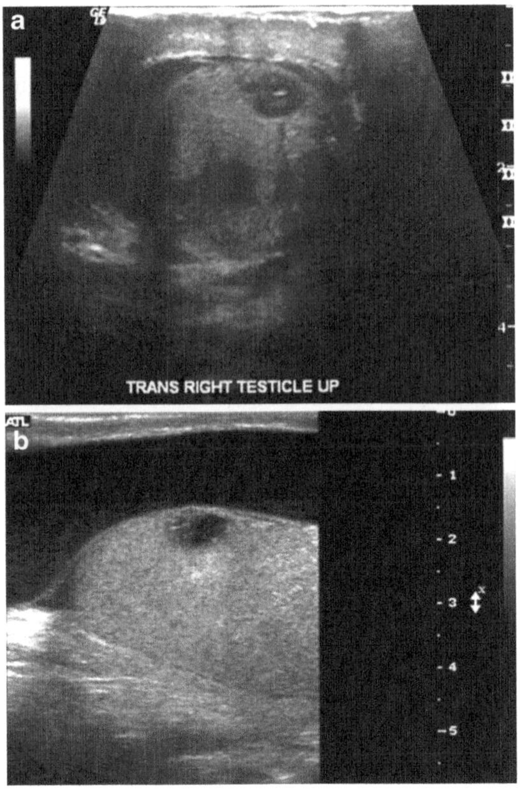

Fig. 17.7 Trauma. Transverse view of the right testis demonstrating several hematomas within the testis, a surrounding hematocele and thickening of the overlying skin following blunt trauma (**a**). The same testis several weeks later demonstrating an isolated remnant hypoechoic area and a large hydrocele (**b**)

Hematoceles are complex fluid collections that separate the visceral and parietal layers of the tunica vaginalis. In the acute setting they appear hyperechoic and become hypoechoic with time [20].

Pyocele/Abscess

Pyoceles are rare in the pediatric population [21]. Its presence is suggested by the clinical history, which usually includes prior surgery or a scrotal or perineal skin infection. Acute pain, fevers, and an elevated white blood cell count are present. The physical findings may include a tender and swollen scrotum, erythema, edema, and a tense hydrocele, which may be confused with an acute torsion of the testicle. An abscess may be suggested radiographically by the presence of complex multiloculated scrotal fluid collection containing debris, thickened tunica vaginalis, and heterogeneous echogenic areas. Color Doppler will demonstrate peripheral hypervascularity without internal blood flow [22]; however, blood flow to the testicle should appear preserved.

Vasculitis

Systemic processes such as Henoch-Schonlein purpura (HSP) may affect the testicle in approximately 15 % of cases. In some patients, scrotal symptoms are the initial clinical manifestation of this disease process. The patient with HSP usually has cutaneous symptoms such as lower extremity petechiae, as well as renal and rheumatologic symptoms. The scrotum is painful and enlarged [23]. Ultrasound examination will reveal enlarged epididymis and thickened scrotal skin, as well as reactive hydroceles. Testicular blood flow is usually maintained or increased (Fig. 17.8). Nuclear scintigraphy is also diagnostic in such cases for epididymo-orchitis, which demonstrate increased perfusion to the testis [23, 24].

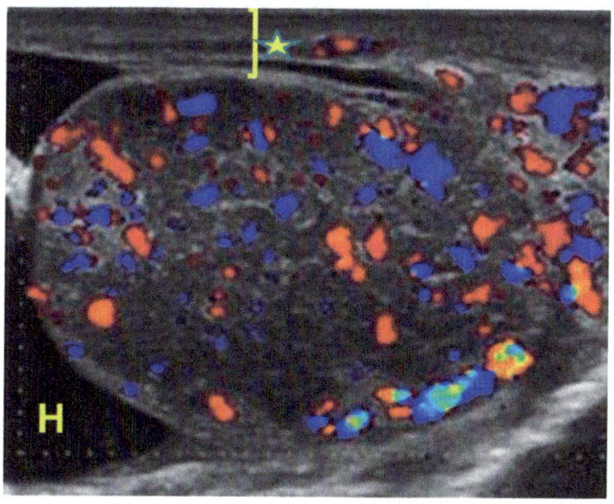

Fig. 17.8 Vasculitis. An 8-year-old boy presented with scrotal pain and a papular rash on the legs. While the diagnosis of Henoch-Schonlein purpura was made, concurrent testicular torsion could not be excluded by history and physical examination. The constellation of ultrasound findings of thickened scrotal skin (*bracket-star*) maintained or increased color Doppler flow, and the presence of a hydrocele (*H*) is all consistent with the diagnosis of HSP

Hydrocele/Hernia

The processus vaginalis is an extension of the parietal peritoneum, which envelops the testicle in two layers as it descends into the scrotum during embryogenesis. The processus vaginalis is normally obliterated in the 7–9 months of gestation, but in approximately 20 % of males the processus vaginalis is patent at birth, resulting in a potential space. In most cases this will resolve by 1 year of age, and many males with a patent processus vaginalis are asymptomatic. Sonographically, the two layers of the tunica vaginalis can appear as isoechoic to hyperechoic linear bands extending from the internal inguinal ring to the scrotum. Pediatric hydroceles are commonly due to an indirect hernia, which is a consequence of a patent processus vaginalis that allows for free communication of peritoneal fluid with the scrotum, and fluid accumulation. Those hydroceles are reducible, and the scrotal sac contents are seen to change in size throughout the day and with different activities. In the noncommunicating variant, the hydrocele sac size is fixed, as it is not in communication with the peritoneal fluid [25]. Hernias may not communicate with the tunica vaginalis, and the fluid may be able to be tracked distally from the groin and seen to end proximal to the testis (Fig. 17.9).

Hydroceles are usually diagnosed clinically, and imaging is not indicated. If imaging is obtained for inconclusive cases, the hernia is sonographically represented by hypoechoic fluid collection within the tunica vaginalis, and the scrotal hydrocele is the peritoneal fluid surrounding the testicle (Fig. 17.10). In the pediatric population these are usually simple fluid collections without septations unless there is a history of infection or trauma. Herniation of bowel via a patent processus vaginalis is more common in the premature infant, in which the inguinal canal is very short as the internal and external rings are almost overlying each other at birth, and the patency of the processus vaginalis is large relative to the abdominal contents. In cases of suspected bowel incarceration, plain radiographs can be use to augment ultrasound findings by detecting bowel gas in the scrotum. Echogenic bowel mucosa or bowel motility can be detected sonographically [26].

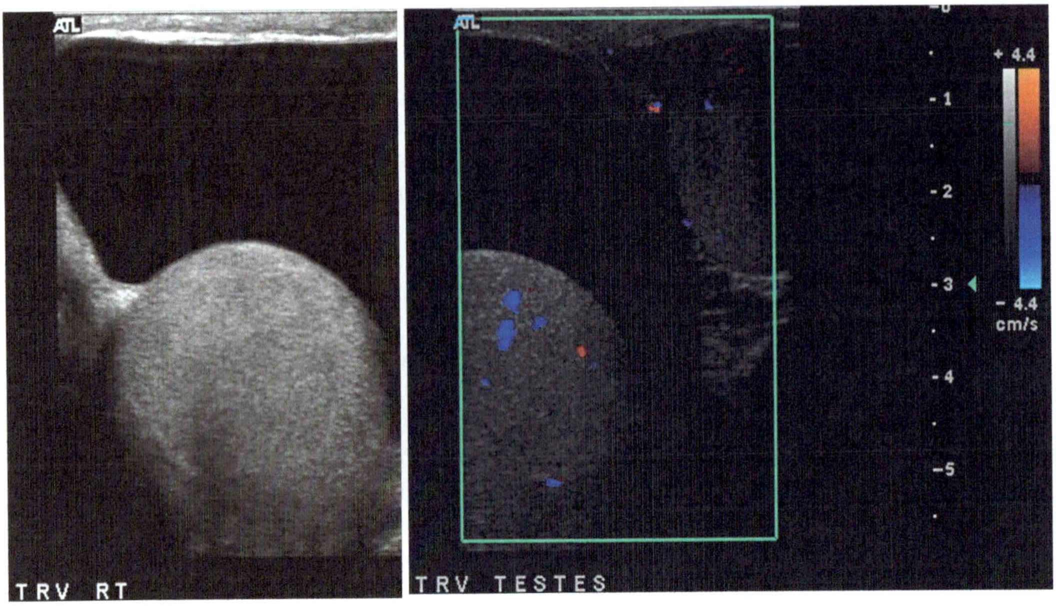

Fig. 17.9 Hydrocele. Anechoic space is seen in the right hemiscrotum that surrounds the testis. The superior margin of this collection was noted

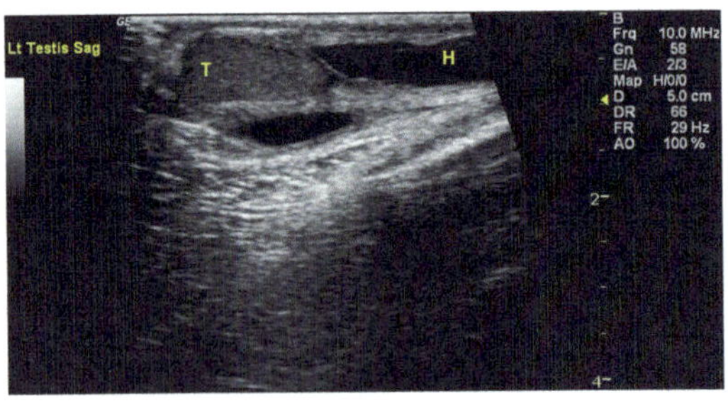

Fig. 17.10 Hernia. Sagittal view of an ultrasound performed in a 6-year-old boy with an inguinal swelling. A longitudinal hypoechoic area (*H*) is noted in the inguinal area superior to the testis (*T*). This was consistent with a left inguinal hernia which was confirmed at surgery

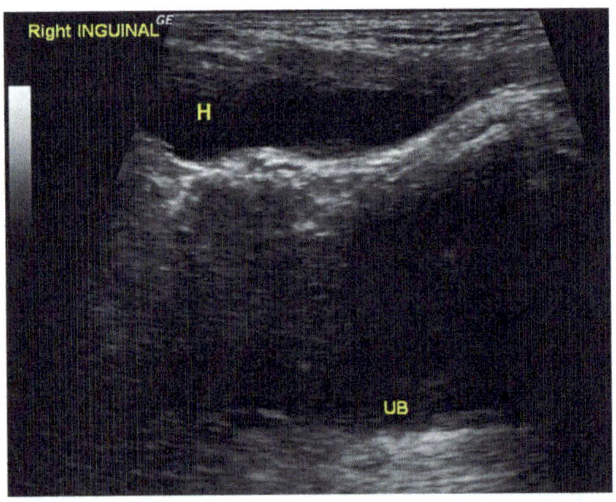

Fig. 17.11 Hydrocele of the spermatic cord. Sagittal view of the inguinal canal in a child who felt a "lump" in the inguinal canal. This area was limited to the spermatic cord on physical examination. The hypoechoic area (*H*) was well defined with normal cord superior and inferior to this area. Bladder (*UB*)

Hydrocele of the spermatic cord may present as an inguinal swelling, with or without pain (Fig. 17.11). It is a rare finding, present is about 1–5 % of cases with inguinal symptoms. Similar to the scrotal hydrocele, the spermatic cord hydrocele emanates from a patent processus vaginalis. This finding may have several variants: the encysted hydrocele, the reducible or funicular hydrocele, and the mixed variety. The encysted hydrocele does not communicate with the peritoneal cavity and therefore cannot be reduced. The funicular hydrocele appears as a peritoneal diverticulum into the inguinal canal that terminates above the scrotum. Occasionally there may be multiple cysts along the spermatic cord, which may appear as beads along the spermatic cord when studied sonographically [25]. In a study assessing the utility of scrotal ultrasound in the diagnosis of a hydrocele of the cord, 3,486 sonograms in 1,743 pediatric patients were reviewed. All patients presented with a mass or swelling of the inguinal region. Of those, 27 patients were diagnosed sonographically with a hydrocele of the cord after finding of an anechoic, avascular mass along the spermatic cord. Only one of these patients was clinically diagnosed with this entity, reflecting the lack of awareness of this diagnosis as well as its rarity [27, 28].

Varicocele

Dilated testicular veins are found in 10–13 % of adolescents and are more common on the left side. Isolated right varicocele or one that does not decompress in the supine position should prompt a workup of an abdominal or pelvic pathology. The association of varicoceles with testicular failure and with infertility is well established; however, the mechanism by which unilateral varicoceles have this bilateral effect remains controversial. This pathology is usually treated in adolescents when hypotrophy of the affected testicle is greater than 20 % as compared to the contralateral testicle. Varicoceles are rarely associated with pain or discomfort, and if severe they may be visible and deform the scrotum. Grade 1 is palpated only on Valsalva; grade 2 is easily palpable, but not visible; grade 3 is visible.

Sonographic evaluation of a varicocele is done both in the supine and standing positions, while performing Valsalva maneuvers. On ultrasound the varicocele appears as an anechoic serpiginous vein greater than 3 mm at rest and retrograde flow with increased vein diameter on Valsalva maneuver (Fig. 17.12). Grading of varicocele depends on sonographic evaluation. Grade 0, subclinical varicocele, is found only on sonogram, but not clinically detectable. High flow rates (>38 cm/s) were strongly associated with testicular volume asymmetry [29].

Ultrasound classification of varicocele grade 1 is characterized by the detection of a prolonged reflux in vessels in the inguinal channel only during Valsalva, while scrotal varicosity is not

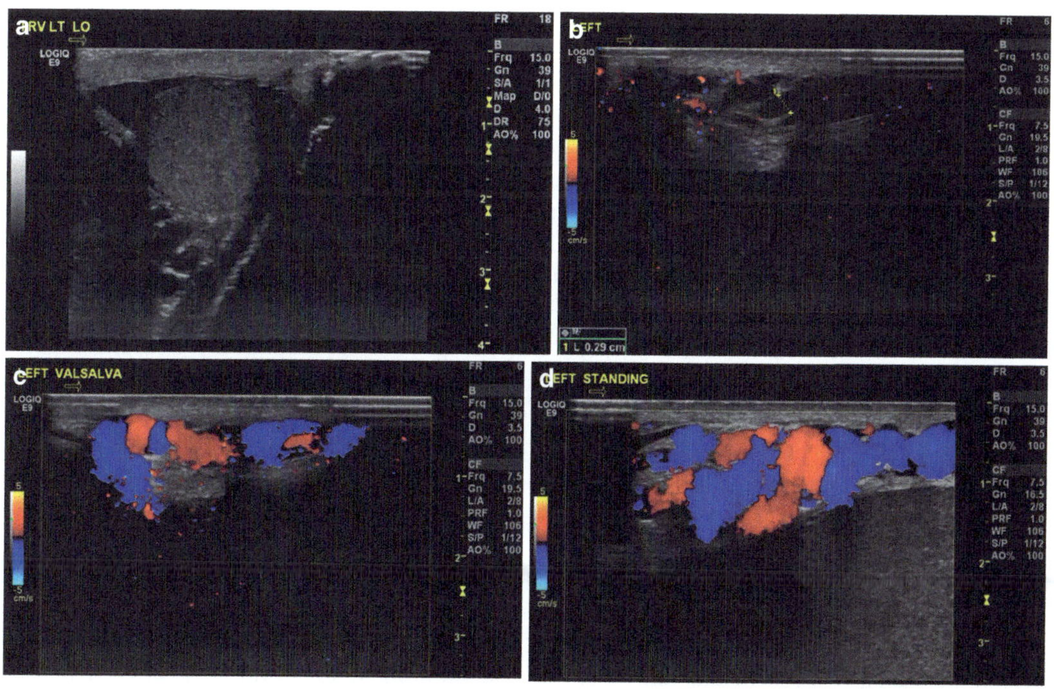

Fig. 17.12 Varicocele. Transverse (**a**) and sagittal (**b**) ultrasound images of the left testis demonstrate hypoechoic spaces inferior and superior to the testis. Color Doppler flow increases considerably with the patent moves from the supine (**c**) to the standing (**d**) position consistent with a varicocele

evident in the previous grayscale study. Grade 2 is characterized by a small posterior varicosity that reaches the superior pole of the testis and whose diameter increases after Valsalva. The ultrasound evaluation clearly demonstrates the presence of a venous reflux in the supratesticular region only during Valsalva. Vessels that appear enlarged at the inferior pole of the testis only when the patient is evaluated in a standing position characterize grade 3. Ultrasound demonstrates a clear reflux only under Valsalva. Grade 4 is diagnosed if vessels appear enlarged, even if the patient is studied in a supine position; dilatation increases in an upright position and during Valsalva. Enhancement of the venous reflux after Valsalva is the criterion that allows the distinction between this grade from the previous and the next one. Hypotrophy of the testis is common at this stage. Grade 5 is characterized by an evident venous dilation even in an upright position. Ultrasound demonstrates the presence of an important basal venous reflux that does not increase after Valsalva [30].

Microlithiasis

Microlithiasis are small (2–3 mm) calcified intratesticular lesions that may be found within the testicular parenchyma. These microcalcifications represent incompletely phagocytized degenerated cellular remnants within the seminiferous tubules. They are usually discovered incidentally when an ultrasound of the scrotum is performed for other reasons including scrotal pain; however, they do not appear to be associated with the etiology of the pain. Furthermore, most likely do not have an association with future testicular malignancy [31]. There is a suggested association with certain pathologies such as Down's syndrome and Klinefelter's syndrome, as well as with infertility and testicular germ cell tumors [32]. Sonographically, they appear as multiple, small (2–3 mm), non-shadowing, echogenic foci found within the testicular parenchyma, defined as the presence of ≥5 echogenic foci per transducer field in one testicle. There occasionally may be a comet tail artifact, which is a form of reverberation artifact seen on grayscale ultrasound of the highly reflective object characteristic of microlithiasis (Fig. 17.13).

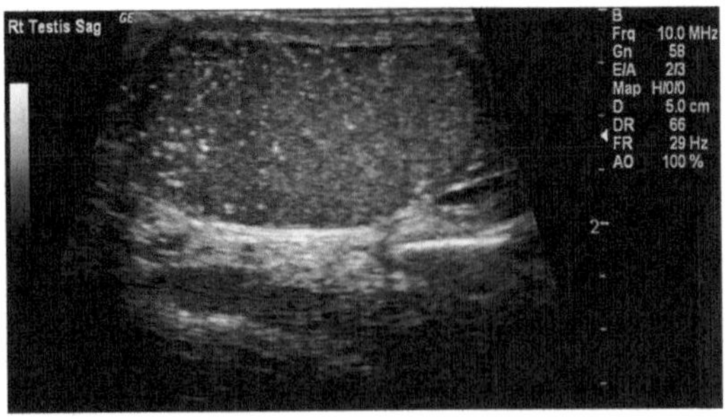

Fig. 17.13 Microlithiasis. Punctate hyperechoic areas are noted primarily in the superior portion of this right testis. Microlithiasis may be present diffusely in the testis or more localized as in this case

Cryptorchidism

The incidence of cryptorchidism is about 3 % at birth and is more common in premature infants and males with Down's syndrome. But by age 1 year, approximately 2/3 of these testes will descend leaving 0.8–1 % of boys requiring management, typically surgical. The incidence of infertility increases when both testes are undescended, when either or both testes are intra-abdominal, and when there is delay in providing descent. After age 2 years, degenerative changes can be seen histologically. In addition, the risk of malignancy is also noted to be higher in cryptorchid testes, and this may improve when early orchidopexy is performed. The undescended testicle is usually smaller from the descended one found in the inguinal canal or pelvis adjacent to the urinary bladder. The judicious use of imaging for localization should be employed as most testes that are beyond the internal inguinal ring should be palpable, except, perhaps the use of ultrasound in the obese child. MR is expensive and does not carry 100 % accuracy thus not precluding subsequent surgical management. If the undescended testis is detected, it is smaller than expected and hypoechoic compared to its partner (Fig. 17.14). An image of the mediastinum testis can serve to distinguish it from the surrounding lymph nodes. Ultrasound is only indicated in cases of ambiguous genitalia [33]. On MR coronal T1-weighted images may reveal the ovoid structure with low signal intensity of the gubernaculum or spermatic cord which can lead to the testes. T2-weighted images will reveal a hyperintense testis located in the abdomen or pelvis (Fig. 17.15)

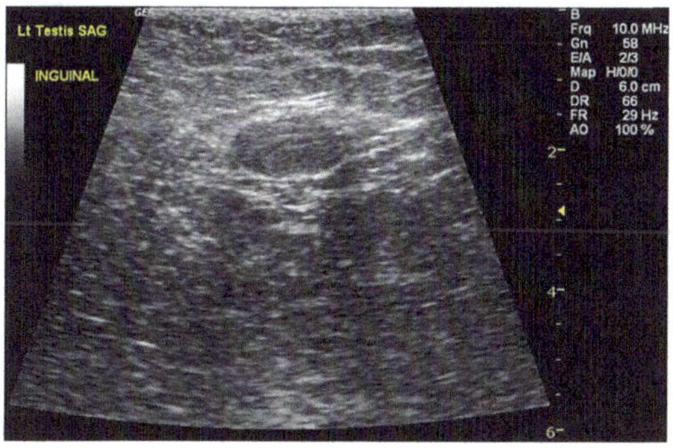

Fig. 17.14 Cryptorchidism. Imaging for an undescended testis may be effective in select cases. Ultrasound may identify (*left*) a testis in the inguinal canal in obese children as an oval homogenous structure that appears very different from the surrounding muscle and fat. MR may be useful in the case of a non-palpable testis

Lymphoma/Leukemia

Infiltrative malignancies such as lymphoma or leukemia may show enhanced vascularity that is similar in pattern to that of orchitis, and therefore the clinical history is of utmost importance in these cases. Leukemic infiltration of the testicle appears as gross enlargement and diffuse hypervascularity. These pathologies can rarely present initially with testicular finding, and therefore a high index of suspicion must be maintained. Sonography will show a diffusely hypoechoic enlarged testis or one with multifocal hypoechoic regions (Fig. 17.16). The process may be bilateral. The testicles are notably a privileged site due to the testis-blood barrier, and therefore recurrence of leukemia is possible posttreatment as chemotherapeutic agents do not cross the barrier effectively [34]. On MRI, one may see similar findings of diffuse replacement of the testicle by infiltrate by tumor, with iso- to hyperintensity on T1-weighted and hypointensity on T2-weighted images [6].

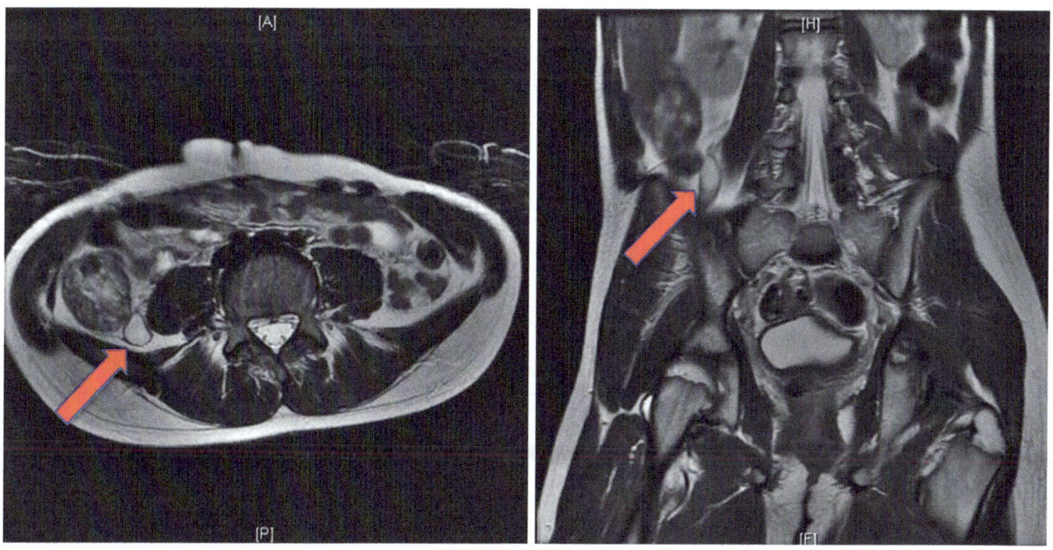

Fig. 17.15 Cryptorchidism. MR may be helpful in identifying an intra-abdominal testis. On these T2-weighted axial (*left*) and coronal (*right*) images, the hyperintense ovoid structure is an undescended testis (*red arrow*) located lateral to the right psoas muscle and adjacent to the mid-ascending colon within the mid-retroperitoneal abdomen

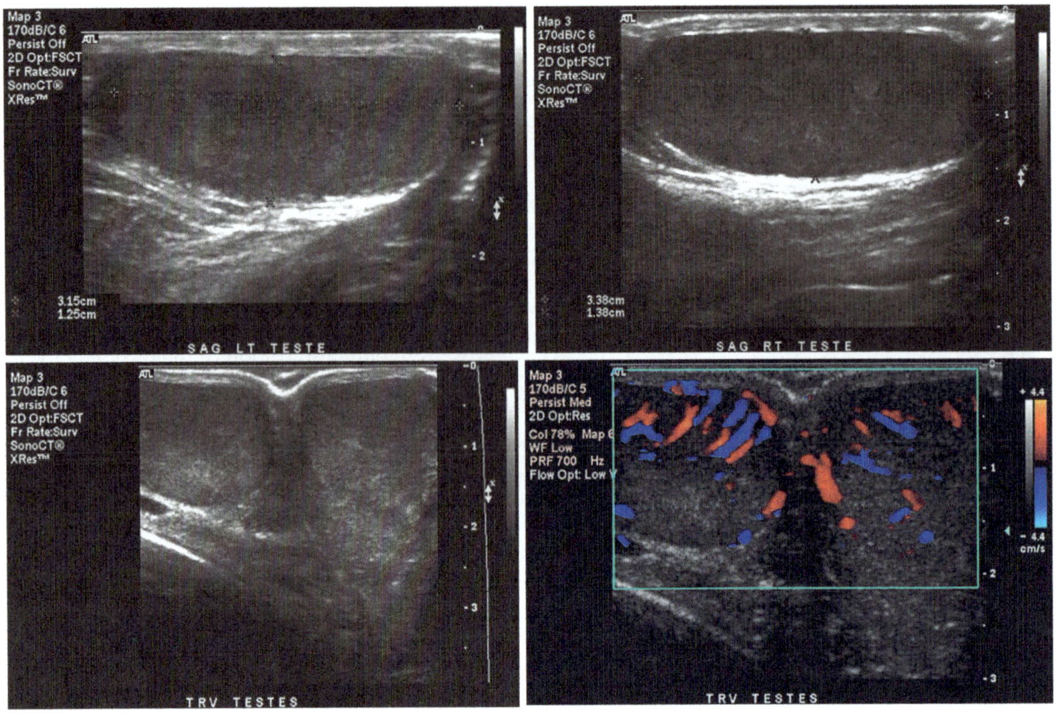

Fig. 17.16 Transverse and sagittal images of the scrotum in a child with acute lymphoblastic leukemia. In this case there is enlargement of both testes with patchy areas of decreased echogenicity and increased color Doppler flow

Masses

Sonograms are commonly used to characterize a testicular mass suspected on physical exam due to the high sensitivity of the test, its availability, and low cost. However, imaging is rarely diagnostic as to the type of tumor and the associated prognosis, which is usually obtained after orchiectomy and pathological analysis. Some patients with certain risk factors such as contralateral testis cancer will have periodical testicular scans to detect masses early, even before the mass is palpable, as sonography can detect masses 3–5 mm in size. Patients with a history of an undescended testicle are at increased risk of developing a malignancy later in life, and some patients may elect to undergo annual sonography for early detection of a tumor, particularly if the position of the testicle was not corrected or corrected after infancy. The incidental finding of microlithiasis in an otherwise normal testis may prompt some practitioners to initiate yearly surveillance for the development of testicular germ cell neoplasia, although this association is controversial.

A testicular mass in a prepubescent child is more likely to be benign, where as a postpubescent child with a testicular mass is highly suspicious for a malignant tumor. Therefore, the clinical history is very important in establishing a diagnosis, as many tumors may appear similar on imaging. In general, the larger the mass, the more vascularized it appears on color Doppler imaging. It is important to note that sonography is not diagnostic for the type of malignancy, and therefore an excisional biopsy or orchiectomy is warranted.

Malignant Germ Cell Tumors

Seminoma

Seminomas are the primary testicular malignancy in the postpubertal population and are not found in the prepubescent population. Sonography may

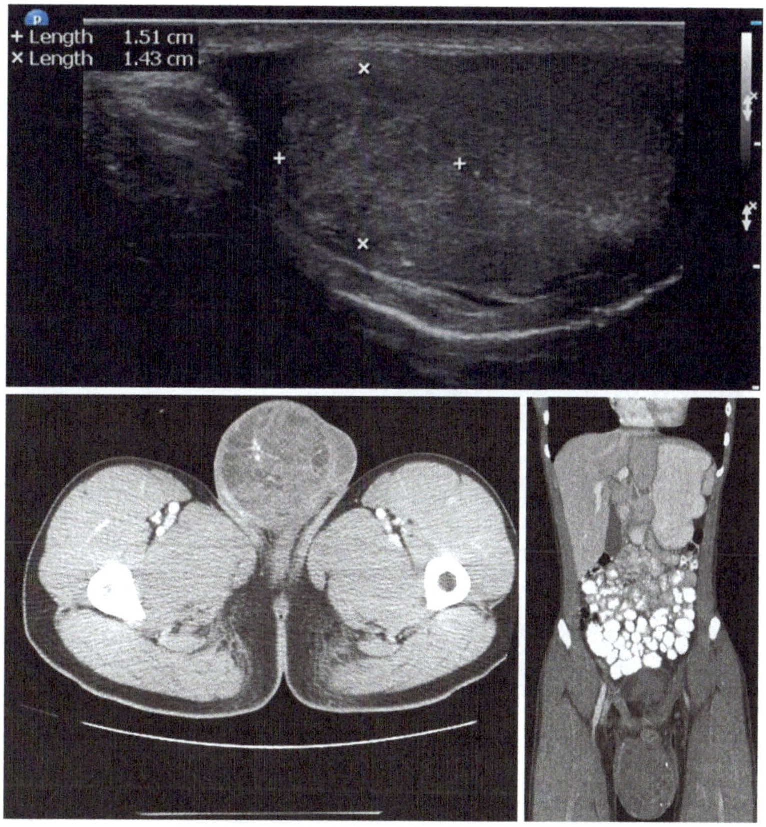

Fig. 17.17 Germ cell tumor found in the right testis. The ultrasound showed a relatively homogeneous and well-circumscribed mass causing enlargement of the testis. Similar findings are seen on the axial and coronal images of the T1-weighted MR

show single or multiple solid hypoechoic masses with homogeneous echotexture. They are usually well circumscribed with lobular margins and are highly vascular. Large masses may cause diffuse testicular enlargement [35]. On MR, seminomas are also homogeneous and usually hypointense to the normal testicular parenchyma on T2-weighted imaging and isointense on T1 [6, 8] (Fig. 17.17).

Nonseminomatous Germ Cell Tumor

In the prepubescent population, yolk sac (endodermal sinus) tumors are the predominant malignant finding. The mean age of diagnosis is 18 months. AFP is elevated in these tumors, which assists with diagnosis as well as response to treatment and long-term follow-up. These lesions are characterized by central necrosis and high degree of vascularity. They may simply enlarge the testicle without a discrete mass. Benign teratomas are probably equally as prevalent as yolk sac tumors (Fig. 17.18). They appear as heterogeneously hypoechoic masses with internal calcifications on US. In the postpubescent population, malignant testicular tumors can include choriocarcinoma, malignant teratoma, and embryonal carcinoma and appear as hypoechoic heterogeneous solid masses (Fig. 17.19). They may contain cystic spaces or densely echogenic foci that result from internal scarring, calcification, or cartilage [32]. On MR, nonseminomatous tumors are usually heterogeneous due to their mixed histology. Areas of increased signal intensity can indicate necrosis or hemorrhage which is often seen in this type of malignancy [6]. They are usually hypointense on T2 and iso- or hyperintense on T1 [8].

Sex Cord-Stromal Tumors

These are rare tumors that have low malignant potential, including Sertoli and Leydig cell tumors. Recently there have been increasing

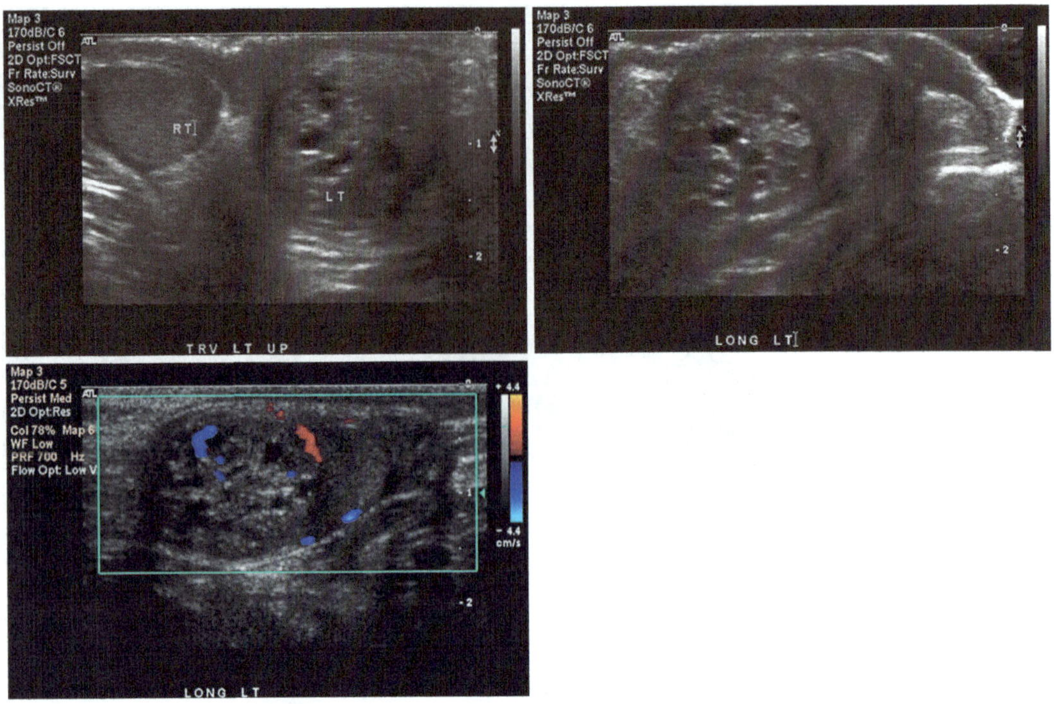

Fig. 17.18 Ultrasound of the testes demonstrates the mass in the right testis with large hypoechoic areas of necrosis and vascularity. The pathologic diagnosis was a benign teratoma

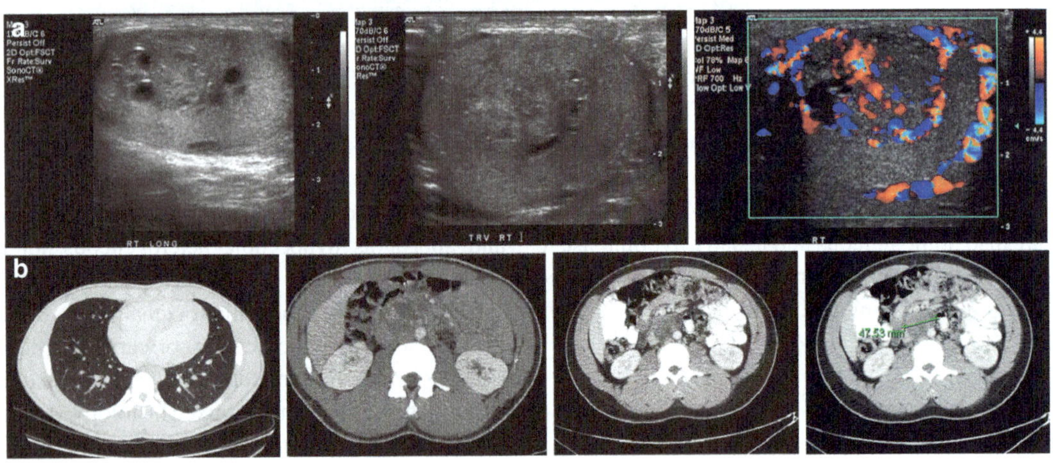

Fig. 17.19 Imaging studies of a palpable testicular mass are useful to characterize the testis tumor and for staging purposes. The pathologic type requires histologic analysis. (**a**) Choriocarcinoma seen on ultrasound as a mainly solid mass with hypoechoic areas (possible necrosis) and hypervascularity on Doppler. (**b**) CT demonstrates metastatic disease to the lung and retroperitoneal lymph nodes

reports of incidentally detected benign tumors, a phenomenon which could be explained by improved imaging techniques and the increase in their use [36, 37]. Approximately 25 % of Leydig cell tumors occur before puberty and may be found on workup for precocious puberty or gynecomastia. Sonographically they appear as a small, hypoechoic, nonhomogeneous nodule with vascularity. Since they are benign in 90 % of cases, partial orchiectomy is advocated (Fig. 17.20).

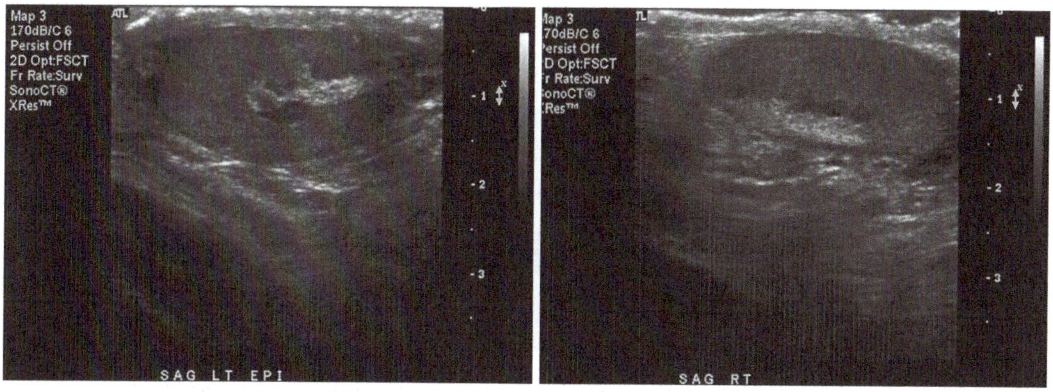

Fig. 17.20 An intratesticular cyst is noted on this transverse ultrasound image. There classic features of a simple cyst are present: imperceptible wall, absence of septations, smooth contour, and through transmission. These are benign

Sertoli cell tumors are found in young men and are usually benign. Sonographically they have increased echogenicity and a characteristic "spoke-wheel" multicystic appearance. Occasionally they contain calcified areas. Sertoli cell tumors have rarely been characterized on MRI; they are described as having a variable appearance and therefore not a recommended diagnostic modality [6].

Benign Intratesticular Tumors

Simple Cysts

As elsewhere, cysts are benign, anechoic, well-circumscribed lesions that may be found arising from the tunica albuginea around the testicle or from within the testicle (Fig. 17.21). These cysts appear as most of these cysts are not palpable and are encountered on ultrasound performed for other reasons. In the absence of symptoms, these cysts do not require treatment.

Adrenal Rests

Testicular adrenal rests tumors (TART) are found in patients with congenital adrenal hyperplasia with 21-hydroxylase deficiency. These are benign lesions that may be implicated in infertility either due to a paracrine effect or due to compression of seminiferous tubules. Sonographically these are

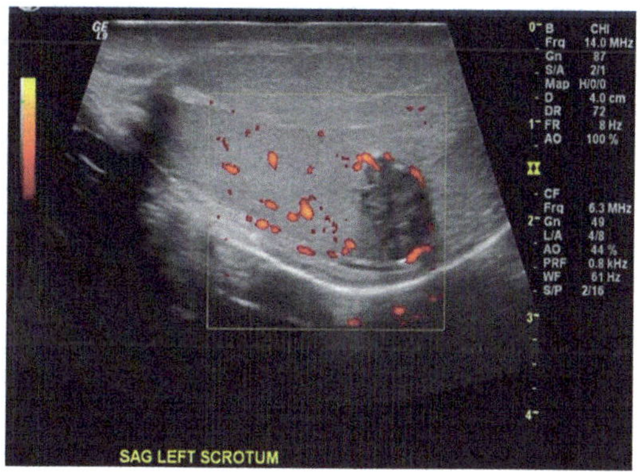

Fig. 17.21 Adrenal rests. Hypoechoic lesions are seen bilaterally in the rete testes of this child with 21-hydroxylase deficiency

hypoechoic lesions located in the rete testis (near the mediastinum) (Fig. 17.22). A study by Cakir et al. attempted to assess the prevalence of TARTs in males with CAH. Sonography of 14 CAH patients detected 2 (14 %) with TART [38]. Another study by Poyrazoglu et al. detected TART in 9/41 (22 %) patients with CAH [39].

Epidermoid Cysts

These are benign intratesticular lesions, with a variable appearance that is related to the ratio of keratin versus calcium. They are associated with the sonographic finding of laminated "onion skin" appearance, surrounded by a hypoechoic or echogenic rim; however, this classic finding is

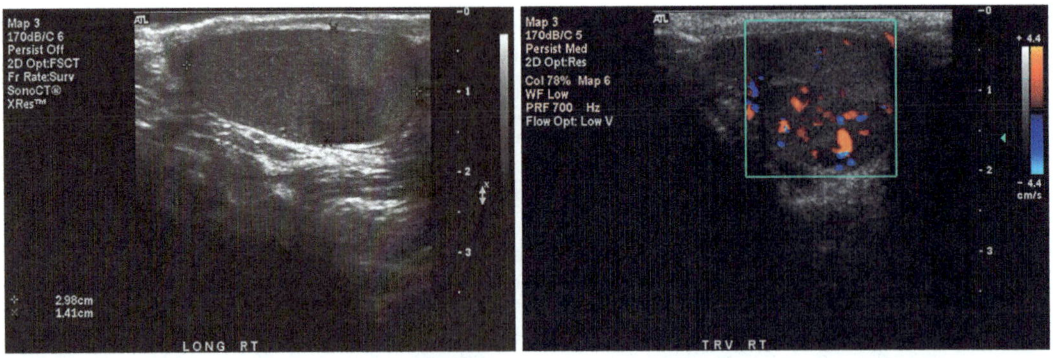

Fig. 17.22 Epidermoid cyst. There is a well-circumscribed lesion in the left testis with "onion skin" appearance of the layers of keratin associated with epidermoid cysts. These benign lesions are amenable to testis-sparing surgery with enucleation of the lesion

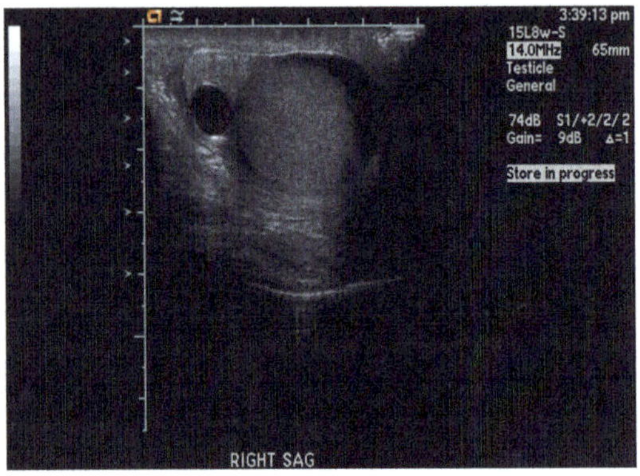

Fig. 17.23 Leydig cell tumor in a prepubertal male with gynecomastia. The ultrasound features include its small size, hypervascularity, and hypoechoic

present only in a minority of cases. Epidermoid cysts uniformly lack color flow on Doppler ultrasound (Fig. 17.23). Real-time elastography shows that these cysts are hard (blue) [40]. On MR imaging, the T2-weighted sequence demonstrates a lesion with increased signal intensity with or without low-intensity signal and surrounded by a low-signal rim. On T1 sequence, there is lack of enhancement [41].

Leydig Cell Hyperplasia

This condition may be the underlying cause for a child presenting with precocious puberty. The testicular parenchyma contains hyperplastic subcentimeter nodules that are usually multiple and bilateral. They are reported to have a variable sonographic appearance, and therefore a scrotal ultrasound is nondiagnostic when the clinical suspicion of Leydig cell hyperplasia is present. MRI is the preferred radiological modality for this entity. On T2 MR imaging these are small hypointense nodules that are contrast enhancing [42].

Paratesticular Masses

The paratesticular space includes the epididymis and the spermatic cord, as well as the investing tunica vaginalis. Pathological conditions in the paratesticular are rare and can be benign or malignant, where the benign conditions are more common. Paratesticular masses are further divided into solid and cystic lesions, all of which can be evaluated sonographically. Benign masses are usually slow growing and may not generate symptoms.

Benign Lesions

Spermatoceles and epididymal cysts are benign lesions that represent the most common causes of paratesticular pathology. Clinically, the patient may be completely asymptomatic or can present with a scrotal mass or induration, which is generally painless (Fig. 17.24).

The epididymal cyst is usually a simple cyst without internal echoes that contains serous fluid. Rarely, they are found to contain septations and calcifications. Some patients present with

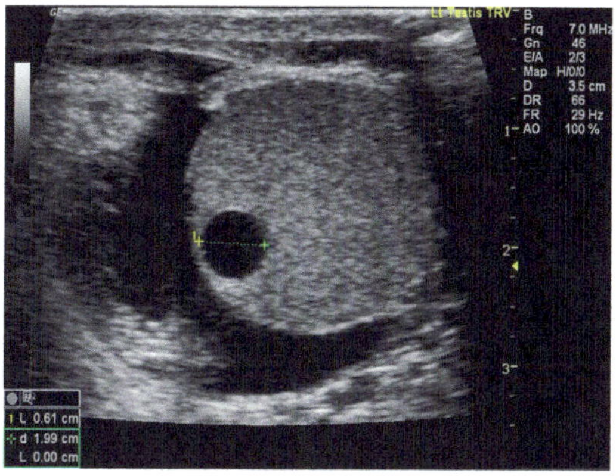

Fig. 17.24 Epididymal cyst. Well-circumscribed hypoechoic lesions in the epididymis or superior to the testis may represent a spermatocele or an epididymal cyst. Both lesions are benign and surgery is rarely indicated

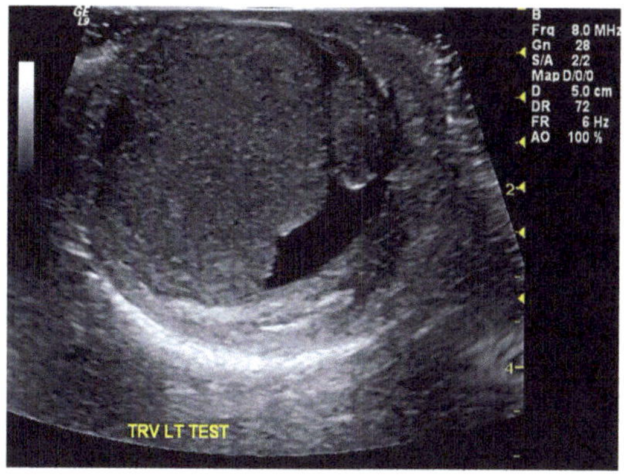

Fig. 17.25 Paratesticular rhabdomyosarcoma. Ultrasound images from a boy presenting with a hard scrotal mass. The mass is heterogeneous with indistinct borders which makes it difficult to determine if it arises from the testis. The pathology demonstrated a paratesticular rhabdomyosarcoma

a multiplicity of cysts and may be found in the appendix testis or appendix epididymis. The spermatocele is a sperm containing outpouching of the epididymis, usually at the level of the epididymal head. It can be differentiated from the epididymal cysts by the low level of internal echoes. Furthermore, it has a thin wall and is generally less taut appearing relative to the epididymal cyst [43, 44]. In a review of all scrotal sonograms done over an 8-year period, 14.4 % of patients had epididymal cysts, questioning the prevailing notion that this is a rare condition. Those were more common in the older pediatric population (35 % in children over age 15) and more common in children with larger testicles [44].

Paratesticular lipomas, which are found along the spermatic cord, and adenomatoid tumors, which arise from the epididymis, are benign masses that may be found in the scrotum. They are homogeneous and lack internal echoes or vascularity on ultrasound. MR imaging of a lipoma demonstrates the presence of fat. Fat suppression sequences can differentiate this entity from hematomas or a proteinaceous cyst. Adenomatoid tumors are the most common benign lesion in young adults, comprising about 30 % of all paratesticular tumors [45]. Sonographically, they are homogeneous round or oval lesions, without increased vascularity. They may have a rim of granulation tissue that is better defined on MR imaging with avid enhancement.

Epididymal cystadenomas are prevalent in patients with von-Hippel-Lindau, as syndrome in which patients are mainly affected by multiple bilateral clear cell renal tumors. The spectrum of clinical manifestations of the disease is broad and includes retinal and central nervous system hemangioblastomas, endolymphatic sac tumors, renal cysts and tumors, pancreatic cysts and tumors, pheochromocytomas, and epididymal cystadenomas.

Malignant Lesions

Malignant extratesticular tumors are very rare. They appear as solid, heterogeneous, hypoechoic masses sonographically due to internal hemorrhage and necrosis [35]. Frequently, they have significantly increased Doppler flow [43]. A malignancy is suspected in cases of a poorly defined solid mass with indistinct borders (Fig. 17.25). Sarcomas of the spermatic cord are the most common malignant extratesticular scrotal tumor. In the pediatric population a rapidly growing extratesticular tumor is suspicious for a rhabdomyosarcoma, while leiomyosarcoma and liposarcoma are usually found in the older population. Mesothelioma and lymphoma are other possible extratesticular malignancies. MR imaging helps in staging as it defines the location and extent of these tumors and their content [8].

References

1. Lam WW, Yap TL, Jacobsen AS, Teo HJ. Colour Doppler ultrasonography replacing surgical exploration for acute scrotum: myth or reality? Pediatr Radiol. 2005;35(6):597–600.
2. Yagil Y, Naroditsky I, Milhem J, Leiba R, Leiderman M, Badaan S, Gaitini D. Role of Doppler ultrasonography in the triage of acute scrotum in the emergency department. J Ultrasound Med. 2010;29(1):11–21.
3. Albrecht T, Lotzof K, Hussain HK, Shedden D, Cosgrove DO, de Bruyn R. Power Doppler US of the normal prepubertal testis: does it live up to its promises? Radiology. 1997;203(1):227–31.
4. Atkinson Jr GO, Patrick LE, Ball Jr TI, Stephenson CA, Broecker BH, Woodard JR. The normal and abnormal scrotum in children: evaluation with color Doppler sonography. AJR Am J Roentgenol. 1992; 158(3):613–17.
5. Parenti GC, Feletti F, Brandini F, Palmarini D, Zago S, Ginevra A, Campioni P, Mannella P. Imaging of the scrotum: role of MRI. Radiol Med. 2009;114(3): 414–24.
6. Cassidy FH, Ishioka KM, McMahon CJ, Chu P, Sakamoto K, Lee KS, Aganovic L. MR imaging of scrotal tumors and pseudotumors. Radiographics. 2010;30(3):665–83.
7. Pinggera GM, Mitterberger M, Bartsch G, Strasser H, Gradl J, Aigner F, Pallwein L, Frauscher F. Assessment of the intratesticular resistive index by colour Doppler ultrasonography measurements as a predictor of spermatogenesis. BJU Int. 2008;101(6):722–6.
8. Kim W, Rosen MA, Langer JE, Banner MP, Siegelman ES, Ramchandani P. US MR imaging correlation in pathologic conditions of the scrotum. Radiographics. 2007;27(5):1239–53.
9. Raman JD, Goldstein M. Intraoperative characterization of arterial vasculature in spermatic cord. Urology. 2004;64(3):561–4.
10. Horstman WG, Middleton WD, Melson GL, Siegel BA. Color Doppler US of the scrotum. Radiographics. 1991;11(6):941–57; discussion 958.
11. Kuijper EA, van Kooten J, Verbeke JI, van Rooijen M, Lambalk CB. Ultrasonographically measured testicular volumes in 0- to 6-year-old boys. Hum Reprod. 2008;23(4):792–6.
12. Goede J, Hack WW, Sijstermans K, van der Voort-Doedens LM, Van der Ploeg T, Meij-de Vries A, Delemarre-van de Waal HA. Normative values for testicular volume measured by ultrasonography in a normal population from infancy to adolescence. Horm Res Paediatr. 2011;76(1):56–64.
13. Barbosa JA, Tiseo BC, Barayan GA, Rosman BM, Torricelli FC, Passerotti CC, Srougi M, Retik AB, Nguyen HT. Development and initial validation of a scoring system to diagnose testicular torsion in children. J Urol. 2013;189(5):1859–64.
14. Vijayaraghavan SB. Sonographic differential diagnosis of acute scrotum: real-time whirlpool sign, a key sign of torsion. J Ultrasound Med. 2006;25(5):563–74.
15. Kalfa N, Veyrac C, Baud C, Couture A, Averous M, Galifer RB. Ultrasonography of the spermatic cord in children with testicular torsion: impact on the surgical strategy. J Urol. 2004;172(4 Pt 2):1692–5; discussion 1695.
16. Kaye JD, Shapiro EY, Levitt SB, Friedman SC, Gitlin J, Freyle J, Palmer LS. Parenchymal echo texture predicts testicular salvage after torsion: potential impact on the need for emergent exploration. J Urol. 2008;180(4 Suppl):1733–6.
17. Nussbaum Blask AR, Bulas D, Shalaby-Rana E, Rushton G, Shao C, Majd M. Color Doppler sonography and scintigraphy of the testis: a prospective, comparative analysis in children with acute scrotal pain. Pediatr Emerg Care. 2002;18(2):67–71.
18. Mueller DL, Amundson GM, Rubin SZ, Wesenberg RL. Acute scrotal abnormalities in children: diagnosis by combined sonography and scintigraphy. AJR Am J Roentgenol. 1988;150(3):643–6.
19. Buckley JC, McAninch JW. Use of ultrasonography for the diagnosis of testicular injuries in blunt scrotal trauma. J Urol. 2006;175(1):175–8.
20. Deurdulian C, Mittelstaedt CA, Chong WK, Fielding JR. US of acute scrotal trauma: optimal technique, imaging findings, and management. Radiographics. 2007;27(2):357–69.
21. Kraft KH, Lambert SM, Snyder 3rd HM, Canning DA. Pyocele of the scrotum in the pediatric patient. J Pediatr Urol. 2012;8(5):504–8.
22. Sung EK, Setty BN, Castro-Aragon I. Sonography of the pediatric scrotum: emphasis on the Ts–torsion, trauma, and tumors. AJR Am J Roentgenol. 2012;198(5):996–1003.
23. Hara Y, Tajiri T, Matsuura K, Hasegawa A. Acute scrotum caused by Henoch-Schonlein purpura. Int J Urol. 2004;11(7):578–80.
24. Huang LH, Yeung CY, Shyur SD, Lee HC, Huang FY, Wang NL. Diagnosis of Henoch-Schonlein purpura by sonography and radionuclear scanning in a child presenting with bilateral acute scrotum. J Microbiol Immunol Infect. 2004;37(3):192–5.
25. Garriga V, Serrano A, Marin A, Medrano S, Roson N, Pruna X. US of the tunica vaginalis testis: anatomic relationships and pathologic conditions. Radiographics. 2009;29(7):2017–32.
26. Munden MM, Trautwein LM. Scrotal pathology in pediatrics with sonographic imaging. Curr Probl Diagn Radiol. 2000;29(6):185–205.
27. Martin LC, Share JC, Peters C, Atala A. Hydrocele of the spermatic cord: embryology and ultrasonographic appearance. Pediatr Radiol. 1996;26(8):528–30.
28. Rathaus V, Konen O, Shapiro M, Lazar L, Grunebaum M, Werner M. Ultrasound features of spermatic cord hydrocele in children. Br J Radiol. 2001;74(885): 818–20.
29. Kozakowski KA, Gjertson CK, Decastro GJ, Poon S, Gasalberti A, Glassberg KI. Peak retrograde flow: a novel predictor of persistent, progressive and new onset asymmetry in adolescent varicocele. J Urol. 2009;181(6):2717–22; discussion 2723.

30. Liguori G, Trombetta C, Garaffa G, Bucci S, Gattuccio I, Salame L, Belgrano E. Color Doppler ultrasound investigation of varicocele. World J Urol. 2004; 22(5):378–81.
31. Chiang LW, Yap TL, Asiri MM, Phaik Ong CC, Low Y, Jacobsen AS. Implications of incidental finding of testicular microlithiasis in paediatric patients. J Pediatr Urol. 2012;8(2):162–5.
32. Hamm B. Differential diagnosis of scrotal masses by ultrasound. Eur Radiol. 1997;7(5):668–79.
33. Tasian GE, Copp HL, Baskin LS. Diagnostic imaging in cryptorchidism: utility, indications, and effectiveness. J Pediatr Surg. 2011;46(12):2406–13.
34. Mazzu D, Jeffrey Jr RB, Ralls PW. Lymphoma and leukemia involving the testicles: findings on gray-scale and color Doppler sonography. AJR Am J Roentgenol. 1995;164(3):645–7.
35. Carkaci S, Ozkan E, Lane D, Yang WT. Scrotal sonography revisited. J Clin Ultrasound. 2010;38(1): 21–37.
36. Leonhartsberger N, Ramoner R, Aigner F, Stoehr B, Pichler R, Zangerl F, Fritzer A, Steiner H. Increased incidence of Leydig cell tumours of the testis in the era of improved imaging techniques. BJU Int. 2011;108(10):1603–7.
37. Carmignani L, Gadda F, Gazzano G, Nerva F, Mancini M, Ferruti M, Bulfamante G, Bosari S, Coggi G, Rocco F, et al. High incidence of benign testicular neoplasms diagnosed by ultrasound. J Urol. 2003;170(5):1783–6.
38. Cakir ED, Mutlu FS, Eren E, Pasa AO, Saglam H, Tarim O. Testicular adrenal rest tumors in patients with congenital adrenal hyperplasia. J Clin Res Pediatr Endocrinol. 2012;4(2):94–100.
39. Poyrazoglu S, Saka N, Agayev A, Yekeler E. Prevalence of testicular microlithiasis in males with congenital adrenal hyperplasia and its association with testicular adrenal rest tumors. Horm Res Paediatr. 2010;73(6):443–8.
40. Patel K, Sellars ME, Clarke JL, Sidhu PS. Features of testicular epidermoid cysts on contrast-enhanced sonography and real-time tissue elastography. J Ultrasound Med. 2012;31(1):115–22.
41. Cho JH, Chang JC, Park BH, Lee JG, Son CH. Sonographic and MR imaging findings of testicular epidermoid cysts. AJR Am J Roentgenol. 2002; 178(3):743–8.
42. Carucci LR, Tirkes AT, Pretorius ES, Genega EM, Weinstein SP. Testicular Leydig's cell hyperplasia: MR imaging and sonographic findings. AJR Am J Roentgenol. 2003;180(2):501–3.
43. Smart JM, Jackson EK, Redman SL, Rutherford EE, Dewbury KC. Ultrasound findings of masses of the paratesticular space. Clin Radiol. 2008;63(8):929–38.
44. Posey ZQ, Ahn HJ, Junewick J, Chen JJ, Steinhardt GF. Rate and associations of epididymal cysts on pediatric scrotal ultrasound. J Urol. 2010;184(4 Suppl):1739–42.
45. Leonhardt WC, Gooding GA. Sonography of intrascrotal adenomatoid tumor. Urology. 1992;39(1):90–2.

Interventional Uroradiologic Procedures in Children

18

Katie Willihnganz-Lawson, Jon C. Kralik, Aseem R. Shukla, and F. Glen Seidel

Introduction

Pediatric interventional radiology (IR) uses the continuously evolving cross-sectional imaging techniques of modern radiology to both diagnose and, when indicated, provide percutaneous access to virtually any body part. There has been a long-standing relationship between urologists and interventional radiologists as both specialties have harnessed these techniques to provide minimally invasive access and therapies. Essential to the growth of both specialties were improvements in cross-sectional imaging including ultrasound (US) and computed tomography (CT), the creation of devices appropriate for children, and the drive for more cost-effective and minimally invasive techniques [1, 2]. Minimally invasive techniques have revolutionized medicine and pediatric practice in recent years, mainly because of perception that they are safer [2]. Interdisciplinary collaboration has led to the development of new techniques and refinement of procedures adopted from adult practice [1]. The aim of this chapter is to discuss the imaging of the clinical entities of the genitourinary tract in children and adolescent patients specifically regarding interventional radiology.

Treating a child instead of an adult requires a specialized set of skills and knowledge, as anatomical structures are more fragile and disease processes vary widely from newborn to adolescent. Imaging of the kidney and urogenital tract in infancy requires dedicated imaging techniques and specific knowledge as well as training of the radiologist. New knowledge and understanding of the pathophysiology and the natural course of many neonatal conditions have altered management approaches requiring adaptation of imaging algorithms [3]. Technical success at minimal risk can be achieved in even the smallest patients by modifying the equipment and by attending to the special needs of the pediatric patient [3]. This

K. Willihnganz-Lawson, MD
Department of Urology, University of Minnesota Medical Center, 420 Delaware St SE MMC394, Minneapolis, MN 55455, USA

Department of Pediatric Urology, University of Minnesota Amplatz Children's Hospital, Minneapolis, MN, USA
e-mail: willi293@umn.edu

J.C. Kralik, MD
Department of Radiology, University of Minnesota, 420 Delaware St. SE, MMC 292, B-212 Mayo, Minneapolis, MN 55455, USA
e-mail: jkralik03@gmail.com

A.R. Shukla, MD (✉)
Department of Surgery, Pediatric Urology, Children's Hospital of Philadelphia, 34th Street and Civic Center Blvd, Philadelphia, PA 19041, USA

Department of Surgery (in Urology), Perelman School of Medicine, University of Pennsylvania, Philadelphia, PA, USA
e-mail: shuklaa@email.chop.edu

F.G. Seidel, MD, FAAP, FACR
Department of Radiology, Pediatric Radiology, Lucille Packard Children's Hospital, MC 5913, 725 Welch Road, Room 1690, Stanford, CA 94304, USA
e-mail: glen@theseidels.net

L.S. Palmer, J.S. Palmer (eds.), *Pediatric and Adolescent Urologic Imaging*,
DOI 10.1007/978-1-4614-8654-1_18, © Springer Science+Business Media New York 2014

chapter should educate the reader as to the principles of each imaging modality and the techniques of the specified procedures regarding the clinical entities encountered in pediatrics.

Care of the Child in Interventional Radiology

Just like in an OR, pediatric patients demand special treatment for radiologic and urologic diagnostic and therapeutic studies. Although most IR procedures will require sedation, allowing the parents to accompany the patient into the room for a minor procedure or prior to sedation helps to reassure the child and parent that all will be well. Child life therapists can reduce stress and eliminate the need for sedation in some cases. Attention to the environment includes child-friendly room designs, colors, and lighting. It is especially important to keep a child warm during the procedure, even if it makes the staff and physicians sweat. Warm blankets may be enough for a short case, but longer cases require use of an external patient warmer.

Anesthetic Considerations in the Pediatric Population

A sedation protocol is essential to establish a successful pediatric interventional practice. Both conscious sedation and general anesthesia may be used, and many factors influence the choice between the two. In healthy patients, sedation can be easier, faster, and more cost-effective than general anesthesia. Since the majority of pediatric IR is inpatient where patient care needs demand same day service, sedation allows much greater flexibility in scheduling and triaging cases. Nevertheless, anesthesia is necessary for critically ill patients, when the procedure is expected to be lengthy or painful, or for patients with a history of failed sedation.

Pediatric radiologists need sedation for many patients who are too young or unable to cooperate with a procedure. This became especially important when computerized tomography (CT) first arrived, because scan times were long for that revolutionary new imaging technique. When MRI arrived a decade later, sedation became even more essential for procedures that routinely lasted 45 min or more and required patients to be motionless throughout a 20 min scan sequence. Similarly, there was increasing need for sedation as more pediatric patients required IR procedures. Most pediatric radiology departments developed their own sedation systems, as anesthesiologists had little time or interest in procedures outside the OR. Initially, the first-line sedation drug was chloral hydrate in doses from 50 to 75 mg/kg as advocated by Kaye et al. for children 3 months to 1 year of age [4, 5]. Although chloral hydrate was popular for many years, it required doses far in excess of the 25 mg/kg recommended by the manufacturer, and even then it was not reliable enough for prolonged IR procedures or MRI exams, and frequently patients slept for hours since the active agent was alcohol. Strain et al. popularized the use of IV Nembutal alone, but again patients might sleep for hours. Others began to use combinations of sedatives, such as a combination of intravenous pentobarbital sodium (Nembutal) 2–3 mg/kg, fentanyl citrate (Sublimaze) 1microg/kg, and midazolam (Versed) 0.05 mg/kg [4]. Some of these medications may be given intramuscularly, orally, or even nasally if needed. Combinations of pentobarbital fentanyl and diazepam (Valium) or midazolam can be used in various combinations with excellent results, sometimes in combination with ketamine. Although modern CT scanners are so fast that the need for sedation has been all but eliminated, MRI remains dependent on an effective sedation system for almost all patients under 6–8 years of age, and IR needs sedation for most pediatric procedures.

Over the past 15 years, the JCAHO has gradually insisted that overall responsibility for hospital-based sedation programs be under the department of anesthesia. As a result, most sedations for pediatric radiology imaging and interventional procedures are now provided by anesthesiologists. Skilled and experienced pediatric nursing support is still essential to assure that patients are appropriately triaged prior to arrival in IR and properly transported to and from IR and that nursing care is maintained during their stay in IR. Since the patients and the case mix in pediatric IR are much different than adult IR, dedicated pediatric IR technologists are also important.

Image Gently and Radiation Exposure

Diagnostic radiology is indispensible for diagnosing pediatric genitourinary abnormalities, influencing treatment courses, and positively impacting patient outcomes. However, the pediatric population presents unique challenges when compared to their adult counterparts. As the population exposure to radiation from medical sources grows, there is increasing concern for children as their tissues are thought to be more sensitive to the effects of radiation, their internal organs receive a greater effective dose for a given radiation level, and they have a longer lifetime for a radiation-related malignancy to manifest. Furthermore, the cancer risk from radiation is thought to be cumulative over a lifetime—each subsequent radiograph, CT, and fluoroscopy study contributes to the lifetime exposure and possibly total risk to a child since many of the radiation-induced cancers will not manifest for decades [6–8].

On January 22, 2008, the Alliance for Radiation Safety in Pediatric Imaging launched the "Image Gently" campaign to "change practice by increasing awareness of the opportunities to promote radiation protection in the imaging of children." This campaign formalized the efforts of many pediatric radiologists to reduce radiation exposures to children. Although initially focused on trying to prevent the use of adult CT radiation dose settings for pediatric CT, the campaign now includes efforts in all aspects of pediatric imaging, including plain films, fluoroscopy, nuclear medicine, and IR.

CT is the major source of radiation from medical imaging to both children and adults. CT represents approximately 5 % of all medical imaging, but accounts for 40–67 % of overall radiation exposure. The utilization of CT has increased in part because the continued improvements in multidetector scanners have decreased acquisition times and improved spatial and temporal resolution, making the imaging of more acutely ill and less cooperative pediatric and adult patients possible without the need for sedation [6, 7]. Initial studies found children being exposed to doses as high as 10–15 mSv per minute, equivalent to 200–300 chest x-rays, for a single CT scan. State of the art CT scanners can be adjusted by concerned radiologists to provide acceptable image quality at radiation doses lower than 20 chest x-rays. Manufacturers are now focusing on reducing dosage for both adults and children. Additionally, radiologists should minimize the use of multiphase scans (i.e., pre- and post-contrast or delayed-phase images), as they rarely add additional benefit to a single phase scan, but can double or triple the radiation dose [8].

Fluoroscopy can deliver doses as high as 5 mSv per minute (100 chest x-rays) in a heavy adult or child, although normal doses are much lower. C-arms are less powerful and usually deliver 2 mSv per minute in continuous fluoroscopy mode which is 30 pulses of radiation per second. There are several techniques that can reduce that dose. First, pulsed fluoroscopy modes will allow reduction of the pulse rate as low as 2 pulses per second on some machines. The radiologist or urologist should ask the technologist to reduce the rate as low as tolerable to still adequately visualize the anatomy, contrast, or device. Eight pulses per second is a standard setting on many C-arms when set in pulsed mode, almost a quarter of the radiation of continuous fluoroscopy on the same machine. Second, coning down the field-of-view to the area of interest limits the amount of radiation exposure. Third, keeping the image intensifier as close as possible to the patient reduces dose to the patient and scatter to the operators. Lastly, it is important to not let a well-intended lead shield be in the radiation beam, as the machine automatically increases the dose in an attempt to penetrate the lead.

Although radiographs and nuclear medicine are both much lower in dose than CT or fluoroscopy, it is still important that the pediatric radiologist and technologist pay attention to techniques to minimize the dose.

Overall, the best way to reduce dose from diagnostic testing is to simply not do the test at all or to substitute ultrasound or MRI when possible. The Image Gently website (www.imagegently.org) offers a wealth of information for physicians, technicians, and families.

Choice of Imaging Modalities

Ultrasound and Fluoroscopy

Ultrasound provides excellent visualization of the urinary tract and retroperitoneum in both adults and children, although visualization becomes more difficult as body size increases. Still, ultrasound provides "real-time" continuous and radiation-free visualization of a needle as it is directed toward the kidney or bladder. As a general rule, the best visualization comes from the highest possible frequency transducer. Unfortunately, the physics of US dictates that penetration and resolution are inversely related, so larger patients will require lower-frequency higher-penetration transducers with lower resolution [9]. Ultrasound guidance is employed for percutaneous nephrostomy, renal biopsy, renal/retroperitoneal abscess drainage, access for ureteral stenting and drug instillation, cyst aspiration, and suprapubic cystostomy.

Fluoroscopy has shifted to a more complementary role with ultrasound for image-guided access with the endorsement of the ALARA principal (as low as reasonably achievable) for radiation exposure in children. Once access has been achieved under US, fluoroscopy becomes the major guidance modality. With a C-arm, the quality of the components of the "imaging chain" (the x-ray tube, the image intensifier that converts the x-rays to an image, the video camera that views the image intensifier, the computers that manipulate the image information, and finally the monitor that display the image) are all lower resolution than a full size IR room. In addition, the "generator power" that drives the x-ray tube is significantly less with a C-arm. That's why the image in a catheterization laboratory or IR suite is much better than a standard C-arm, especially for small catheters and wires in small kidneys and ureters. As patient sizes increase, the C-arm also struggles because it doesn't have the same penetrating power as a full size room. C-arm manufacturers can use image smoothing and frame averaging to improve the image in adults where most objects are larger and don't move very much. But in children these same processing techniques blur the image and make it difficult to see small wires and catheters, so most pediatric IR would prefer to use the IR suite for every procedure, if at all possible.

Magnetic Resonance Imaging

Over the past decade, there have been continuous improvements to MRI imaging, especially in the body, so evaluation of the kidney and retroperitoneum with MRI has become more popular [10]. MRI provides superb soft tissue detail and multiplanar imaging with no radiation. Magnetic resonance urography creates both superb imaging and some functional measurements using a precise hydration and imaging algorithm.

Use of MRI for guidance for IR procedures is an emerging field as devices and needles appropriate for MRI continue to be developed. It provides unequaled soft tissue visualization and resolution without radiation, but access to the patient inside the magnet and imaging coils remains problematic. Currently, its greatest use is in the adult population as a guidance modality in ablative therapies for renal malignancies. Primary disadvantages of MR are its susceptibility to motion, high cost, scanner limitations on procedural manipulations, the need for MR compatible equipment, and limited availability [10]. Still, if the lesion, most likely a small tumor or cyst in the kidney or retroperitoneum, can only be seen by MRI, then MRI safe devices are available to allow needle placement in MRI. In the future, MRI will likely play an increasing role in IR and urologic procedures.

Computed Tomography

The GU tract is the second most common injured organ system in a child. CT is the imaging modality of choice for evaluation of abdominal trauma because multidetector CT (MDCT) provides improved spatial resolution and multiplanar reconstructions that give clear images of the entire abdomen and pelvis with near instantaneous acquisition speeds. It is also used when there is a strong suspicion of urolithiasis, infection, or masses that are not well demonstrated on ultrasound [11].

CT as a guidance modality is much less commonly used in children because of its high radiation dose relative to US or fluoroscopy. Still, as patient size increases with adolescence, ultrasound becomes more limited. CT is helpful for indications such as renal or retroperitoneal abscess drainage or ablation procedures. Although many modern CT scanners have "CT fluoroscopy" capabilities, they are much higher dose than conventional fluoroscopy. In addition, CT fluoroscopy only provides "real-time" imaging of a single slice or two of the patient. As a result, it is cumbersome to try to place a guidewire or catheter into a small space with CT guidance alone. Still, CT can be essential for imaging a small structure in a large patient that can't be well demonstrated by ultrasound. Disadvantages are, again, radiation exposure and high cost [8].

Urinary Tract Interventions

Evaluation of the Hydronephrotic Kidney and Ureter

Although nuclear medicine renography with furosemide is easy to perform, results in a dilated collecting system can be unreliable, even if care is taken to make sure the patient is adequately hydrated and the bladder is drained. Indeterminate results can leave the radiologist and urologist uncertain whether obstruction is playing a role in the deteriorating function of a kidney, especially kidneys that have been previously operated on for UPJ or UVJ obstruction (Figs. 18.1 and 18.2). Intravenous pyelography rarely provides sufficient visualization of structures in a dilated col-

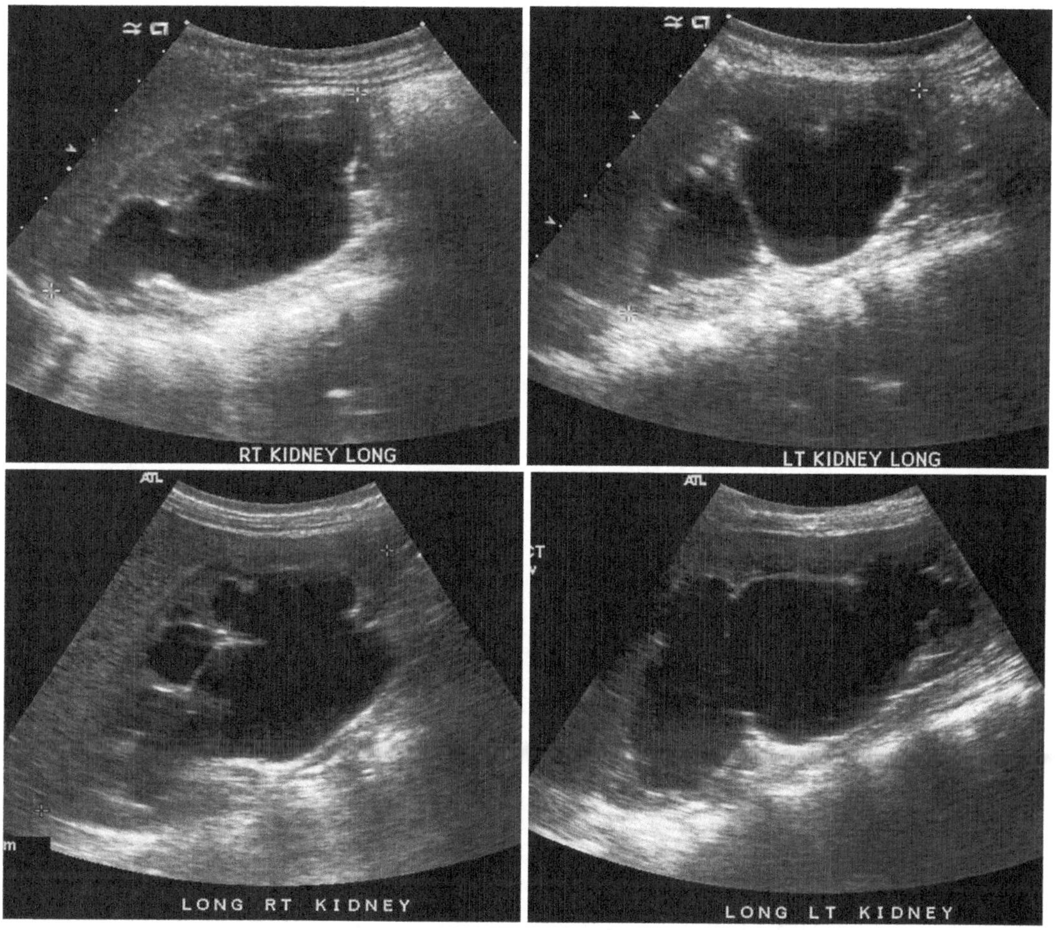

Fig. 18.1 A 2 ½-year-old with a history of "megaureter" being followed for upper tract dilation. There is significant progression of left-sided dilation between September 30, 2008 (*top*), and February 23, 2009 (*bottom*)

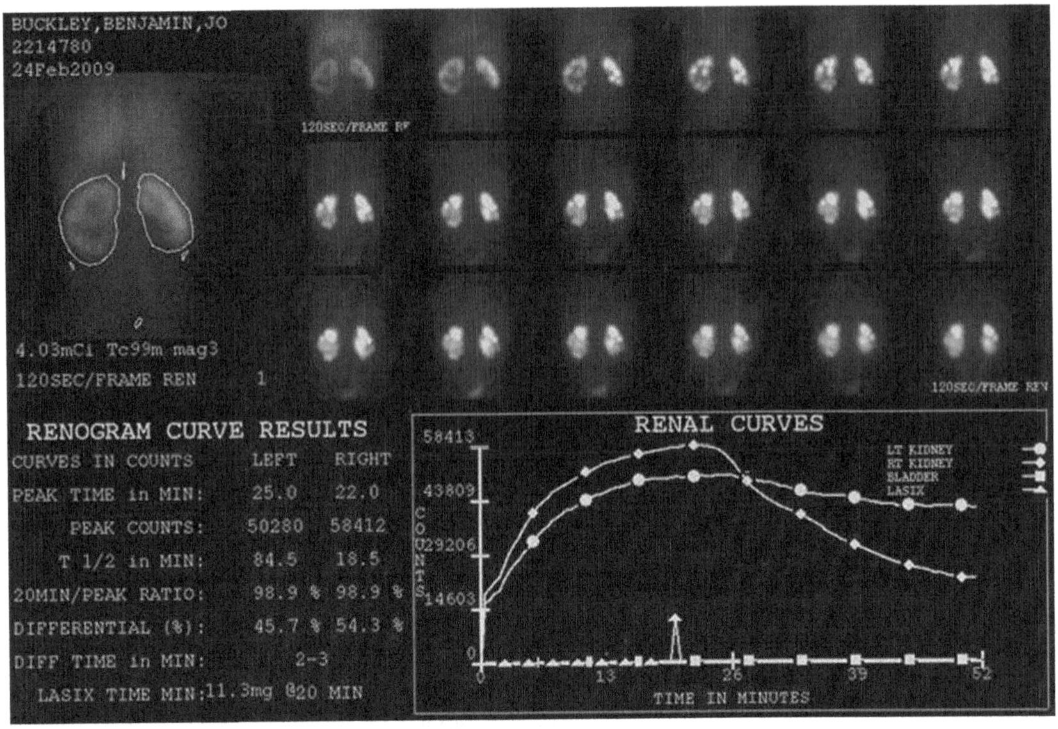

Fig. 18.2 DTPA renogram with furosemide at 20 min shows slow uptake and excretion bilaterally. The slope of the curve is flatter on the *left*. Does this mean obstruction?

lecting system because of the large amount of unopacified urine in the collecting system. Antegrade pyelography, or direct injection of more radiopaque contrast into the kidney, allows detailed visualization of the dilated collecting system. Use of a C-arm allows visualization of the point of narrowing from multiple angles, and use of a higher-resolution angiographic room provides even better imaging.

The Whitaker Test

The classic Whitaker test combines a urodynamic study with an antegrade pyelogram to differentiate patients with residual or recurrent obstruction from nonobstructive dilation secondary to musculature changes. The Whitaker is performed by percutaneous puncture of the renal pelvis with or without placement of a nephrostomy tube. The upper tract is then perfused at rate of 5, 10, and 15 ml/min with saline or dilute contrast, while serial pressures are monitored in the renal pelvis and bladder. Obstructed systems will have a progressive rise in renal pelvis pressure above 12 cm H_2O, while nonobstructed systems will tolerate the increased volumes without rise in pressure [12]. Today, the Whitaker test is performed far less frequently than in the past, as other less invasive testing has become available for defining renal obstruction. The Whitaker antegrade pressure flow study is an invasive procedure with significant limitations, especially in infants whom normal data has not been established [13]. Still, the combination of a detailed antegrade pyelogram with direct pressure measurements can be helpful in problem cases (Fig. 18.3, for Whitaker study images on same infant presented in Figs. 18.1 and 18.2).

MR Urography

MR urography has emerged over the past decade as an effective, noninvasive method for the evaluation of obstructive uropathy in the pediatric patient. MR urography combines excellent spatial resolution and high temporal resolution as it tracks the passage of contrast through the kidney giving both excellent anatomic and functional information in one exam without exposing the patient to ionizing radiation. Using a three-dimensional sequence to follow contrast through the kidneys, it is possible to calculate the renal

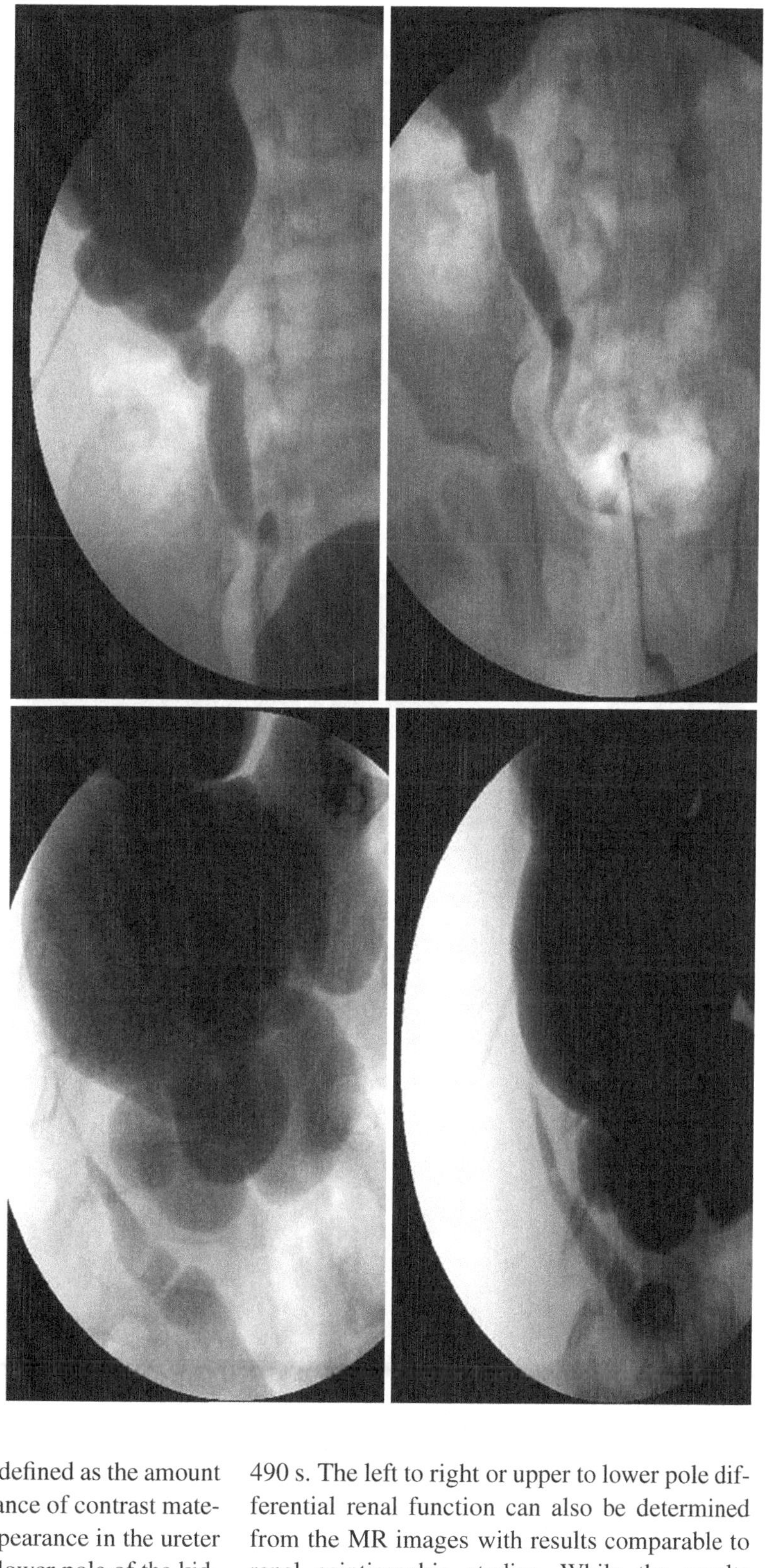

Fig. 18.3 AP and lateral images from antegrade pyelogram show tight narrowing at the UPJ. The Whittaker test showed an opening pressure of 17 cm of water. Following 10 min at 5 cc per minute, the pressure was approximately 35 cm of water. Following 10 min at 10 cc per minute, the pressure fell to 22 cm of water, and did not change at 15 cc per minute. This suggests significant but compensated left UPJ obstruction

transit time (RTT) which is defined as the amount of time between the appearance of contrast material in the kidney and its appearance in the ureter at or below the level of the lower pole of the kidney. A normal RTT is less than 245 s, and unequivocal obstruction is a RTT greater than 490 s. The left to right or upper to lower pole differential renal function can also be determined from the MR images with results comparable to renal scintigraphic studies. While the results between the two methods are comparable, MR urography has a significant advantage secondary to its greater resolution, contrast, and rendering of three-dimensional anatomic detail. The primary disadvantages of MR urography are its requirement for extensive post-processing and its susceptibility to motion, often requiring conscious sedation or even general anesthesia in the pediatric population in order to minimize the motion artifact. High costs and limited availability are other current disadvantages of MR utilization. However, its advantages still far exceed its limitations, and MRU utilization will likely continue to because of its unique combination of functional imaging and high-resolution detail without any ionizing radiation [14–17] (Fig. 18.4 is MR urogram for same infant discussed in Figs. 18.1, 18.2, and 18.3).

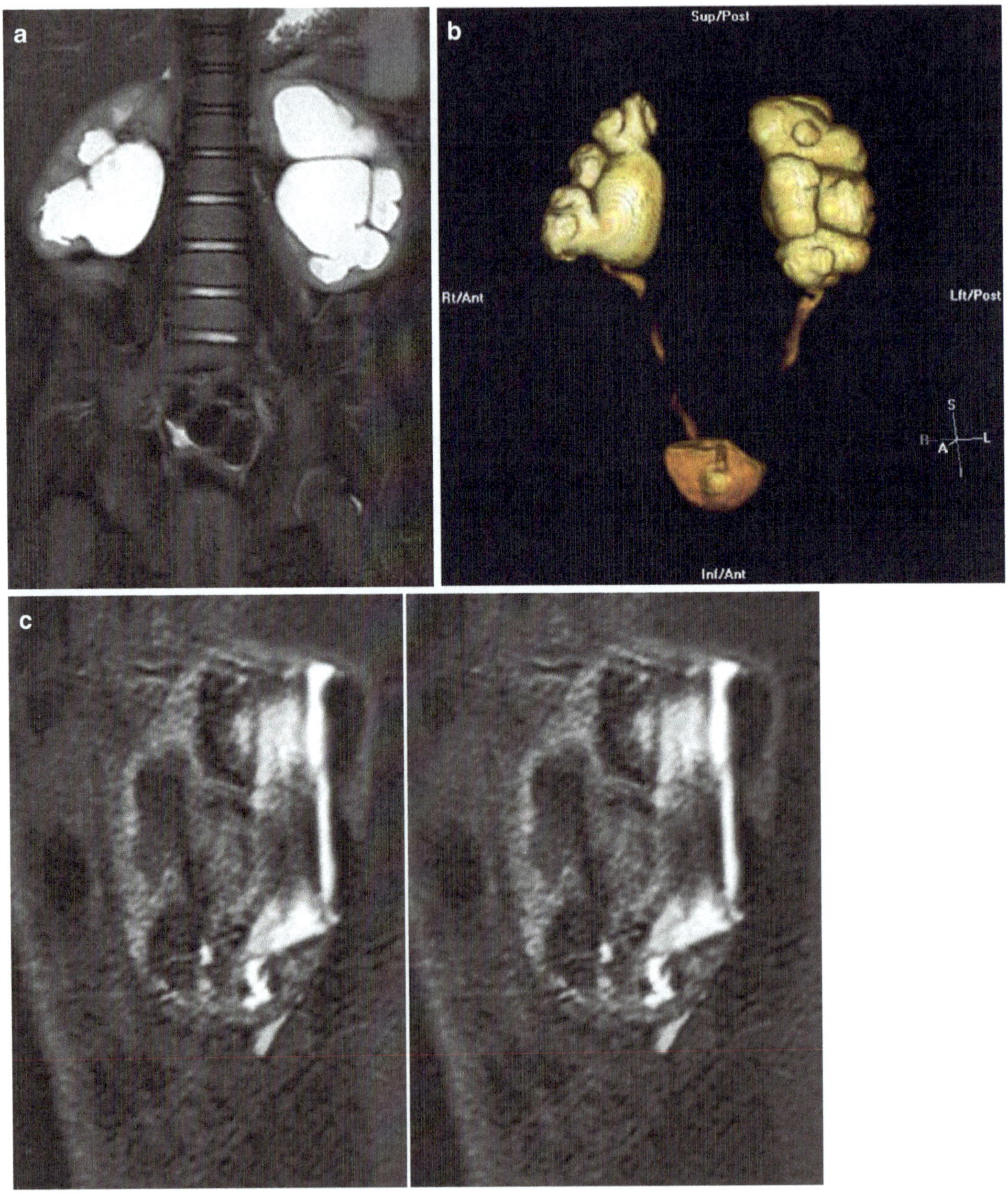

Fig. 18.4 Coronal T2 (**a**) and 3D (**b**) reconstructions show detail available on MRU. Thin slice lateral views of the left kidney show the narrowing of the ureter as it enters the pelvis, similar to the antegrade pyelogram (**c**)

Basic Techniques of Renal Access with Emphasis on the Child and Infant

The basic technique for renal access is the same in adults and children. In fact, it is much easier to visualize the infant kidney by US than in adults, because there is very little intervening soft tissue. Still, kidney sizes are very small, ranging from 25 mm in a premature infant to 50 mm in a full-term infant. Even a hydronephrotic collecting system may be only a cm or two in diameter. In addition, the kidneys are very mobile in the infant and young child, tending to move away from the needle or especially the dilator or catheter if you are not careful [18].

Just as in adults, it is not necessary for the patient to be completely asleep for a nephrostomy, just adequately sedated. Unlike adults who can cooperate if only partially asleep, most children and infants become frightened, agitated, and uncooperative when they are lightly sedated. As a result, moderate to deep sedation is required, and many anesthesiologists feel it is safer to incubate small children who are moderately sedated.

Needle Placement and Antegrade Pyelography

Once the patient is adequately sedated, they are positioned either prone (for bilateral nephrostomies) or partially on their side with the kidney needing access somewhat above the spine [19]. A preliminary US is helpful to locate the kidney and identify a safe access point and mark it on the skin. After standard sterile prep and drape, with the US in a sterile probe cover, after local anesthesia, an echo tip 22 G needle is advanced under US guidance into the kidney (Figs. 18.5 and 18.6). Like adults, use of a mid or upper pole calyx is recommended if ureteral access is planned. Generally, the needle can be well seen by US all the way into the kidney and calyx. If hydronephrosis is present, urine usually drips from the needle when the stylet is removed. A small amount of contrast is injected to demonstrate the collecting system and the position of the needle in the kidney. If necessary, the needle can be repositioned using US or fluoroscopy, or both [20]. Although an antegrade pyelogram can be performed with a needle only, we usually prefer to place a small catheter or dilator to provide more flexible and secure access.

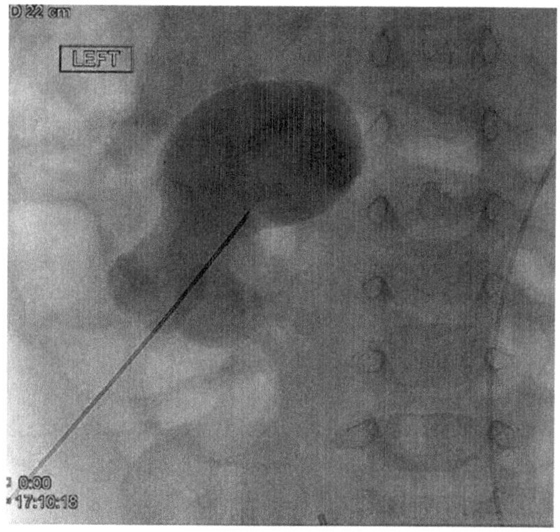

Fig. 18.5 Percutaneous access with needle to lower pole calyx is obtained

Nephrostomy Tube Placement

Once the needle is in place, a 60 cm 0.018 in. guidewire can then be advanced into the renal pelvis and ideally down the ureter. Generally, a stainless steel mandril or nitinol wire can be positioned, with the stainless steel wire offering the greatest stiffness for subsequent dilation and catheter placement. Occasionally, a 0.018 in. hydrophilic guidewire (Glidewire) may be needed to either coil in the renal pelvis or maneuver into the ureter, but this wire is both too long (150–180 cm) and too flexible to easily allow advancement of dilators and the catheter. We routinely cut a Glidewire shorter, but this can leave a burr on the end making it harder to advance a dilator or catheter over the wire. Especially in infants, sequential dilation starting with a 4 Fr dilator is suggested, followed by a 5 or 6 Fr dilator or a "micropuncture" access kit allowing placement of a larger wire if needed, but larger wires are rarely helpful in small patients (Fig. 18.7).

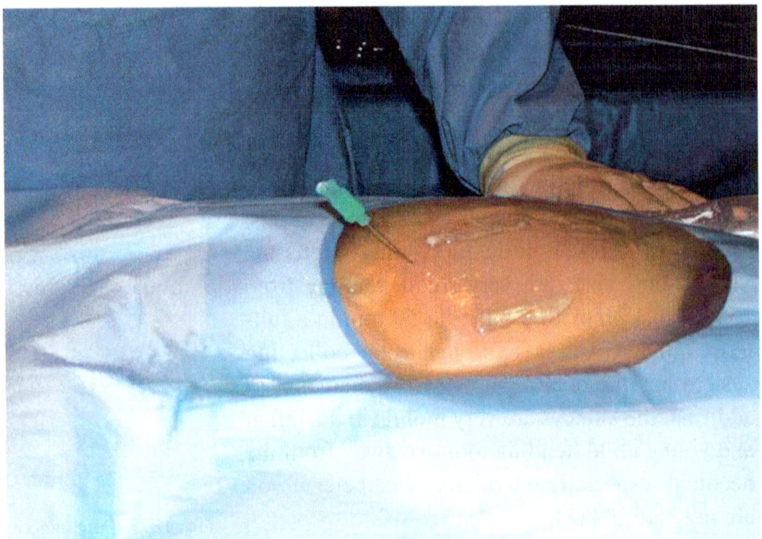

Fig. 18.6 Prone position of patient at time of percutaneous access is demonstrated. Ultrasound-guided access to kidney using micropuncture needle is obtained

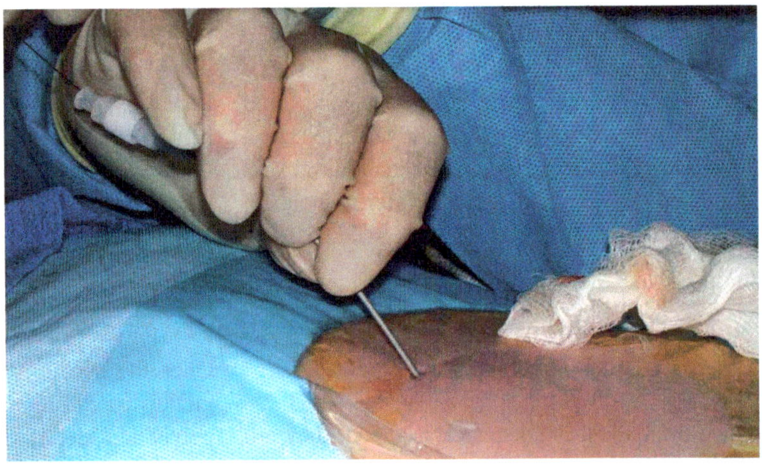

Fig. 18.7 Using Seldinger technique, dilator is passed over guidewire that was inserted through access needle

For infant nephrostomies, a 5 or 6 Fr drainage catheter is sufficient. Because the renal pelvis is small in an infant or child, use of a smaller loop catheter such as the Cook Dawson Mueller catheter is preferred. Hopefully, the renal pelvis is large enough to allow the catheter to form, but this can be problematic, especially if the wire cannot be advanced down the ureter or coiled in the renal pelvis [21]. This is where a Glidewire can help because it will usually coil more easily in the renal pelvis. Use caution if you use a Glidewire with the small drainage catheters because the plastic coating can be torn by the internal metal stiffener, making deploying the catheter difficult or impossible. The 5 Fr drain and stiffener requires a 0.018 in wire, the 6 Fr a 0.025in wire, and the 7 Fr a 0.032in wire. Generally, the 5 and 6 Fr catheters can be advanced over the 0.018in wire, while the 7 Fr will track better with a larger wire. This is where it becomes necessary to use a micropuncture access set to allow a larger wire. Still, we generally use only 5 or 6 Fr catheters in smaller patients.

The infant kidney can be pushed off the end of the guidewire by the dilator or catheter, especially if the guidewire could not be advanced down the ureter. Use of US to confirm that the dilators and catheter are inside the collecting system is frequently helpful because injecting contrast into a drain that is external to the collecting system makes it even harder to regain access [22]. In that situation, repuncture of the now decompressed collecting system under US is challenging but usually possible. Once the catheter is in place, the catheter is secured with one or two nylon sutures and a secure dressing and drainage bag applied.

Nephroureteral Stent Placement

Although infant-sized "double J" stents are now available, it is sometimes easier or desirable to place a nephroureteral stent. This allows external drainage for a time to treat infection or renal failure. Once infection or renal failure has improved, the external portion of the catheter can be capped to allow internal drainage. This has the advantage of relatively easy placement at the time of initial nephrostomy as compared to the antegrade placement of double J stents. In addition, it allows easy access for follow-up antegrade pyelograms to check ureteral stenosis or leak. Finally, it is easy to exchange these catheters should they become clogged, and it is usually easy to remove them at the completion of therapy.

Once renal access has been achieved, a guidewire is advanced down the ureter and hopefully into the bladder. If a UPJ or UVJ obstruction is present, or if there is marked ureteral tortuosity, use of an angiographic catheter and various guidewires may be needed. Once the wire is in the bladder, the UVJ, UPJ, or stricture can be dilated by angiographic catheter directly, or a coronary balloon advanced into position. Once the stricture is dilated as desired, the length of the ureter is measured by guidewire from the bladder to the renal pelvis. A standard drainage catheter is then modified with additional side holes measured so that they are within the kidney and ureter. This allows precise placement of the catheter so that excess catheter length in the bladder or kidney is not an issue. The modified catheter is then advanced over the wire into the bladder. Careful contrast injection to make sure all of the side holes are in the renal pelvis is essential. The catheter is secured in place and a drainage bag attached. Once external drainage is completed, the catheter is capped. If the patient exhibits signs of infection or obstruction after discharge from the hospital, the family can reopen the drain to external drainage at home. This allows trials of capping on an outpatient basis.

When removal is needed, it is preferred to remove catheters under fluoroscopy. Advance a guidewire down the catheter into the bladder to straighten the loop, and then remove the catheter and apply a dressing.

Antegrade Ureteral Stent Placement

Placement of a conventional double J (JJ) ureteral stent from above is also possible, although deployment of the catheter can be technically challenging, especially in a relatively non-dilated upper tract. Preferably, renal access is achieved into a mid or upper pole calyx. Placement of a small peel-away sheath helps to stabilize access to the kidney. A guidewire and catheter are advanced down the ureter and the ureteral length estimated with a guidewire. The conventional JJ stent can then be pushed down the guidewire into the bladder. Getting the proximal J to deploy properly can be challenging, and withdrawing the catheter back into the renal pelvis difficult, although the peel-away sheath allows the proximal string on the catheter to be withdrawn (Fig. 18.8). It is important to make sure the prox-

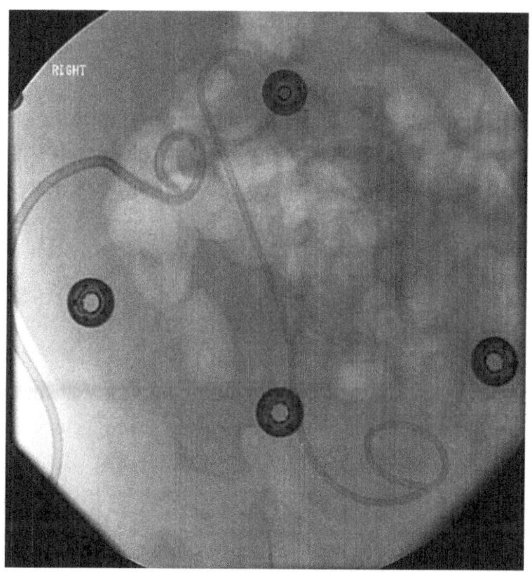

Fig. 18.8 Successful antegrade placement of double J stent via percutaneous renal access

imal end of the stent is not left in the renal parenchyma because pain and bleeding may occur. The nephrostomy tube can be left in for a day or two, especially in an infected system. Removal of the stent can be done from above, but is usually done from the bladder. Reliable estimation of a JJ stent length is often obtained by utilizing the formula of 10 + age of patient = length of JJ stent in cm [23].

Endopyelotomy/UPJ Balloon Dilation

Balloon dilation of the ureteropelvic junction in adults was first described in 1982 and is now well established and commonly performed using a retrograde approach by urologists. When retrograde catheterization of the ureter proves difficult, an antegrade approach via nephrostomy is employed. The complication rate of the procedure is low, and success rates up to 85 % have been reported [24]. Diagnosis of ureteropelvic junction obstruction in children is now frequently suspected on fetal ultrasound, but it may also remain undetected until infection is detected. Later presentations may include pain, hematuria, or stone formation. DTPA renal scan with furosemide assesses the degree of impairment of renal function. It can then be treated by surgical pyeloplasty. However, a minimally invasive technique by balloon dilation may be used to treat as well, either retrograde via nephrostomy or antegrade via cystoscopy. This technique is also commonly used to treat restenosis after pyeloplasty, especially when there has been more than one attempt at surgical correction [24].

Percutaneous Nephrolithotomy

The incidence of urolithiasis in pediatrics varies worldwide with geography and socioeconomic factors, but stones occur in children of all ages without gender predominance. Overall incidence of appears to be increasing globally, likely reflecting westernized lifestyle and dietary changes, including higher salt intake in processed food and decreased water consumption [25]. Anatomic abnormalities, urinary tract infections, and metabolic disturbances increase the risk for stone development, with hypercalciuria and hypocitraturia as most common metabolic risk factors [26].

Renal calculi in neonates and younger children are often diagnosed with ultrasound. Although location and presence of hydronephrosis can be accurately assess with this, 40 % of stones may be missed on ultrasound. Though computed tomography (CT) is more sensitive compared to ultrasound, concerns regarding radiation exposure limit its use in young children. Typically, asymptomatic calculi incidentally found are followed with serial US or plain films to minimize exposure. CT noncontrast is the diagnostic choice in older children, or younger children symptomatic with stone in which plain films or US are nondiagnostic [27].

Stones are treated conservatively, as long as pain is well controlled, the patient is tolerating liquids, and stone size is consistent with high chance of spontaneous passage. In cases of urinary tract infection, significant hydronephrosis with renal colic, or uncontrolled nausea and vomiting, a ureteral stent or nephrostomy may be placed to decompress the urinary system and allow resolution of edema before endourologic management is undertaken, usually 1–2 weeks later.

Percutaneous nephrolithotomy (PCNL) is indicated in children whose therapy with shock wave lithotripsy or ureteroscopy has failed and in those with anatomic abnormalities that impair urinary drainage and stone clearance, such as ureteropelvic junction obstruction, ureteroenteric anastomosis, previous ureterovesical surgery, infundibular stenosis, and caliceal diverticulae [28]. Special considerations in children include preserving renal development and function, limitation of radiation exposure, and minimizing need for retreatment and, if the latter does become necessary in the future, to not limit or preclude any possible treatment options [29].

The first PCNL series was reported in 1985 by Woodside et al. and included seven children with a mean age of 14 years, treated using instruments for adults with no significant complications [30]. Unsal et al. compared the morbidity and success differences in use of adult versus pediatric-sized devices for PCNL for two groups of children, those less than 7 and greater than 7 years old. Pediatric instruments were used in preschool children and children without dilated collecting systems and small stone burden, and adult instruments and techniques in older children with dilated collecting systems achieved equal results. There was less postoperative bleeding if the degree of dilation was less. Small instrument size did not increase the operative time and resulted in the same success rates as adult-sized devices [31].

Over time, many standardized adult stone treatment options have proven efficacious and safe in treating children. With age no longer a limiting risk factor, recent reports have shown that almost any version of PCNL can be applied safely in children as well. The Clinical Research Office of the Endourological Society (CROES) presented retrospective data review of 24 centers treating children under age of 14 years old, demonstrating the differences between pediatric age groups (<1 year old infants, 1–4 years old preschool children and 5–14 years old school age children) and adults in the indications, complications, and outcomes of treatment with PCNL. The preferred method for determining postoperative stone-free status was ultrasound in preschool children over KUB abdominal x-ray in school age children and adults (>15 years old). Although there were no significant differences between the age subgroups for operative details, the mean sheath size and nephrostomy tube size were larger in school age children compared to younger subgroups [32].

PCNL procedure is performed under general anesthesia, with antibiotic prophylaxis after preoperative urinary cultures demonstrate sterile urine. The patient is initially placed in the lithotomy position for stent or catheter placement, and a retrograde pyelogram is performed to outline the collecting system. The patient is then repositioned in the prone position. The desire calyx is the selected, either by ultrasound guidance or under fluoroscopy using biplane orientation—the ideal tract provides the shortest most direct access to the stone. After access is confirmed, a flexible guidewire is then placed into the collecting system and directed down the ureter into the bladder. A small skin incision is made with a No. 11 blade, and then coaxial dilators, 8F and 10F, are passed into the collecting system. Next an Amplatz Super Stiff guidewire is placed as the working wire, the previous wire clamped to the drape and saved as safety wire. Serial dilators, a balloon dilator, or a small peel-away sheath and trocar are placed over the wire into the calyx under fluoroscopic guidance (Figs. 18.9 and 18.10). Once adequate dilation has been achieved, depending on the size of the sheath, rigid or flexible nephroureteroscopes can be employed to identify the stone, and working ports within the scopes are used to pass either lasers or lithotripters to break up the stones. Fragments are then removed by irrigation or stone basketing. The outer diameter of nephroscopes range from 17 to 26F, and flexible nephroscopes are 15F with 6F working channel. Offset cystoscopes 7 and 8F with 5F working ports can also be used. Flexible ureteroscopes 7–9F can be used through 11 F sheath, with enough clearance to allow low-pressure irrigation. Electrohydraulic, ultrasonic, and pneumatic lithotripsy, as well as holmium

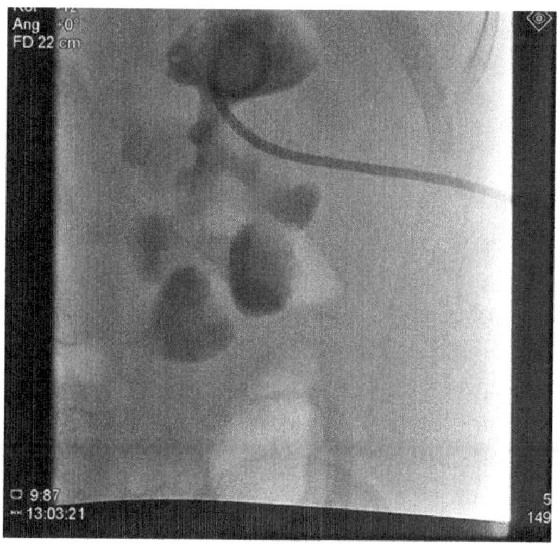

Fig. 18.9 Percutaneous access, in preparation for percutaneous nephrolithotomy (*PCNL*) is obtained into upper pole calyx with antegrade pyelography. A 1.5 cm renal pelvis stone is seen (More visible in Fig. 18.10)

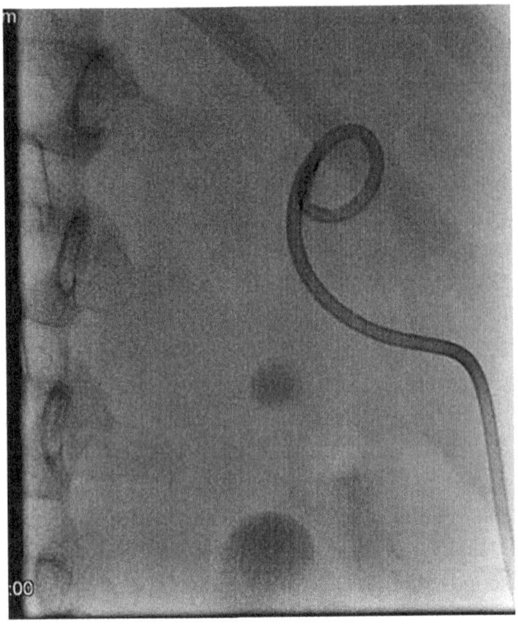

Fig. 18.10 A 1.5 cm renal stone is seen in position of renal pelvis while successful access to upper poly calyx already accomplished as in Fig. 18.9

laser lithotripsy, is effective for stone fragmentation. Finally, after the stone has been adequately treated, postoperative drainage of collecting system with stenting ("tubeless") or placement of a nephrostomy tube will be performed, with imaging assessment to follow [30].

Mini-perc is a novel percutaneous renal access technique developed using an 11F peel-away vascular access sheath, the system passed over a single wire. This was developed in an effort to decrease the morbidity of percutaneous nephrolithotomy, hoping to minimize blood loss and damage to nephrons. In the Jackman study, seven renal units underwent the "mini-perc" procedure, with three take backs for second look resulting in overall stone-free rate of 85 %. No transfusion or urosepsis complications were reported. 7F rigid pediatric cystoscope or 9F flexible ureteroscope was used in most cases, and stones fragmented with electrohydraulic lithotripsy probes [33].

Residual stone fragments are associated with adverse clinical outcome, and every attempt should be made to achieve a stone-free status. In effort to reduce the number of tracts and associated morbidity, some centers choose to follow primary PCNL with adjunctive shock wave lithotripsy (SWL) to clear residual fragments. After SWL sandwich therapy, the stone-free rate increases to 100 % [29]. Second-look nephroscopy through the original tract to ensure stone-free status is another alternative, done at the same hospital admission rather than another admission and procedure.

Percutaneous Cystostomy

Direct percutaneous bladder drainage is rarely needed in children. Bladder outlet obstruction is usually due to congenital urethral obstruction from posterior, or less commonly anterior, urethral valves. This is generally managed by cystoscopic fulguration of the valves. If the bladder needs short-term drainage, a Foley catheter is used. For longer-term decompression, cystostomy can be performed. The technique is similar to nephrostomy placement or abscess drainage from an anterior suprapubic approach.

Retroperitoneal Interventions

Renal and Perirenal Abscesses and Fluid Collections

Perirenal fluid collections usually resolve spontaneously, but when they become infected or are producing significant mass effect, percutaneous drainage can be helpful. Guidance is almost always by US, although CT can be helpful in larger patients. The basic technique is the same as the nephrostomy tube placement and is generally easier since the collection is usually larger than the collecting system and the point of needle access less critical. Care needs to be taken to avoid adjoining bowel (usually the ascending or descending colon). Once the needle is in place, a sample of the fluid is obtained before contrast injection if possible. A guidewire is passed into the collection and the tract dilated. Finally, a suitable-size drainage catheter is placed. If the fluid is simple, such as a urinoma or lymphocele, a relatively small catheter is appropriate. If it is infected or hemorrhagic, catheters of at least 10 Fr should be placed (Fig. 18.11). An attempt to

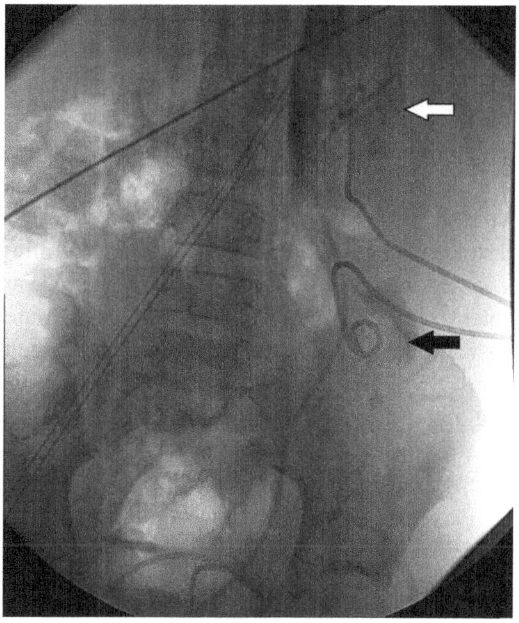

Fig. 18.11 This child underwent ureteroureterostomy following ureteral transection during exploratory laparotomy which subsequently developed an anastomotic leak. After percutaneous access was obtained to the right lower pole calyx (*top white arrow*), ultrasound show a bilobed collection at the right flank within the retroperitoneum. Under ultrasound guidance, a 21 gauge needle was advanced into the collection and urine immediately drained. Over a 0.018 wire, serial exchanges were performed to 7 Fr. A 7 Fr pigtail catheter was placed and 5 cc of diluted contrast injected to confirm its placement (*lower black arrow*)

aspirate as much of the fluid as possible should be performed, confirming placement of catheter with US and fluoroscopy. Occasionally, it is necessary to maneuver the catheter into a better position to assure complete drainage. The catheter is sutured in place and a drainage system applied. Postoperative lymphoceles may require sclerotherapy to prevent recurrence. Agents such as doxycycline or absolute alcohol can be used. If a perinephric urine collection continues to drain, placement of a nephrostomy or stent may be needed to control the leak from the renal collecting system. In infected spaces, drainage catheters are usually left in place until the drainage is clear and less than 10–20 cc/day. Irrigation of catheters left in infected spaces to assure patency with 5–10 cc of normal saline 2–4 times daily is recommended.

Percutaneous Drainage of a Renal, Retro-, or Intraperitoneal Abscess

Percutaneous image-guided drainage of retro- or intraperitoneal abscesses or fluid collections can be considered a first-line treatment for infected or symptomatic fluid collections that are causing pressure, pain, or obstruction. Treatments of fluid collections with percutaneous drainage in children are comparable to adults, with a success rate of 85–90 % even though the etiology of the fluid collection may differ slightly. Appendiceal abscess is the most common etiology of fluid collections, but pyelonephritis, inflammatory bowel disease or adjoining osteomyelitis in the spine or pelvis are other known causes. Again, the technique is similar to nephrostomy access, with US with subsequent fluoroscopy preferred but CT when the collection cannot be visualized by US. Once the needle is in place, a guidewire is passed, the tract is dilated, and a drainage catheter is placed. Simple fluid collections can be drained by 7 or 8 Fr catheters, but more complex fluid should be drained by a 10–14 Fr catheter, even in small patients. Although manufacturers supply the drainage catheters with internal trocars to allow single step direct puncture of fluid collections, it is generally much more controlled to use the Seldinger technique with a needle followed by guidewire, tract dilation, and final catheter placement. Percutaneous drainage of fluid collections is a safe and effective treatment with complications occurring in less than 5 % of pediatric patients and major complications, including sepsis and fistula formation, occurring in less than 1 % of cases [34–36].

Biopsy of Retroperitoneal Mass

Most intraabdominal tumors are biopsied surgically, perhaps because of concerns that the tissue samples are inadequate for accurate diagnosis, that no safe access will be possible, or that a second procedure and anesthesia would be required if the biopsy yields inconclusive results. However, with improvements in imaging and new molecular diagnostic techniques, several studies have demonstrated that retroperitoneal percutaneous biopsy is a safe and effective means by which to obtain an accurate histopathologic diagnosis and staging of many types of tumors [37–42]. It is especially useful for those masses that would benefit from neoadjuvant chemotherapy or radiation and when the masses are not easily resectable, such as advanced stages of neuroblastoma or Wilms' tumor. Other tumors can also be biopsied if a safe access route is available. Consultation with oncologists and surgeons to be sure that a biopsy will not result in "upstaging" a tumor by violating tissue planes or the peritoneum, and with a pathologist to be sure that tissue volume will be sufficient to allow a confident diagnosis is certainly recommended before embarking on a biopsy.

Pre-biopsy imaging will demonstrate the tumor margins and the degree of vascularity and necrosis of the lesion. Once the patient is positioned, repeat imaging with CT or US is needed to confirm the position of the lesion and surrounding structures. Children under the age of 7–10 will typically require general anesthesia for the procedure. After skin marking, sterile draping, local anesthesia administration, and skin incision is made, the tip of the guiding needle is positioned at the proximal margin of the lesion under US or CT guidance. Needle size will vary by the size and location of the lesion and its proximity to vital structures, but generally a coaxial technique with a 16 or 17 gauge thin-walled guiding needle with an 18 or 19 gauge cutting-edge core biopsy needle can be utilized without significant complications compared to smaller needles, such as those used in FNA, while increasing the tissue sample size and, therefore, its diagnostic capabilities. The biopsy needle is then inserted, and the stylet and the probe notch are released. If CT guidance is used, the lesion is localized with contiguous 5–10 mm thick slices. 3–6 passes or more of the biopsy needle are typical, but will depend on the size of the lesion. Needle angulation and rotation can be slightly varied to obtain the repeat biopsy samples. Gelfoam pledgets or a microfibrillar collagen solution can be injected into the coaxial needle track as the needle is withdrawn to prevent tumor seeding or bleeding. Advantages of the coaxial technique are that precise needle placement is required only once, which reduces the potential for complications, the light-weight guidance needle is easier to handle than the biopsy needle itself, and it offers a large amount of tissue for histopathology. FNA should only be considered if the pathologist is confident that they can make a diagnosis off of cytology alone. Contraindications to performing a percutaneous retroperitoneal biopsy include an uncorrectable coagulopathy, no safe access route, or if the pathologist is not confident that needle biopsy will be sufficient [38, 39]. Complications are minor and include bleeding from the biopsy site, retroperitoneal hematomas, transient pain at the puncture site, and infection.

Percutaneous retroperitoneal biopsies are a useful tool in the diagnostic work-up of pediatric malignancies that can replace some surgical biopsies. It is minimally invasive with a low rate of complications and can be highly accurate. It also can decrease treatment costs, length of stay, and delays in initiation of therapy waiting for surgical incisions to heal. It is especially useful in advanced stage disease when systemic chemotherapy and/or radiation will be utilized to reduce tumor bulk prior to definitive surgical treatment and in the treatment of lymphoma or metastasis of solid tumors (e.g., germ cell tumors) resection [37–42].

Renal Biopsy

At most institutions, renal biopsies are performed by nephrologists. Therefore, the role of the interventional radiologist or pediatric urologist is typically reserved for special circumstances. Nephrologists at our institution prefer the radiologists to perform biopsies in intraabdominal transplants because the kidney is not stabilized by the retroperitoneum, patients with hydronephrosis or cysts, or if CT guidance is needed. Pediatric urologists may be tasked with performing a laparoscopic renal biopsy in cases where coagulopathy or renal anatomy—such as horseshoe or ectopia—precludes percutaneous access alone.

Minor hematuria and a small hematoma are common complications following a renal biopsy and usually resolve without need of further intervention. In less than 1 % of patients, significant complications can occur including hemorrhage requiring transfusion, a large subcapsular hematoma that could produce sizeable clots that leads to urinary obstruction, or a symptomatic arteriovenous fistula (gross hematuria and elevated blood pressure) where percutaneous embolization may be indicated. There is also a small possibility it can upstage an isolated mass contained to the kidney, since the biopsy violates Gerota's fascia and the soft tissues of the back. Overall, renal biopsy is a safe, accurate, and reliable procedure that is a useful option for managing indeterminate and suspicious lesions, or generalized renal disease that often guides or changes clinical management [42, 43].

Biopsy of a native kidney can be painful and requires good patient cooperation, often necessitating general anesthesia in younger children. The patient should be positioned in the prone or ipsilateral side down decubitus position to limit the respiratory motion of the kidney. The coaxial technique can then be employed using a 17 gauge guidance needle—which allows the passage of an 18 gauge or smaller biopsy needle—which is advanced into the lesion or beneath the capsule for a non-focal biopsy in generalized parenchymal disease (Fig. 18.12). Biopsy of the capsule instead of the cortex may increase the risk of hemorrhage. Typically, 2–3 samples are obtained with an 18 gauge cutting core biopsy needle depending on the size of the lesion. If a cystic component is present, a 21 or 22 gauge needle can be used to obtain fluid for cytology, followed by biopsy. The advantage of using a coaxial technique is that it limits the number of times that the renal capsule is punctured, which decreases the bleeding risk [42, 43]. Gelfoam pledgets can sometimes be deployed to further reduce the risk of bleeding.

Renal Angiography and Embolization

Conventional catheter angiography (CA) was once the only way to image the arterial and venous anatomy of the body, but it has largely been replaced by CT angiography and MR angiography for basic diagnostic needs. While invasive, CA still offers the greatest spatial resolution (below 200 μm) as compared to CTA (perhaps 500 μm) or MRA (1–2 mm in a body coil). CA also offers the best temporal resolution with frame rates as high as 30–60 frames per second if needed, as compared to MRA or CTA (about 5 s). So CA remains the gold standard for imaging the renal arteries of a hypertensive child because the incidence of treatable renal artery stenosis is much higher and the incidence of essential hypertension relatively lower than in an adult. Still, MRA and CTA remain sufficient to screen for main renal artery stenosis and both modalities may adequately demonstrate the first-order branches [44, 45]. But if hypertension is significant, CA is still

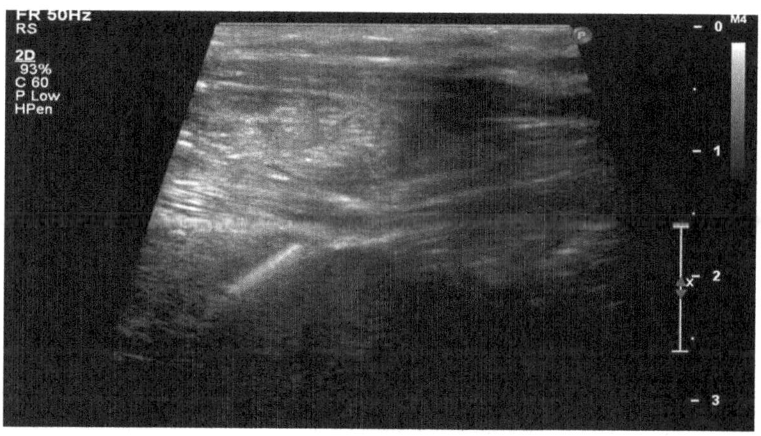

Fig. 18.12 A coaxial needle system is used to obtain percutaneous renal biopsy of transplant kidney. The coaxial system limits the need for multiple passages to obtain biopsy cores and can substantially increase the number of glomeruli obtained

indicated to search for treatable renal artery stenosis. Modern coronary balloons make it possible to treat stenosis in even 2nd- or 3rd-order branches with excellent results.

Bookstein and Goldstein first described renal artery embolization (RAE) in 1973 for control of a post-biopsy arteriovenous fistula. Although iatrogenic hemorrhaging post-percutaneous renal procedures, such as nephrolithotomy, endopyelotomy, or a renal biopsy, remain the most common indications for RAE, they can be useful in other situations, including trauma or treatment of an isolated renal artery aneurysm. Patients with tuberous sclerosis develop angiomyolipomas as they reach adolescence. These tumors can cause severe hematuria and/or a retroperitoneal hemorrhage. As a result, many authors advocate prophylactic embolization of these tumors when they reach 5 cm in size.

RAE is almost always performed from a femoral approach. Using digital subtraction angiography, selective arteriography can be accomplished by advancing a 4 or 5F Cobra, Simmons, or double renal curve catheter into the renal artery. The catheter is then advanced over a nontraumatic guidewire to as close proximity with the lesion as possible. Although embolization can be performed through the larger guiding catheter, a microcatheter is more often advanced more peripherally into the kidney. There are several embolization agents that can be used without a significant advantage of one material over another. For post-biopsy fistulas, microcoils are relatively inexpensive and can be easily deployed to block only a single feeding vessel, although a Gelfoam pledget can also be deployed. Tumor embolization uses more permanent agents such as polyvinyl alcohol particles or acrylic microspheres. Trauma embolization most commonly can be treated with a temporary agent such as Gelfoam. Angiographic nephrectomy or intentional partial nephrectomy of a portion of a kidney is usually accomplished with absolute ethanol. Once the embolization material has been injected, the catheter is withdrawn into the main renal artery, and an angiogram is obtained to confirm that the embolized segment has absent flow and to evaluate the remaining vessels (Figs. 18.13 and 18.14).

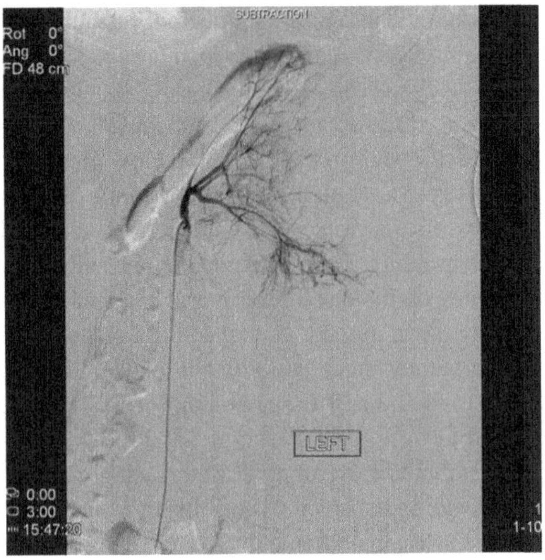

Fig. 18.13 A 21 gauge needle was advanced into the right common femoral artery. The needle was exchanged over a wire a 4 Fr vascular sheath through which a 4 Fr catheter was advanced into the left renal artery. Selective left renal arteriogram demonstrates a large area of tumor vascularity arising off of the second-order branch supplying the lower pole and confirmed by subselective arteriography

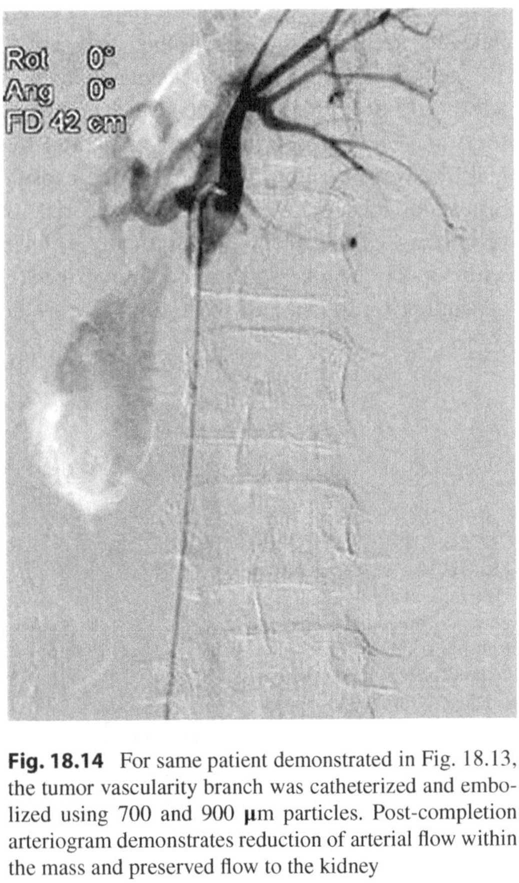

Fig. 18.14 For same patient demonstrated in Fig. 18.13, the tumor vascularity branch was catheterized and embolized using 700 and 900 μm particles. Post-completion arteriogram demonstrates reduction of arterial flow within the mass and preserved flow to the kidney

Improvement in embolic materials and delivery systems, as well as imaging capabilities, has led to more effective treatments with fewer complications since its inception in 1973. The most common complication is the post-infarct syndrome consisting of nausea, fever, transient leukocytosis, and flank pain that typically resolves in a few days. Other short-term complications include incomplete embolization, coil or particle migration, and groin hematomas. Delayed morbidity can present with renal failure and hypertension.

The efficacy of therapeutic renal embolization has been shown to be between 82 and 100 % in numerous studies [44, 45], demonstrating that RAE warrants an attempt in a hemodynamically stable patient with significant renal hemorrhage before submitting them to the morbidity associated with a laparotomy and possible nephrectomy. RAE is a highly effective procedure with excellent renal preservation and minimal short and long term morbidity.

Genital Interventions

Varicocele Ablation

A varicocele is an abnormal dilation of the pampiniform venous plexus secondary to either an incompetent valve with venous reflux into the internal spermatic vein, or aberrantly fed vessels with the left side being the most commonly affected. Symptoms range from scrotal swelling to discomfort and dysuria. The importance of early treatment in children is to prevent testicular atrophy and male infertility.

Typically, varicocele ablation is performed by accessing the right common femoral vein, but the right internal jugular vein can also be used for equivalent access. A 4–5Fr hydrophilic catheter is advanced over a hydrophilic guidewire to just beyond the spermatic vein ostium in the left renal vein. A left renal venogram is preformed while having the patient perform the Valsalva maneuver (if the patient is awake) to illicit reflux down the spermatic vein. The catheter is then advanced into the spermatic vein and contrast is again injected during Valsalva to induce retrograde flow toward the testes and visualize the size of the vein and positioning of all parallel collaterals. There are several techniques for embolization, with two of the more common ones being coil embolization and sclerotherapy. Coil embolization is completed using metallic coils that are appropriately sized for the desired occlusion level within the spermatic vein (usually 0.035 in. or 0.038 in., but smaller are available if necessary). All coils are placed with the patient performing Valsalva to cause maximum expansion of the coils, reducing the risk of migration. Four levels of coils are placed with the first being near the superior pubic ramus or just below the level of the lowest draining collateral. Two other levels of coils are placed at the level of the upper third of the pelvis, and the fourth is placed 2–3 cm from the junction of the internal spermatic vein with the left renal vein. Contrast is injected after the occlusion to assess for new collaterals with higher pressure now in the occluded spermatic vein. Since persistent collaterals could result in failure of the procedure, they have to be occluded. This can be done either directly if the collateral is large enough, or at its origin with the spermatic vein. Coils should now be placed every 3–5 cm along the length of the spermatic vein with the last coil placed in the most cephalad portion of the spermatic vein, exercising care to prevent extension into the renal vein (Figs. 18.15 and 18.16).

Sclerotherapy causes embolization of the spermatic vein by producing a local thrombophlebitis that leads to thrombosis. Examples of sclerosants that can be used are Aethoxysklerol and Na tetradecyl sulfate, usually opacified with contrast to make it visible fluoroscopically. The catheter is advanced with tip positioned at the lower edge of the ischiopubic ramus. A rubber band is applied at the highest level of the scrotum, and contrast is injected during Valsalva to check that there is no reflux in the pampiniform plexus below the rubber band. The sclerosant is injected in the anterior pampiniform plexus during Valsalva while having the patient in reverse Trendelenburg. Elastic compression of the scrotum is continued for 1 min and then released to prevent posterior pampiniform phlebitis. If the sclerosant remains in the anterior pampiniform plexus, the procedure is complete; otherwise, sclerotherapy is repeated at 10-min intervals until sclerosis is achieved.

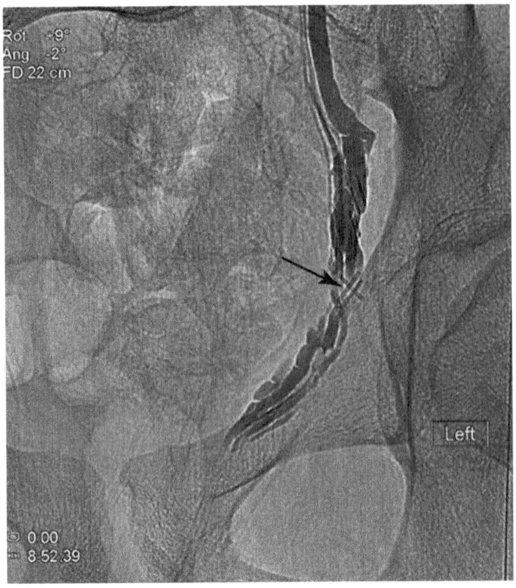

Fig. 18.15 For embolization of left varicocele, the IVC was accessed through the right femoral vein initially using a 21 gauge micropuncture needle. The sheath was advanced into the left renal vein, and the left gonadal vein was accessed via a 2.8 Fr microcatheter. Gonadal venography showed cutoff of the left gonadal vein in the region of surgical clips (*block arrow*). Small collateral veins opacified the multiple gonadal vein tributaries with reflux identified to the level of the scrotum

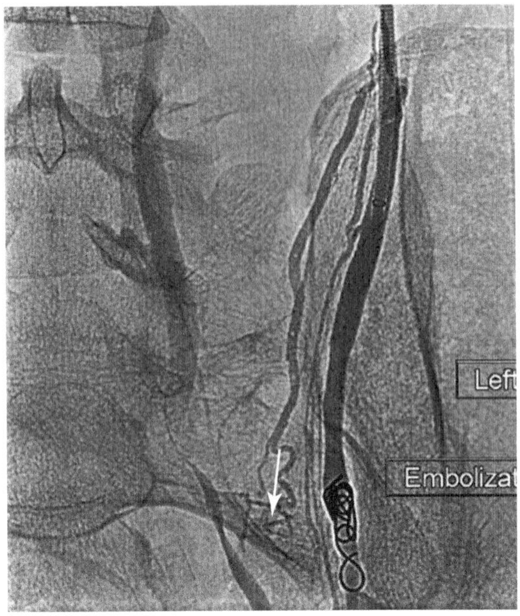

Fig, 18.16 For same patient in Fig. 18.15, access was gained to the dilate veins distally as described, and 3 6 mm embolization coils deployed distal to the clips (*white arrow*). An additional 6 mm coil and a 7 mm coil were deployed just proximal to the clips

Complications of varicocele embolization include coil migration into the central venous circulation, venous perforation, migration of the sclerosant centrally, and hemoglobinuria with higher levels (>15 ml) of sclerosant. The results of varicocele embolization are comparable to surgical ligation while avoiding general anesthesia and postoperative surgical morbidity with a return to normal activity the following day [46–51].

Scrotal and Testicular Biopsy

Ultrasound is considered the imaging modality of choice for the scrotum. However, despite its high sensitivity, it has a low specificity for scrotal and testicular lesions with a high rate of false positives. Although percutaneous biopsy is possible, it is rarely performed in children. In adults, the advantages are that it can be performed on an outpatient basis, requires only local anesthesia, and is minimally invasive. Complications are minimal, mainly consisting of minor hemorrhage and pain. There has been no convincing evidence that violation of the scrotum leads to tumor seeding secondary to the differential lymphatic drainage of the testes and scrotal skin. Percutaneous scrotal and testicular biopsy is, again, a safe, accurate, and cost-effective means to diagnose indeterminate lesions on imaging to appropriately guide subsequent management [52–56].

Conclusion

Percutaneous access to the kidney revolutionized pediatric urology by obviating exclusive reliance on open surgery to treat upper urinary tract obstruction or infection. Even as miniaturization of fiberoptic technology allows more versatility in approaching the kidney and proximal ureter from the bladder, a pediatric interventionalist remains a critical ally to the urologist for providing imaging interpretation and minimally invasive access to the kidney, ureter, and retroperitoneum in many circumstances. US and fluoroscopy are the mainstays of imaging guidance, and MRI may someday supplant CT in cases requiring comprehensive imaging and functional estimations. Consideration of radiation exposure during imaging will increasingly drive radiological exams, and something radiologists and urologists will necessarily contend with. Percutaneous surgery conjoined the specialties of interventional radiology and pediatric urology—and that relationship must remain the cornerstone of comprehensive urological health care into the future.

References

1. Reddy PP. Recent advances in pediatric uroradiology. Indian J Urol. 2007;23(4):390–402.
2. Uppot RN, Gervais DA, Mueller PR. Interventional uroradiology. Radiol Clin North Am. 2008;46(1):45–64. vi.
3. Riccabona M, Sorantin E, Hausegger K. Imaging guided interventional procedures in paediatric uroradiology–a case based overview. Eur J Radiol. 2002;43(2):167–79.
4. Kaye RD, Sane SS, Towbin RB. Pediatric intervention: an update–part I. J Vasc Interv Radiol. 2000; 11(6):683–97.
5. Kaye R, Sane SS, Towbin RB. Pediatric intervention: an update–part II. J Vasc Interv Radiol. 2000;11(7): 807–22.
6. Frush DP, Donnelly LF, Rosen NS. Computed tomography and radiation risks: what pediatric health care providers should know. Pediatrics. 2003;112(4):951–7.
7. Brenner D, Elliston C, Hall E, Berdon W. Estimated risks of radiation-induced fatal cancer from pediatric CT. AJR Am J Roentgenol. 2001;176(2):289–96.
8. Feng S. Radiation dose and cancer risk from pediatric CT examinations on 64-slice CT: a phantom study. Eur J Radiol. 2010;76(2):19.
9. Ginat D. Ultrasound-guided therapeutic urological procedures. Ultrasound Clin. 2010;5(3):401.
10. Kirsch AJ, McMann LP, Jones RA, Smith EA, Scherz HC, Grattan-Smith JD. Magnetic resonance urography for evaluating outcomes after pediatric pyeloplasty. J Urol. 2006;176(4 Pt 2):1755–61.
11. Riccabona M. Urinary tract imaging in infancy. Pediatr Radiol. 2009;39 Suppl 3:436–45.
12. Jaffe RB, Middleton Jr AW. Whitaker test: differentiation of obstructive from nonobstructive uropathy. AJR Am J Roentgenol. 1980;134(1):9–15.
13. Kandarpa K, Aruny J. Handbook of interventional radiologic procedures. 3rd ed. Philadelphia: Lippincott Williams & Wilkins; 2002.
14. Jones RA, Easley K, Little SB, Scherz H, Kirsch AJ, Grattan-Smith JD. Dynamic contrast-enhanced MR urography in the evaluation of pediatric hydronephrosis: part 1, functional assessment. AJR Am J Roentgenol. 2005;185(6):1598–607.
15. McDaniel BB, Jones RA, Scherz H, Kirsch AJ, Little SB, Grattan-Smith JD. Dynamic contrast-enhanced MR urography in the evaluation of pediatric hydronephrosis: part 2, anatomic and functional assessment of uteropelvic junction obstruction. AJR Am J Roentgenol. 2005;185(6):1608–14.
16. Calder AD, Hiorns MP, Abhyankar A, Mushtaq I, Olsen OE. Contrast-enhanced magnetic resonance angiography for the detection of crossing renal vessels in children with symptomatic ureteropelvic junction obstruction: comparison with operative findings. Pediatr Radiol. 2007;37(4):356–61.
17. Fennessy FM, Tuncali K, Morrison PR, Tempany CM. MR imaging-guided interventions in the genitourinary tract: an evolving concept. Magn Reson Imaging Clin N Am. 2010;18(1):11–28.
18. Ebel KD. Uroradiology in the fetus and newborn: diagnosis and follow-up of congenital obstruction of the urinary tract. Pediatr Radiol. 1998;28(8):630–5.
19. Ball Jr WS, Towbin R, Strife JL, Spencer R. Interventional genitourinary radiology in children: a review of 61 procedures. AJR Am J Roentgenol. 1986;147(4):791–6.
20. Barnacle AM, Wilkinson AG, Roebuck DJ. Paediatric interventional uroradiology. Cardiovasc Intervent Radiol. 2011;34(2):227–40.
21. Gupta S, Gulati M, Suri S. Ultrasound-guided percutaneous nephrostomy in non-dilated pelvicaliceal system. J Clin Ultrasound. 1998;26(3):177–9.
22. Hogan MJ, Coley BD, Jayanthi VR, Shiels WE, Koff SA. Percutaneous nephrostomy in children and adolescents: outpatient management. Radiology. 2001;218(1):207–10.
23. Palmer JS, Palmer LS. Determining the proper stent length to use in children: age plus 10. J Urol. 2007;178(4 Pt 2):1566–9.
24. Wilkinson AG, Azmy A. Balloon dilatation of the pelviureteric junction in children: early experience and pitfalls. Pediatr Radiol. 1996;26(12):882–6.
25. Yavascan O, Aksu N, Erdogan H, Aydin Y, Kara OD, Kangin M, et al. Percutaneous nephrostomy in children: diagnostic and therapeutic importance. Pediatr Nephrol. 2005;20(6):768–72.
26. Porowski T, Kirejczyk JK, Konstantynowicz J, Kazberuk A, Plonski G, Wasilewska A, Laube N. Correspondence between Ca(2+) and calciuria, citrate level and pH of urine in pediatric urolithiasis. Pediatr Nephrol. 2013;28(7):1079–84. doi:10.1007/s00467-013-2420-0.
27. Mandeville JA, Nelson CP. Pediatric urolithiasis. Curr Opin Urol. 2009;19(4):419–23.
28. Koral K, Saker MC, Morello FP, Rigsby CK, Donaldson JS. Conventional versus modified technique for percutaneous nephrostomy in newborns and young infants. J Vasc Interv Radiol. 2003;14(1): 113–16.

29. Smaldone MC, Docimo SG, Ost MC. Contemporary surgical management of pediatric urolithiasis. Urol Clin North Am. 2010;37(2):253–67.
30. Woodside JR, Stevens GF, Stark GL, Borden TA, Ball WS. Percutaneous stone removal in children. J Urol. 1985;134(6):1166–7.
31. Unsal A, Resorlu B, Kara C, Bozkurt OF, Ozyuvali E. Safety and efficacy of percutaneous nephrolithotomy in infants, preschool age, and older children with different sizes of instruments. Urology. 2010;76(1):247–52.
32. Guven S, Frattini A, Onal B, Desai M, Montanari E, Kums J, et al. Percutaneous nephrolithotomy in children in different age groups: data from the Clinical Research Office of the Endourological Society (CROES) Percutaneous Nephrolithotomy Global Study. BJU Int. 2013;111(1):148–56.
33. Jackman SV, Hedican SP, Peters CA, Docimo SG. Percutaneous nephrolithotomy in infants and preschool age children: experience with a new technique. Urology. 1998;52(4):697–701.
34. Arellano RS, Gervais DA, Mueller PR. CT-guided drainage of abdominal abscesses: hydrodissection to create access routes for percutaneous drainage. AJR Am J Roentgenol. 2011;196(1):189–91.
35. Gervais DA, Brown SD, Connolly SA, Brec SL, Harisinghani MG, Mueller PR. Percutaneous imaging-guided abdominal and pelvic abscess drainage in children. Radiographics. 2004;24(3):737–54.
36. Arani K, Nandalur K, Tucker CM, Bloom DA. Image-guided percutaneous drainage in the pediatric population: a primer for radiologists. J Clin Imaging Sci. 2011;1:31.
37. Tomozawa Y, Inaba Y, Yamaura H, Sato Y, Kato M, Kanamoto T, et al. Clinical value of CT-guided needle biopsy for retroperitoneal lesions. Korean J Radiol. 2011;12(3):351–7.
38. Garrett KM, Fuller CE, Santana VM, Shochat SJ, Hoffer FA. Percutaneous biopsy of pediatric solid tumors. Cancer. 2005;104(3):644–52.
39. Guimaraes AC, Chapchap P, de Camargo B, Chojniak R. Computed tomography-guided needle biopsies in pediatric oncology. J Pediatr Surg. 2003;38(7):1066–8.
40. Sklair-Levy M, Lebensart PD, Applbaum YH, Ramu N, Freeman A, Gozal D, et al. Percutaneous image-guided needle biopsy in children–summary of our experience with 57 children. Pediatr Radiol. 2001;31(10):732–6.
41. Hussain HK, Kingston JE, Domizio P, Norton AJ, Reznek RH. Imaging-guided core biopsy for the diagnosis of malignant tumors in pediatric patients. AJR Am J Roentgenol. 2001;176(1):43–7.
42. Parker SH, Hopper KD, Yakes WF, Gibson MD, Ownbey JL, Carter TE. Image-directed percutaneous biopsies with a biopsy gun. Radiology. 1989;171(3):663–9.
43. Wood BJ, Khan MA, McGovern F, Harisinghani M, Hahn PF, Mueller PR. Imaging guided biopsy of renal masses: indications, accuracy and impact on clinical management. J Urol. 1999;161(5):1470–4.
44. Jacobson AI, Amukele SA, Marcovich R, Shapiro O, Shetty R, Aldana JP, et al. Efficacy and morbidity of therapeutic renal embolization in the spectrum of urologic disease. J Endourol. 2003;17(6):385–91.
45. Schwartz MJ, Smith EB, Trost DW, Vaughan Jr ED. Renal artery embolization: clinical indications and experience from over 100 cases. BJU Int. 2007;99(4):881–6.
46. Cahill AM, Nijs EL. Pediatric vascular malformations: pathophysiology, diagnosis, and the role of interventional radiology. Cardiovasc Intervent Radiol. 2011;34(4):691–704.
47. Wunsch R, Efinger K. The interventional therapy of varicoceles amongst children, adolescents and young men. Eur J Radiol. 2005;53(1):46–56.
48. Clarke SA, Agrawal M, Reidy J. Percutaneous transfemoral testicular vein embolisation in the treatment of childhood varicocoele. Pediatr Radiol. 2001;31(7):515–17.
49. Sivanathan C, Abernethy LJ. Retrograde embolisation of varicocele in the paediatric age group: a review of 10 years' practice. Ann R Coll Surg Engl. 2003;85(1):50–1.
50. Jaganathan S, Gamanagatti S, Mukund A, Dhar A. Bleeding scrotal vascular lesions: interventional management with transcatheter embolization. Cardiovasc Intervent Radiol. 2011;34 Suppl 2:S113–16.
51. Iaccarino V, Venetucci P. Interventional Radiology of Male Varicocele: Current Status. Cardiovasc Intervent Radiol. 2012;35(6):1263–80.
52. Shaida N, Berman LH. Percutaneous testicular biopsy for indeterminate testicular lesions. Br J Radiol. 2012;85(1):S54–6.
53. Sung T, Riedlinger WF, Diamond DA, Chow JS. Solid extratesticular masses in children: radiographic and pathologic correlation. AJR Am J Roentgenol. 2006;186(2):483–90.
54. Heikkila R, Heilo A, Stenwig AE, Fossa SD. Testicular ultrasonography and 18G biopty biopsy for clinically undetected cancer or carcinoma in situ in patients with germ cell tumours. Br J Urol. 1993;71(2):214–16.
55. Fossa SD, Aass N, Heilo A, Daugaard G, Skakkebaek NE, Stenwig AE, et al. Testicular carcinoma in situ in patients with extragonadal germ-cell tumours: the clinical role of pretreatment biopsy. Ann Oncol. 2003;14(9):1412–18.
56. Pai D, Coletti MC, Elkins M, Ladino-Torres M, Caoili E. Diffuse uterine leiomyomatosis in a child. Pediatr Radiol. 2012;42(1):124–8.

Exstrophy-Epispadias Complex (Epispadias Classic Bladder Exstrophy and Cloacal Exstrophy), Prune-Belly Syndrome, and Bladder Augmentation

19

Heather N. Di Carlo, Jane E. Benson, and John P. Gearhart

Abbreviations

EEC	Exstrophy-epispadias complex
CBE	Classic bladder exstrophy
CE	Cloacal exstrophy
OEIS	Omphalocele-exstrophy-imperforate anus-spinal defects
PBS	Prune-belly syndrome
CT	Computed tomography
MRI	Magnetic resonance imaging
VUR	Vesicoureteral reflux
VCUG	Voiding cystourethrography
PUV	Posterior urethral valves
MAG-3	Tc-99 m mercaptoacetyltriglycine
DMSA	Dimercaptosuccinic acid
CIC	Clean intermittent catheterization

H.N. Di Carlo, MD (✉) • J.P. Gearhart, MD, FAAP
James Buchanan Brady Urological Institute, The Johns Hopkins Children's Center, 1800 Orleans St., Baltimore, MD 21287, USA

Robert T. Jeffs Division of Pediatric Urology, Johns Hopkins University School of Medicine, 1800 Orleans St., Suite 7304, Baltimore, MD 21287, USA
e-mail: hdicarl1@jhmi.edu; jgearha2@jhmi.edu

J.E. Benson, MD
Robert T. Jeffs Division of Pediatric Urology, Johns Hopkins University School of Medicine, Zayed Tower, Room 4174, 1800 Orleans St., Baltimore, MD 21287, USA

Introduction

Radiologic imaging for the initial diagnosis, treatment planning, and follow-up is essential in the complex conditions of pediatric urology including classic bladder exstrophy (CBE), cloacal exstrophy (CE), prune-belly syndrome (PBS), and in patients requiring bladder augmentation. Many of the indications and protocols for imaging in these disease processes are based upon anecdotal evidence, small series, and individual clinical scenarios. The authors seek to review and establish guidelines for imaging in each diagnosis.

Imaging modalities applied in these conditions include plain film radiography, fluoroscopy, ultrasonography, computed tomography (CT), magnetic resonance imaging (MRI), and nuclear scintigraphy. Each has associated pros and cons, as well as variable relative cost (Table 19.1).

Latex sensitization and latex allergy are concerns for all patients undergoing many diagnostic tests and surgical procedures due to increased exposure to the latex antigen. The patients described in this chapter fit these criteria. All patients in this category should be treated with full latex precautions from the beginning of their care [1].

Genital ambiguity is present in some patients discussed in this chapter, particularly those in the exstrophy-epispadias complex (EEC). Radiologists are often called upon to assist in establishing gender in the fragile neonate through the use of portable ultrasound to detect pelvic

L.S. Palmer, J.S. Palmer (eds.), *Pediatric and Adolescent Urologic Imaging*, DOI 10.1007/978-1-4614-8654-1_19, © Springer Science+Business Media New York 2014

Table 19.1 Summary of imaging modalities

Modality	Pro	Con	Relative expense
Radiography	Universally available	Small radiation dose	$
Fluoroscopy	Physiologic, dynamic visualization of anatomy	Higher radiation dose	$$
Ultrasound	No radiation, dynamic visualization of anatomy	Operator dependent	$$$
CT	Anatomy easily understood	High radiation dose	$$$
MRI	High level of anatomic detail; exam can be protocolled to target-specific questions; comprehensive evaluation of multiple systems including CNS	Poor imaging of bone, calcifications; general anesthesia required for young children/long exams (more detailed protocols), not universally available	$$$$
Nuclear imaging	Small radiation dose; physiologic, dynamic imaging	Not universally available	$$$$ (particularly when radiotracer is not made at institution)

organs (e.g., uterus) and characterize the gonads. Early gender assignment helps parents cope with their child's diagnosis and bond with the child.

Exstrophy-Epispadias Complex

Clinical Overview

EEC comprises a spectrum of congenital genitourinary abnormalities ranging in severity from epispadias to CBE to CE. These conditions all affect the genitalia, infraumbilical abdomen, and pelvic ring. EEC is a multisystem birth defect involving the genitourinary tract, musculoskeletal system, pelvic floor, bony pelvis, and anus.

Epidemiology of EEC

CBE is the most common form of EEC. The incidence is estimated to be between 1 in 10,000–50,000 live births [2], while the International Clearinghouse for Birth Defects estimates 3.3 per 100,000 live births [3]. CE is the rarest manifestation of EEC with incidence approximated at 1 per 200,000 live births. EEC is most common in Caucasians, and the male to female ratio ranges from 2.3:1 to 6:1 [3]. It is also more common in infants born to younger mothers and multiparous women. Maternal tobacco exposure is associated with more severe forms (e.g., CE). There is evidence to suggest an increased incidence of this complex of abnormalities in pregnancies utilizing assisted reproductive technologies [4].

Epispadias

Epispadias affects the genitalia and pubic symphysis. The pubic symphysis is diastatic with divergent distal rectus abdominis muscles. In males, the phallus is short and broad with a dorsal chordee. The glans is open along the dorsal surface and shaped like a spade. The dorsal foreskin is absent. The urethral meatus is located along the dorsal penile shaft, between the peno-pubic angle and the proximal glans. In females, the clitoris is bifid with superiorly divergent labia, and the distal dorsal aspect of the urethra is open with a patulous bladder neck (Figs. 19.1 and 19.2). Prolapse of bladder mucosa can sometimes occur.

Classic Bladder Exstrophy

CBE presents with an open bladder exposed through a triangular-shaped fascial defect on the infraumbilical abdomen (Fig. 19.3). The umbilicus is low set and located on the upper edge of the bladder plate. In both sexes, the distance between the umbilicus and anus is shortened. The anatomy of the levator ani and puborectalis muscles is distorted, leading to varying degrees of

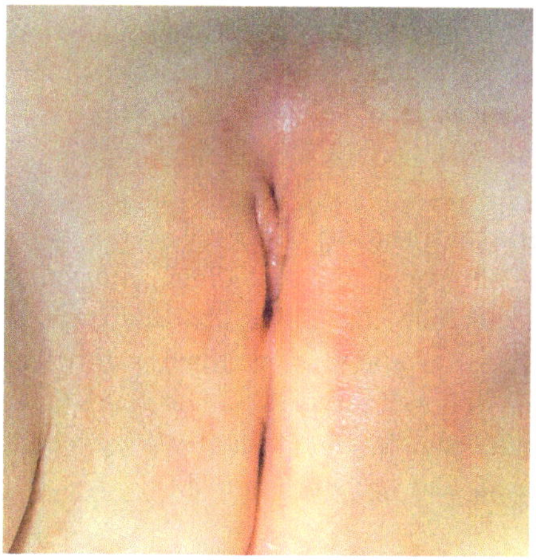

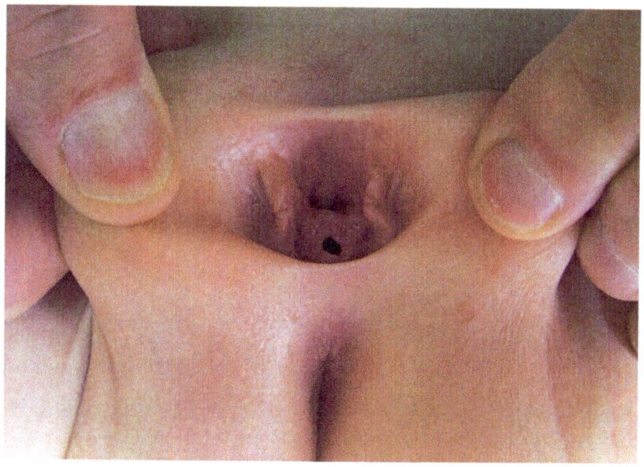

Figs. 19.1 and 19.2 Epispadias in a 2-year-old female patient. Note bifid clitoris and superiorly divergent labia

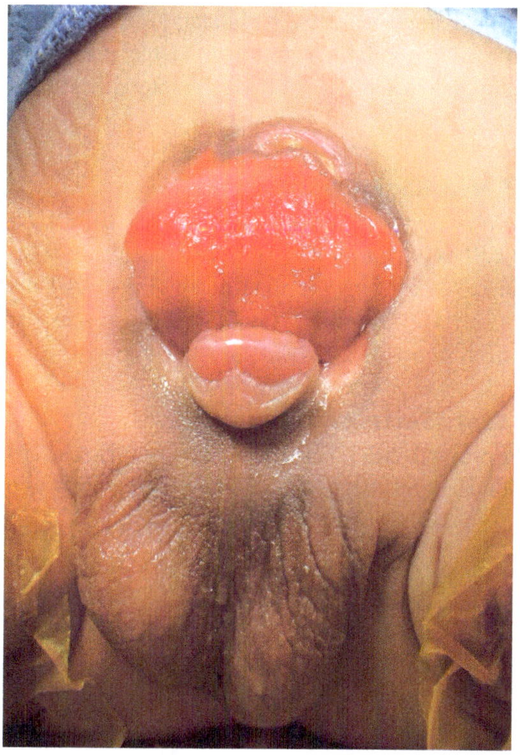

Fig. 19.3 Classic bladder exstrophy in a 1-week-old male patient. Note features of epispadias including a shortened phallus with dorsal chordee, spade-shaped glans, and dorsal meatal opening

fecal incontinence and rectal prolapse. The pubic symphysis is widely diastatic with distally divergent rectus abdominis muscles, which is the result of outward rotation of the innominate bones. There is outward and downward rotation of the anterior pelvic ring ultimately resulting in the classic waddling gait [5–7]. Indirect inguinal hernias are common secondary to wide inguinal rings and short inguinal canals [8, 9].

In males, genital features of epispadias are also present as described above. The urethral and bladder plates are in continuity along the lower abdominal wall and onto the dorsal surface of the penis. The verumontanum and prostatic ducts are present and visible along the prostatic urethral plate. Females also have the same genital features of epispadias, and the open urethral plate is in continuity with the bladder plate. There is anterior displacement of the vagina, which is short.

Cloacal Exstrophy

As in CBE, the bladder is widely open on the infraumbilical abdominal wall but separated into two distinct halves in CE. Cecum is present in between both halves of the bladder. Two appendices may be seen within the cecal plate, and the terminal ileum may prolapse between the hemibladders resulting in the so-called "elephant trunk sign". Most patients with CE have an associated omphalocele.

The pelvic ring has a similar configuration to CBE. 65 % of these patients can have major deformities of the lower extremity, such as clubfoot. Up to 75 % have vertebral anomalies and neural tube defects [10, 11]. In males, the phallus is small and bifid, with a hemi-glans caudal to each hemi-bladder. Females have a bifid clitoris and two hemivaginas. The uterus is most commonly bicornuate, but there are varying degrees of Müllerian duplication [12, 13].

Embryology of EEC

A definite cause of EEC has not yet been elucidated. It is hypothesized that early in fetal development (approximately during the fourth gestational week) there is an abnormal overdevelopment of the cloacal membrane, which results in failure of the medial migration of mesenchyme between the ectodermal and endodermal layers of the lower abdominal wall, thus preventing the normal development of the lower abdominal wall [14]. This occurrence makes the cloacal membrane unstable and prone to early rupture (before it migrates into its normal caudal location during gestational weeks 6–8). The stage of development when this premature rupture occurs will determine the severity along the EEC spectrum. When rupture occurs after complete separation of the genitourinary and gastrointestinal tracts via descent of the urorectal septum, CBE results. When rupture occurs prior to this event, externalization of the lower urinary tract and distal gastrointestinal tract occurs, resulting in CE [15].

Prenatal Imaging of EEC

Transabdominal ultrasonography is the mainstay of prenatal imaging. Although not utilized routinely, there is a role for fetal MRI, which provides more anatomic detail, particularly when anomalies are detected but not fully elucidated on ultrasonography.

CBE: Prenatal Imaging

Prenatal ultrasonographic findings suggestive of CBE include the repeated failure to visualize the filled bladder, a lower abdominal wall echogenic mass that increases in size with an increase of the intra-abdominal viscera, a low-set umbilicus, abnormal or diminutive genitalia, an increased pelvic diameter, and widening of the pubic symphysis [16–18].

CE: Prenatal Imaging

Prenatal ultrasonographic findings compatible with CE include the above characteristics of CBE, as well as a lower abdominal wall defect, herniation of bowel between bladder plates ("elephant trunk sign"), limb abnormalities, neural tube defects, and vertebral anomalies.

Postnatal Imaging Modalities for EEC

The diagnosis of EEC is clinical, yet radiographic imaging modalities can help detect associated anomalies and better define the internal anatomy of the patient.

Pelvic Radiography

Pubic diastasis is noted in patients with EEC, as well as outward rotation of the innominate bones and squaring of the iliac notch (Figs. 19.4 and 19.5). Hip dysplasia is not typically seen as part of this complex.

Cross-Sectional Imaging

Postnatal MRI has been increasingly used to understand the pelvic anatomy in patients with

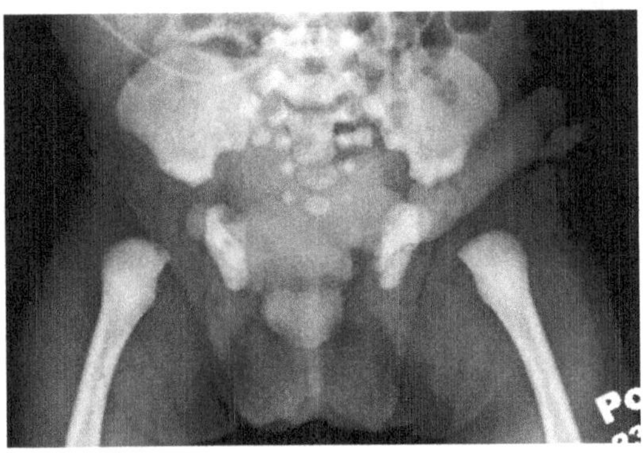

Fig. 19.4 AP plain radiograph of the pelvis in a newborn male with classic bladder exstrophy. Note diastasis of the symphysis pubis. Soft tissue density over the pelvis represents the bladder plate and the scrotum. The umbilical cord stump passes to the patient's left

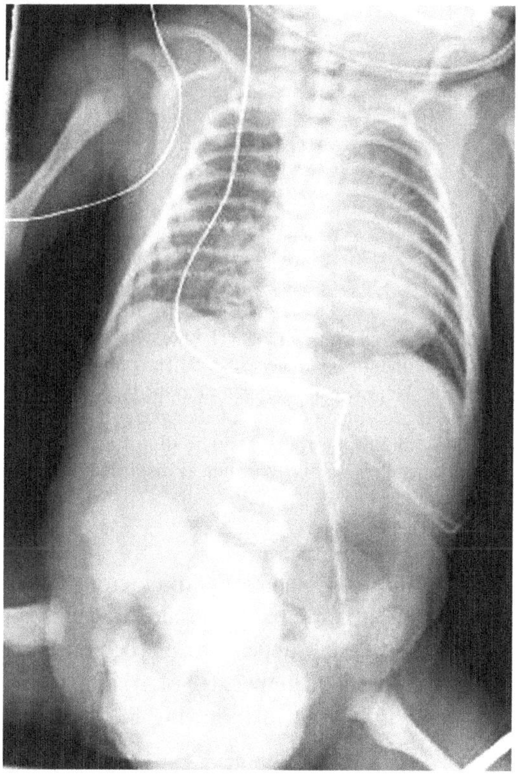

Fig. 19.5 AP plain radiograph of the abdomen and pelvis in a newborn male patient with cloacal exstrophy. Soft tissue density overlies the lower abdomen and pelvis, representing omphalocele. Splayed pelvic bones and dysplastic sacrum are present, but nearly obscured, as is often the case

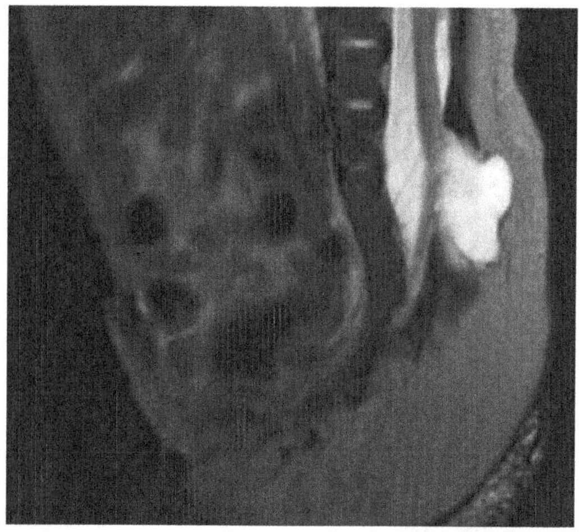

Fig. 19.6 T2-weighted midline sagittal MRI of the pelvis and spinal cord in a 5-day-old male with cloacal exstrophy. Soft tissue plate on the anterior abdominal wall represents bladder; lipomeningocele is seen at L5/S1

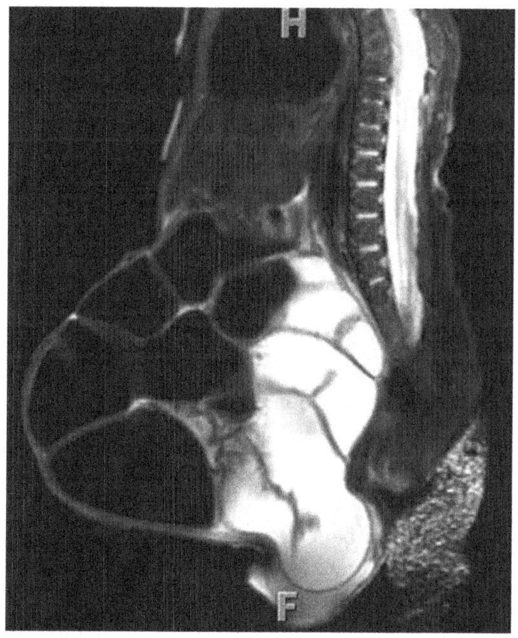

Fig. 19.7 Midline sagittal T2-weighted abdomen and pelvis MR of a 4-day-old male with cloacal exstrophy demonstrates large omphalocele. Included spine suggests anomalies, but these are better demonstrated on dedicated spine MR obtained in the same session

EEC. These patients have a wider pelvic diameter with pubic diastasis, externally rotated sacroiliac joints, a flatter pelvic floor with a more laterally placed levator ani complex, an anteriorly displaced anus, and shorter anterior corporal bodies [19]. Given its myriad of protocol possibilities, imaging of the spine can also be included in the same examination (Figs. 19.6, 19.7, and 19.8). MRI, however, has the constraint of requiring general anesthesia for obtaining quality images, as well as being time consuming (especially with more complex protocols).

Bony and soft tissue pelvic anatomy can also be studied utilizing CT (Fig. 19.9).

Cystourethrography

Post-closure gravity cystography is performed in the operating suite under general anesthesia in patients with CBE and CE to look for vesicoureteral reflux (VUR), which is present in nearly all patients after closure, due to the anatomy of the

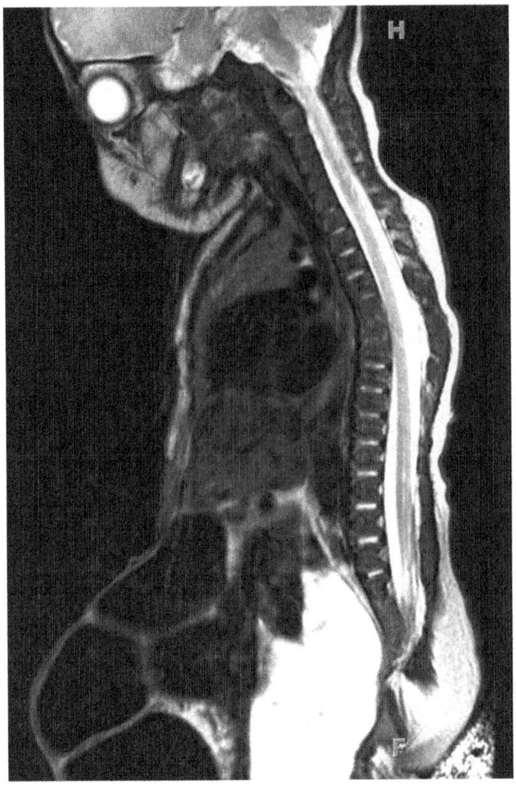

Fig. 19.8 Sagittal T2-weighted spine MR in same patient shows mid-thoracic dyssegmentation and kyphosis, short sacrum, and low cord with spinal canal lipoma

ureterovesical junction (Figs. 19.10 and 19.11). This imaging modality is also used to assess bladder capacity in preparation for bladder neck reconstruction and continence surgery.

Additionally, voiding cystourethrography (VCUG) using fluoroscopy in the radiology suite is useful to evaluate the bladder neck and proximal urethra in patients with epispadias.

Renal Ultrasonography

Baseline renal ultrasonography should be obtained when the clinical diagnosis along the spectrum of EEC has been made. Associated congenital anomalies of the upper urinary tract are rare with epispadias and CBE but are more common in patients with CE. These can include renal agenesis, renal ptosis, and multicystic dysplastic kidney.

Virtually all patients will develop VUR after bladder closure. Increased intravesical pressure

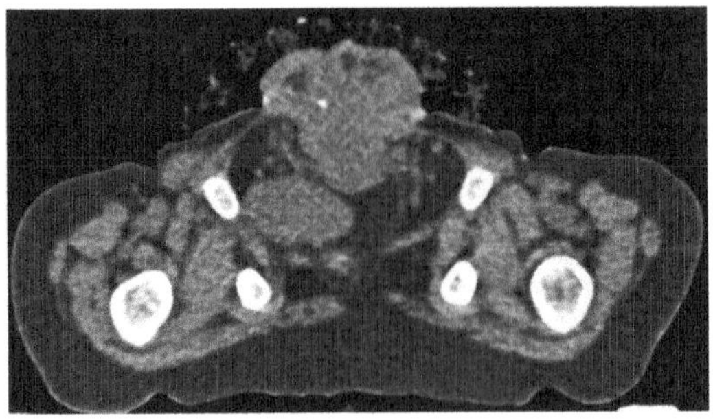

Fig. 19.9 Axial non-contrast CT image through the pelvis in a 19-month-old male with CE. The pubic bones are outwardly rotated and the open anterior bladder plate is shown. The cartilaginous tip of the coccyx is displaced anteriorly and to the right. The left slip of the pubococcygeus muscle is visible; the right is displaced by a loop of pelvic bowel

after closure can lead to hydroureteronephrosis with upper urinary tract pressure transmission and subsequent upper tract deterioration. Therefore, baseline knowledge of existing hydronephrosis is helpful in following these patients postoperatively.

Imaging of the Spine

Spinal ultrasonography should be performed in all neonates with cloacal exstrophy, as spinal dysraphism must be diagnosed when present.

Spinal MRI can be performed in patients with cloacal exstrophy to detect occult spinal cord anomalies that could lead to tethering of the cord with growth of the child (Figs. 19.6 and 19.8).

Differential Diagnosis of EEC

The differential diagnosis of EEC includes patent urachus, omphalocele, gastroschisis, persistent cloaca and cloacal malformation, as well as the common variants of EEC. These include superior vesical fissure, pseudoexstrophy, duplicate exstrophy, covered exstrophy, and the omphalocele-exstrophy-imperforate anus-spinal defects (OEIS) complex.

Exstrophy variants all have a widely diastatic pubic symphysis with distally divergent rectus abdominis muscles. A low-set umbilicus is common. There may be a small bladder opening or

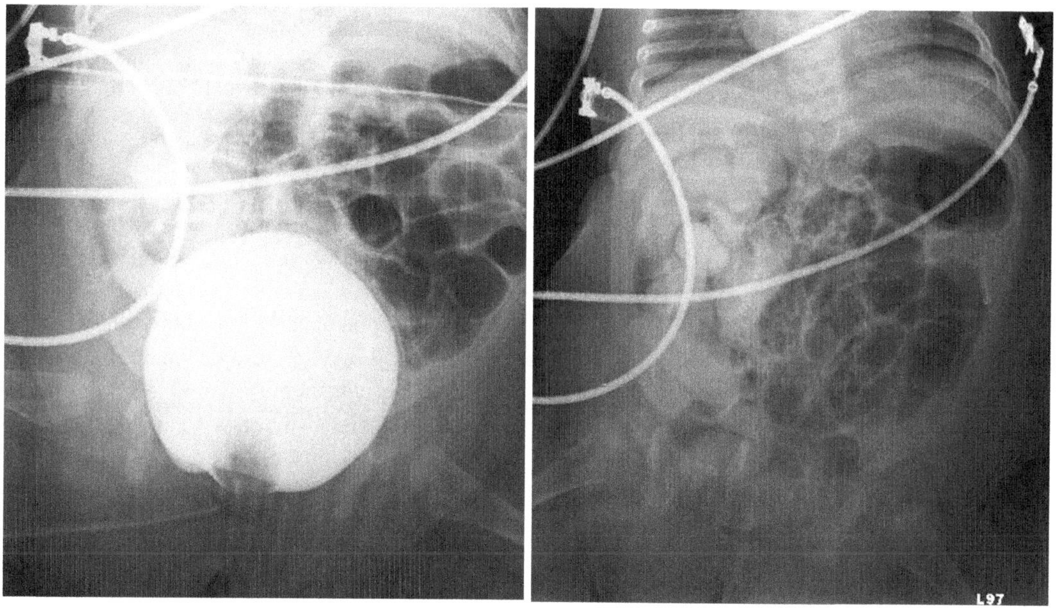

Figs. 19.10 and 19.11 Cystogram in a 4-month-old male patient with skin covered exstrophy variant. Fig. 19.10: AP pelvis radiograph shows Grade V vesicoureteral reflux into the right collecting system. Fig. 19.11: Post-emptying AP abdominal radiograph demonstrates persistence of reflux in the right collecting system and ureter

patch of isolated bladder mucosa as seen in superior vesical fissure.

The OEIS complex is the most severe form of EEC and is characterized by an omphalocele, imperforate anus or anal atresia, spinal dysraphism with incomplete development of the lumbosacral vertebrae, and exstrophy of a common cloaca that receives ureters, ileum, and a rudimentary hindgut. There is also failure of fusion of the genital tubercles and pubic rami, epispadias in males and Müllerian duct anomalies in females. There is a wide spectrum of urinary tract malformations, including supernumerary kidney [20].

Treatment of EEC

Patients undergo surgical correction, urinary diversion, or urinary augmentation as treatment of CBE. Planning for surgical correction can be complex and is tailored to the individual patient.

Surgical correction can be performed by the modern staged repair, which involves primary bladder closure with or without pelvic osteotomy within 72 h of birth, epispadias repair between 6 and 12 months of age, and bladder neck reconstruction at 4–5 years of age. Epispadias repair allows for increase in bladder outlet resistance and subsequent increase in bladder capacity. Ureteral reimplantation for VUR is almost universally indicated at the time of bladder neck reconstruction.

Complete primary repair, an alternative approach, encompasses primary bladder closure and genital reconstruction in one operation [21–23]. Because of the advantage of early bladder cycling, some patients have not required additional bladder neck reconstruction to achieve early continence, yet some evidence suggests an increased number of surgical procedures and complications in these patients [24, 25].

Some EEC patients have a bladder plate that is too small for closure or do not develop adequate bladder capacity (>85 mL). These patients may be treated with bladder augmentation with a continent catheterizable stoma (e.g., Mitrofanoff, Monti) or urinary diversion [12, 26].

Follow-Up Imaging in EEC

All EEC patients that have been reconstructed or diverted should be monitored with periodic renal and bladder ultrasonography to assess for evidence of obstruction, upper tract deterioration, or calculus formation.

Prune-Belly Syndrome

Prune-belly syndrome (PBS) is characterized by deficient or absent abdominal wall musculature, dilation of the urinary tract, and intra-abdominal testes [27]. It has a number of other names, including Eagle-Barrett syndrome, triad syndrome, mesenchymal dysplasia syndrome, and abdominal musculature deficiency syndrome, to mention a few. PBS is the most commonly used name, given its evocative nature.

These patients have a wrinkled abdomen (like a prune), secondary to the lack of abdominal musculature, and males have an empty scrotum due to undescended testes (Fig. 19.12). The incidence ranges from 1:35,000 to 50,000 live births [28]. This is increased in twins, blacks, and patients born to younger mothers. PBS rarely occurs in females [29], but its clinical manifestation in these patients includes the abdominal wall deficiency and urinary tract dysmorphism without any gonadal abnormality [30, 31].

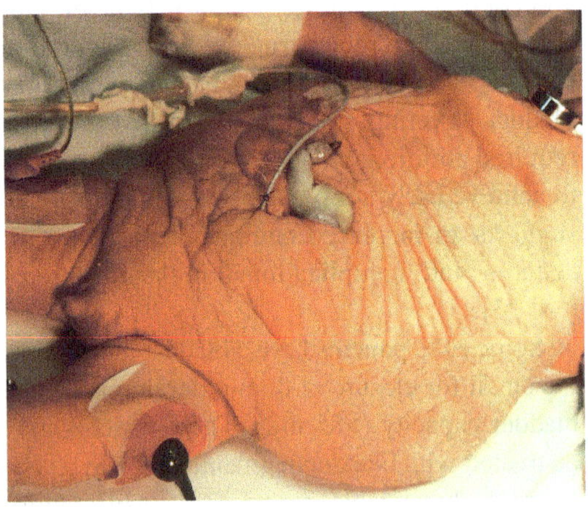

Fig. 19.12 Newborn male with prune-belly syndrome

There are two dominant theories regarding the pathogenesis of PBS yet the exact mechanism is unknown. The obstructive theory suggests that urethral obstruction—either atresia or transient obstruction during a critical period in fetal development [29, 32, 33]—results in bladder distension, hydroureteronephrosis, and atrophy of the abdominal musculature. The mesodermal defect theory proposes a defect in lateral plate mesoderm development early in embryogenesis and is supported by related mesenchymal defects (e.g., prostatic hypoplasia in PBS) [34, 35].

Similar to EEC discussed earlier, there is a spectrum of severity associated with PBS. PBS can be categorized into three main groupings, first classified by Woodard in 1978 [36]. Category I patients have urethral obstruction, pulmonary hypoplasia, oligohydramnios, renal dysplasia, and Potter's facies. These patients are among the most seriously affected group and usually suffer an early death from pulmonary hypoplasia. Category II patients have mild renal dysfunction or dysplasia and hydroureteronephrosis. These patients may go on to develop progressive renal failure [37]. Category III patients have normal renal function and a mild degree of uropathy. The single most predictive factor in survival of the patient with PBS is the severity of renal dysplasia.

Histologically, the proximal ureters are more normal than their distal portions, containing more smooth muscle proximally and more fibrous connective tissue distally [38, 39]. This contributes to the poor ureteral peristalsis seen in PBS patients [40]. Similar to the ureters, the bladder tends to have a higher collagen to smooth muscle ratio [41]. The trigone is widened and the ureteral orifices are displaced laterally, potentially contributing to VUR.

Extragenitourinary manifestations of PBS affect the cardiac, pulmonary, gastrointestinal, and musculoskeletal systems, necessitating more extensive multisystem imaging (such as MRI). Ten percent of patients can have cardiac anomalies, such as patent ductus arteriosus, ventricular and atrial septal defect, and tetralogy of Fallot. These are often more pressing in the newborn period than the genitourinary manifestations.

Prenatal Imaging

PBS is most commonly diagnosed in the second trimester with prenatal transabdominal ultrasonography [42]. Diagnostic features of PBS on prenatal imaging include bilateral hydroureteronephrosis, a distended, thin-walled bladder, and oligohydramnios [43]. Lung volume can be estimated, and cardiac anomalies, if suspected, can be characterized more fully with echocardiography.

Differential diagnosis of PBS on prenatal imaging includes any cause of bladder outlet obstruction, including posterior urethral valves (PUV) as well as megacystis microcolon intestinal hypoperistalsis syndrome [44].

The potential therapeutic role for antenatal intervention with vesicoamniotic shunting has yet to be clarified. Numerous case reports have demonstrated survival of fetuses treated with vesicoamniotic shunting for lower urinary tract obstruction, but whether or not that was truly the result of intervention is yet to be revealed [45, 46]. The results of the PLUTO trial (percutaneous shunting for lower urinary tract obstruction: a randomized controlled trial) will hopefully provide guidance in the use of antenatal intervention in the PBS patient [46].

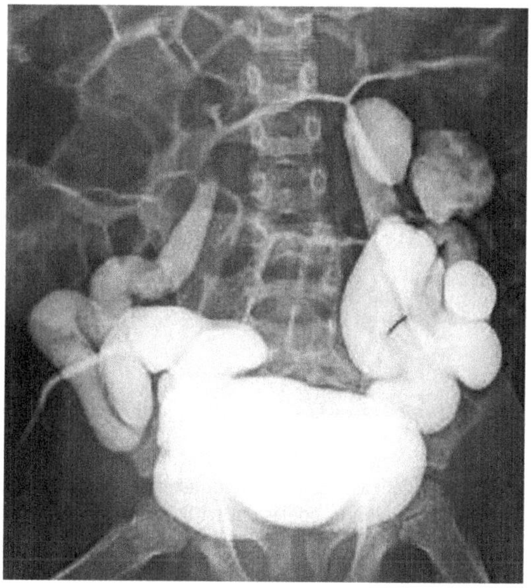

Fig. 19.13 AP pelvis radiograph from cystogram in a 4-year-old male patient with prune-belly syndrome demonstrating severe bilateral vesicoureteral reflux into grossly ectatic ureters. Note the large flaccid bladder

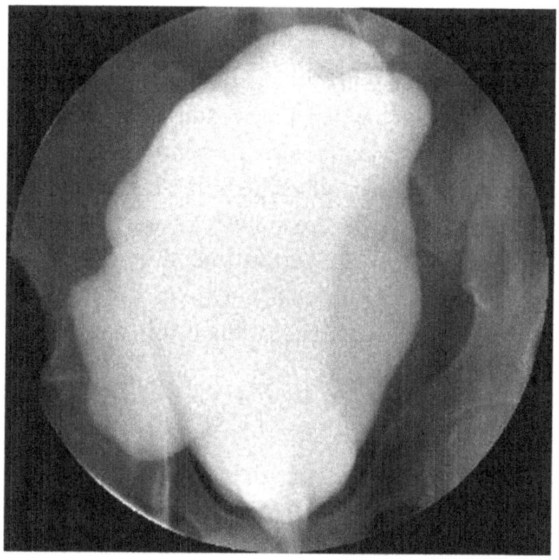

Fig. 19.14 Fluoroscopic image from cystogram in a 16-year-old male patient with prune-belly syndrome with capacious, lobulated bladder

Imaging of PBS

Chest radiography, renal and bladder ultrasonography, VCUG, and renal scintigraphy are critical in the evaluation of the patient with PBS. A chest radiograph is obtained to evaluate for the associated conditions of pulmonary hypoplasia, pneumothorax, and pneumomediastinum. Utilizing ultrasonography, renal parenchyma can be assessed for thickness, echogenicity suggestive of renal disease, and cortical cysts consistent with renal dysplasia. The ability of the bladder to empty can also be assessed.

VCUG is a vital imaging modality for the PBS patient. Care must be taken to place the patient on prophylactic antibiotics before the procedure as bacteria introduced into a potentially stagnant urinary tract can produce profound sepsis. The bladder is capacious and often a urachal diverticulum is visualized (Figs. 19.13, 19.14, and 19.15). When urethral atresia is present, a patent urachus will be found. This allows drainage of

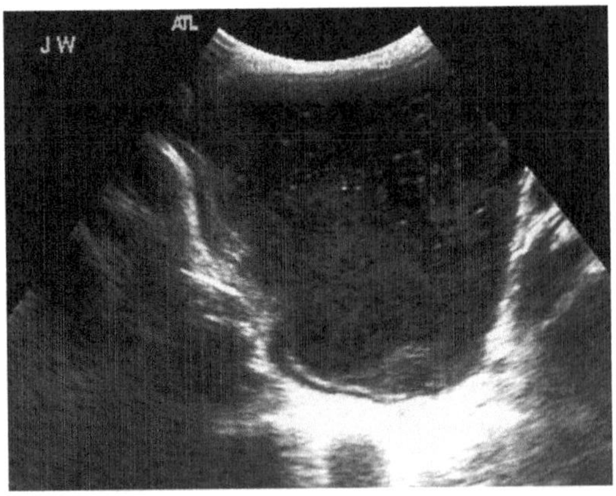

Fig. 19.15 Sagittal midline bladder sonogram image of the same patient as Fig. 19.14 demonstrating large amount of intravesical debris, consistent with cystitis

the urinary tracts, without which bilateral renal atresia results, leading to perinatal fetal demise. The prostatic urethra is wide and appears to taper as the membranous urethra traverses the urogenital diaphragm. Anterior urethral abnormalities are common in PBS, particularly mild dilation (70 %) and megalourethra [36, 47, 48]. VUR is present in 75 % of patients with PBS [49].

Nuclear renal imaging using Tc-99 m mercaptoacetyltriglycine (MAG-3) and furosemide is necessary to evaluate the differential renal function and assess for adequate upper tract drainage. Although there is commonly severe hydroureteronephrosis in PBS, upper tract drainage is usually adequate. Additionally, a dimercaptosuccinic acid (DMSA) scan can evaluate for renal parenchymal scarring.

Treatment of Genitourinary Manifestations of PBS

PBS patients need reconstruction of the urinary tract. This can include ureteral reimplantation with or without remodeling, reduction cystoplasty, and anterior urethral reconstruction. Abdominal wall reconstruction and orchidopexy are also necessary but can be delayed until other issues are resolved. Temporary urinary diversion (via nephrostomy or ureterostomy) can be performed in the very ill, young, or small child.

Follow-Up Imaging of PBS

Long-term follow-up, including upper tract surveillance with periodic ultrasonography, is important in PBS patients. The functional urodynamics of their bladders may change over time, causing deterioration of their upper tracts, necessitating further intervention.

Bladder Augmentation

Bladder augmentation is the surgical process of supplementing the bladder volume using a native structure such as a segment of bowel or redundant ureter. It is a treatment option for patients with noncompliant, low-capacity bladders. Neurogenic bladder is a common cause in the pediatric urologic population, as well as EEC discussed earlier.

Augmentation is performed by isolation of a chosen segment of bowel, detubularizing the segment, and anastomosing it to the bladder. The bladder is drained in the immediate postoperative period, and irrigation via a catheter with normal saline is performed to remove mucus. Bladder augmentation necessitates clean intermittent catheterization (CIC) to allow for adequate emptying.

Imaging of the Augmented Bladder and Its Complications

Routine surveillance of the upper urinary tract with ultrasonography is performed at 6 weeks postoperatively, 6 months postoperatively, and yearly thereafter, looking for hydronephrosis, increased post-void residual volume, and calculi. Cystoscopy is recommended yearly beginning 5 years postoperatively particularly in immunosuppressed patients (transplant recipients) or EEC/CBE patients managed with bladder augmentation because of an increased risk of malignancy along the anastomotic line between bladder and bowel [50, 51]. Imaging via ultrasonography, CT of the pelvis, or MRI of the pelvis may detect a lesion in the bladder, but does not replace direct visualization with cystoscopy.

Calculi in the augmented bladder may form as a result of inadequate irrigation of mucus and

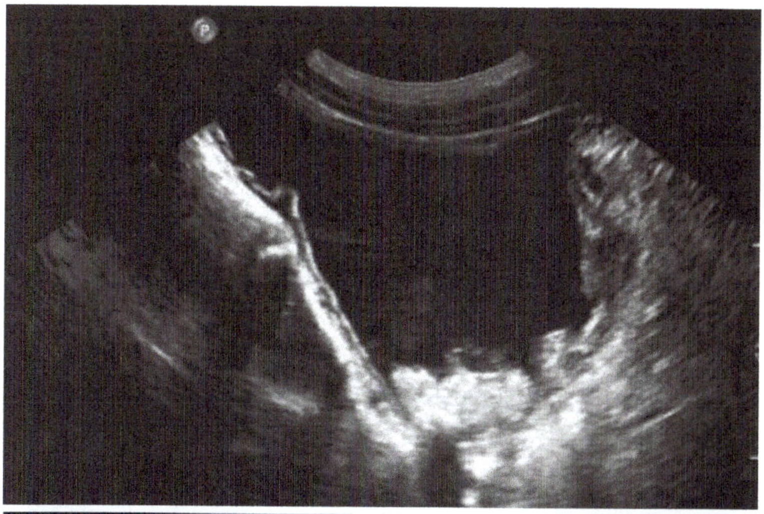

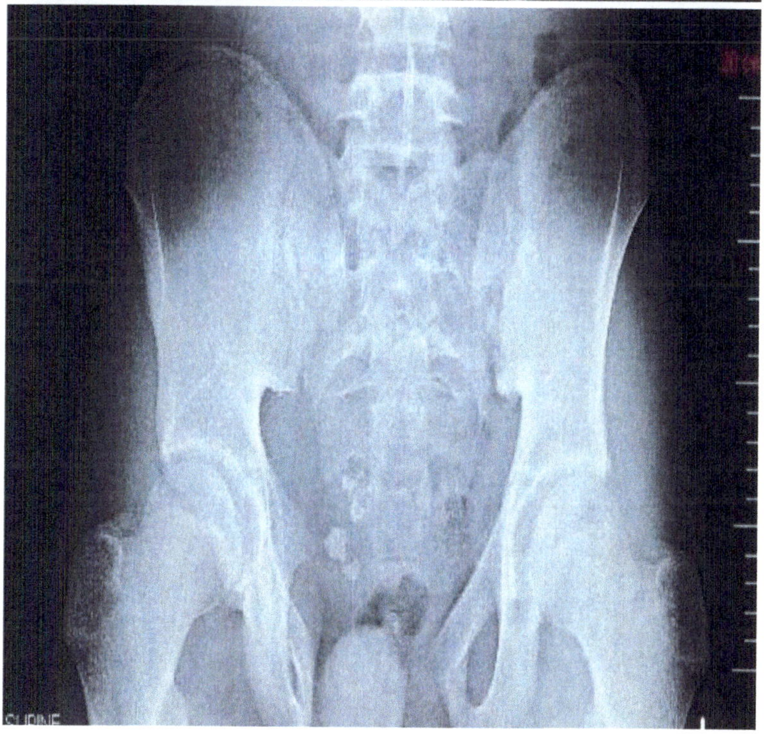

Figs. 19.16 and 19.17 A 15-year-old boy with classic bladder exstrophy who underwent augmentation cystoplasty at age 6 years. He developed recurrent urinary tract infections and some difficulty in performing intermittent catheterization. A bladder sonogram (*left*) demonstrated debris in the bladder with hyperechoic areas at the base that shadow, consistent with stones. A KUB (*right*) better demonstrates the stone burden as there are several radiopaque stones in the pelvis

incomplete emptying. Mucus acts as a nidus for calculus formation, allowing for heterogeneous nucleation and calcification. Additionally, they may form as a result of urine stagnation and subsequent infection. Calculi may be visualized on plain radiograph, ultrasound, and non-contrast CT (Figs. 19.16 and 19.17).

Perforation of an augmented bladder can occur acutely (anastomotic leak) or in delayed fashion. The latter is thought to be a result of inadequate emptying with subsequent pressure necrosis of the augmented bowel. Perforation is a clinical diagnosis, which can be confirmed with conventional or CT cystography [52–54] showing leakage of contrast from the bladder. Ultrasonography can also be utilized, which can demonstrate free fluid in the abdomen and pelvis. This is a surgical emergency.

Table 19.2 Summary of imaging findings in EEC, PBS, and augmented bladder

Disease	Prenatal	Plain film	Ultrasound	CT/MRI	Cystourethrogram
Epispadias	N/A	*Pelvis*—pubic diastasis, outward rotation of the innominate bones, squaring of the iliac notch	*Renal*—normal	*Pelvis*—pubic diastasis, outward rotation of the innominate bones, squaring of the iliac notch, divergent distal rectus abdominis muscles, divergent corpora cavernosa	Dorsal urethral meatus, bladder neck incompetence
CBE	*Ultrasound*—nonvisualization of bladder (non-filling), lower abdominal wall echogenic mass, low-set umbilicus, diminutive genitalia, pubic diastasis (all characteristics seen more clearly on fetal MRI)	*Pelvis*—pubic diastasis, outward rotation of the innominate bones, squaring of the iliac notch	*Renal*—no definite associated anomalies; possible hydroureteronephrosis (post-closure, secondary to VUR)	*Abdomen/pelvis*—findings associated with epispadias, PLUS divergent distal rectus abdominis muscles, open bladder on lower abdomen, anterior displacement of pelvic organs; possible indirect inguinal hernias; possible hydroureteronephrosis	Dorsal urethral meatus; post-closure bladder neck incompetence, VUR, variable bladder capacity
Cloacal exstrophy	*Ultrasound*—findings associated with CBE, PLUS herniation of bowel between bladder plates; possible limb abnormalities, neural tube defects, and vertebral anomalies (all characteristics seen more clearly on fetal MRI)	*Pelvis*—pubic diastasis, outward rotation of the innominate bones, squaring of the iliac notch	*Renal*—possible hydroureteronephrosis (post-closure, secondary to VUR)	*Abdomen/pelvis*—findings associated with CBE, PLUS herniation of hindgut between bladder plates; possible duplicate appendix	Findings associated with CBE
PBS	*Ultrasound/MRI*—protuberant abdomen, bilateral hydroureteronephrosis, distended bladder; possible oligohydramnios, Potter's facies, pulmonary hypoplasia, renal dysplasia	*Chest*—possible pulmonary hypoplasia, pneumothorax, pneumomediastinum	*Renal/bladder*—large-capacity bladder, bilateral hydroureteronephrosis; possible renal dysplasia *Scrotum*—absent testes (undescended)	*Abdomen/pelvis*—large-capacity bladder, bilateral hydroureteronephrosis, intra-abdominal testes, possible renal dysplasia	*VCUG*—bilateral VUR, large-capacity bladder *Nuclear renal scintigraphy*—differential renal function, assess for appropriate upper tract drainage, parenchymal scarring
Augmented bladder	N/A	N/A	*Renal/bladder*—possible thickened bladder; increased incidence of tumor at anastomotic line between bowel and bladder; monitor for development of hydronephrosis	*Abdomen/pelvis*—possible thickened bladder; increased incidence of tumor at anastomotic line between bowel and bladder; monitor for development of hydronephrosis	Possible VUR *Cystography (conventional or CT)*—extravasation of contrast = bladder perforation

Summary

Radiologic imaging is crucial in EEC, PBS, and in the patient with an augmented bladder as summarized in Table 19.2. There are numerous imaging modalities useful in these diagnoses, including ultrasonography (prenatal and postnatal), plain film radiography, CT, MRI (fetal and postnatal), cystourethrography, and nuclear renal scintigraphy. These diagnoses are clinical, yet these imaging modalities allow for assessment of anatomy and aide in the diagnosis and treatment planning.

Key Points

- Plain film radiography, ultrasonography (prenatal and postnatal), CT, MRI (fetal and postnatal), cystourethrography, and nuclear renal scintigraphy can be utilized in assessing EEC patients, PBS patients, and those with bladder augmentation.
- The patient's clinical scenario will dictate the necessity for particular imaging modalities, with one of the important goals being to detect other anomalies (e.g., spinal in CE) and evaluate the genitourinary tract for evidence of VUR or obstruction.
- EEC is a spectrum of anomalies affecting the bony pelvis, pelvic musculature, and genitourinary tract with severity increasing as one moves from epispadias to CBE to CE.
- PBS patients may present with multiple anomalies affecting the musculoskeletal, pulmonary, and cardiac systems.
- Patients that have been treated with bladder augmentation need surveillance for development of hydronephrosis and calculi, as well as to evaluate for adequate emptying.

References

1. Ricci G, Gentili A, Di Lorenzo F, Righetti F, Pigna A, Masi M, et al. Latex allergy in subjects who had undergone multiple surgical procedures for bladder exstrophy: relationship with clinical intervention and atopic diseases. BJU Int. 1999;84(9):1058–62. Epub 1999/11/26.
2. Lattimer JK, Smith MJ. Exstrophy closure: a followup on 70 cases. J Urol. 1966;95(3):356–9. Epub 1966/03/01.
3. Siffel C, Correa A, Amar E, Bakker MK, Bermejo-Sanchez E, Bianca S, et al. Bladder exstrophy: an epidemiologic study from the International Clearinghouse for Birth Defects Surveillance and Research, and an overview of the literature. Am J Med Genet C Semin Med Genet. 2011;157C(4):321–32. Epub 2011/10/18.
4. Wood HM, Babineau D, Gearhart JP. In vitro fertilization and the cloacal/bladder exstrophy-epispadias complex: a continuing association. J Pediatr Urol. 2007;3(4):305–10. Epub 2008/10/25.
5. Stec AA, Pannu HK, Tadros YE, Sponseller PD, Fishman EK, Gearhart JP. Pelvic floor anatomy in classic bladder exstrophy using 3-dimensional computerized tomography: initial insights. J Urol. 2001;166(4):1444–9. Epub 2001/09/08.
6. Stec AA, Pannu HK, Tadros YE, Sponseller PD, Wakim A, Fishman EK, et al. Evaluation of the bony pelvis in classic bladder exstrophy by using 3D-CT: further insights. Urology. 2001;58(6):1030–5. Epub 2001/12/18.
7. Sponseller PD, Bisson LJ, Gearhart JP, Jeffs RD, Magid D, Fishman E. The anatomy of the pelvis in the exstrophy complex. J Bone Joint Surg Am. 1995;77(2):177–89. Epub 1995/02/01.
8. Connolly JA, Peppas DS, Jeffs RD, Gearhart JP. Prevalence and repair of inguinal hernias in children with bladder exstrophy. J Urol. 1995;154(5):1900–1. Epub 1995/11/01.
9. Husmann DA, McLorie GA, Churchill BM, Ein SH. Inguinal pathology and its association with classical bladder exstrophy. J Pediatr Surg. 1990;25(3):332–4. Epub 1990/03/01.
10. Hendren WH. Pediatric rectal and perineal problems. Pediatr Clin North Am. 1998;45(6):1353–72. Epub 1999/01/16.
11. Mathews R, Jeffs RD, Reiner WG, Docimo SG, Gearhart JP. Cloacal exstrophy–improving the quality of life: the Johns Hopkins experience. J Urol. 1998;160(6 Pt 2):2452–6. Epub 1998/11/17.
12. Schober JM, Carmichael PA, Hines M, Ransley PG. The ultimate challenge of cloacal exstrophy. J Urol. 2002;167(1):300–4. Epub 2001/12/18.
13. Lund DP, Hendren WH. Cloacal exstrophy: a 25-year experience with 50 cases. J Pediatr Surg. 2001;36(1):68–75. Epub 2001/01/11.
14. Muecke EC. The role of the cloacal membrane in exstrophy: the first successful experimental study. J Urol. 1964;92:659–67. Epub 1964/12/01.
15. Ambrose SS, O'Brien 3rd DP. Surgical embryology of the exstrophy-epispadias complex. Surg Clin North Am. 1974;54(6):1379–90. Epub 1974/12/01.
16. Gearhart JP, Ben-Chaim J, Jeffs RD, Sanders RC. Criteria for the prenatal diagnosis of classic bladder exstrophy. Obstetr Gynecol. 1995;85(6):961–4. Epub 1995/06/01.
17. Mirk P, Calisti A, Fileni A. Prenatal sonographic diagnosis of bladder exstrophy. J Ultrasound Med. 1986;5(5):291–3. Epub 1986/05/01.

18. Verco PW, Khor BH, Barbary J, Enthoven C. Ectopia vesicae in utero. Australas Radiol. 1986;30(2):117–20. Epub 1986/05/01.
19. Silver RI, Yang A, Ben-Chaim J, Jeffs RD, Gearhart JP. Penile length in adulthood after exstrophy reconstruction. J Urol. 1997;157(3):999–1003. Epub 1997/03/01.
20. Janda GM, Nepple KG, Cooper CS, Austin JC. Supernumerary kidney in a child with OEIS complex. Urology. 2009;74(2):305–7. Epub 2009/04/18.
21. Grady RW, Mitchell ME. Complete primary repair of exstrophy. Surgical technique. Urol Clin North Am. 2000;27(3):569–78, xi. Epub 2000/09/14.
22. Grady RW, Mitchell ME. Complete primary repair of exstrophy. J Urol. 1999;162(4):1415–20. Epub 1999/09/24.
23. Grady RW, Carr MC, Mitchell ME. Complete primary closure of bladder exstrophy. Epispadias and bladder exstrophy repair. Urol Clin North Am. 1999;26(1):95–109, viii. Epub 1999/03/23.
24. Cervellione RM, Husmann DA, Bivalacqua TJ, Sponseller PD, Gearhart JP. Penile ischemic injury in the exstrophy/epispadias spectrum: new insights and possible mechanisms. J Pediatr Urol. 2010;6(5):450–6. Epub 2010/06/15.
25. Schaeffer AJ, Stec AA, Purves JT, Cervellione RM, Nelson CP, Gearhart JP. Complete primary repair of bladder exstrophy: a single institution referral experience. J Urol. 2011;186(3):1041–6. Epub 2011/07/26.
26. Baradaran N, Stec A, Wang MH, Cervellione RM, Luskin J, Gearhart JP. Urinary diversion in early childhood: indications and outcomes in the exstrophy patients. Urology. 2012;80(1):191–5. Epub 2012/04/21.
27. Hassett S, Smith GH, Holland AJ. Prune belly syndrome. Pediatr Surg Int. 2012;28(3):219–28. Epub 2011/12/27.
28. Tonni G, Ida V, Alessandro V, Bonasoni MP. Prune-belly syndrome: case series and review of the literature regarding early prenatal diagnosis, epidemiology, genetic factors, treatment, and prognosis. Fetal Pediatr Pathol. 2012;31(1):13–24. Epub 2012/04/18.
29. Wheatley JM, Stephens FD, Hutson JM. Prune-belly syndrome: ongoing controversies regarding pathogenesis and management. Semin Pediatr Surgery. 1996;5(2):95–106. Epub 1996/05/01.
30. Rabinowitz R, Schillinger JF. Prune belly syndrome in the female subject. J Urol. 1977;118(3):454–6. Epub 1977/09/01.
31. Reinberg Y, Shapiro E, Manivel JC, Manley CB, Pettinato G, Gonzalez R. Prune belly syndrome in females: a triad of abdominal musculature deficiency and anomalies of the urinary and genital systems. J Pediatr. 1991;118(3):395–8. Epub 1991/03/01.
32. Hutson JM, Beasley SW. Aetiology of the prune belly syndrome. Austr Paediatr J. 1987;23(5):309–10. Epub 1987/10/01.
33. Stephens FD, Gupta D. Pathogenesis of the prune belly syndrome. J Urol. 1994;152(6 Pt 2):2328–31. Epub 1994/12/01.
34. Ives EJ. The abdominal muscle deficiency triad syndrome–experience with ten cases. Birth Defects Orig Artic Ser. 1974;10(4):127–35. Epub 1974/01/01.
35. Popek EJ, Tyson RW, Miller GJ, Caldwell SA. Prostate development in prune belly syndrome (PBS) and posterior urethral valves (PUV): etiology of PBS–lower urinary tract obstruction or primary mesenchymal defect? Pediatr Pathol. 1991;11(1):1–29. Epub 1991/01/01.
36. Woodard JR. The prune belly syndrome. Urol Clin North Am. 1978;5(1):75–93. Epub 1978/02/01.
37. Reinberg Y, Manivel JC, Pettinato G, Gonzalez R. Development of renal failure in children with the prune belly syndrome. J Urol. 1991;145(5):1017–19. Epub 1991/05/01.
38. Palmer JM, Tesluk H. Ureteral pathology in the prune belly syndrome. J Urol. 1974;111(5):701–7. Epub 1974/05/01.
39. Berdon WE, Baker DH, Wigger HJ, Blanc WA. The radiologic and pathologic spectrum of the prune belly syndrome. The importance of urethral obstruction in prognosis. Radiol Clin North Am. 1977;15(1):83–92. Epub 1977/04/01.
40. Gearhart JP, Lee BR, Partin AW, Epstein JI, Gosling JA. A quantitative histological evaluation of the dilated ureter of childhood. II: ectopia, posterior urethral valves and the prune belly syndrome. J Urol. 1995;153(1):172–6.
41. Workman SJ, Kogan BA. Fetal bladder histology in posterior urethral valves and the prune belly syndrome. J Urol. 1990;144(2 Pt 1):337–9. Epub 1990/08/01.
42. Papantoniou N, Papoutsis D, Daskalakis G, Chatzipapas I, Sindos M, Papaspyrou I, et al. Prenatal diagnosis of prune-belly syndrome at 13 weeks of gestation: case report and review of literature. J Matern Fetal Neonatal Med. 2010;23(10):1263–7. Epub 2010/05/28.
43. Chen L, Cai A, Wang X, Wang B, Li J. Two- and three-dimensional prenatal sonographic diagnosis of prune-belly syndrome. J Clin Ultrasound. 2010;38(5):279–82. Epub 2009/12/17.
44. Osborne NG, Bonilla-Musoles F, Machado LE, Raga F, Bonilla Jr F, Ruiz F, et al. Fetal megacystis: differential diagnosis. J Ultrasound Med. 2011;30(6):833–41. Epub 2011/06/03.
45. Morris RK, Kilby MD. An overview of the literature on congenital lower urinary tract obstruction and introduction to the PLUTO trial: percutaneous shunting in lower urinary tract obstruction. Austr N Z J Obstet Gynaecol. 2009;49(1):6–10. Epub 2009/03/14.
46. Kilby M, Khan K, Morris K, Daniels J, Gray R, Magill L, et al. PLUTO trial protocol: percutaneous shunting for lower urinary tract obstruction randomised controlled trial. BJOG. 2007;114(7):904–5, e1-4. Epub 2007/06/15.
47. Shrom SH, Cromie WJ, Duckett Jr JW. Megalourethra. Urology. 1981;17(2):152–6. Epub 1981/02/01.
48. Kroovand RL, Al-Ansari RM, Perlmutter AD. Urethral and genital malformations in prune belly syndrome. J Urol. 1982;127(1):94–6. Epub 1982/01/01.

49. Kinahan TJ, Churchill BM, McLorie GA, Gilmour RF, Khoury AE. The efficiency of bladder emptying in the prune belly syndrome. J Urol. 1992;148(2 Pt 2):600–3. Epub 1992/08/01.
50. Husmann DA. Malignancy after gastrointestinal augmentation in childhood. Ther Adv Urol. 2009;1(1):5–11. Epub 2009/04/01.
51. Husmann DA, Rathbun SR. Long-term follow up of enteric bladder augmentations: the risk for malignancy. J Pediatr Urol. 2008;4(5):381–5; discussion 6. Epub 2008/07/26.
52. Braverman RM, Lebowitz RL. Perforation of the augmented urinary bladder in nine children and adolescents: importance of cystography. AJR Am J Roentgenol. 1991;157(5):1059–63. Epub 1991/11/01.
53. Rosen MA, Light JK. Spontaneous bladder rupture following augmentation enterocystoplasty. J Urol. 1991;146(5):1232–4. Epub 1991/11/01.
54. Bauer SB, Hendren WH, Kozakewich H, Maloney S, Colodny AH, Mandell J, et al. Perforation of the augmented bladder. J Urol. 1992;148(2 Pt 2):699–703. Epub 1992/08/01.

Trauma

20

Benjamin Whittam, Boaz Karmazyn, and Mark Cain

Abbreviations

MVA	Motor vehicle accident
AAST	American Association for Surgery of Trauma
RBC	Red blood cells
UA	Urinalysis
US	Ultrasonography
UPJ	Ureteropelvic junction
IVP	Intravenous pyelogram
RGP	Retrograde pyelogram
IP	Intraperitoneal
EP	Extraperitoneal
RUG	Retrograde urethrogram

Introduction

Trauma-related injuries are the leading cause of death in children older than 1 year old. Injuries are responsible for approximately 20,000 deaths in children each year in the United States [1]. Pediatric trauma is twice as prevalent in boys than girls across all ages [2]. Pediatric injuries typically occur from falls and bicycle and motor vehicle accidents. These types of injuries usually result in a blunt trauma, which account for 80–90 % of all pediatric traumas. Incidence of penetrating trauma secondary to assault increases in teenage boys [2].

Trauma to the urogenital system is present in approximately 3 % of all significant pediatric injuries evaluated at pediatric trauma centers [1]. Imaging is used to evaluate the extent of the injuries and to direct their management. The armamentarium of radiographic modalities is available for imaging the traumatized genitourinary tract, but interestingly, specific modalities are best suited for specific types of injuries. CT scanning is the cornerstone and most comprehensive imaging modality for evaluation for abdominal trauma in children. Angiography is performed selectively to diagnose and treat active bleeding. Ultrasound is the imaging modality of choice for evaluation of scrotal trauma and is used selectively in follow-up of renal injuries. Retrograde urethrogram is mainly used in children with meatal hematuria to evaluate for urethral injury. The vast majority of urogenital trauma is managed conservatively with only active observation. The challenge is to promptly diagnose the few injuries requiring emergent intervention to save life or to preserve organ function.

Radiographic imaging is essential for diagnosing, staging, and management of urogenital trauma. The focus of this chapter is imaging evaluation of pediatric urogenital trauma. Traumatic

B. Whittam, MD • M. Cain, MD (✉)
Division of Pediatric Urology, Riley Hospital for Children, 705 Riley Hospital Drive, Indianapolis, IN 46202, USA
e-mail: bwhittam@iupui.edu; mpcain@iupui.edu

B. Karmazyn, MD
Department of Pediatric Radiology and Imaging Sciences, Riley Hospital for Children at IU Health, 705 Riley Hospital Drive, Suite 1053, Indianapolis, IN 46202, USA
e-mail: bkarmazy@iupui.edu

L.S. Palmer, J.S. Palmer (eds.), *Pediatric and Adolescent Urologic Imaging*,
DOI 10.1007/978-1-4614-8654-1_20, © Springer Science+Business Media New York 2014

injuries of the adrenal, kidney, ureter, bladder, urethra, and testicle will be reviewed in systematic fashion enhanced with clinically relevant radiographic images. The relative indications for imaging injuries to the urogenital system and common radiographic findings will be discussed as well as general clinical management.

Adrenal

Adrenal trauma is uncommon with reported incidence of between 0.5 and 3.0 % of all pediatric traumas and is almost always the result of blunt force trauma [3]. This correlates well with the low incidence of adult adrenal trauma [4–6]. The most common etiology is motor vehicle accidents (MVA) followed by pedestrian versus automobile and falls. Adrenal injuries are typically the result of a major trauma (Fig. 20.1). Nearly 90 % of pediatric patients suffering from adrenal trauma have severe associated injuries, typically to other abdominal organs, head or brain, and long bones [3]. In both pediatric and adult patients, the right adrenal gland is injured greater than 75 % of time, while bilateral injuries occur in less than 5 % of patients [3, 4].

Adrenal injuries are believed to be a result of direct compression and increase in venous pressure caused by compression of the inferior vena cava (IVC). The vascular anatomy of the adrenal gland causes any increase in pressure in the adrenal vein to be immediately transferred to small venules, which cannot accommodate the rapid pressure increase resulting in rupture. It is hypothesized that the short right adrenal vein poorly accommodates (compared to the left adrenal vein) a rapid rise in pressure caused by traumatic compression of the IVC, thus resulting in the predominance of right-sided adrenal injuries [3, 4].

Adrenal injuries are almost exclusively diagnosed by CT scan [3]. The most common finding is an oval or rounded enlarged adrenal gland (Fig. 20.1). Other findings on CT include hematoma that obscures the adrenal outline, stranding of the periadrenal fat, and hemorrhage in adjacent retroperitoneum [3, 4, 7]. A unilateral adrenal injury is typically of minimal clinical significance. In a series of 41 pediatric patients, none required endovascular or surgical intervention for their adrenal [3]. Even the pediatric patients with isolated adrenal injuries (no other injuries identified during trauma evaluation) did not require intervention. Rarely is adrenal replacement required, but clinicians should maintain high suspicion in patients with bilateral adrenal injuries.

Neonatal adrenal hemorrhage may result from birth trauma and increased abdominal pressure and is associated with ischemia and septicemia (Fig. 20.2). The incidence of neonatal adrenal hemorrhage is 0.2–3 % of live births [8]. The

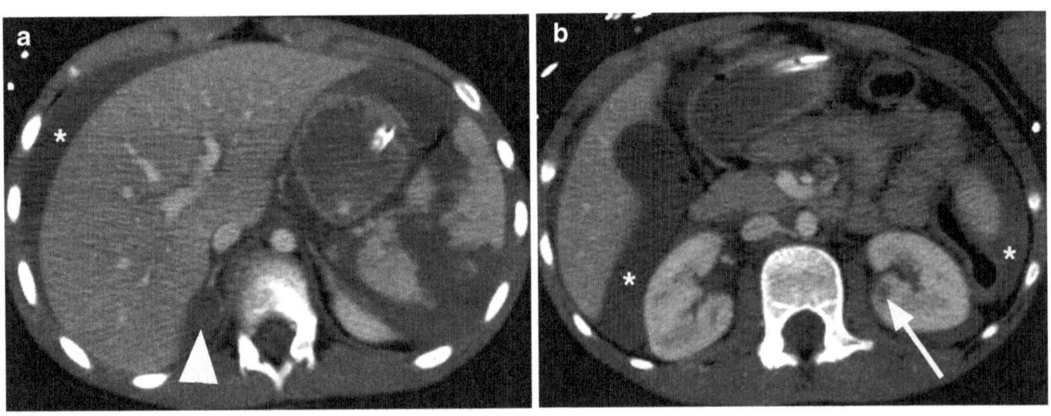

Fig. 20.1 Right adrenal hematoma and right Grade II renal injury in an 8-year-old boy pedestrian in a car struck by a train. CT scan of the abdomen (**a**) demonstrates shattered spleen, right adrenal hematoma (*arrowhead*), and (**b**) superficial laceration of the right kidney. In addition there was large hemoperitoneum (*)

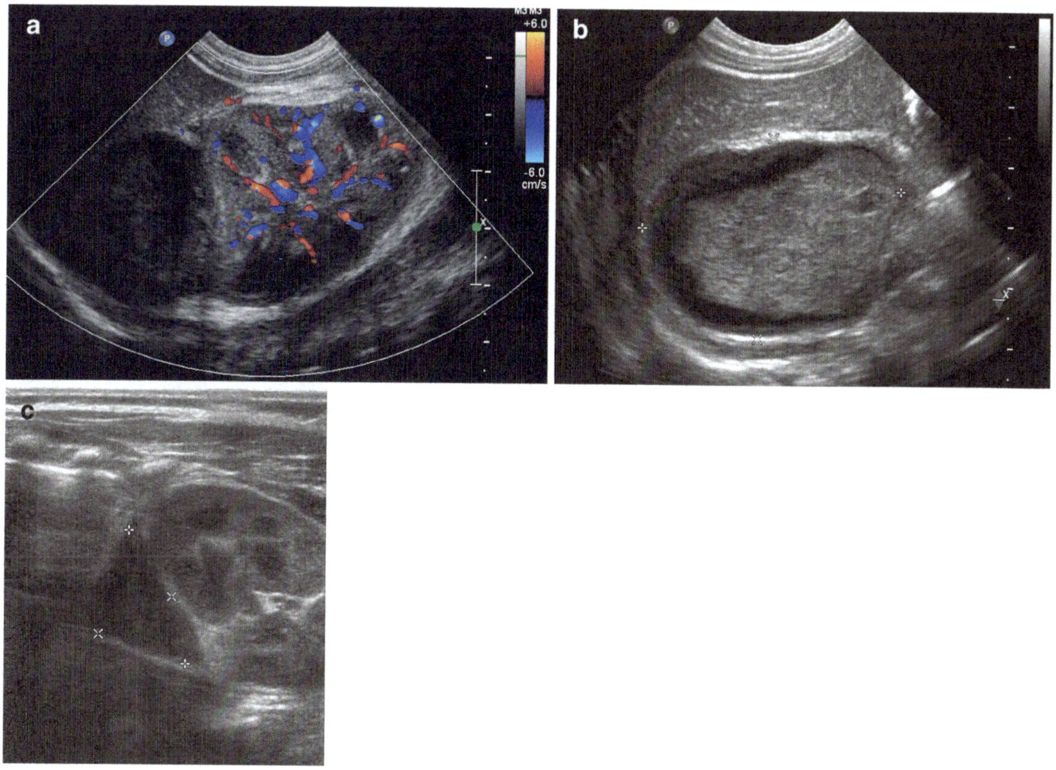

Fig. 20.2 Neonatal adrenal hemorrhage in a large for gestational age term infant post vacuum-assisted vaginal delivery who presented with jaundice, anemia, and suspicion of right renal mass on physical examination. (**a**) Longitudinal Doppler US demonstrates avascular suprarenal mass with a maximal diameter of 4.4 cm (**b**). The mass is better delineated on high-resolution linear transducer and demonstrates a well-defined rounded shape with complex fluid. (**c**) Follow-up US demonstrates marked decrease of the suprarenal mass with a maximal diameter of 2.4 cm, compatible with evolving adrenal hemorrhage

typical presentation is the presence of an abdominal mass and anemia and/or jaundice due to reabsorption of the hematoma, although many children are asymptomatic and there are rare cases complicated with hypovolemic shock due to anemia. Diagnosis is primarily made by ultrasound, which shows a well-defined complex cystic enlargement of the adrenal. The other main possible diagnosis is neuroblastoma. Follow-up imaging is indicated to confirm its involution.

Kidney

The kidney is the most frequently injured genitourinary organ, typically as a result of blunt trauma and present in 2–3 % of all pediatric trauma-related injuries. The pediatric kidney is at increased susceptibility to trauma secondary to multiple anatomic protective factors: softer rib cage, less mature torso musculature, proportionally larger kidneys extending below the protection of the rib cage, and less cushioning perinephric fat [9]. There has been a steady shift over the past 30 years toward conservative therapy for renal trauma, with intervention reserved only for selected patients. Multiorgan trauma is common and present in 50–80 % of patients with any renal injury [10, 11].

Congenitally abnormal kidneys are more susceptible to trauma. Unrecognized renal anomalies are far more common in children and are present in approximately 10 % of children with renal injuries (Figs. 20.3 and 20.4). The most common congenital abnormalities associated with trauma are hydronephrosis, horseshoe

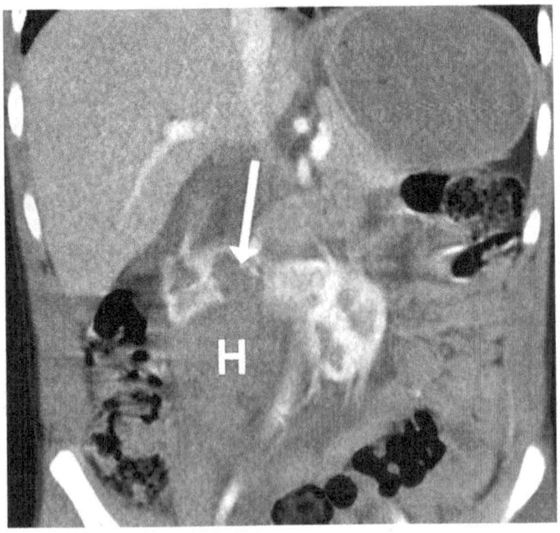

Fig. 20.3 A Grade III renal injury in a 7-year-old boy with a horseshoe kidney who had handlebar injury from a bike. Coronal post-early IV contrast CT scan demonstrates the laceration (*arrow*) and perirenal hematoma (*H*)

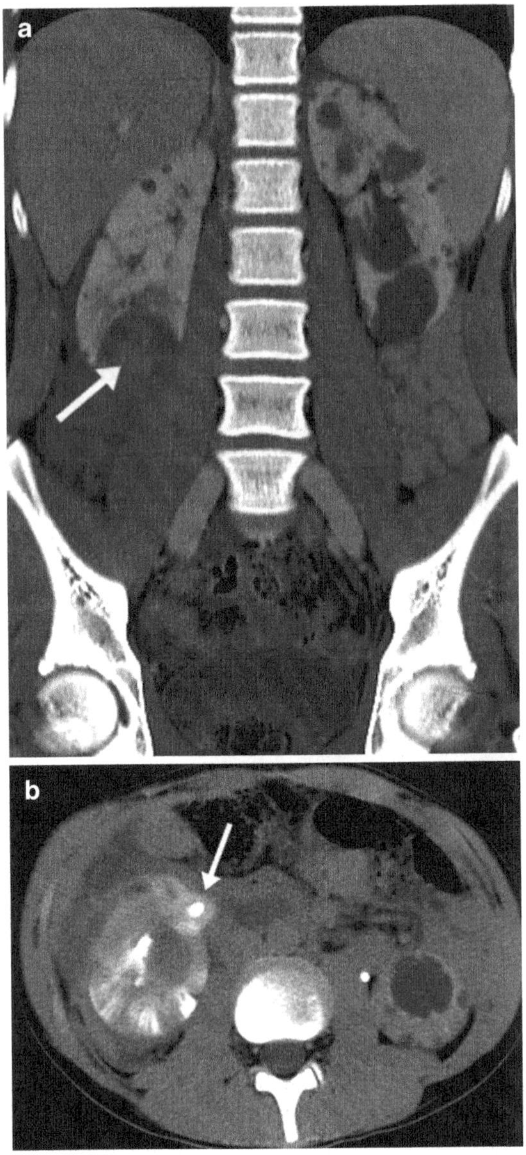

Fig. 20.4 A right Grade IV renal injury in a 14-year-old who had football injury. (**a**) Coronal post-early IV contrast discovered bilateral polycystic renal disease with laceration in the lower pole and hematoma in a right lower pole cyst (*arrow*). (**b**) Axial post-delayed IV contrast demonstrates contrast extravasation (*arrow*)

kidney, and renal ectopia [12–14]. Despite making the kidney more prone to injury, there does not appear to be an increase in morbidity or mortality [15, 16].

Since the late 1980s CT scan has become the imaging modality of choice for the initial evaluation of suspected renal trauma. CT allows for assessment of injury to the renal parenchyma and hilum, extent of renal hemorrhage, extravasation of urine, as well as associated injuries to other abdominal organs and vasculature structures.

The American Association for the Surgery of Trauma (AAST) has developed a universally accepted grading scale (I–V) to quantify the severity of renal trauma and the likelihood of surgical intervention (Fig. 20.5). There is no consensus on an imaging algorithm for the evaluation of the pediatric trauma patients [17]. The most comprehensive and most algorithm was proposed by McAninch in 2004 and based on observation and management of 374 pediatric patients [18]. This algorithm utilizes the etiology of blunt or penetrating trauma, stability of patient, coupled with the number of red blood cells (RBCs) found on urinalysis (UA) to determine if abdominal CT scan is warranted. They concluded that Abdominal CT scan should be performed in all stable patients with penetrating trauma who have greater than five RBCs on UA and selectively in stable patients with blunt abdominal trauma greater than 50 RBC on UA. The selection criteria to obtain a abdominal CT scan in patients with blunt abdominal trauma, include positive clinical findings of renal trauma (e.g., flank pain, ecchymosis) and rapid

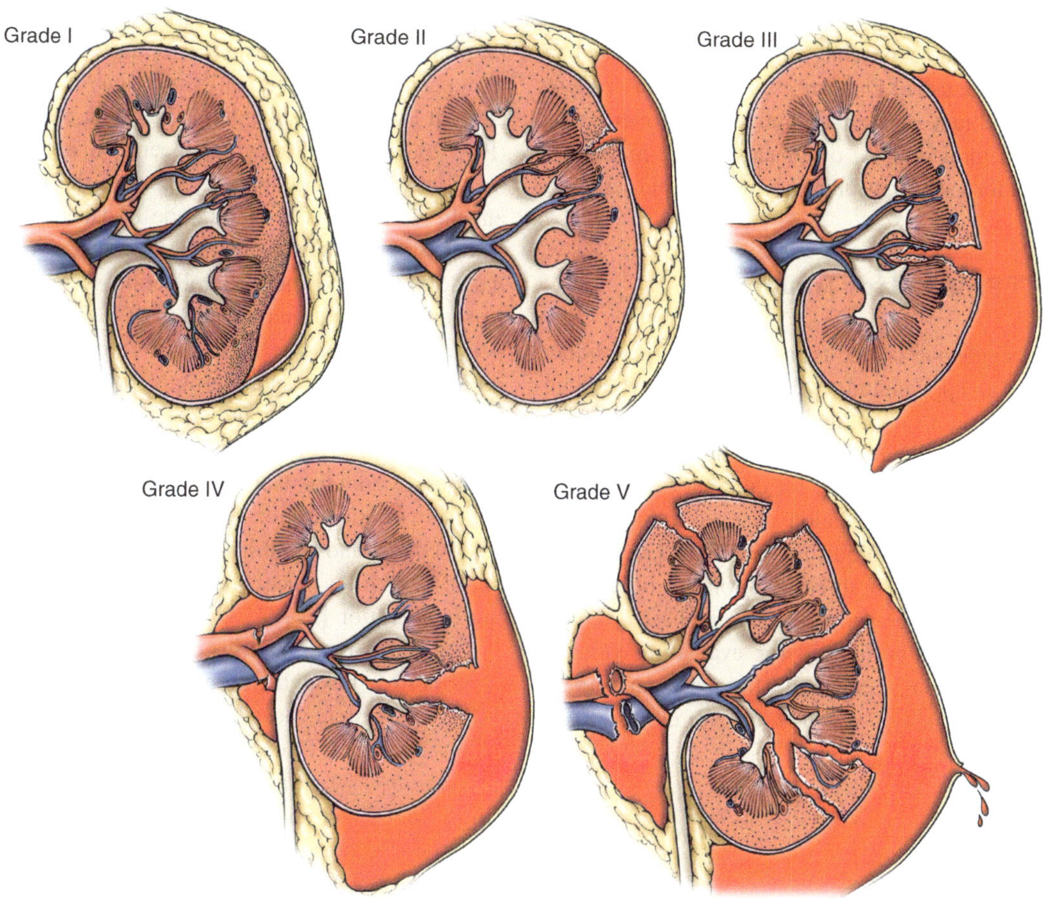

Fig. 20.5 American Association for the Surgery of Trauma (*AAST*) organ injury scaling for kidney injury, Grade I–V (From Vanni and Wessells [51], www.acssurgery.com. Reprinted with permission. Copyright Decker Publishing)

deceleration injury. Management of unstable patients depends on the expertise of the medical center. In level 1 trauma center more patients are treated with conservative or minimally invasive procedures (e.g., angiographic embolization, nephrostomy, ureteral stent) as compared to abdominal exploration and nephrectomy. This approach results in a sensitivity for detecting Grade II or greater injuries in over 98 % of blunt trauma and greater than 95 % of penetrating trauma [18]. However, the yield of abdominal CT scan in pediatric patients with microscopic hematuria is very small, and its use should be considered carefully in these patients [19].

Some groups have raised concerns that this approach (CT scan for microscopic hematuria >5 RBC/hpf) results in the performance of many unnecessary CT scans which have no impact on clinical course. These groups support the use of established adult trauma criteria for CT scan in the pediatric population; i.e., CT scan is reserved for patients with gross hematuria or are that are clinically unstable [19, 20]. A study simulating this approach in 27 children with microscopic hematuria after blunt trauma showed that only one patient had a Grade IV injury; the kidney was found to be uninjured at surgery [11] and in retrospect misdiagnosed by CT scan.

Ultrasonography (US) evaluation for renal injuries is enticing, as it does not require radiation and can be performed at the bedside, but it lacks sensitivity for detecting solid-organ and vascular injuries. However, if the decision is made to limit CT scanning only to children with gross hematuria, major trauma, or clinical instability, then one may consider use of Doppler US for screening patients with blunt abdominal trauma and microscopic hematuria [19]. At our institution we mainly use US for long-term follow-up of renal injuries.

CT Protocol for Trauma

A single portal venous phase IV contrasts abdominal and pelvis study is performed for any abdominal trauma including for renal trauma. If any renal injury is detected, 5 min delayed CT scan is performed to evaluate for contrast extravasation. To reduce the radiation dose, a split-bolus CT urographic technique has been introduced [21]. It is possible to use three split contrast boluses and scan only once and get all three phases which is our current preference for evaluating vascular, parenchymal, and collecting system injuries (Fig. 20.6) and for follow-up. We use three contrast phases in a single CT scan (Fig. 20.7).

Grading

Grade I injuries are defined as hematuria with a normal CT, renal parenchymal contusion, or nonexpanding subcapsular hematoma without parenchymal laceration. This is the least severe renal injury and accounts for approximately 80 % of all renal injuries [18]. Typical CT findings consist of ill-defined or discrete areas of decreased contrast enhancement or with subcapsular hematoma. A subcapsular hematoma is found between the renal capsule and the parenchyma and demonstrates a crescent or elliptical shape, often deforming the parenchyma beneath. A large subcapsular hematoma may cause severe enough compression to impair renal perfusion, resulting in hypertension and a "Page" kidney. Patients with Grade I renal injuries may be observed but frequently do not require admission, bed rest, or any serial laboratory investigations. No follow-up imaging is typically necessary [22–24].

More severe renal injuries occur when the parenchyma tears or splits and include both Grade II and III injuries, determined by depth of laceration. A Grade II injury is defined as either a nonexpanding perirenal hematoma or renal cortical laceration that extends less than one cm (Fig. 20.1). A parenchymal laceration appears as a linear or wedge-shaped defect in the renal enhancement. On CT scan Grade III lacerations extend greater than 1 cm into the renal cortex but do not extend into the collecting system. A perinephric hematoma appears on CT as an ill-defined, high-density fluid collection between renal parenchyma and Gerota's fascia, rarely deforming the renal contour (Figs. 20.3, 20.8, and 20.9). Throughout multiple series Grade I–III injuries account for over 90 % of all renal injuries and are without question managed conservatively, e.g., bed rest and serial laboratory investigations, and do not often necessitate follow-up imaging nor intervention [22–24].

Grade IV renal injuries extend through the renal cortex, through the medulla, and into the collecting system, possibly resulting in urinary extravasation. CT delayed phase may show extravasation of urine into the perirenal space (Figs. 20.4, 20.6, and 20.10). Urinary extravasation does not necessitate surgical intervention as over 80 % spontaneously resolve. Follow-up by US can be performed to evaluate change in the extrarenal fluid collection (Fig. 20.9). An injury to the hilum, either venous or arterial, is also considered a Grade IV renal injury. Grade IV injuries including thrombosis, dissection, or injury to the renal vasculature result in segmental infarcts. CT scan may demonstrate active arterial extravasation, which can be managed with angiographic embolization (Fig. 20.10). Infarcts appear as well-circumcised linear or wedge-shaped areas without enhancement.

Grade IV renal injuries involve any injury to collecting system, including the renal pelvis. Ureteropelvic junction (UPJ) disruption is more commonly seen in pediatric patients, typically resulting from a deceleration injury. A complete UPJ avulsion is diagnosed by lack of contrast in the distal ureter, but a partial UPJ avulsion may demonstrate ureteral contrast. Contrast-laden urine located medial to the renal pelvis and UPJ is often seen in injury to UPJ or the renal pelvis.

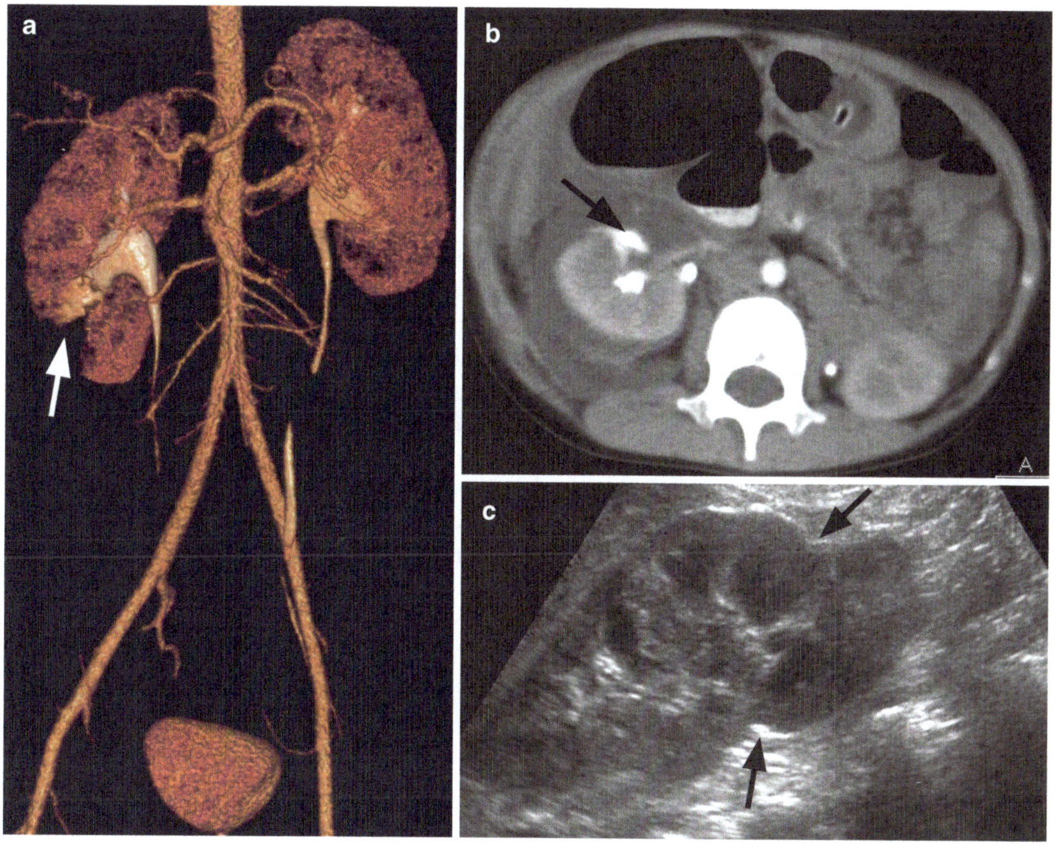

Fig. 20.6 Right Grade IV renal injury in a 5-year-old boy who fell landing on his right flank. He later developed hematuria. Initial CT scan demonstrated Grade IV right renal laceration. A follow-up post-IV contrast CT scan was performed with three-phase technique (arterial, parenchymal, and excretion) in one scan. Volume rendering (**a**) and axial view demonstrate good opacification of the aorta and major branches including the renal arteries. (**b**) In the right kidney there is inferior pole triangular-shaped laceration with contrast extravasation (*arrows*). A 7-month follow-up ultrasound (**c**) demonstrates lower pole scarring (*arrows*) and atrophy

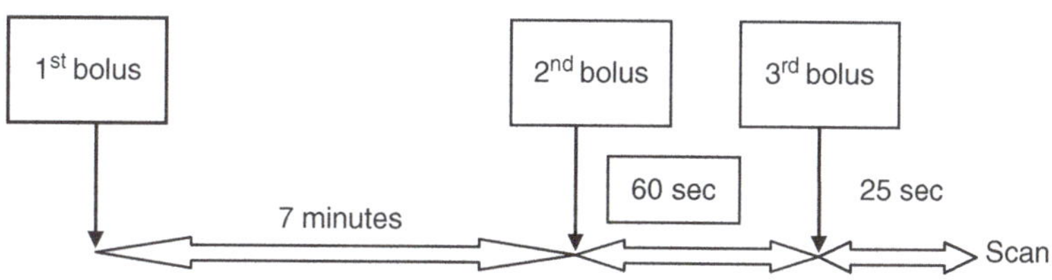

Fig. 20.7 *Protocol.* Contrast volume = 2 mL/kg body weight
1st bolus = 0 s, 20 % contrast volume
2nd bolus = 420 s after the start of the 1st bolus, 35 % of contrast volume
3rd bolus = 60 s after the start of the 2nd bolus, 45 % of contrast volume
Scan after 25 s from the start of the 3rd bolus

Treatment of nonvascular Grade IV renal injury varies, but most can be managed conservatively and will not require intervention. Urinomas may require a ureteral stent or percutaneous drainage in approximately 15 %, while only 10 % require open surgical exploration. One study has shown that medial urinary extravasation on initial CT scan increases risk for necessitating urologic

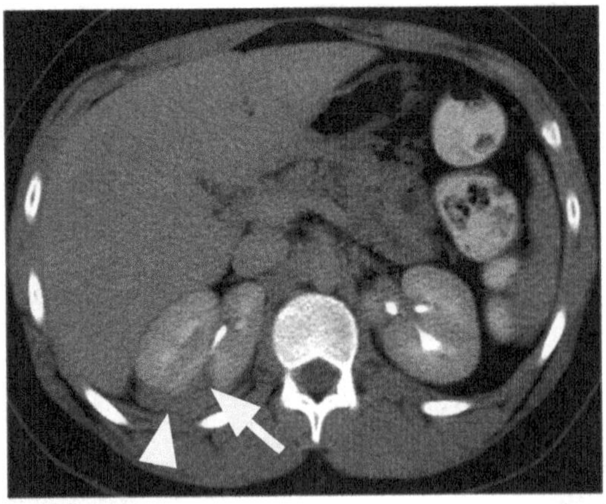

Fig. 20.8 Right Grade III renal injury in a 15-year-old boy stabbed with crooked hook accidentally while playing with his sister at home. Delayed post-contrast CT scan of the abdomen demonstrates a laceration in the right kidney (*arrow*) with small perirenal hematoma (*arrowhead*). There is no contrast extravasation

intervention. This same study suggested that lack of filling of the ipsilateral ureter is concerning for UPJ disruption, which likely will require surgical intervention.

Grade V injuries denote a shattered or devascularized kidney or complete avulsion of the renal hilum resulting in devascularization of the kidney. Radiographic appearance of a shattered kidney demonstrates multiple Grade IV injuries, with infarcted, devitalized areas coupled with urinary extravasation secondary to trauma to the collecting system (Fig. 20.11).

Injuries to the renal hilum may not result in hematuria but are almost always associated with significant injuries to other organs. The most common hilar injury is renal artery occlusion secondary to acute stretching of the renal artery causing intimal tearing, arterial dissection, and vessel occlusion. CT will demonstrate a well-defined segment or global absence of renal enhancement but reniform contour is maintained (Figs. 20.12 and 20.13). Right renal artery injuries may also demonstrate retrograde filling of the right renal vein from the inferior vena cava. Collateral perfusion may result in enhancement to the capsule and subcapsular areas, also known as the cortical rim sign, but several hours are required for the appearance of this sign. Isolated renal vein injuries are particularly uncommon, and renal vein thrombosis is often seen in concert with arterial or parenchymal injuries. CT will show renal enlargement, decreased early nephrogram, and prolonged corticomedullary nephrogram with delayed or absent opacification of the collecting system. Laceration of the renal vein demonstrates medial or circumferential subcapsular or perinephric hematoma.

The management of a Grade V renal injury is complex and should be tailored to each patient, as each individual represents a unique injury. Conservative management is possible in Grade V renal injuries, but often an interventional radiology or surgical intervention is necessary. Follow-up imaging is necessary to assess for expanding hematoma or urinoma. Findings on early follow-up imaging may necessitate percutaneous drains, percutaneous nephrostomy tubes, or ureteral stents for further management. Nephrectomy may be required for unstable patients or unsalvageable renal injuries; however, renorrhaphy should always be attempted prior to nephrectomy.

Vascular injuries seen in Grade IV and Grade V renal trauma may necessitate renal angiography (Fig. 20.10). CT scan remains the initial study of choice, unless the patient is too unstable and requires immediate operative intervention. Vascular extravasation may be detected on CT scan; however, it is less sensitive compared to angiography. Angiography with transcatheter embolization may be required in patients with arteriovenous fistula, pseudoaneurysm, or an active arterial bleeding [25].

Currently no consensus exists regarding subsequent imaging after initial CT scan in this population, and a follow-up CT scan may be necessary during hospitalization for Grade IV and V injuries. In the past a repeat CT scan was routinnely obtained at 48 h to assess for persistent urinary extravasation [26]. This practice is evolving and at our institution we use renal US for routine follow-up to evaluate for change in

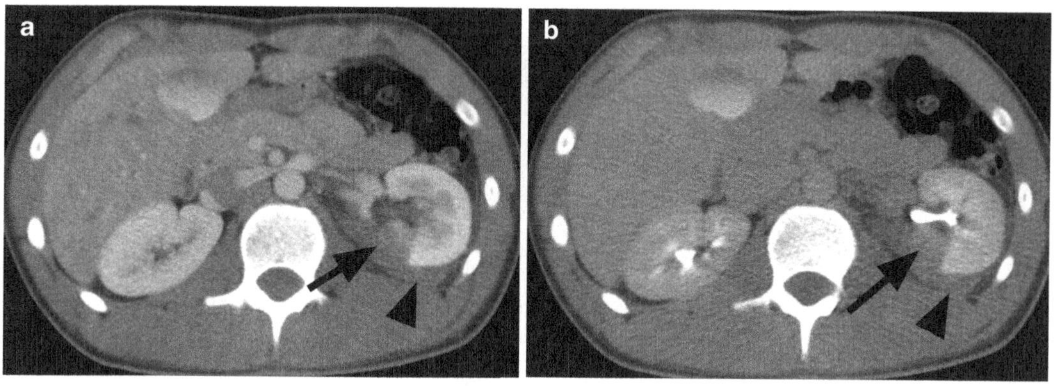

Fig. 20.9 Left Grade III renal injury in a 15-year-old boy with a history of factor IX deficiency who was hit on the left flank during football practice and subsequently began having increased abdominal pain. (**a**) Initial and (**b**) delayed post-contrast IV contrast CT scans demonstrated left renal laceration (*arrow*) with perirenal hematoma (*arrowhead*). (**b**) Delayed CT scan did not demonstrate contrast extravasation

perirenal hematoma and urinoma (Fig. 20.10). Repeat CT scans are used selectively in the presence of persistent ileus, fever, worsening flank pain, hemodynamic instability, increasing pain, fever, leukocytosis, decreasing hematocrit, enlarging hematoma as urinoma or increasing blood transfusion requirements [24].

Long-term follow-up imaging after Grade IV or V renal injuries with a renal ultrasound is often necessary to determine resolution of hematoma or urinoma. No definitive follow-up protocol exists, but we typically repeat ultrasounds every few months until complete or near resolution of renal defect, hematoma, or urinoma. Patients should undergo routine blood pressure evaluation for hypertension screening. A nuclear renogram should be obtained if a devascularization injury occurred to determine residual renal function or if post-trauma hypertension is present [27, 28].

Unstable trauma patients that require immediate surgical exploration should undergo an intraoperative intravenous pyelogram (IVP) to assess for presence of enhanced kidneys and collecting system. It can help determine if renal or ureteral intervention is necessary. Intraoperative IVP is performed by intravenous injection of 1.5–2.0 mL/kg dose of intravenous contrast and abdominal X-ray at 10–15 min.

Ureter

Isolated traumatic pediatric ureteral injuries are exceedingly rare and are often the result of penetrating injury or severe blunt trauma where there is significant deceleration injury. The ureter is well protected by the psoas muscle and bony pelvis throughout its course in the retroperitoneum. The upper ureter is susceptible to injury despite the ureter being protected by the vertebral column and paraspinal muscles. The ureter is small, flexible, and mobile making injury more likely by penetrating trauma than blunt trauma. Blunt ureteral trauma from severe deceleration injuries may result in avulsion of the ureter from the renal pelvis secondary to extreme hyperextension. Hematuria is a poor predictor of ureteral injury; one study showed less than 20 % of patients with ureteric injury had hematuria[29].

An opacified ureter on delayed post-contrast CT scan makes a ureteral injury unlikely. Findings of ureteral injury include contrast extravasation and large fluid collection in the perinephric space without contrast in the ureter (Fig. 20.14). Unstable patients requiring emergent operative intervention can be evaluated with an intraoperative single-shot IVP [25]. No published evidence supports the use of US in evaluation for acute ureteric trauma [30].

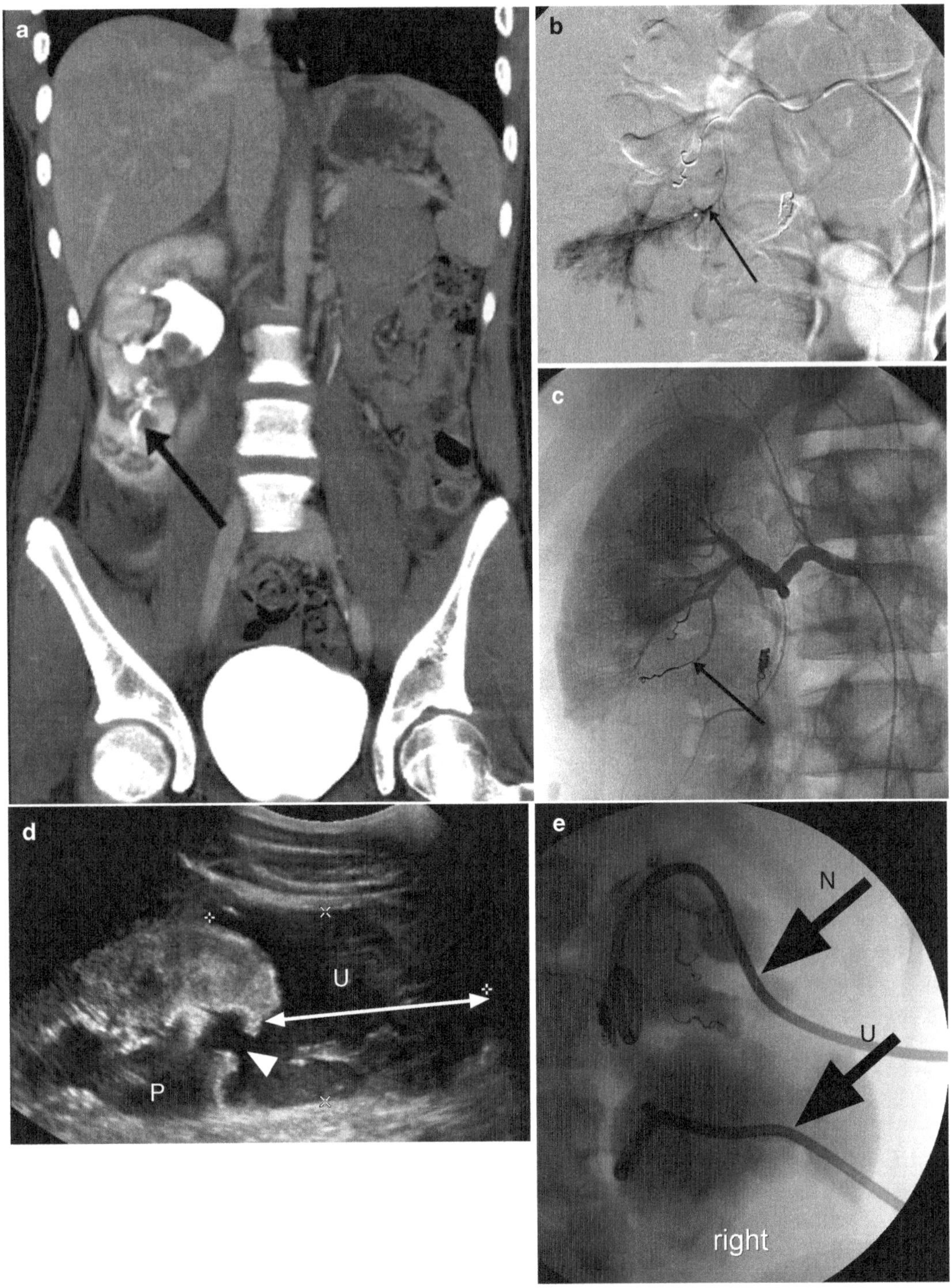

Fig. 20.10 Right Grade IV renal injury in a 15-year-old boy that was crashing into a tree while mountain biking. (**a**) Post-IV contrast CT scan demonstrates laceration of the lower pole of the right kidney with massive retroperitoneal leak of contrast (contrast in the renal system was secondary to prior outside CT scan). Hemoglobin drop in the second day of admission led to renal angiography study. (**b**) Selective catheterization of a second-order branch of the lower pole demonstrated small extravasation from terminal arteries (*arrow*). (**c**) Three terminal branches were successfully embolized with microcoils. (**d**) Two-week follow-up ultrasound demonstrated right renal hydronephrosis with moderate dilation of the renal pelvis (*P*), lower pole laceration (*arrowhead*), and large (an *arrow* with *two arrowheads*) urinoma. (**e**) Nephrostomy (*arrow*, *N*) and pigtail drainage to the urinoma (*arrow*, *U*) were placed

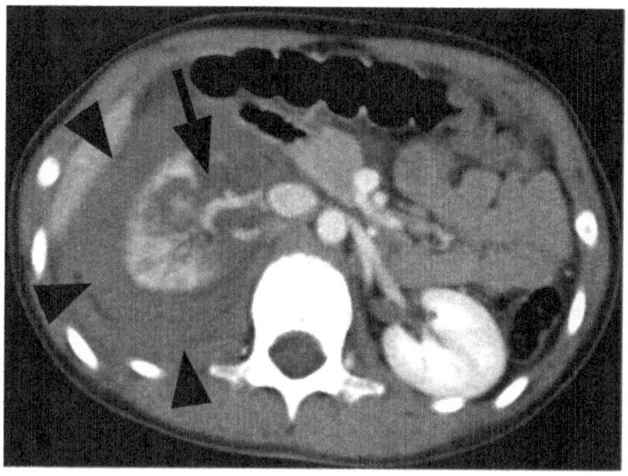

Fig. 20.11 Right Grade V renal injury to the upper pole in a 10-year-old girl who fell from a dresser. Axial post-contrast CT scan shows shattered right upper pole (*arrow*) with a large (*arrowheads*) retroperitoneal hematoma

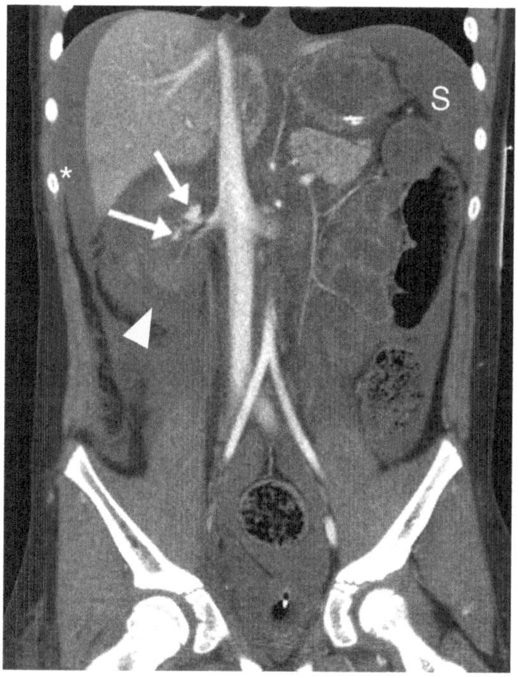

Fig. 20.12 Right Grade V renal trauma, pancreatic and liver lacerations, and severe brain contusion in an 11-year-old boy who had motor vehicle accident. Coronal post-contrast CT scan demonstrates devascularization of the right kidney with active extravasation at the renal pelvis (*arrows*) and moderate perirenal hematoma (*arrowhead*). There is large hemoperitoneum (*) and the spleen is devascularized (*S*)

Cystoscopy and retrograde pyelogram (RGP) should be performed when CT urogram is inconclusive. The diagnosis of a ureteral injury is made by extravasation of contrast (RGP). Direct visualization of the ureter at laparotomy and retrograde pyelogram are most definitive in diagnosing a ureteral injury. Ureteral injuries are often missed on initial trauma evaluation possibly secondary to late presentation from devascularization or suboptimal CT scan without delayed post-contrast phase. The surgeon must remain vigilant in the pediatric patients with high-risk penetrating injuries or severe blunt trauma [30, 31].

CT imaging, antegrade nephrostogram, and RGP are useful to evaluate for a ureteral injury. CT scan may demonstrate ascites, localized fluid collections or urinomas, hydronephrosis, and contrast extravasation. Antegrade nephrostogram and RGP will show extravasation of contrast with instillation of ureteral contrast.

Ureteral injuries range from simple contusions to complex lacerations or avulsions, all necessitating variable interventions depending upon the location of the injury. These surgical decisions are heavily impacted by the location of injury, amount of ureteral tissue loss, and stability of the patient. Regardless, these complex ureteral injuries will require internal ureteral stenting and bladder drainage [30]. Initially, percutaneous drainage via nephrostomy tubes or percutaneous drainage of the associated urinoma may suffice for certain injuries. For contusions and minor lacerations, ureteral stenting and primary repair are paramount, but large ureteral tissue loss may require a ureteral reimplantation, psoas bladder hitch, Boari flap, nephropexy, or a combination of the above. In extensive ureteral injury, complete ureteral replacement with intestine may be necessary.

In adults iatrogenic ureteral injuries occur more frequently then traumatic injuries; however, in the pediatric population the reverse is true [32]. Iatrogenic injuries most frequently occur during pelvic surgery. Intraoperative injury identification and repair is ideal. However, if one suspects a ureteral injury, an intraoperative retrograde pyelogram can assess for ureteral injury. If presentation is delayed, a CT urogram may be useful to diagnosis ureteral injury, but RGP remans the gold standard [30, 32, 33].

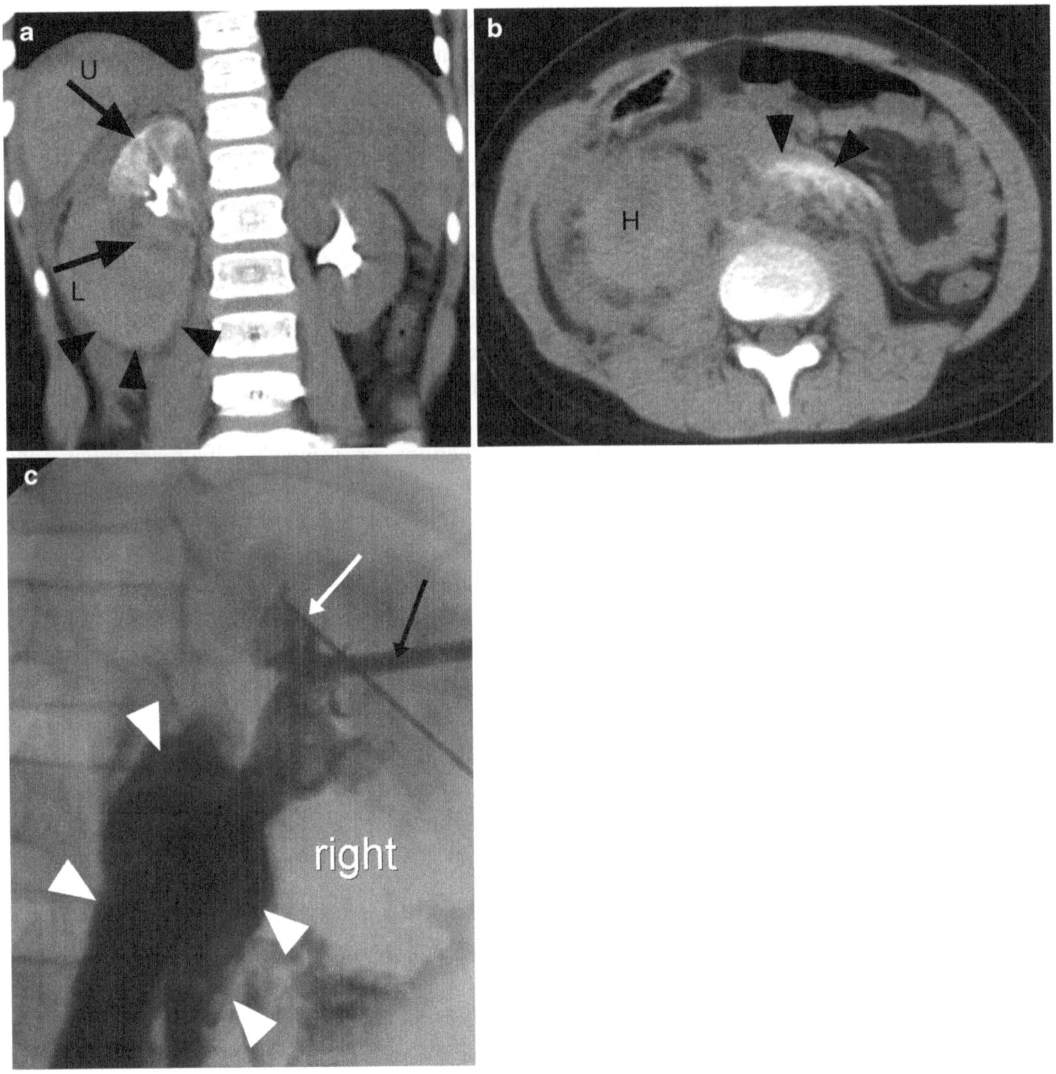

Fig. 20.13 Right Grade V renal accident to the lower pole in a 7-year-old girl who had sledding accident. (**a**) Delayed coronal post-contrast CT scan demonstrates devascularization of the lower pole of the right kidney (*arrow*, *L*) and large perirenal hematoma (*arrowheads*). The upper pole (*arrow*, *U*) is obstructed with delayed nephrographic phase. (**b**) Axial delayed post-contrast CT scan at the level of the lower abdomen demonstrates the perirenal hematoma (*H*) and a central retroperitoneal dense material compatible with contrast extravasation from the collecting system. (**c**) Nephrostogram was performed using Seldinger technique with 22 gauge Chiba needle (*white arrow*) and fluoroscopic guidance. An 8.5 French locking drain (*black arrow*) was placed in the renal pelvis

Bladder

Pediatric bladder injuries are rare and often the result of blunt trauma. The adult bladder resides deep in the pelvis and is well protected by the bony pelvis and rectus musculature. Anatomically the pediatric bladder has a larger portion lying within the abdominal cavity, making it more susceptible to blunt trauma, particularly when it is full [34]. Traumatic bladder injuries should be suspected in the pediatric patient with significant lower abdominal blunt trauma, gross hematuria, and pelvic fracture [34].

Trauma X-ray series include frontal radiograph of the pelvis which is useful to identify pelvic fractures which are associated with a bladder

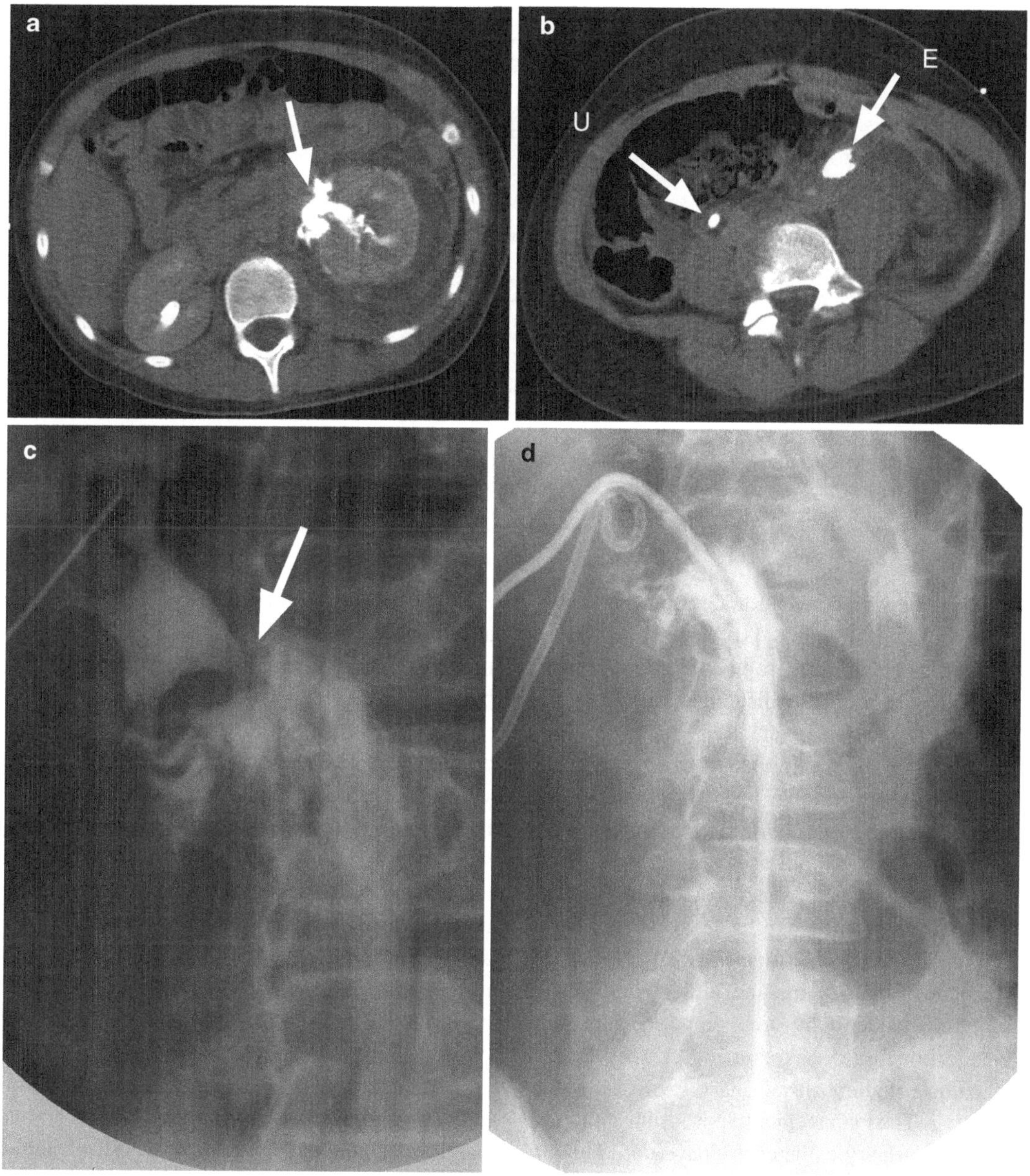

Fig. 20.14 Left ureteral injury at the ureteropelvic junction (*UPJ*) and Grade IV renal injury in an 11-year-old girl that was knocked by a dog. (**a**) Delayed post-contrast CT scan demonstrates extravasation of contrast at the UPJ (*arrow*) and in the lower abdomen (**b**) enhanced right ureter (*arrow-U*) and left extravasated retroperitoneal contrast (*arrow-E*). The left ureter was not enhanced. (**c**) US-guided percutaneous left nephrostomy to the posterior lower calyx was performed. Contrast injected while the patient in prone position demonstrates disruption of the UPJ with contrast extravasation. (**d**) Nephroureteral stent was successfully placed over a wire

rupture [35]. Ultrasound is capable of showing hematomas or free fluid but unable to identify bladder injury.

Suspected bladder trauma should be evaluated by cystography via contrast filling of the bladder through either a suprapubic or urethral catheter. We recommend urethral evaluation prior to urethral catheterization in any patient with a severe pelvic fracture, given the frequent association with urethral injuries in this population. Imaging

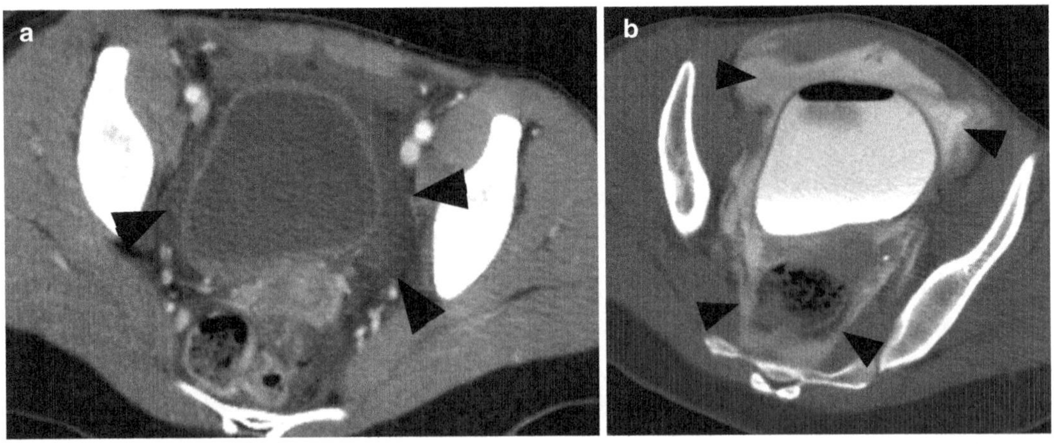

Fig. 20.15 Intraperitoneal bladder rupture in a 16-year-old girl who was in a backseat in a motor vehicle accident. (**a**) Post-contrast CT scan of the pelvis demonstrates fluid (*arrowheads*) in the pelvis around the bladder. (**b**) CT cystography demonstrated large bladder leak (*arrowheads*) to the peritoneum

can be done with conventional retrograde cystography or CT cystography [16, 36–38]. In conventional retrograde cystography, the bladder needs to be imaged both fully distended, obliquely, and emptied to maximize sensitivity and specificity. We use 5 % diluted iodinated contrast solution hung 24 in. above table level. In children older than 10 years, we administer contrast until amount reaches 350 ml or flow stops [39]. If the child is younger than age 10, we use a maximal volume per patent's age as follows: volume of contrast in milliliters = (age + 2) × 30.

Bladder injuries include either contusion or rupture. Bladder contusions represent damage to bladder mucosa or detrusor muscle, resulting in hematuria without any urinary extravasation on imaging. The management approach is conservative with urinary catheter drainage until hematuria resolves, and no follow-up imaging is required if the patient voids normally. Traumatic bladder ruptures are classified as either intraperitoneal (IP) or extraperitoneal (EP). On cystogram an IP bladder rupture is diagnosed by contrast within the peritoneal cavity and outlining loops of bowel (Fig. 20.15). EP bladder ruptures are thought to have a high association with pelvic fracture and appear as contrast extravasation into the perivesical soft tissue in a flame pattern (Fig. 20.16).

Patients with IP bladder rupture will typically have abnormal serum chemistries, including elevated creatinine and potassium from peritoneal absorption of urine. Treatment of IP rupture is immediate surgical exploration and repair of the bladder defect, coupled with maximal urinary drainage. Treatment of EP bladder rupture is typically conservative with catheter drainage of bladder via either urethra or suprapubic catheter. Operative intervention is warranted for EP bladder injuries, when bony fragments are in the bladder, injury to the bladder trigone, severe hematuria resulting in obstruction of the urethral catheter, or plan for operative intervention for other injuries (e.g., vaginal or rectal injury). A follow-up cystogram should be performed after 7–14 days of catheter drainage or operative repair, and prior to removal of catheter.

Patients with bladder augmentation or surgically created urinary reservoir represent a unique population and risk group for bladder trauma. Many of these patients have spinal dysraphism or other neurologic deficits resulting in abnormal sensation and thus may not present with abdominal pain. A high index of suspicion for bladder perforation in this population should be maintained and CT cystogram performed with any abdominal blunt trauma. Bladder perforations in this population are always intraperitoneal and require immediate surgical exploration and repair. To reduce the risk of trauma these children should be instructed to empty their bladder/reservoir prior to any participation in sports [40, 41].

Urethra

Pediatric urethral injuries occur in about 3 % of all genitourinary traumas [34]. Urethral injury should be suspected in the presence of pelvic fractures, straddle injuries or penetrating perineal trauma. Clinical symptoms include blood at the urethral meatus, inability to void, high-riding prostate, and perineal, scrotal, or labial hematomas. A "butterfly" hematoma is classic for urethral injury distal to the urogenital diaphragm [42] (Fig. 20.17).

Plain films and CT scan of the abdomen and pelvis may show a pelvic fracture which may suggest urethral injury. An elevated contrast-filled bladder can be a sign of urethral disruption and accumulating hematoma and/or urinoma.

Retrograde urethrogram (RUG) is the imaging modality of choice. Depending on the age, 6 or 12 French Foley catheter is placed with the balloon portion in the fossa navicularis and contrast injected. In young children we secure the catheter with a tape along the dorsal surface of the penis, and we gently pinch the distal penis at the fossa navicularis with the thumb and index finger. In older children we inflate the balloon with 1–1.5 mL of water. Commonly there is a spasm of the external sphincter, which can be overcome by a constant mild pressure. Radiographs are taken when any extravasation is detected, or the bladder is filled with contrast. The child is positioned obliquely with the penis stretched laterally to visualize the entire urethra including the bladder neck.

Stretching of the posterior urethra represents the mildest injury to the urethra (Fig. 20.16). More severe injuries to the urethra result in contrast extravasation. Depending on the level of injury, contrast extravasation can either below or above the urogenital membrane (Fig. 20.18). It is important to see retrograde opacification of the bladder to ensure complete visualization of the entire urethra and exclude injury above the prostatic urethra [42].

Radiographic evaluation of the female urethra is difficult given its short length. CT scan and cystogram may suggest a urethral injury, e.g., soft tissue injuries or bone fragments. Diagnosis is usually confirmed via cystoscopy and should be considered in any bladder trigonal injury or vaginal injury [43].

Male urethral injuries are typically classified as either bulbar or posterior urethral with different etiologies and management. Bulbar urethral injuries usually caused by isolated straddle injuries that most commonly cause edema and inflammation and rarely result in urethral lacerations or disruption. These injuries can typically be managed with urethral catheterization. However, posterior urethral injuries are more severe injuries, often characterized by loss of urethral continuity [44]. The adult male posterior urethra is protected by mature, well-developed prostate; the pediatric prostate provides little support resulting in more frequent partial or complete avulsion of the posterior urethra [44].

Management of posterior urethral injury is dependent upon location, severity of the injury, and physician preference. Urethral realignment should be attempted for partial urethral injury but requires cystoscopy and suprapubic tube placement to facilitate drainage of the bladder. More significant proximal urethral disruption will usually be managed by proximal diversion with a suprapubic tube and delayed reconstruction.

Testes

Scrotal trauma represents less than 1 % of all trauma-related injuries and is usually the result of blunt trauma secondary to sport injury or motor vehicle accident [45]. The testicles are protected by their mobility and elasticity of the scrotal skin. Testicular rupture or fractured testicle refers to a disruption of the tunica albuginea and extrusion of testicular content. Testicular rupture results from a direct blow to the testicle when the testicle is trapped between the pubic bone and a crushing force. In blunt trauma unilateral testicular injury is common, whereas penetrating trauma often injures both testicles [46].

On physical exam, the involved hemiscrotum is edematous, swollen, and tender and may show the following signs of trauma: laceration, ecchymosis, abrasions, or avulsions of scrotal

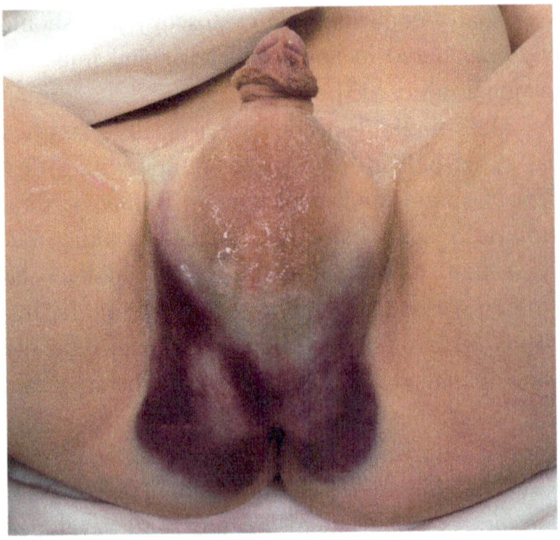

Fig. 20.16 Urethral injury with retroperitoneal bladder leak in a 12-year-old boy who had a motor vehicle accident in which his pelvis was crushed. Retrograde urethrography shows multiple pubic fractures (arrowheads), a stretched posterior urethra (*arrow U*), pear-shaped bladder, and extraperitoneal extravasation of contrast (*arrow, E*)

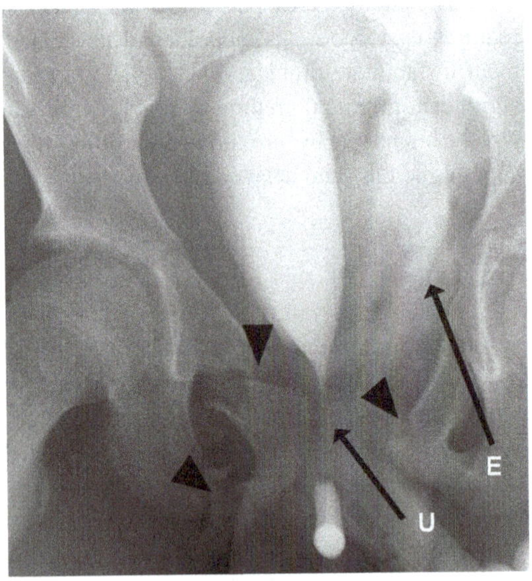

Fig. 20.17 "Butterfly hematoma" in an 8-year-old boy after sustaining a straddle injury; patient had a negative retrograde urethrogram

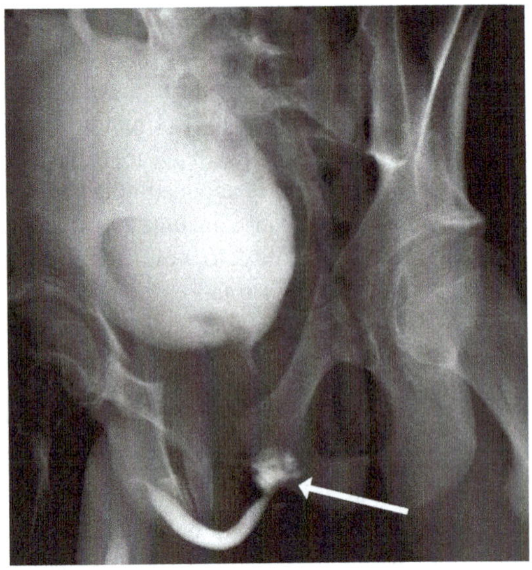

Fig. 20.18 Urethral injury with intact urogenital diaphragm in a 15-year-old boy driver of an ATV that rolled over. He was unable to urinate and had blood in the meatus. Retrograde urethrography shows an area of contrast extravasation (*arrow*) below the symphysis pubis. The bladder is well opacified. This indicates an injury to the posterior urethra with an intact urogenital diaphragm

skin. Physical examination is limited in evaluation of testicular injury. Severe testicular injury may be suspected when the testicle have lost its normal smooth contour. Concomitant testicular torsion is more common in children and should be suspected when there is abnormal lie of the testicle and absence of cremasteric reflex [47].

Scrotal US is the gold standard for evaluation of scrotal trauma and guides whether conservative or surgical management is appropriate. Scrotal US can diagnose intra- and extratesticular hematoma, a defect in the tunica albuginea, testicular rupture, and testicular contusion (Figs. 20.19, 20.20, and 20.21). Color Doppler US allow evaluation of testicular perfusion and diagnose an associated testicular torsion [48].

Management depends on the mechanism and severity of injury. Penetrating scrotal trauma requires immediate scrotal exploration, due to high proportion of testicular injury and testicular salvage surgeries [49, 50]. Blunt trauma can be managed conservatively if US and exam do not show any evidence of testicular fracture; however if testicular fracture is suspected, exploration should be performed [45].

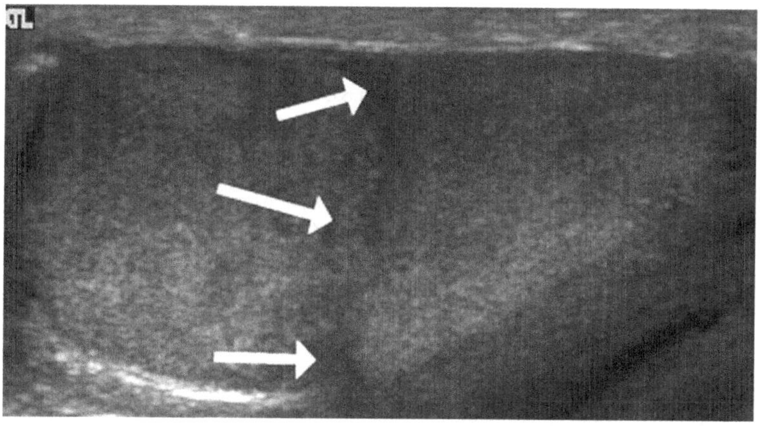

Fig. 20.19 Right testicular fracture in a 17-year-old boy who was a pedestrian struck by a car. Longitudinal view of the right testis shows a midtransverse linear hypodensity compatible with a fractured testis

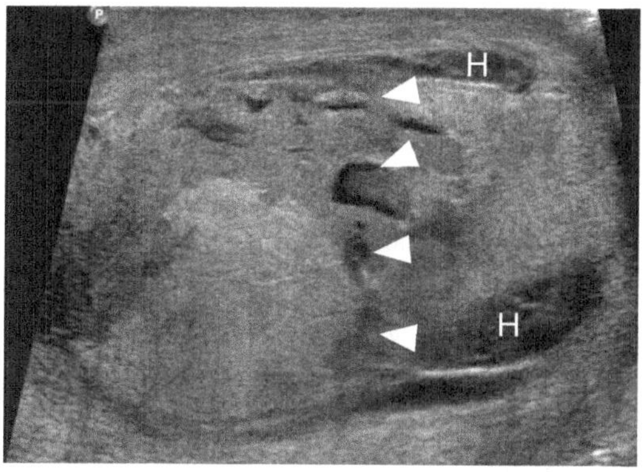

Fig. 20.20 Right testicular fracture and hematoma in a 15-year-old boy who was injured in a basketball game. Longitudinal view of the right testis shows a midtesticular fracture (*arrowheads*). In the lower pole there are hypoechoic areas representing hematoma (*H*)

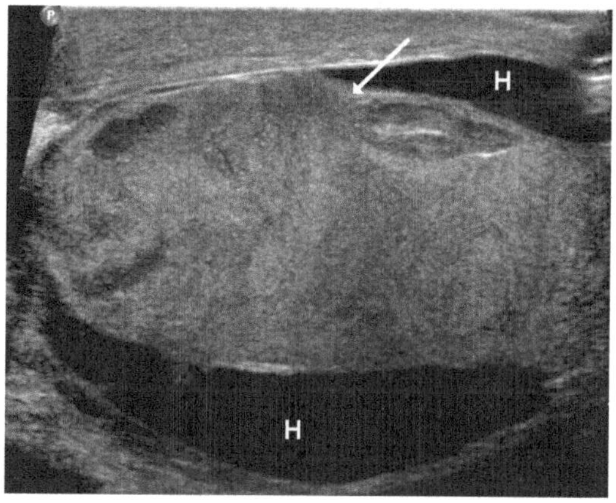

Fig. 20.21 Right testicular rupture with testicular hematoma and hematocele in a 17-year-old boy who had a stick injury to the right scrotum. Longitudinal ultrasound of the right testis demonstrates budging, swelling heterogenicity, and changes in the upper pole contour suggestive of a rupture. In addition there is a moderate hematocele (*H*)

References

1. Alterman DMR, Daley BM, Kennedy AM, Raju R, Lee S. Considerations in pediatric trauma. In: Geibel J, editor. 2011. http://emedicine.medscape.com/article/435031-overview.
2. Guice KS, Cassidy LD, Oldham KT. Traumatic injury and children: a national assessment. J Trauma Inj Infect Crit Care. 2007;63(Suppl):S68–80.
3. Figler BD, Webman R, Ramey C, Kaye J, Patrick E, Kirsch A, et al. Pediatric adrenal trauma in the 21st century: children's hospital of atlanta experience. J Urol. 2011;186(1):248–51.
4. Mehrazin R, Derweesh IH, KINcade MC, Thomas AC, Gold R, Wake RW. Adrenal trauma: Elvis Presley Memorial Trauma Center experience. Urology (Internet). 2007;70(5):851–5. Available from http://linkinghub.elsevier.com/retrieve/pii/S009042950701816X.
5. Burks DW, Mirvis SE, Shanmuganathan K. Acute adrenal injury after blunt abdominal trauma: CT findings. AJR Am J Roentgenol. 1992;158(3):503–7.
6. Sivit CJ, Ingram JD, Taylor GA, Bulas DI, Kushner DC, Eichelberger MR. Posttraumatic adrenal hemorrhage in children: CT findings in 34 patients. AJR Am J Roentgenol. 1992;158(6):1299–302.
7. Pinto A, Scaglione M, Guidi G, Farina R, Acampora C, Romano L. Role of multidetector row computed tomography in the assessment of adrenal gland injuries. Eur J Radiol. 2006;59(3):355–8.
8. Abdu A, Kriss V, Bada H, Reynolds E. Adrenal hemorrhage in a newborn. Am J Perinatol. 2009;26(08):553–7.
9. Rathaus V, Pomeranz A, Shapiro-Feinberg M, Zissin R. Isolated severe renal injuries after minimal blunt trauma to the upper abdomen and flank: CT findings. Emerg Radiol. 2004;10(4):190–2.

10. He B, Lin T, Wei G, He D, Li X. Management of blunt renal trauma: an experience in 84 children. Int Urol Nephrol. 2011;43(4):937–42.
11. Broghammer JA, Langenburg SE, Smith SJ, Santucci RA. Pediatric blunt renal trauma: its conservative management and patterns of associated injuries. Urology. 2006;67(4):823–7.
12. Molina Escudero R, Cancho Gil MJ, Husillos Alonso A, Lledo Garcia E, Herranz Amo F, Ogaya Pinies G, et al. Traumatic rupture of horseshoe kidney. Urol Int. 2012;88(1):112–14.
13. Hannay RS, Dente CJ, Nicholas JM, Wyrzykowski AD, Feliciano DV. Trauma to a horseshoe kidney. Am Surg. 2010;76(6):E54–6.
14. Dominguez K, Ekeh AP. Blunt trauma causing transection of a horseshoe kidney. J Trauma Inj Infect Crit Care. 2011;71(2):517.
15. Chopra P, St-Vil D, Yazbeck S. Blunt renal trauma[mdash]blessing in disguise? J Pediatr Surg. 2002;37(5):779–82.
16. Horstman WG, McClennan BL, Heiken JP. Comparison of computed tomography and conventional cystography for detection of traumatic bladder rupture. Urol Radiol. 1991;12(4):188–93.
17. Yeung LL, Brandes SB. Contemporary management of renal trauma: differences between urologists and trauma surgeons. J Trauma Acute Care Surg. 2012;72(1):68–75. discussion75–7.
18. Buckley JC, McAninch JW. Pediatric renal injuries: management guidelines from a 25-year experience. J Urol. 2004;172(2):687–90.
19. Raz O, Haifler M, Copel L, Lang E, Abu-Kishk I, Eshel G, et al. Use of adult criteria for slice imaging may limit unnecessary radiation exposure in children presenting with hematuria and blunt abdominal trauma. Urology. 2011;77(1):187–90.
20. Santucci RA, Langenburg SE, Zachareas MJ. Traumatic hematuria in children can be evaluated as in adults. J Urol. 2004;171(2 Pt 1):822–5.
21. Kekelidze M, Dwarkasing RS, Dijkshoorn ML, Sikorska K, Verhagen PCMS, Krestin GP. Kidney and urinary tract imaging: triple-bolus multidetector CT urography as a one-stop shop–protocol design, opacification, and image quality analysis. Radiology. 2010;255(2):508–16.
22. Bent C, Iyngkaran T, Power N, Matson M, Hajdinjak T, Buchholz N, et al. Urological injuries following trauma. Clin Radiol. 2008;63(12):1361–71.
23. Dunfee BL, Lucey BC, Soto JA. Development of renal scars on CT after abdominal trauma: does grade of injury matter? AJR Am J Roentgenol. 2008;190(5): 1174–9.
24. Malcolm JB, Derweesh IH, Mehrazin R, DiBlasio CJ, Vance DD, Joshi S, et al. Nonoperative management of blunt renal trauma: is routine early follow-up imaging necessary? BMC Urol. 2008;8(1):11.
25. Lee YJ, Oh SN, Rha SE, Byun JY. Renal trauma. Radiol Clin North Am. 2007;45(3):581–92.
26. Blankenship JC, Gavant ML, Cox CE, Chauhan RD, Gingrich JR. Importance of delayed imaging for blunt renal trauma. World J Surg. 2001;25(12):1561–4.
27. Moog R, Becmeur F, Dutson E, Chevalier-Kauffmann I, Sauvage P, Brunot B. Functional evaluation by quantitative dimercaptosuccinic acid scintigraphy after kidney trauma in children. J Urol. 2003;169(2):641–4.
28. Heyns CF. Renal trauma: indications for imaging and surgical exploration. BJU Int. 2004;93(8):1165–70.
29. Helmy TE, Sarhan OM, Harraz AM, Dawaba M. Complexity of non-iatrogenic ureteral injuries in children: single-center experience. Int Urol Nephrol. 2010;43(1):1–5.
30. Brandes S, Coburn M, Armenakas N, McAninch J. Diagnosis and management of ureteric injury: an evidence-based analysis. BJU Int. 2004;94(3): 277–89.
31. Best C, Petrone P, Buscarini M, Demiray S, Kuncir E, Kimbrell B, et al. Traumatic ureteral injuries: a single institution experience validating the american association for the surgery of trauma-organ injury scale grading scale. J Urol. 2005;173(4):1202–5.
32. Elliott SP, McAninch JW. Ureteral injuries from external violence: the 25-year experience at San Francisco General Hospital. J Urol. 2003;170(4 Pt 1):1213–16.
33. Ghali AM, El Malik EM, Ibrahim AI, Ismail G, Rashid M. Ureteric injuries: diagnosis, management, and outcome. J Trauma Inj Infect Crit Care. 1999;46(1):150–8.
34. Tarman GJ, Kaplan GW, Lerman SL, McAleer IM, Losasso BE. Lower genitourinary injury and pelvic fractures in pediatric patients. Urology. 2002;59(1):123–6. discussion 126.
35. Burke CJ, Thomas RH, Owens E, Howlett D. The role of plain films in imaging major trauma. Br J Hosp Med (Lond). 2010;71(11):612–18.
36. Quagliano PV, Delair SM, Malhotra AK. Diagnosis of blunt bladder injury: a prospective comparative study of computed tomography cystography and conventional retrograde cystography. J Trauma Inj Infect Crit Care. 2006;61(2):410–21. discussion 421–2.
37. Deck AJ, Shaves S, Talner L, Porter JR. Computerized tomography cystography for the diagnosis of traumatic bladder rupture. J Urol. 2000;164(1):43–6.
38. Peng MY, Parisky YR, Cornwell 3rd EE, Radin R, Bragin S. CT cystography versus conventional cystography in evaluation of bladder injury. AJR Am J Roentgenol. 1999;173(5):1269–72.
39. Chan DPN, Abujudeh HH, Cushing GLJ, Novelline RA. CT cystography with multiplanar reformation for suspected bladder rupture: experience in 234 cases. AJR Am J Roentgenol. 2006;187(5):1296–302.
40. Metcalfe PD, Casale AJ, Kaefer MA, Misseri R, Dussinger AM, Meldrum KK, et al. Spontaneous bladder perforations: a report of 500 augmentations in children and analysis of risk. J Urol. 2006;175(4): 1466–71.
41. DeFoor W, Tackett L, Minevich E, Wacksman J, Sheldon C. Risk factors for spontaneous bladder perforation after augmentation cystoplasty. Urology. 2003;62(4):737–41.

42. Pichler R, Fritsch H, Skradski V, Horninger W, Schlenck B, Rehder P, et al. Diagnosis and management of pediatric urethral injuries. Urol Int. 2012;89(2):136–42.
43. Perry MO, Husmann DA. Urethral injuries in female subjects following pelvic fractures. J Urol. 1992;147(1):139–43.
44. Koraitim MM. Posttraumatic posterior urethral strictures in children: a 20-year experience. J Urol. 1997;157(2):641–5.
45. Buckley JC, McAninch JW. Use of ultrasonography for the diagnosis of testicular injuries in blunt scrotal trauma. J Urol. 2006;175(1):175–8.
46. Pogorelić Z, Jurić I, Biočić M, Furlan D, Budimir D, Todorić J, et al. Management of testicular rupture after blunt trauma in children. Pediatr Surg Int. 2011;27(8):885–9.
47. Buckley JC, McAninch JW. Diagnosis and management of testicular ruptures. Urol Clin North Am. 2006;33(1):111–16. vii.
48. Bhatt S, Dogra VS. Role of US in testicular and scrotal Trauma1. Radiographics. 2008;28(6):1617–29.
49. Simhan J, Rothman J, Carter D, Reyes J, Jaffe W, Pontari M, et al. Gunshot wounds to the scrotum: a large single-institutional 20-year experience. BJU Int. 2012;109(11):1704–7.
50. Phonsombat S, Master VA, McAninch JW. Penetrating external genital trauma: a 30-year single institution experience. J Urol. 2008;180(1):192–6.
51. Vanni JA, Wessells H. Injuries to the urogenital tract. In: Ashley SW, editors. ACS surgery. 2013. http://www.acssurgery.com/acssurgery/institutional/tableOfContent.action#.

Disorders of Sexual Differentiation, Gynecological, and Anorectal Abnormalities

21

Konrad M. Szymanski, Boaz Karmazyn, and Richard C. Rink

Abbreviations

CAH	Congenital adrenal hyperplasia
CAIS	Congenital androgen insensitivity syndrome
CT	Computed tomography
DSD	Disorders of sexual differentiation
MRI	Magnetic resonance imaging
MRKH	Mayer-Rokitansky-Kuster-Hauser syndrome
PET	Positron emission tomography
US	Ultrasound
VACTERL	Vertebral abnormalities anal atresia, cardiac abnormalities, tracheoesophageal fistula, renal abnormalities, and limb defects
VCUG	Voiding cystourethrogram

K.M. Szymanski, MD, MPH
R.C. Rink, MD, FAAP, FACS (✉)
Pediatric Urology, Riley Hospital for Children at IU Health, 705 Riley Hospital Drive ROC4230, Indianapolis, IN 46202, USA
e-mail: szymanko@iupui.edu
rrink@iupui.edu;

B. Karmazyn, MD
Department of Radiology and Imaging Sciences, Riley Hospital for Children at IU Health, 705 Riley Hospital Drive, Suite 1053, Indianapolis, IN 46202, USA
e-mail: bkarmazy@iupui.edu

Introduction

An effective approach to abnormalities of the female genital tract, intersex conditions, and anorectal malformations requires a clear understanding of the embryology of the genital, urinary, and gastrointestinal systems. Paired Müllerian, or paramesonephric, ducts develop laterally to the mesonephric ducts, which form the trigone, ureters, renal pelvis, and calyces. In the female, Müllerian ducts fuse medially to form the fallopian tubes, uterus, and proximal 1/3 of the vagina. The close proximity of these two duct systems explains the common association of paramesonephric abnormalities and ipsilateral renal anomalies. The urogenital sinus canalizes in a caudal-to-cranial direction to form the distal 2/3 of the vagina. In the male, the utricle is the distal remnant of the Müllerian ducts and a homologue of the vagina. It is a small, midline diverticulum in the ventral prostatic urethra and is usually asymptomatic. Rarely, it can be quite large and associated with urinary tract infections, stone formation, abnormal voiding, and infertility.

General Concepts in Imaging for Patients with Gynecological, Disorders of Sexual Differentiation, and Anorectal Abnormalities

Imaging modalities for patients with gynecological, disorders of sexual differentiation, and anorectal abnormalities are chosen to allow proper

L.S. Palmer, J.S. Palmer (eds.), *Pediatric and Adolescent Urologic Imaging*,
DOI 10.1007/978-1-4614-8654-1_21,

diagnosis, guide treatment, and detect possible associated anomalies in other organ systems. Not surprisingly, they are often individualized to the particular clinical scenario. Ultrasound (US) is the primary imaging modality for evaluation of internal genital anatomy and abnormalities. Genitography and voiding cystourethrography (VCUG) have a role in evaluation of the vagina, cervical impression, urethra, urethrovaginal confluence, and fistulas. Magnetic resonance imaging (MRI) is used in select cases to better delineate anatomy and pathology. It has a larger field of view and better contrast resolution, which may improve the identification of internal gonads and Müllerian structures [1–3]. Additional information can be gained by examination under anesthesia, cystoscopy, vaginoscopy, hysteroscopy, and laparoscopy.

Ultrasonography

US is the primary modality for identifying and characterization of gonads and Müllerian structures, as well as any associated upper urinary tract anomalies. US has the advantage of being a readily available study that does not involve ionizing radiation or injection of contrast material and is performed without the need for sedation. A pelvic US examination should include screening of the kidneys and adrenals [1–3]. The normal adrenal limb is less than 4 mm in width in a newborn [4]. In patients with ambiguous genitalia, the groins need to be evaluated for undescended or herniated gonads. Identifying only one ovary, or being unable to identify either ovary, with US may not represent a pathology. In 40 % of patients, only one ovary is detected, while neither ovary is seen in 16 % [5]. A perineal approach should be used for evaluation of vaginal masses.

Genitography

Genitography is mainly used to evaluate the urethra, Müllerian remnants, or vagina in patients with ambiguous genitalia [1–3]. In patients with a urogenital sinus or a cloacal malformation, we typically place separate 8-Fr feeding tubes in the bladder, vagina, and rectum. Contrast material is then injected in a retrograde direction. Another method involves retrograde filling via an 8-Fr Foley catheter, with the balloon inflated outside the common opening. This method is most useful when it is not possible to selectively place separate catheters in each anatomical location. Optimally, the location of the common orifice is delineated with a metallic marker.

Genitography can assess the degree of urethral virilization by its length, the presence of a verumontanum, and a distinct separation between anterior and posterior urethra [1–3]. In a normal male, this ratio is approximately 3:2 [2]. In patients with a cloacal malformation or a urogenital sinus, the level of the confluence (where the urethra and the vagina join) should be evaluated. Presence of a cervical impression should be noted as it is typically identified in the vagina while it is absent in a Müllerian remnant in males [1–3].

MRI

MRI sequences, with their multiplanar capability and superior tissue characterization, can provide detailed anatomic information. In addition to axial and sagittal planes, we also perform coronal oblique planes following the main axis of the uterus [6, 7]. MRI is more sensitive than US in the detection of Müllerian duct structures and gonads [8]. Streak gonads are difficult to detect with any imaging modality, including MRI, and are typically identified laparoscopically. Foci of high signal intensity in streak gonads at T2-weighted imaging are suggestive of malignant changes [7]. MRI does not expose patients to radiation and is considered the "gold standard" for determining internal pelvic anatomy, particularly the presence of a cervix and functioning endometrium [9–11].

Both MRI and computed tomography (CT) scans have a role in evaluation and staging of gonadal tumors secondary to disorders of sex development [12].

Gynecological Anomalies

Interlabial Masses

The differential diagnosis for a girl with an interlabial mass is broad. It includes labial adhesions, introital cysts, hymenal disorders, a prolapsed urethra, a prolapsed ureterocele, a urethral polyp, and botryoides rhabdomyosarcoma. Particularly if a lesion appears to involve the urethra, workup should always include a renal bladder US. Several of the lesions described below deserve particular radiological attention.

Introital Cysts

Introital cysts in the newborn can represent a mesonephric ductal remnant (Gartner's duct cyst), a paraurethral cyst (Skene's duct cyst), or a covered ectopic ureter. Mesonephric ductal cysts can be found along the anteromedial wall of the vagina [13]. Paraurethral glands are located just inside the urethral meatus and are homologues of the male prostatic gland. The two largest glands are known as Skene's glands. In the newborn, paraurethral ducts can become obstructed with mucus produced in response to maternal estrogen stimulation, forming cysts. Paraurethral cysts typically displace the urethral meatus, causing an eccentric urinary stream. If the urethral meatus is completely separate from the mass, radiologic evaluation may not be needed to confirm diagnosis [14]. Paraurethral cysts usually rupture spontaneously, but can be drained by a small needle at the bedside. Prenatally, an ectopic ureter (usually from the upper pole of a duplicated system) can insert into the mesonephric system and spontaneously rupture, draining into the vagina. If, on the other hand, the surface epithelium does not rupture, a urine-filled cyst will remain in the vaginal wall.

A retrograde injection of contrast into the cystic structure can be diagnostic (Figs. 21.1 and 21.2). Transvaginal incision relieves the obstruction, but the dysplastic renal moiety may continue to produce urine. A nephrectomy (single system) or upper pole heminephrectomy or ureteropyelostomy (duplicated system) may be indicated if urine production from the dysplastic segment leads to incontinence or there is infection.

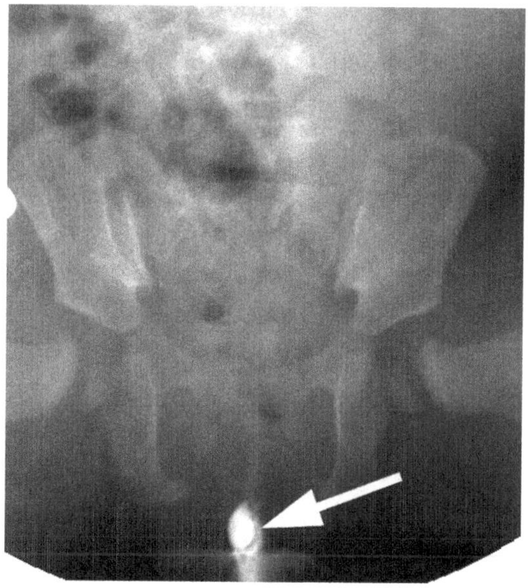

Fig. 21.1 Introital cyst. A 10-month-old girl with a persistent vaginal cyst. Intraoperative injection of contrast demonstrated the vaginal cyst (*arrow*). The cyst was unroofed

Imperforate Hymen

Imperforate hymen is likely the most common congenital obstructive anomaly in the female reproductive tract. The diagnosis of hydrometrocolpos, or accumulation of fluid in the vagina and uterus, is typically made shortly after birth. The distended hymen presents as a whitish bulge in the posterior introitus and/or a suprapubic mass may be palpable. Whitish vaginal secretions build up in the vagina secondary to maternal estradiol stimulation of the child's cervical glands. If the diagnosis is delayed after the newborn period, the mucus might be reabsorbed and the bulging hymen no longer evident. If a patient presents in adolescence, it is often with primary amenorrhea, possible cyclic abdominal pain, or a bluish bulging hymen.

Abdominal and pelvic US allows for visualization of the vagina and uterus, as well as the upper urinary tract, which can be obstructed by a dilated vagina (Fig. 21.3). Reimaging is needed to confirm upper tract decompression after an incision of the hymen.

Repair in the newborn consists of a transverse incision of the hymenal tissue. A longitudinal incision would risk injury to the urethra and

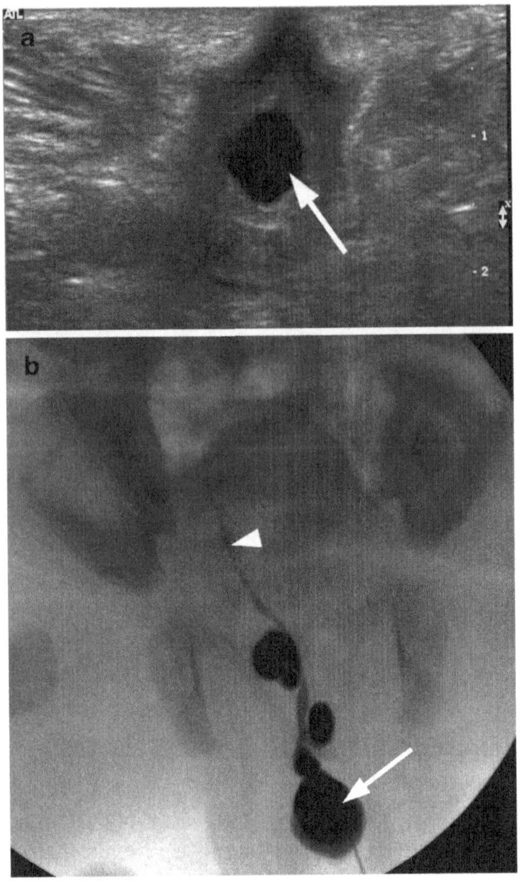

Fig. 21.2 Ectopic ureterocele. A 2-week-old girl with an ectopic ureterocele presented at delivery as an interlabial mass. (**a**) Transperineal transverse ultrasound demonstrated a cystic mass (*arrow*) at the introitus. The vagina was not distended. Both kidneys were normal. (**b**) Intraoperative fluoroscopy with contrast injection to the cystic structure demonstrated an ectopic ureterocele (*arrow*) and a highly tortuous cystic dysplastic atretic ureter (*arrowhead*) likely to represent the ureter of an involuted right upper pole

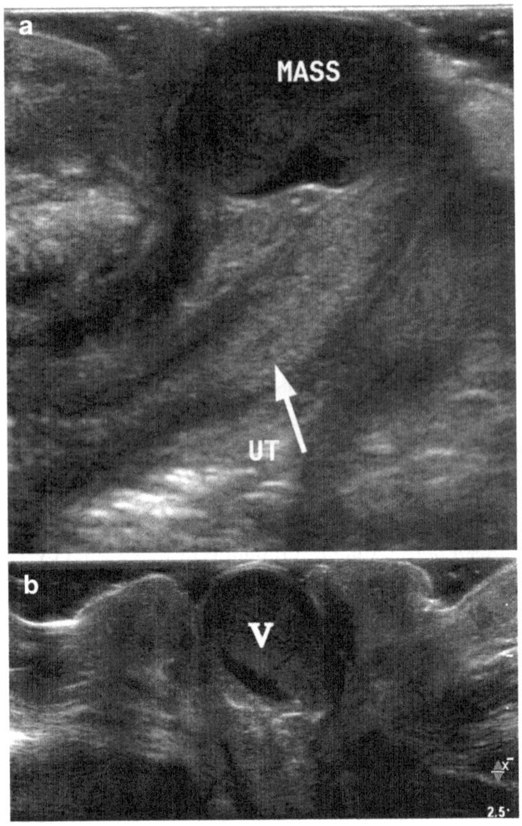

Fig. 21.3 Imperforate hymen. A 1-day-old girl with imperforate hymen presented as a round pink mass protruding through the vagina. (**a**) High-resolution longitudinal ultrasound demonstrated the uterus (*arrow*, *UT*) and a distended vagina appearing as a rounded cystic mass (*mass*) with echogenic debris. (**b**) Transverse perineal high-resolution ultrasound demonstrated the distended vagina and the hymen bulging through the introitus

rectum. Simple aspiration is inadequate as incompletely evacuated material may become infected. In pubertal girls, a hymenectomy of excess tissue may be needed. This condition does not appear to predispose to primary infertility or fetal loss.

Prolapsed Ureterocele

A ureterocele is a cystic dilation of the distal ureter. It is classified as ectopic when it extends distal the bladder neck. If it is large enough, an ectopic ureterocele can prolapse through the urethra, making visualization of the meatus and vagina difficult. With time, the mucosa prolapsing through the urethral meatus changes from pink to congested, dusky purple. In infancy, the ureterocele can prolapse during voiding, resulting in secondary bladder outlet obstruction, urinary retention, and a urological emergency [15]. Management of a prolapsed ureterocele involves manual reduction, often under anesthesia and urethral catheterization for several days. Treatment consists of needle decompression or incision with reduction followed by urethral catheterization. Later, definitive surgical therapy may be required.

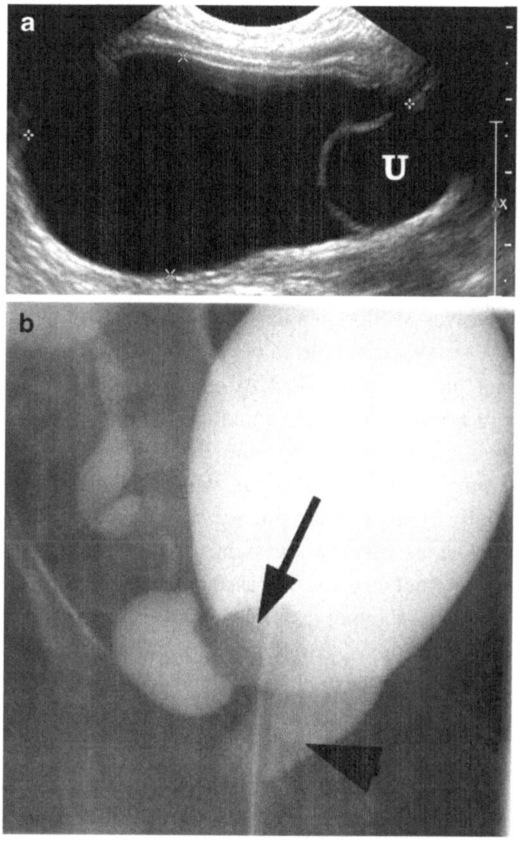

Fig. 21.4 Ectopic ureterocele. A 1-week-old girl with a prolapsed cecoureterocele of right hydronephrotic upper pole kidney. (**a**) Right longitudinal ultrasound demonstrated distended bladder with ureterocele (*U*) at the bladder base. (**b**) VCUG demonstrated a partially everted right ureterocele (*arrow*) that has prolapsed through the bladder neck to the urethra (*arrowhead*)

About 90 % of ectopic ureteroceles drain the upper pole of a duplicated collecting system. A renal bladder US in the setting of a prolapsed ureterocele is performed to assess for collecting system duplication and upper pole hydronephrosis (Fig. 21.4). Retrograde pyelography can help delineate the relevant anatomy. Subsequent evaluation of the ureterocele also includes a VCUG to rule out concomitant vesicoureteral reflux and bladder abnormalities, as well as a nuclear medicine scan to determine split renal function.

Botryoides Rhabdomyosarcoma Tumor

Rhabdomyosarcoma is the fifth most common malignancy of childhood, accounting for 4–8 % of malignant disease in children under 15 years old [16]. Tumors arise from embryonal mesenchyme, a precursor of striated muscle. Histologic classification includes favorable histology, namely, embryonal rhabdomyosarcoma, with botryoid and spindle cell variants, as well as unfavorable histology, including alveolar, anaplastic, or undifferentiated [17]. About 29 % of cases of rhabdomyosarcoma are genitourinary in origin and most are embryonal [17]. Its botryoid variant has the best prognosis, with a 95 % 5-year survival [17]. Vaginal primary has the best prognosis of all female genital tract primary tumors, owing to favorable histology and early detection [18].

These tumors typically occur in children younger than 4 years old [17]. The classic, and most common, presentation of sarcoma botryoides is an interlabial, prolapsing mass arising from the vagina, bladder, or, rarely, cervix, resembling a “bunch of grapes.” Other presentations include an abdominal mass, bladder outlet obstruction, vaginal discharge, hematuria, bleeding, or passing of tumor fragments [17].

Workup involves a thorough history, physical exam, serum tests, and imaging. Initial imaging is performed with a US to confirm the tumor (Fig. 21.5). Cross-sectional imaging with CT or MRI is recommended to assess the tumor, lymph node involvement, and possible metastases. CT may be superior in assessing abdominal lymphadenopathy, although MRI is often recommended because it lacks ionizing radiation [19]. Limitations of MRI include the following: edema after radiotherapy can be misinterpreted as residual disease in 20 % of cases [20], bright urine on T2 imaging may obscure bladder wall tumors, and, on a delayed post-intravascular contrast scan, gadolinium can confuse interpretation when it layers in the bladder. Therefore, we perform multiphase post-contrast MRI in the evaluation of pelvic masses, which include an arterial, venous, and delayed phase [21]. Importantly, the same modality needs to be used for follow-up after therapy. Contrast cystograms and IVPs are rarely required today. Bone marrow biopsy and bone scintigraphy can

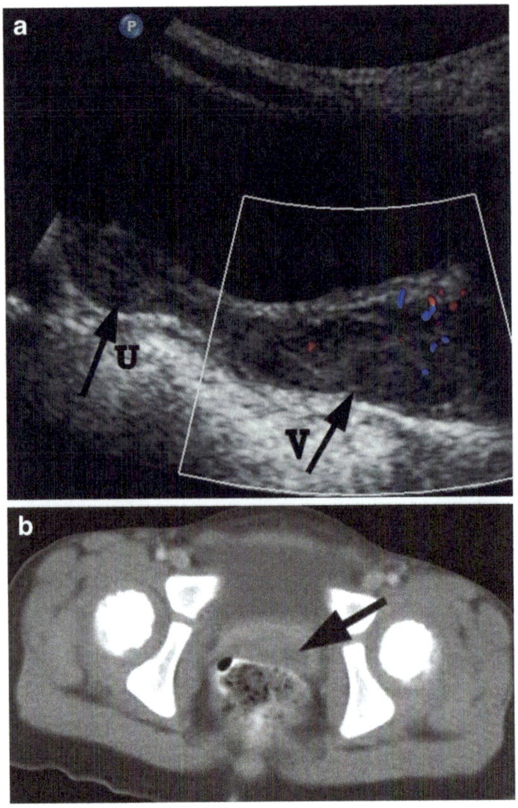

Fig. 21.5 Rhabdomyosarcoma. A 2-year-old girl with a botryoid rhabdomyosarcoma of the vagina presented with a mass protruding from the vagina. (**a**) *US*. Longitudinal ultrasound demonstrated a distended vagina (*arrow V*) with a heterogeneous hypoechogenic solid mass with mild vascularity. The uterus (*arrow U*) is normal. (**b**) *CT*. Post-contrast CT scan demonstrated the vaginal mass (*arrow*). There was no evidence for lymphadenopathy

assess distant spread. PET is not considered a standard staging modality for rhabdomyosarcoma [22].

Diagnosis requires adequate biopsy, preferably by endoscopy, which is less invasive than percutaneous biopsy and avoids needle tract seeding. If endoscopic biopsy is not possible, percutaneous core biopsy with a Tru-Cut needle or surgical biopsy can also be considered. Fine-needle biopsy is often inadequate. Treatment is multimodal, involving multi-agent chemotherapy, surgical excision, and possible adjuvant radiation. Therapy is aimed at preserving function, especially of the bladder, without affecting survival.

Internal Gynecological Abnormalities

Vaginal Agenesis, or Mayer-Rokitansky-Kuster-Hauser (MRKH) Syndrome

Vaginal, or Müllerian, agenesis is a congenital absence of the proximal vagina in a phenotypically, chromosomally, and hormonally normal female. It is also known as the Mayer-Rokitansky-Kuster-Hauser (MRKH) syndrome. Etiology involves Müllerian aplasia secondary to failure of the sinovaginal bulb to develop and form a vaginal plate. On physical exam, external genitalia are normal. A small vaginal pouch and hymenal fringe are usually present, as they are derived from the urogenital sinus which develops normally. Patients often present with primary amenorrhea, usually without pain.

Vaginal agenesis is associated with variable absence or hypoplasia of the cervix, uterus, and fallopian tubes. An obstructed, normal, or rudimentary uterus with functional endometrium is found in only 10 % of patients [23, 24]. The majority of girls have a solid rudimentary uterus and rudimentary fallopian tubes. Although occasionally cystic, the ovaries are almost always present and functional [25].

Two types of MRKH have been described. In typical (Type A) MRKH, patients have symmetric uterine remnants and normal fallopian tubes, without abnormalities in other body systems. Atypical (Type B) MRKH is characterized with an asymmetric uterus and abnormal fallopian tubes. The atypical form is associated with renal anomalies, such as agenesis or ectopia, and skeletal abnormalities, including scoliosis, cervical vertebrae, and hand and facial abnormalities including scoliosis, cervical vertebral fusion (Klippel-Feil syndrome) as well as hand and fascial abnormalities [26]. The anomalies are part of the Müllerian duct aplasia, renal aplasia, and cervical somite dysplasia (MURCS) association. Unlike cloacal anomalies, vaginal agenesis is not associated with lumbosacral spinal disorders [26].

Surgical management has traditionally included vaginal dimple invagination and skin graft neovagina. Today, vaginal dilation is typically the first line of management, prior to considering surgery. Modern techniques involve vaginal substitution using intestine, made of either sigmoid or ileum [27, 28].

Abnormalities of Vertical Fusion

Transverse vaginal septum is caused by a failure of fusion and/or canalization of the urogenital sinus and Müllerian ducts. Patients present with primary amenorrhea and other symptoms of obstruction, such as abdominal discomfort or pain. Septa are usually less than 1 cm thick and have a small central or eccentric perforation [29]. They most commonly occur in the upper (46 %) and middle (40 %) vagina [30]. Hematometrocolpos from retained menses needs to be treated to improve symptoms and preserve fertility. Patients with a history of transverse vaginal septum have a higher risk of spontaneous abortions, endometriosis, and infertility [31]. Rarely is the etiology of hydrometrocolpos, as seen on US, not obstructive. In our experience, severe vaginal voiding with distension of the vagina with accumulated urine can mimic hydrometrocolpos, with the characteristic resolution once the distended vagina drains by changing body position [32] (Fig. 21.6).

Transperineal, transrectal, and abdominal US and MRI may help establish the diagnosis and delineate the thickness and location of the septum [9, 10]. In addition, MRI can help determine whether a cervix is present, to differentiate a high septum from a congenital absence of the cervix.

Surgical treatment includes simple incision or excision of the septum with approximation of upper and lower mucosal edges [31] and Z-plasties [33]. Skin grafts to enlarge the vagina carry a higher risk of subsequent vaginal stenosis [34].

Vaginal atresia occurs when the urogenital sinus fails to contribute to the formation of the lower (distal) portion of the vagina. This condition differs from vaginal agenesis or androgen insensitivity syndrome in that the upper vagina, uterus, fallopian tubes, and ovaries are normal. A shallow dimple caudad to the urethral meatus and a distended vagina and uterus may be noted on physical examination. Patients present with primary amenorrhea and pain or a mass secondary to retained menses.

US and/or MRI evaluation is needed to delineate the Müllerian anatomy. Surgical treatment involves a transverse incision at the level of the hymenal ring. After drainage of retained menstrual blood, the vaginal mucosa is identified and a vaginal pull-through performed to bring the distended vagina to the introitus, with possible use of skin flaps and vaginal mobilization.

Abnormalities of Lateral Fusion

Failure of Mullerian duct lateral fusion leads to a spectrum of anomalies of duplicated reproductive structures. True uterine duplication is rare and the two uteri more often present as uterine horns. They range from complete uterine and cervical duplication (*didelphys uterus*) with or without a longitudinal vaginal septum leading to two vaginas (Figs. 21.7, 21.8, and 21.9), through two uterine horns and one cervix (*bicornuate uterus*) (Fig. 21.10), to a single uterus with a midline septum and a single cervix (*septate uterus*).

Most patients are asymptomatic, with the exception of uterus didelphys with unilateral vaginal obstruction. Although the patient might experience cyclic or chronic abdominal pain, she does not present with primary amenorrhea because the contralateral vagina is not obstructed. Abdominal US and MRI are excellent modalities to outline these anatomical variants. Renal anomalies, particularly renal agenesis followed by ectopia, are common on the ipsilateral side of the obstructed or maldeveloped system [35] (Fig. 21.8d). Treatment involves a wide transvaginal marsupialization of the vaginal septum to release trapped menstrual blood.

Anomalies in Disorders of Sexual Differentiation

Disorders of sexual differentiation (DSD) require a multidisciplinary approach. A thorough and timely workup allows for appropriate diagnosis, management of any acute medical problems, parental counseling, and gender assignment. It includes the physical exam, imaging, karyotyping,

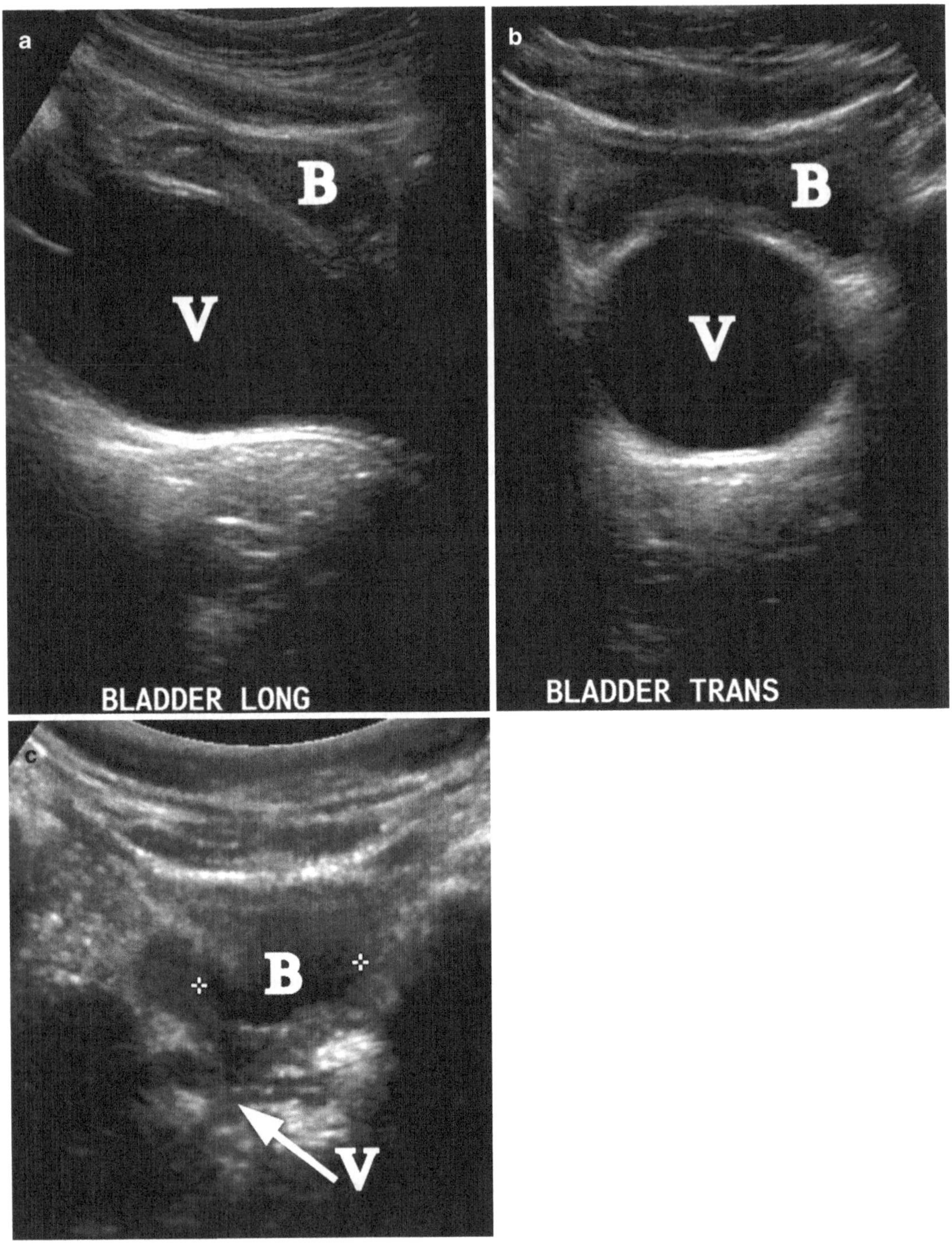

Fig. 21.6 Vesicovaginal reflux. A 6-year-old girl with a UTI and reflux of urine to the vagina mimicking hydrocolpos. Longitudinal (**a**) and transverse (**b**) ultrasound demonstrated distension of the vagina (*V*). The bladder (*B*) is nearly empty. (**c**) Repeated post-void ultrasound demonstrated that the vagina (*arrow V*) was completely emptied (B-bladder)

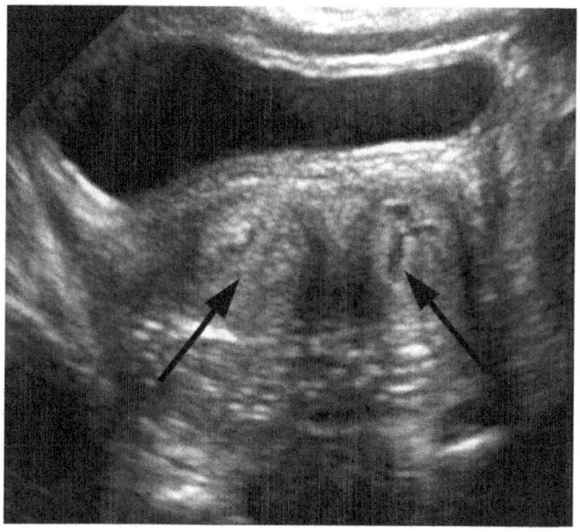

Fig. 21.7 Didelphys uterus. A 1-day-old girl with solitary right kidney and didelphys uterus. Transverse ultrasound demonstrated two separate cervices (*arrow*)

biochemical and hormonal testing, as well as possible laparotomy or laparoscopy with tissue biopsy.

Gonads in individuals with DSD and a Y chromosome are at an elevated risk of developing gonadoblastoma and dysgerminoma. Management involves either a gonadectomy or, with appropriate counseling in children raised male, an orchidopexy. This allows for an early detection of possible malignant transformation (Fig. 21.11).

Complete Androgen Insensitivity Syndrome

Complete androgen insensitivity syndrome (CAIS), formerly known as testicular feminization syndrome, is characterized as a phenotypic female with a 46XY karyotype. Patients present in infancy either with an inguinal hernia or a palpable gonad which turns out to be a testicle or in adolescence with primary amenorrhea. Pubic hair is sparse or absent and the vagina is short and blind-ending without a cervix. Internal female organs are absent. The testes are located along the tract of testicular descent, being intra-abdominal, inguinal or in the labia majora.

The absence of internal female organs can be confirmed with US. Detection of epididymal cysts on an abdominal-pelvic MRI can help in localization and characterization of the gonads (Fig. 21.12). Given a predisposition to gonadal tumors (Fig. 21.13), follow up imaging (US or MRI) is advocated. Other option is surgical exploration offers the benefit of diagnosis with a possible simultaneous prophylactic orchiectomy.

Ovotesticular Disorder of Sexual Differentiation

Individuals with ovotesticular disorders of sexual differentiation, traditionally known as true hermaphrodites, have both testicular tissue with well-developed seminiferous tubules and ovarian tissue with primordial follicles. Dysgenetic testicular tissue lacks spermatogonia, the ovarian tissue is typically normal. Most commonly, a normal gonad presents on one side and an ovotesticle on the other (Fig. 21.14), but gonads can take the form of one ovary and one testis or two ovotestes [36]. Patients present before puberty with abnormal external genitalia [37], but some present later in life with normal, or almost normal, male or female phenotype [38]. Undescended gonads and inguinal hernias are common.

In general, laparoscopy, rather than imaging, is recommended to delineate gonadal anatomy. Gonadal biopsy, either by laparotomy or laparoscopically, allows for tissue diagnosis, but should be performed only if the findings would influence the gender of rearing. A deep incision should be made in the gonad, since the ovarian component of the ovotesticle may completely surround the testicular component or be found at the poles [39].

Treatment and sex assignment depends on the age at diagnosis and anatomical considerations. Male sex assignment is considered when there is good phallic size with a correctable hypospadias and sufficient testicular tissue which can be brought down to the scrotum. Testicular tissue preservation may allow spontaneous puberty, but not fertility. Female sex assignment is considered if internal female organs are present, particularly if ovarian tissue can be preserved. These patients are potentially fertile.

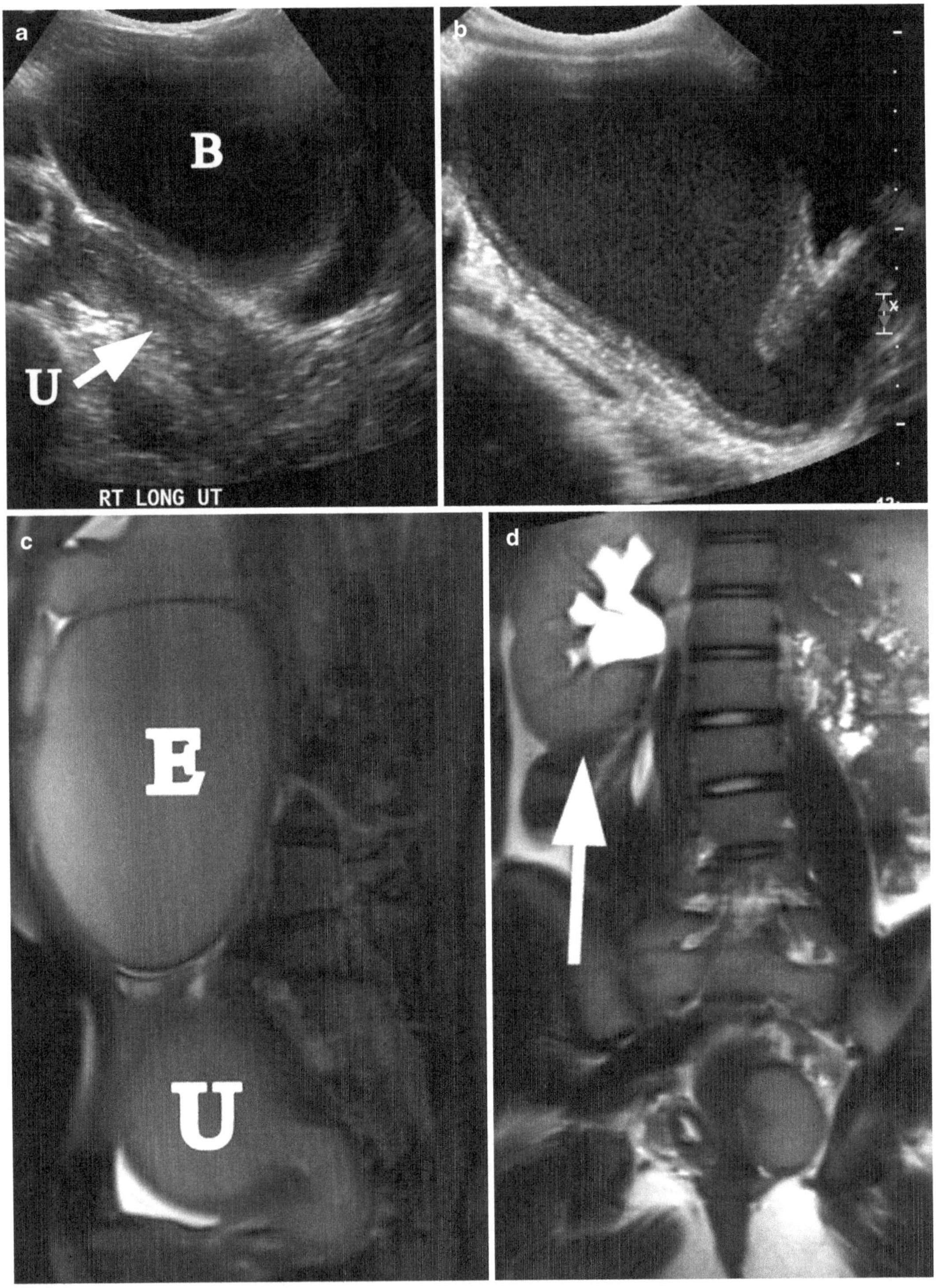

Fig. 21.8 Didielphys uterus and hydrometrocolpos. A 15-year-old girl with uterus didelphys and left hydrometrocolpos due to distal vaginal agenesis. She presented with abdominal mass and painful menses. (**a**) Right longitudinal ultrasound demonstrated normal right uterus (*arrow*, *U*) and bladder (*B*). (**b**) Left longitudinal ultrasound demonstrated hydrometrocolpos. (**c**) Left sagittal T2 MRI demonstrated left hydrometrocolpos (*U*) and a large endometrioma cyst (*E*). (**d**) Coronal T2 MRI shows a solitary right kidney (*arrow*)

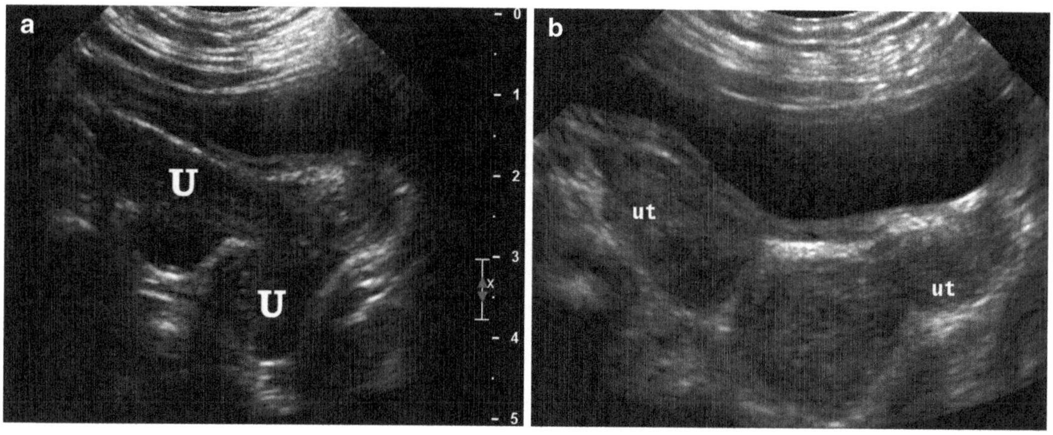

Fig. 21.9 Didelphys uterus. A 6-month-old girl with didelphys uterus and VACTERL association. Longitudinal (**a**) and transverse (**b**) ultrasound demonstrated 2 uteri (*U*, *ut*)

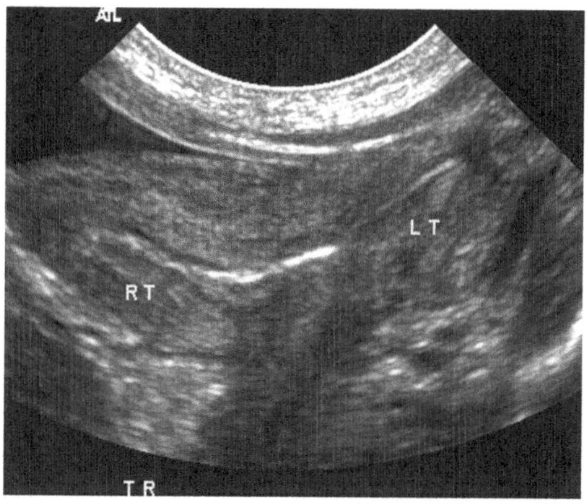

Fig. 21.10 Bicornucate uterus. A 1-day-old girl with bicornuate uterus, imperforate anus, cloacal malformation, and solitary right kidney. Transverse ultrasound demonstrated the bicornuate (*Rt* and *Lt*, right and left, respectively) uterus

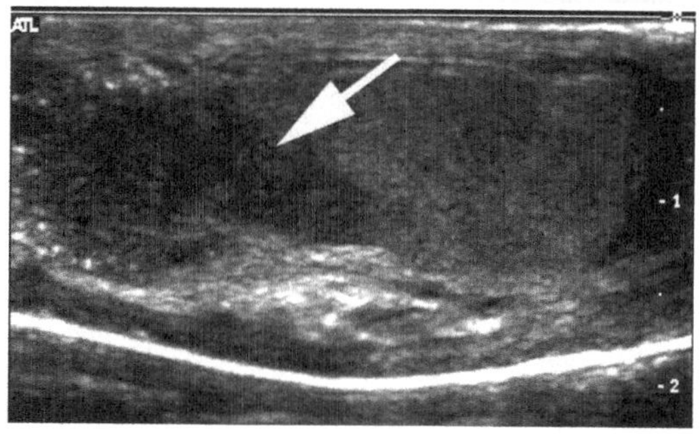

Fig. 21.11 Mixed gonadal dysgenesis with testicular lesion. A 14-year-old child with mixed gonadal dysgenesis and 46XY/45XO mosaicism was raised male and developed intratubular germ cell neoplasm in the right testis. Longitudinal ultrasound of the right testis demonstrated a hypoechogenic mass (*arrow*)

Urogenital Sinus

In urogenital sinus anomalies, the vagina and the urinary tract communicate and exit on the perineum as a single channel. Although the communication can occur in any location between the bladder neck and the urethral meatus, most cases involve the distal two thirds of the urethra. Rather than the length of the common channel, the most important clinical variable in surgical management is the location of the confluence of the urinary and genital tracts in relation to the bladder neck [40]. A urogenital sinus is found in genital ambiguity states (most commonly in CAH), in pure urogenital sinus (with normal external genitalia), in cloacal anomalies (with additional rectal involvement), and in female exstrophy.

Urogenital sinus in genital ambiguity deserves special mention. These DSD states are most often secondary to CAH. The most common enzymatic defect in CAH is 21-hydroxylase deficiency, with 67–75 % of these patients having significant salt wasting [41, 42]. On the other hand, children with an 11β-hydroxylase deficiency can be hypertensive. Initial management involves fluid and electrolyte monitoring, karyotype, hormonal levels for CAH to allow for an accurate diagno-

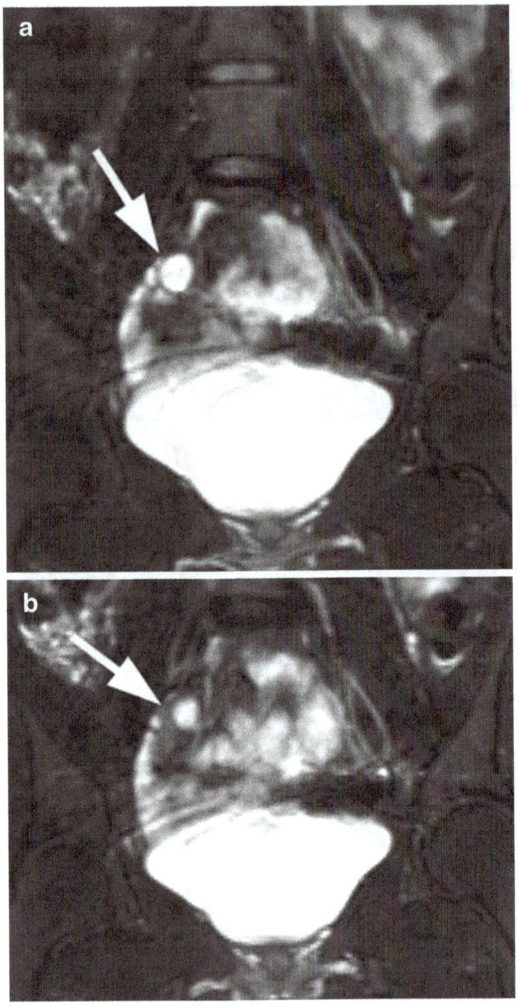

Fig. 21.12 Androgen insensitivity syndrome. An 18-year-old child with androgen insensitivity syndrome and female rearing with multiple epididymal cysts. (**a** and **b**) Coronal T2 fat suppression MRI demonstrated the right testis with multiple epididymal cysts (*arrows*)

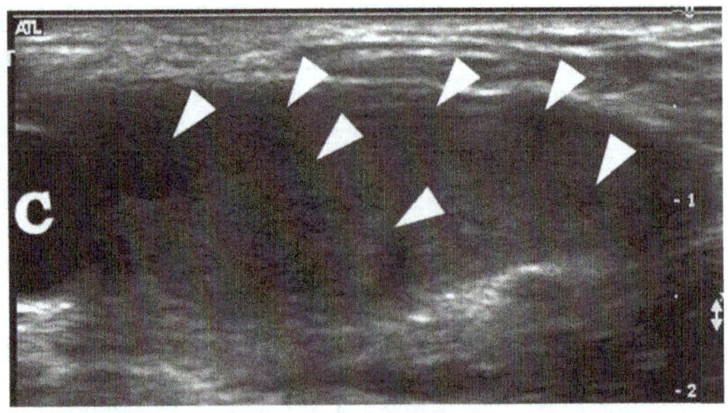

Fig. 21.13 Androgen insensitivity syndrome. An 11-year-old child with androgen insensitivity syndrome and female rearing developed Sertoli cell nodular hyperplasia of the left testis. Longitudinal ultrasound of the left groin demonstrated markedly heterogeneous testis with multiple nodules (*arrowheads*) and an epididymal cyst (*c*). Epididymal cysts are commonly seen in patients with AIS

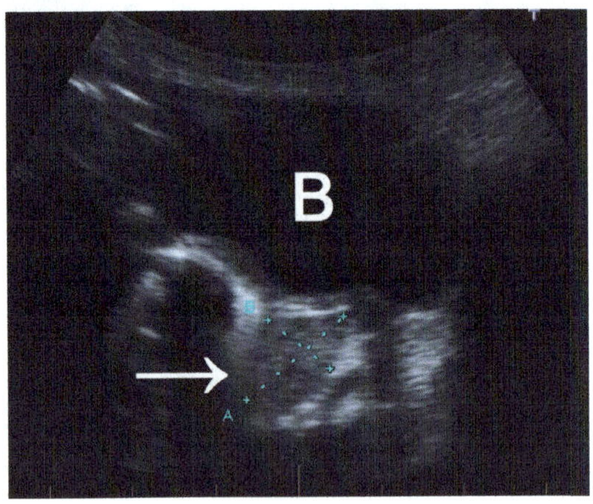

Fig. 21.14 Ovotesticular disorder of sexual differentiation (DSD). A 2-month-old child with ovotesticular DSD, 46XY karyotype, uterus, vagina, and non-palpable gonads. Sagittal ultrasound demonstrated a right pelvic gonad (*arrow*) behind the bladder (*B*). Both gonads were confirmed to be an ovotesticles on laparoscopic biopsy and subsequently removed because the biopsy also revealed gonadoblastoma (Courtesy of Mohamed El Sherbini, Division of Urology, Montreal Children's Hospital, McGill University, Montreal, Quebec, Canada)

sis, and proper gender evaluation. Medical management involves oral steroids with possible salt supplementation. Surgical treatment is individualized and may involve clitoroplasty, urethroplasty, vaginoplasty, and labiaplasty.

Mixed, or asymmetric, gonadal dysgenesis is a less frequent condition associated with urogenital sinus. This syndrome is characterized by an abnormal testis on one side and a rudimentary gonad, streak, or no gonad on the other. The most common karyotype is 46XY/45XO mosaicism, with ambiguous or asymmetric external genital and persistent Müllerian structures. Development of the genital tract follows gonadal differentiation, and Müllerian ducts are present on the side of the streak gonad. A contralateral vas deferens may develop.

Children with a urogenital sinus may present with an abdominal/suprapubic mass. This mass may represent a distended bladder, hydrometro-

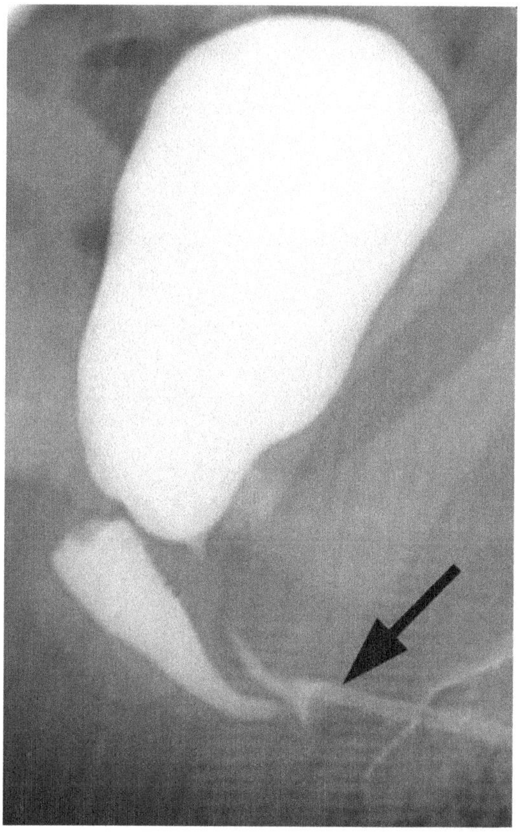

Fig. 21.15 Mixed gonadal dysgenesis. A 2-day-old child with mixed gonadal dysgenesis, 46XY/45XO mosaicism, male rearing, left cryptorchidism, normal right testicle, and perineal hypospadias. He had a normal uterus and vagina, as well as a urogenital sinus. Genitogram was performed with balloon occlusion (*arrow*) of the urogenital sinus, demonstrating a female-shaped urethra with distal confluence of a normal-appearing vagina to the distal urogenital sinus

colpos, or both. Hydrometrocolpos is a common initial sign and possibly the only finding in pure urogenital sinus abnormalities. A genital exam should be performed, particularly to determine if palpable gonads are present. Girls with CAH present with varying degrees of virilization, clitoromegaly, and labial fusion. The location of the anus is usually normal, but it can be anteriorly displaced. It is absent in a cloacal anomaly. The lower back should be examined for any evidence of spinal cord abnormalities, which can be seen in children with pure urogenital sinus or cloacal abnormalities. Findings may include a sacral dimple, hair patch, abnormal pigmentation, asymmetrical buttock crease, or flattened buttocks, as a result of sacral agenesis.

A genitogram and endoscopic evaluation is used to delineate the length of the common urogenital sinus, the location of the vaginal confluence, the distance to the bladder neck, the size and number of vaginas, the presence of cervix, and the anatomy of the urethra and bladder [40, 43, 44]. A genitogram is performed by filling the entire bladder, urethra, vagina, and sinus with contrast (Figs. 21.15 and 21.16). A Foley catheter balloon is used to occlude the perineal meatus prior to injecting contrast. If a catheter can be passed into the bladder, it is useful to perform a VCUG. A cervical impression at the vaginal dome suggests that internal female organs are normal.

A US of the abdomen and pelvis is mandatory, to assess the location of kidneys, ovaries, and uterus. Vaginal, bladder, or intestinal distension should be noted (Fig. 21.17). A cribriform appearance with bilateral enlargement of the adrenals suggests CAH (see "The Adrenal Gland" chapter) (Fig. 21.18).

Anorectal Anomalies

Imperforate Anus

Imperforate anus is associated with a congenital rectourethral fistula in the male (Fig. 21.19) or a rectovaginal fistula in the female (Fig. 21.20). It can be diagnosed on a VCUG or a fistulogram through the mucocutaneous fistula via a diverting colostomy. In addition, it can be visualized endoscopically and studied in a retrograde fashion. Calcifications on plain abdominal film form by the mixing of urine with meconium (Fig. 21.21).

Cloaca

Cloacal anomalies involve urinary, vaginal, and rectal communication, with a single perineal orifice. It affects 1 in 40,000–50,000 patients [45]. They represent 14 % of the anorectal malformations and are the most challenging ones to manage

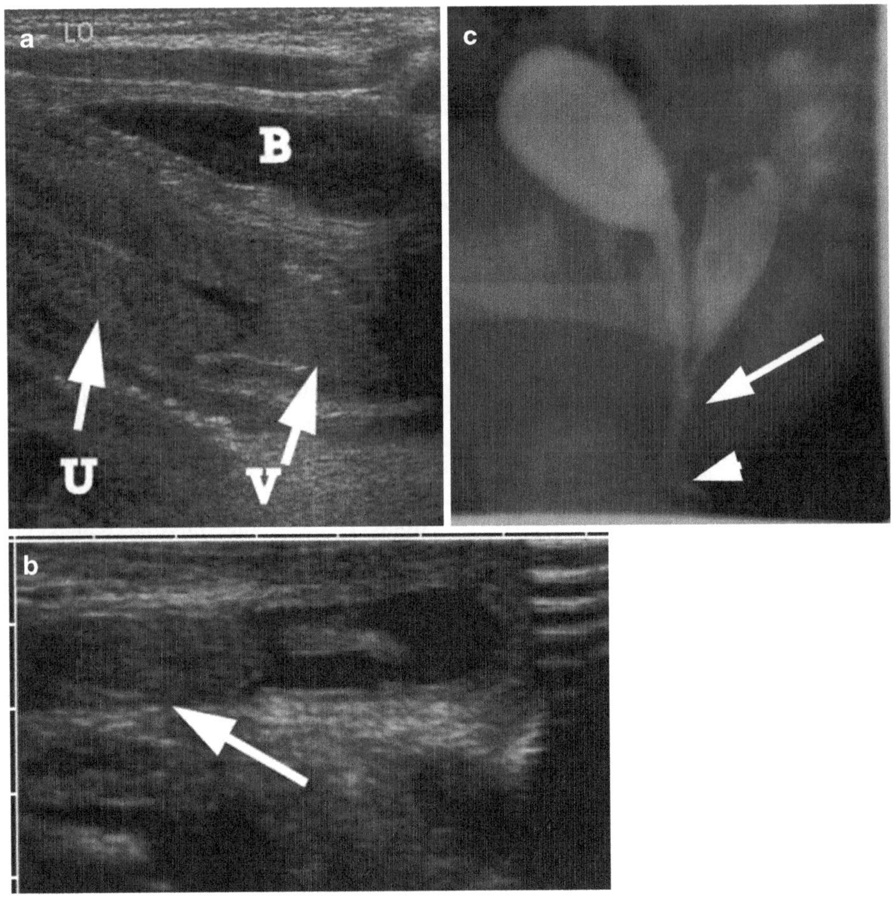

Fig. 21.16 Mixed gonadal dysgenesis. A 2-day-old child with mixed gonadal dysgenesis, 46XY/45XO mosaicism, and female rearing. (**a**) Pelvic ultrasound demonstrated a normal uterus (*arrow U*), vagina (*arrow V*), and bladder (*B*). (**b**) Inguinal ultrasound demonstrated an undescended right testis (*arrow*) in the inguinal canal. (**c**) Genitogram demonstrated the confluence (*arrow*) of the vagina to the urogenital sinus and the common opening at the perineum (*arrowhead*)

[46]. Children can present with a spectrum of physical findings, ranging from a nearly normal female appearance, to genital transposition, a phallic structure or blank-appearing, or doll-like, perineum. Even with a phallic structure, children with cloacal malformations have a 46XX karyotype and ovaries [47].

In cloacal anomalies, abdominal distension may be severe due to hydrometrocolpos, a distended bladder or bowel. Hydrometrocolpos is caused by a preferential flow of voided urine into the vagina, or vaginas, and subsequent poor drainage. Cervical glands produce mucus due to maternal estrogen stimulation, further contributing to the distension. Intestinal distension secondary to urinary flow into the rectum can cause edematous, cyanotic lower extremities, respiratory distress, and metabolic acidosis [48]. Endoscopy should be performed early as a separate procedure in order to decompress the vagina and help define anatomy.

Cloacal anomalies carry a high risk of concomitant anomalies in other organ systems. Many have the VACTERL association: vertebral abnormalities, anal atresia, cardiac abnormalities, tracheoesophageal fistula with or without esophageal atresia, renal agenesis and dysplasia, and limb defects. Echocardiography needs to be performed. Sacral anomalies are present in half of the cases. Spinal cord abnormalities are commonly associated with cloacal anomalies and detected in 35–48 % of patients [43, 49]. An MRI

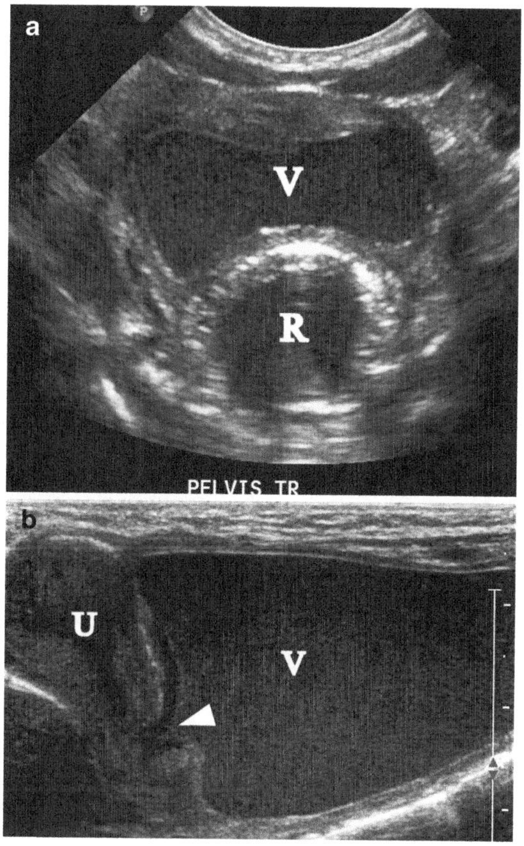

Fig. 21.17 Urogenital sinus. A 1-day-old girl with urogenital sinus and hydrocolpos. (**a**) Transverse pelvis ultrasound demonstrated midline cystic mass. The bladder is empty. (**b**) Sagittal ultrasound demonstrated distended vagina (*V*), cervix (*arrowhead*), and uterus (*U*)

allows the evaluation of the lumbosacral spine, anatomy, and musculature.

Cloacal anomalies have been detected on antenatal US as early as 19 weeks' gestation. Antenatal findings include bilateral hydronephrosis, oligohydramnios, transient fetal ascites, and a solitary, bilobed, or trilobed pelvic cystic mass between the rectum and bladder, representing the distended vagina or vaginas [50].

Postnatal evaluation includes a chest radiograph and a plain abdominal film. The abdominal film can reveal a pelvic mass, linear calcifications from urinary ascites, and granular calcification along the rectum as a result of meconium calcified by coming into contact with urine [43].

Abdominal and pelvic US helps detect distension of the bladder, vagina, or rectum while

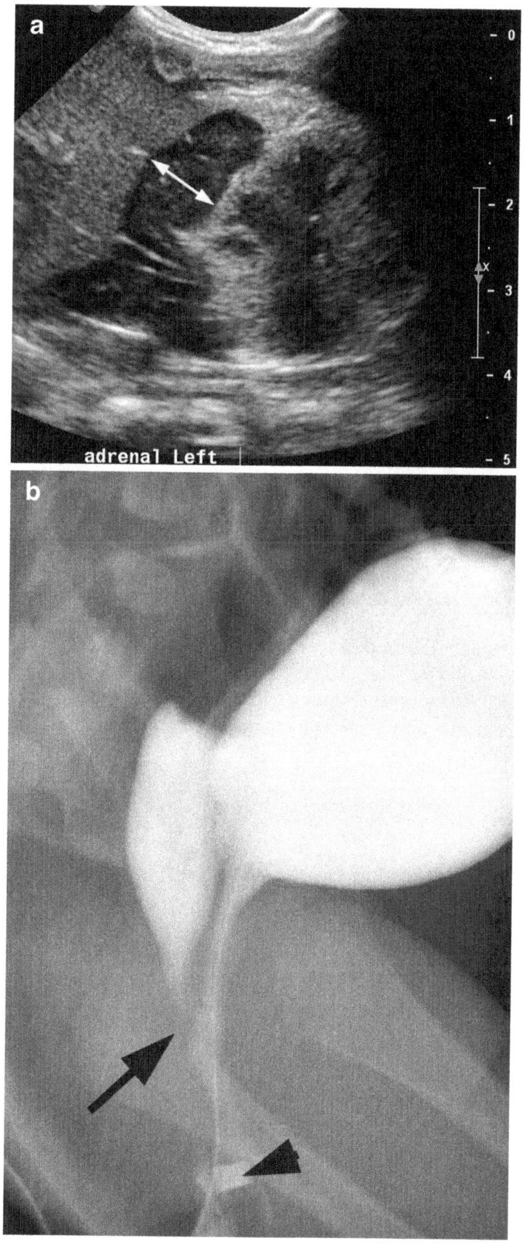

Fig. 21.18 Urogenital sinus in congenital adrenal hyperplasia (CAH). A One-day-old girl with CAH due to17-hydroxylase deficiency. (**a**) Longitudinal high-resolution ultrasound demonstrated marked thickening (9 mm) of the left adrenal limb (*double head arrow*). (**b**) Voiding cystourethrogram during voiding phase demonstrated reflux to the vagina and the confluence (*arrow*) at the urogenital sinus. The common opening at the perineum has been marked (*arrowhead*)

delineating pelvic and renal anatomy. It may show hydronephrosis, possibly either due to bladder outlet, or even ureteral, obstruction by

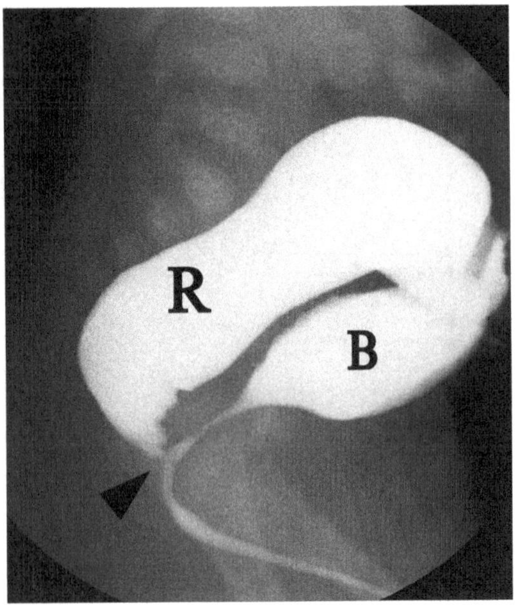

Fig. 21.19 Male imperforate anus. A 3-day-old boy with imperforate anus and meconium in the urine, without any other anomalies. Voiding cystourethrogram demonstrated a rectourethral fistula (*arrowhead*) (*R*: rectum, *B*: bladder)

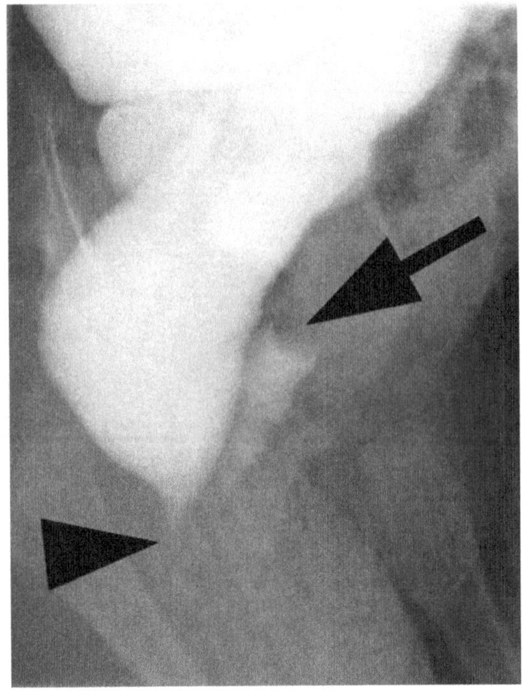

Fig. 21.20 Female imperforate anus. A 3-week-old girl with imperforate anus and rectovaginal fistula. Her mother noted stool coming from the vagina. She had diverting colostomy. Antegrade enema study through the colonic mucous fistula demonstrated a short perineal fistula (*arrowhead*) and contrast in the vagina. *Arrow* indicates cervix impression on the vagina vault

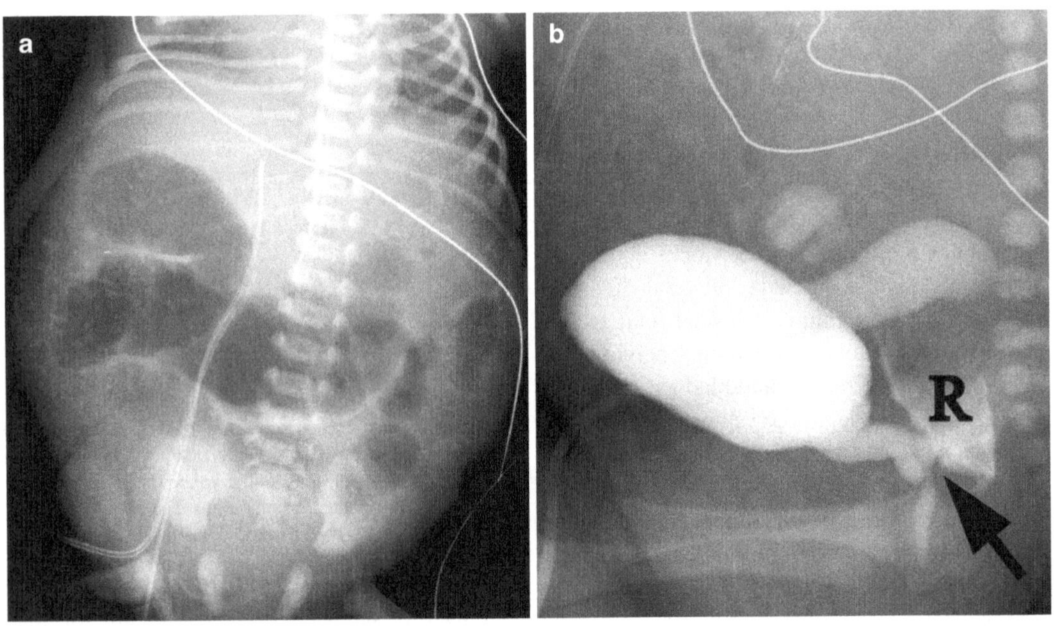

Fig. 21.21 Male imperforate anus. A 1-day-old boy with imperforate anus, vesicorectal fistula, and VACTERL association. (**a**) Plain abdominal radiograph shows punctuated calcifications along the colon suggesting rectourethral fistula which was confirmed in a voiding cystourethrogram study (**b**). The fistula is indicated by the arrow (*R*-rectum)

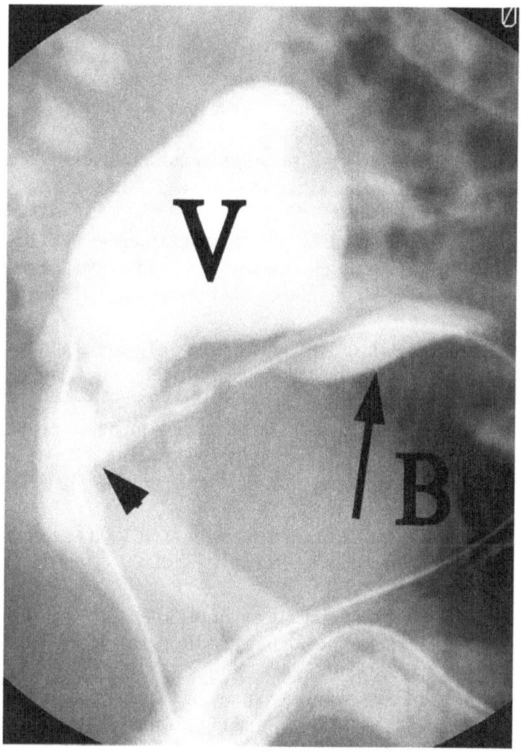

Fig. 21.22 Cloacal malformation. A 5-day-old girl with cloacal malformation and VACTERL association including single right kidney, tracheoesophageal fistula, tethered cord, and imperforate anus. Genitogram demonstrated the bladder (*arrow B*) which was opacified using a suprapubic catheter, dilated vagina (*V*), with high confluence (*arrowhead*) to the common channel. The bowel was not visualized on this study

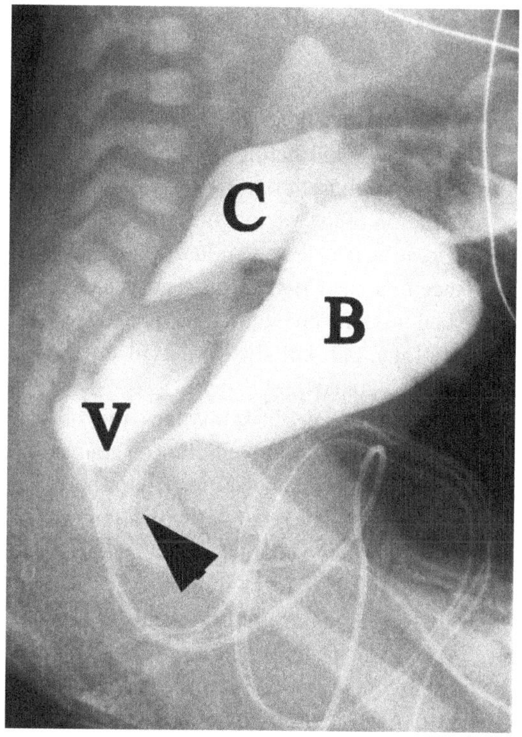

Fig. 21.23 Cloacal malformation. A 1-day-old girl with cloacal malformation. Genitogram demonstrated the bladder (*B*), vagina (*V*), and colon (*C*) with the confluence to the cloacal opening (*arrowhead*)

hydrometrocolpos. Renal anomalies have been reported in 33–83 % of patients and include dysplasia, fusion anomalies, ectopia, ureteropelvic junction, and duplication [51].

A genitogram can help further define cloacal anatomy (Figs. 21.22 and 21.23). Just as with a urogenital sinus, the confluence between the urethra and vagina needs to be evaluated, with the addition of assessing the rectal confluence. Vaginal duplication is quite common, although solitary or absent vagina are also reported. Vaginal anatomy varies, with most vaginas entering side by side with a single opening into the cloaca, although they may also enter by separate openings. A cervix is typically present with the vagina. Uterine anatomy typically parallels vaginal anatomy, although a uterus may be present in the setting of an absent vagina.

The rectal confluence is most commonly located at the level of the vaginal confluence, within the septum of the duplicated vagina [52]. The rectal opening can vary in size and can even enter the vagina or bladder without direct communication to the cloaca.

Prior to considering surgical treatment, a child born with a cloacal anomaly needs to be medically stabilized. Distended abdominal organs need to be decompressed by a variety of methods, including clean intermittent catheterizations, a vaginostomy, a vesicostomy, and a diverting colostomy. Management involves four steps: gastrointestinal tract decompression, genitourinary tract decompression, repair of associated other pathology, as well as a definitive cloacal malformation repair. A definitive repair of the cloaca should address all its aspects. An isolated rectal pull-through without vaginal reconstruction should be always avoided.

Key Points to Remember

- Ultrasound (US) is the primary imaging modality for evaluating internal genital anatomy and abnormalities. Genitography and voiding cystourethrography have a role in the evaluation of the vagina, urethra, urethrovaginal confluence, and fistulas. Magnetic resonance imaging (MRI) is used in selected cases to better delineate internal pelvic anatomy and pathology, particularly Müllerian duct structures and gonads.
- If an interlabial mass involves the urethra, workup should always include a renal bladder US. Sarcoma botryoides (rhabdomyosarcoma) needs to be ruled out with all interlabial masses and has a characteristic appearance of an interlabial "bunch of grapes" prolapsing from the vagina or urethral meatus.
- Gynecological abnormalities of vertical fusion most frequently lead to an obstructed vagina and patients presenting with hydrometrocolpos and primary amenorrhea. Abnormalities of lateral fusion consist of varying degrees of uterine, cervical, and vaginal duplication. These patients occasionally present with unilateral obstruction, but possibly without amenorrhea, since one of the vaginas is not obstructed. Both can benefit from US and MRI evaluation.
- Anomalies in disorders of sexual differentiation require a multidisciplinary approach. US can help screen for Müllerian duct structures, intra-abdominal gonads, and hyperplastic adrenal glands. MRI can help delineate internal pelvic anatomy. Genitography is particularly useful in a urogenital sinus or a cloacal anomaly, helping to delineate the length of the common channel, urethra, and vagina as well as location of the confluence.
- Radiographic investigation of a particular anomaly must include imaging evaluation of associated malformations. Depending on the anomaly, and particularly in cloacal malformation, this may include spinal cord, anal, cardiac, tracheoesophageal, genitourinary, and skeletal anomalies.

References

1. Chavhan GB, et al. Imaging of ambiguous genitalia: classification and diagnostic approach. Radiographics. 2008;28(7):1891–904.
2. Garel L. Abnormal sex differentiation: who, how and when to image. Pediatr Radiol. 2008;38 Suppl 3: S508–11.
3. Moshiri M, et al. Evaluation and management of disorders of sex development: multidisciplinary approach to a complex diagnosis. Radiographics. 2012;32(6): 1599–618.
4. Al-Alwan I, et al. Clinical utility of adrenal ultrasonography in the diagnosis of congenital adrenal hyperplasia. J Pediatr. 1999;135(1):71–5.
5. Cohen HL, et al. Normal ovaries in neonates and infants: a sonographic study of 77 patients 1 day to 24 months old. AJR Am J Roentgenol. 1993;160(3): 583–6.
6. Secaf E, et al. Role of MRI in the evaluation of ambiguous genitalia. Pediatr Radiol. 1994;24(4): 231–5.
7. Gambino J, et al. Congenital disorders of sexual differentiation: MR findings. AJR Am J Roentgenol. 1992;158(2):363–7.
8. Kanemoto K, et al. Accuracy of ultrasonography and magnetic resonance imaging in the diagnosis of non-palpable testis. Int J Urol. 2005;12(7):668–72.
9. Fedele L, et al. Magnetic resonance imaging in Mayer-Rokitansky-Kuster-Hauser syndrome. Obstet Gynecol. 1990;76(4):593–6.
10. Lang IM, Babyn P, Oliver GD. MR imaging of paediatric uterovaginal anomalies. Pediatr Radiol. 1999;29(3):163–70.
11. Russ PD, et al. Mayer-Rokitansky-Kuster-Hauser syndrome diagnosed by magnetic resonance imaging in a 15-year-old girl. J Pediatr Adolesc Gynecol. 1997;10(2):89–92.
12. Shah RU, et al. Imaging of pediatric pelvic neoplasms. Radiol Clin North Am. 2011;49(4):729–48, vi.
13. Pradhan S, Tobon H. Vaginal cysts: a clinicopathological study of 41 cases. Int J Gynecol Pathol. 1986;5(1):35–46.
14. Nussbaum AR, Lebowitz RL. Interlabial masses in little girls: review and imaging recommendations. AJR Am J Roentgenol. 1983;141(1):65–71.
15. Gingell JC, Gordon IR, Mitchell JP. Acute obstructive uropathy due to prolapsed ectopic ureterocele. Case report. Br J Urol. 1971;43(3):305–8.
16. Pizzo PA, Poplack DG. Principles and practice of pediatric oncology. 3rd ed. Philadelphia: Lippincott-Raven; 1997. xxii, 1522 p., [1] leaf of plates.
17. Qualman SJ, et al. Intergroup Rhabdomyosarcoma Study: update for pathologists. Pediatr Dev Pathol. 1998;1(6):550–61.
18. Hays DM, et al. Clinical staging and treatment results in rhabdomyosarcoma of the female genital tract among children and adolescents. Cancer. 1988;61(9): 1893–903.

19. McHugh K, Boothroyd AE. The role of radiology in childhood rhabdomyosarcoma. Clin Radiol. 1999; 54(1):2–10.
20. Atra A, et al. Conservative surgery in multimodal therapy for pelvic rhabdomyosarcoma in children. Br J Cancer. 1994;70(5):1004–8.
21. Agrons GA, et al. From the archives of the AFIP. Genitourinary rhabdomyosarcoma in children: radiologic-pathologic correlation. Radiographics. 1997;17(4):919–37.
22. Breitfeld PP, Meyer WH. Rhabdomyosarcoma: new windows of opportunity. Oncologist. 2005;10(7): 518–27.
23. Singh J, Devi YL. Pregnancy following surgical correction of nonfused mullerian bulbs and absent vagina. Obstet Gynecol. 1983;61(2):267–9.
24. Bates GW, Wiser WL. A technique for uterine conservation in adolescents with vaginal agenesis and a functional uterus. Obstet Gynecol. 1985;66(2):290–4.
25. Salvatore CA, Lodovicci O. Vaginal agenesis: an analysis of ninety cases. Acta Obstet Gynecol Scand. 1978;57(1):89–94.
26. Gunderson CH, et al. The Klippel-Feil syndrome: genetic and clinical reevaluation of cervical fusion. Medicine (Baltimore). 1967;46(6):491–512.
27. Hendren WH, Atala A. Use of bowel for vaginal reconstruction. J Urol. 1994;152(2 Pt 2):752–5; discussion 756–7.
28. Hensle TW, Reiley EA. Vaginal replacement in children and young adults. J Urol. 1998;159(3):1035–8.
29. Suidan FG, Azoury RS. The transverse vaginal septum: a clinicopathologic evaluation. Obstet Gynecol. 1979;54(3):278–83.
30. Lodi A. Clinical and statistical study on vaginal malformations at the Obstetrical and Gynecological Clinic in Milano, 1906–50. Ann Ostet Ginecol. 1951;73(9):1246–85.
31. Rock JA, et al. Pregnancy success following surgical correction of imperforate hymen and complete transverse vaginal septum. Obstet Gynecol. 1982;59(4):448–51.
32. Snyder EM, et al. Vesicovaginal reflux mimicking obstructive hydrocolpos. J Ultrasound Med. 2007; 26(12):1781–4.
33. Garcia RF. Z-plasty for correction of congenital transferse vaginal septum. Am J Obstet Gynecol. 1967; 99(8):1164–5.
34. Garcia J, Jones Jr HW. The split thickness graft technic for vaginal agenesis. Obstet Gynecol. 1977;49(3): 328–32.
35. Rock JA, Azziz R. Genital anomalies in childhood. Clin Obstet Gynecol. 1987;30(3):682–96.
36. Bouvattier C. Disorders of sex development: endocrine aspects. In: Gearhart JP, Rink RC, Mouriquand DE, editors. Pediatric urology. Philadelphia: Saunders Elsevier; 2010. p. 459–75.
37. van Niekerk WA. True hermaphroditism: an analytic review with a report of 3 new cases. Am J Obstet Gynecol. 1976;126(7):890–907.
38. Montero M, et al. True hermaphroditism and normal male external genitalia: a rare presentation. Acta Paediatr. 1999;88(8):909–11.
39. Hensle T, Kennedy WAI. Surgical management of intersexuality. Philadelphia: W.B. Saunders; 1998.
40. Rink RC, Adams MC, Misseri R. A new classification for genital ambiguity and urogenital sinus anomalies. BJU Int. 2005;95(4):638–42.
41. Merke DP, Bornstein SR. Congenital adrenal hyperplasia. Lancet. 2005;365(9477):2125–36.
42. Speiser PW, White PC. Congenital adrenal hyperplasia. N Engl J Med. 2003;349(8):776–88.
43. Jaramillo D, Lebowitz RL, Hendren WH. The cloacal malformation: radiologic findings and imaging recommendations. Radiology. 1990;177(2):441–8.
44. Rink RC, Adams MC. Feminizing genitoplasty: state of the art. World J Urol. 1998;16(3):212–18.
45. Karlin G, et al. Persistent cloaca and phallic urethra. J Urol. 1989;142(4):1056–9.
46. Fleming SE, et al. Imperforate anus in females: frequency of genital tract involvement, incidence of associated anomalies, and functional outcome. J Pediatr Surg. 1986;21(2):146–50.
47. Levitt MA, Pena A. Pitfalls in the management of newborn cloacas. Pediatr Surg Int. 2005;21(4): 264–9.
48. Raffensperger JG. The cloaca in the newborn. Birth Defects Orig Artic Ser. 1988;24(4):111–23.
49. Pena A. The surgical management of persistent cloaca: results in 54 patients treated with a posterior sagittal approach. J Pediatr Surg. 1989;24(6): 590–8.
50. Cilento Jr BG, Benacerraf BR, Mandell J. Prenatal diagnosis of cloacal malformation. Urology. 1994;43(3):386–8.
51. Rink RC, et al. Upper and lower urinary tract outcome after surgical repair of cloacal malformations: a three-decade experience. BJU Int. 2005;96(1):131–4.
52. Rink RC, Kaefer M. Surgical management of intersexuality, cloacal malformation and other abnormalities of the genitalia in girls. In: Retik AB, Walsh P, Vaugh EP, Wein AJ, editors. Campell's urology. Philadelphia: W.B. Saunders; 2002. p. 2428–67.

Index

L.S. Palmer, J.S. Palmer (eds.), *Pediatric and Adolescent Urologic Imaging*,
DOI 10.1007/978-1-4614-8654-1, © Springer Science+Business Media New York 2014

O

P

S

CPSIA information can be obtained at www.ICGtesting.com
Printed in the USA
LVOW01*1914031014

407171LV00002B/61/P

9 781461 486534